THE ENCYCLOPEDIA OF

SLEEP AND SLEEP DISORDERS

Second Edition, Updated and Revised

Michael J. Thorpy, M.D.
and
Jan Yager, Ph.D.

Facts On File, Inc.

The Encyclopedia of Sleep and Sleep Disorders, Second Edition, Updated and Revised

Facts On File, Inc.
11 Penn Plaza
New York, NY 10001

Library of Congress Cataloging-in-Publication Data

Thorpy, Michael J.
The encyclopedia of sleep and sleep disorders /
Michael J. Thorpy and Jan Yager.—2nd, ed., updated and rev.
p. cm.
Includes bibliographical references and index.
ISBN 0-8160-4089-3 (alk. paper)
1. Sleep disorders—Dictionaries. 2. Sleep—Dictionaries. I. Yager, Jan, 1948– II. Title.
RC547 .Y34 2001
616.8′498′03—dc21 00-064028

Text and cover design by Cathy Rincon

Printed in the United States of America

MP FOF 10 9 8 7 6 5 4 3 2 1

This book is printed on acid-free paper.

CONTENTS

PREFACE TO THE SECOND EDITION

Since the first edition of *The Encyclopedia of Sleep and Sleep Disorders* was published in 1991, there has been a great expansion in the national awareness of sleep disorders and an increase in services for patients. Terms such as *narcolepsy, insomnia, sleep apnea* and *excessive daytime sleepiness* are commonly used and understood by a greater percentage of the population than before. Laypersons have become more aware that there is help available if they suffer from a sleep disorder. This increased awareness is a positive development. Better understanding of the symptoms and features of a sleep disorder leads to more rapid recognition and treatment of the disorder.

The Encyclopedia of Sleep and Sleep Disorders has been updated to reflect the current science and understanding of sleep disorders and includes the addition of numerous entries that reflect new terms, drugs and procedures introduced in the last decade. Recent advances in the understanding of the pathophysiology of sleep and wakefulness, including the recognition of a neurochemical system involved in the control of sleep and wakefulness, the orexin system, are covered in this second edition. Revised entries reflect the advances in our understanding and treatment of disorders such as sleep apnea, insomnia and narcolepsy. Modafinil, recently approved in the United States, is a major breakthrough medication for the treatment of disorders of tiredness, fatigue, sleepiness and narcolepsy. This medication is being used to treat obstructive sleep apnea syndrome and other disorders that produce tiredness and fatigue, such as multiple sclerosis.

Along with the increased availability of sleep specialists, sleep disorders centers and current treatments for sleep disorders, there has been growth in public knowledge of sleep disorders, in part through the efforts of such national organizations as the National Sleep Foundation (NSF). The NSF has helped to propagate information on innovative advances in sleep medicine as well as helping corporate America understand the implications of sleep disorders and sleepiness in the workplace.

Appendix II, the American Academy of Sleep Medicine (AASM)—Member Sleep Centers and Laboratories, is an updated list. (Further updates are available at the AASM's website: http://www.aasmnet.org.) Sources that provide further information about sleep disorders have been updated with website addresses, if available. The entries and bibliography have also been updated with new popular and scholarly books and articles that have been published since the first edition.

In the A to Z section, words or terms in SMALL CAPITAL LETTERS within an entry indicate that there is a separate entry for that term, concept or disorder. For further information, you are directed to that separate entry, arranged alphabetically.

—Michael J. Thorpy, M.D.
—Jan Yager, Ph.D.

PREFACE TO THE FIRST EDITION

The Encyclopedia of Sleep and Sleep Disorders is intended for laypersons as well as health care professionals. We have tried to use clear, understandable language, without distorting the meanings of the terms and conditions we describe. We hope this volume is useful to laypersons who are experiencing a sleep-related problem, or who have a family member or friend who has sleep concerns; to students at a variety of undergraduate and graduate levels; to the administrative staff and technicians of sleep disorder centers, psychologists, and specialists in sleep disorders medicine as well as physicians of all specialties.

Sleep is an area of increasing interest as the connection between physical and mental well-being and sleep disorders becomes clearer to clinicians and laypersons alike. Such problems as insomnia or excessive sleepiness affect a large percentage of the population and are of concern not only to patients but also to family members and employers. The relationship among alcohol, alertness, alcohol-related driving accidents, and sleep and sleep disorders affects the community as a whole.

This volume contains descriptions of the most common as well as the more obscure sleep-related disorders. We have described the most commonly prescribed medications and "home" remedies for sleep and alertness, listing their advantages and disadvantages. Also included are case histories for common sleep disorders, among them, insomnia, elderly sleep, anxiety disorders, narcolepsy, sleepwalking, sleep terrors and obstructive sleep apnea syndrome.

Although this volume is intended to stand alone, it appears as a new volume in a well-regarded series, begun by Facts On File, Inc., that now includes *The Encyclopedia of Alcoholism* by Robert O'Brien and Dr. Morris Chafetz; *The Encyclopedia of Drug Abuse* by Robert O'Brien and Dr. Sidney Cohen, M.D.; *The Encyclopedia of Suicide* by Glen Evans and Norman Fabrow, M.D.; *The Encyclopedia of Child Abuse* by Robin Clark and Judith Freeman Clark; *The Encyclopedia of Marriage, Divorce and the Family* by Margaret DiCanio, Ph.D., among other titles.

We have tried to be as up-to-date in our information as possible. However, any project of this kind is a continuing effort, as new information is acquired and new treatment modalities are developed and put into practice. New research studies will provide additional knowledge or refute or confirm previously held ideas. Future editions will take into account any additional information on sleep and sleep disorders unavailable or unknown at this time.

We have included lists of sleep centers and laboratories that are members of the American Sleep Disorders Association (ASDA) and of organizations and agencies that provide additional sleep-related information, as well as a bibliography of popular and scholarly books, journal or magazine articles and newspaper references, to help readers to further explore this key subject.

—Michael J. Thorpy, M.D.
—Jan Yager, Ph.D.

ACKNOWLEDGMENTS

An enormous project like this rests upon the efforts of more than the authors alone. First and foremost, we want to thank James Chambers, our editor for this second edition, as well as his assistant, Regina Sampogna, and project editor Dorothy Cummings. In the first edition, we thanked Howard Epstein, former president of Facts On File, Inc., as well as our former editor, Kate Kelly, for her enthusiasm and commitment to this project from the start, and for the competence and attention to detail with which she followed the project, and to Neal Maillet, who saw it through to its publication.

Sleep experts from around the world kindly provided their curriculum vitae and lists of publications to help in the creation of their biographical entries; they then checked over these entries for accuracy. A collective thanks is offered to all those individuals in this country as well as in France, England, Scotland, Canada, Japan, Israel and Italy.

The American Academy of Sleep Medicine (formerly the American Sleep Disorders Association) based in Rochester, Minnesota, and its membership director, Gregory Mader, have been especially helpful in granting permission to reprint in the Appendix the International Classification of Sleep Disorders, the Diagnostic Classification of Sleep and Arousal Disorders as well as a list of member sleep centers and laboratories.

We would also like to thank Arthur J. Spielman, Ph.D., and Paul B. Glovinsky, Ph.D., of the Department of Psychology of the City College of New York and Paul D'Ambrosio of the Department of Psychology of the City College of New York, who contributed to the essay for the second edition, for providing their original essay on the psychology of sleep that follows Dr. Thorpy's introductory essay, "History of Sleep and Man."

Dr. Yager would especially like to thank Dr. Thorpy, who provided the majority of the content of this encyclopedia based on his enormous knowledge, experience and research in the field of sleep and sleep disorders medicine.

Dr. Thorpy appreciates, in preparing his introductory essay, the careful review by Dr. William Dement and Dr. Steven Martin, the library assistance of Vernon Bruette, Josephina Lim, Deborah Green and Andreas Lamerz, and the secretarial assistance of Elaine Ullman.

Finally, we would both like to thank our families for their patience while we completed this vast undertaking as well as this revised and updated edition, a decade after the first edition was published. To get from the first entry to the more than 800 completed entries—and the numerous drafts back and forth of each and every entry—required sacrifice and selflessness on their parts, as this project consumed much of our time and concentration.

IMPORTANT NOTE AND DISCLAIMER

This book is not intended to take the place of medical advice from a medical professional or psychological or psychiatric advice from a therapist. Readers are advised to consult a physician, psychologist, psychiatrist or other qualified health or psychological professional regarding treatment of any sleep, health or psychological problems. Neither the publisher nor the authors take any responsibility for any possible consequences from any treatment, action or application of medicine or preparation by any person reading or following the information in this book.

Before you make any changes in your or someone else's sleep or health care regimens, or take any medications described in this book, make sure you consult a licensed physician, preferably a sleep expert. While this book provides general information on sleep strategies and disorders, since every person is unique, it is not intended to be a substitute for appropriate medical or psychological diagnosis or treatment. If you or someone you know has a sleep-related concern or a persistent problem, consult your physician or a physician/qualified health care professional at one of the accredited sleep disorder centers listed in Appendix II or at the website for the American Academy of Sleep Medicine (AASM), which continually updates its list of accredited sleep disorders centers (http://www.aasmnet.org).

Throughout this book, you will find street addresses for associations or organizations, phone numbers, fax numbers, e-mail addresses or websites. Since this information may change at any time, including even the name of the association or the existence of a website on the Internet, neither the publishers nor the authors take any responsibility for the accuracy of any listings.

HISTORY OF SLEEP AND MAN

Michael J. Thorpy, M.D.

"Sleep; King of all the gods and of all mortals,
hearken now, prithee, to my word;
and if ever before thou didst listen, obey me now,
and I will ever be grateful to thee all my days."

—Homer, Fourteenth Book of the *Iliad*

Few physiological conditions have received as much attention through the ages by poets, novelists, scholars and scientists as sleep. From Aristotle and Ovid, to Shakespeare and Dante, writers have been fascinated with sleep and its impact upon emotions, behavior and health. The cause and reason for sleep have been pondered by some of the world's greatest minds, including Hippocrates and Freud, who attempted explanations of the physiological basis of sleep and dreams. Not only has sleep and waking behavior changed through the ages but the environment for sleep has also undergone a change. From communal sleeping rooms with beds of twigs, straw or skins, the bedroom has evolved in the 21st century into a private place with electronic equipment, including computers, remote-controlled television, thermostats and lighting.

A rudimentary understanding of insomnia and sleepiness was known in ancient times, but specific sleep disorders, such as narcolepsy, began to be recognized only in the late 19th century. Differentiation between causes of sleepiness and insomnia has reached a peak within the last 50 years since the development of sophisticated technology for the investigation of sleep.

Although most sleep disorders have probably been present since man evolved, modern society has inadvertently produced several new disorders. Thomas Edison's electric light bulb has allowed the light of day to be extended into night so that shift work can now occur around the clock—but at the expense of circadian rhythm disruption and sleep disturbance. Similarly, international travel by plane has enabled the rapid crossing of time zones, which also can lead to a disruption of circadian rhythms and sleep disturbance.

Scientific investigation has produced more information on the physiology and pathophysiology of sleep in recent years than ever before. This rapid advance in sleep research and the development of sleep disorders medicine is producing answers to questions that date from antiquity regarding the third of our day that is spent in the mysterious state of sleep.

Sleep in Prehistoric and Ancient Times

"Sleep's the only medicine that gives ease."

—Sophocles, *Philoctetes*

The sleep patterns and sleep disorders of prehistoric man are unknown, and therefore we must speculate from the comparative physiology of animals and from evidence of other behaviors and illnesses. Theories on the phylogenetic development of sleep stages in mammals have been developed from information available on the mammal-like reptiles. The earliest form of life developed about 600 million years ago in the pre-Cambrian period, and mammal-like reptiles evolved approximately 250 million years ago. It was about 180 million years ago, when slow wave sleep is believed to have appeared, that the monotremes (egg-laying mammals) evolved as a separate line from the therian (live-bearing) mammals; REM sleep (paradoxical sleep) appeared about 50 million years later. Recent sleep research on one of the three surviving monotremes, the Australian short-nosed echidna, has provided some of the evidence for the evolution of sleep stages. The echidna does not have paradoxical sleep, which suggests that the reptilian ancestors also may not have had paradoxical sleep.

The pattern of sleep and waking behavior in prehistoric man can be deduced from studies of nonhuman primates, such as apes and Old World monkeys, the animal groups phylogenetically closest to man. Sleep-wake patterns in non-primates consist mainly of polyphasic episodes of rest and activity with frequent (up to 12) cycles of wakeful activity throughout the 24-hour day. Man has the most developed monophasic pattern, with one episode of consolidated sleep and one main episode of wakefulness. Some animals have a biphasic sleep-wake pattern, with a nap taken during the daytime, the pattern present, for instance, in the chimpanzee. The chimpanzee has a rather prolonged sleep episode from dusk to dawn of approximately 10 hours; however, during this time there are frequent, brief awakenings. The daytime is characterized by two long episodes of wakefulness and an approximately five-hour midday nap, which also includes frequent brief wakefulness episodes.

An early polyphasic sleep pattern seems likely to have been characteristic of earliest man, particularly if man also attempted to sleep between dusk and dawn. There would have been frequent awakenings during the major sleep episode, as a single sleep episode of more than 10 hours appears unlikely. It is reasonable to predict that man first began to develop a monophasic sleep-wake pattern in the Neolithic period (since 10,000 B.C.). The chimpanzee's sleep pattern probably was similar to that present in man prior to the Neolithic period; Neanderthal Man (70,000 to 40,000 B.C.) may well have been in a transitional stage between a polyphasic sleep pattern and the monophasic pattern seen today.

There is evidence from studies of animal fossils that disease was present even before humans evolved. It is known that dinosaurs and prehistoric bears commonly suffered arthritic changes in their bones (called "Cave Gout"). Changes suggestive of tuberculosis have also been seen in Neolithic bones. However, although it must have occurred, there is no evidence of disease outside of the skeleton in humans, as no soft tissue parts have been discovered that are earlier than 4,000 years B.C. Medical evidence of illnesses such as pneumonia, arteriosclerosis and parasitic disease has been found in the mummies of early Egypt, and it is reasonable to expect that the presence of disease in early man was associated with changes in sleep and wakefulness in a similar manner as is seen today. However, evidence also suggests that man's lifetime was much shorter during the Paleolithic and early Neolithic periods, averaging only about 30 to 40 years. The sleep disturbances of concern to the elderly today may not have been a problem in prehistoric man.

It seems reasonable that prehistoric man would have attempted to treat sleep disturbances, but how early man treated these disorders is unknown. Therapy probably resembled that utilized by sick animals, such as the removal of infective agents, eating various plants to induce emesis, and possibly even bloodletting. Certainly, bloodletting became an increasingly frequent therapeutic means for treating disease, including sleep disorders, in more advanced ancient civilizations. Primitive societies, even today, consider many illnesses and diseases to be caused by gods, magic and spirits, and therefore various forms of divination, such as the casting of bones, moving of beads, charms, fetishes, chanting or the use of elaborate ceremonies, are invoked for therapeutic reasons. Such forms of treatment probably were applied by prehistoric man for disturbances of sleep and wakefulness.

Mesopotamians (ca. 3000 B.C.) thought illness was produced by irate gods, and so their gods were named for specific diseases, such as Tiu, the god of headache, and Nergel, the god of fever. Treatment largely consisted of determining what misdeed had been committed by the sufferer, and then performing divination in an attempt to appease the gods. Plants, oils, minerals and animal substances were ingested, inhaled or given as suppositories or enemas. These agents were usually administered by a priest/physician, and strict codes for payment of medical services were established, as well as physician punishment for a failure to treat disease adequately. It is likely that many punishments were administered for failure to relieve sleep disorders that would have been chronic and often difficult to cure, such as insomnia and narcolepsy.

The ancient medical papyruses of Egypt provide most of our current knowledge of ancient Egyptian medicine. The Chester Beatty papyrus, which was written around 1350 B.C., contains information on the interpretation of dreams. Dreams were regarded as being contrary predictions, for example, a dream of death meant a long life. However, the Georg Ebers papyrus (1600 B.C.), an extensive text on a variety of medical subjects, including treatment, has not been reported to contain any information on sleep disturbances. Ancient Egyptian medical practice consisted largely of praying to the gods and invoking the help of these divine healers. Thoth, who was a physician to the gods, and Imhotep were important gods of healing at that time. The ancient Egyptians were known for their attention to hygiene and cleanliness, and it is likely that such attention was also paid to sleeping habits.

Medical opinion at the time held that the body was made up of a system of channels (Metu), which conveyed air to all parts of the body. Because they believed that bodily fluids could enter this system of channels, the ancient Egyptians were particularly concerned about feces entering the Metu. Hence the treatment of many illnesses was carried out by purging and enemas. Infective illnesses, including malaria, parasitic infections, smallpox and leprosy, were common at that time. Wine and other mildly alcoholic drinks (as compared to distilled alcoholic products) were consumed in large amounts and were probably the earliest treatments for insomnia but also may have been important in its development. Medicinal plants were utilized, particularly the product of the opium poppy (*papaver somniferum*), and hyoscyamine and scopolamine, derived from belladonna and nightshade. (The word "opium" is derived from the Greek word for "juice," as the drug is derived from the juice of the poppy. *Papaver somniferum* was coined at a much later date; *somniferum* was derived from the Latin word *somnus* [the Roman god of sleep]. In subsequent periods in history opium [laudanum] was widely used as a treatment for insomnia, and it is likely that it was used as far back as the Sumerian age, which suggests that opium may have been the first hypnotic medication used.)

Bloodletting was commonly performed by the ancient Egyptians for the treatment of a variety of ailments and illnesses and was likely to have been used for sleep disorders, particularly for those disorders that produced excessive sleepiness or stupor. Medical treatment was widely available; the names of several hundred physicians have been documented in ancient Egypt. Herodotus (fifth century B.C.) wrote of the Egyptians:

> Medicine with them is distributed in the following way: every physician is for one disease and not for several, and the whole country is full of physicians for the eyes; others of the head; others of the teeth; others of the belly, and others of obscure diseases.

It appears likely that some physicians specialized in insomnia, and possibly even in disorders that produced excessive sleepiness. There certainly were physicians who specialized in dream interpretation, for example Artemidorus of Daldis who wrote the major work on dreams, *Oneirocritica.*

Other civilizations that developed around the same time were those of ancient India and China. Early Indian medicine mainly consisted of magical and religious practices but also featured soundly based, rational treatments. Over 700 Indian vegetable medicines have been documented from ancient times and include the plant called *Rauwolfia serpentina* (reserpine). Rauwolfia was used for the treatment of anxiety, among other disorders, and is likely to have been used to treat insomnia. In India, as in Egypt, infective illnesses were common, and therefore physicians, who were largely from the Brahman or priestly caste, were viewed with great importance. Effective treatment of most illnesses is reported to have been dependent upon four major factors: the physician, the patient, the medicine and the nurse. Asoka (273–232 B.C.), a ruler of the Mauryan dynasty, reported that hospitals were established as early as the third century B.C.

The ancient Chinese believed in the importance of the universe and environment in producing all things, including behavior and health. The basic principles of life were thought to derive from the interplay of two basic elements in nature, the active, light, dry, warm, positive, masculine *Yang*, and the passive, dark, cold, moist, negative *Yin*. The proportions of Yin and Yang determined the *Tao* (the way), which determined right and wrong, good and bad, health or illness, etc. The basic Yin-Yang symbol is attributed to Fu Hsi (ca. 2900 B.C.), who originated the concept of eight interacting conditions, the "Pa kua." The Yin-Yang has since become the symbol for sleep and wakefulness. (This Yin-Yang symbol has been adopted by the American Academy of Sleep Medicine as its emblem.) Chinese views on physiology were similar to those of the ancient Greeks; they also believed in a humoral system of physiology. The palpation of the pulse was important in the diagnosis of disease, and in order to determine whether a patient had upset the Tao, not only were the patient's symptoms taken into consideration but also the social and economic status, the weather and particularly the patient's dreams, as well as the dreams of other family members.

The most important medical compendium of the time was that produced by Yu Hsiung (ca. 2600 B.C.), the *Nei Ching* ("Canon of Medicine"), which mentioned five important methods of treatment: curing the spirit, nourishing the body, the administration of medications, treating the whole body and the use of acupuncture and moxibustion (counter-irritation by moxa, a combustible substance that is burned on the skin). It is most likely that these latter forms of therapy were applied to the sleep disorders. Massage and breathing exercises were also commonly employed, in a manner similar to that of Yoga. Herbal medicines were plentiful and consisted of extracts of virtually anything available, including minerals and metals, animal-derived products and waste products.

Two important Chinese remedies existed. One was ephedra (Ma Huang), a stimulant that contained ephedrine, derived from the "horsetail" plant and first described by the Red Emperor, Shen Nung (ca. 2800 B.C.). The second common medicinal herb was ginseng (a man-shaped root), which was used for stimulation as well as sedating purposes. Although opium was commonly employed by the Greeks at this time it does not appear to have been used in ancient China. Acupuncture was widespread and is believed to have been developed by the Yellow Emperor (Huang Ti) around 2600 B.C. Acupuncture and moxibustion were used for treating virtually every illness and symptom and therefore are likely to have been administered for sleep disorders.

In ancient China, physicians were also highly regarded and were grouped into five categories, the chief physician, food physicians, physicians for simple diseases, ulcer physicians and physicians for animals. They were rated according to their treatment results, and each doctor had to report his therapeutic successes and failures. Sleep was regarded by the Chinese as a state of unity with the universe and therefore was regarded as very important for health. The Chinese philosopher Chuang-Tzu (300 B.C.) said "everything is one; during sleep the soul, undistracted, is absorbed into the unity; when awake, distracted, it sees the different beings."

Much of what we know about early Greek medicine is derived from the *Iliad* and *Odyssey* of Homer, a collection of traditions, legends and epic poems. Homer (ca. 900 B.C.) based his epic works on the life of the ancient Greeks in the days of the Mycenaean Citadel of about 1200 B.C. The Mycenaeans, who came from mainland Greece about 1600 B.C., conquered the Minoans, who had established a well-developed civilization in Crete at Knossus. This civilization was the setting for Homer's epics, which concerned an earlier period, but his writings included medical details that were probably derived from his own era. However, Homer's view of medicine in early Greece, called Homeric medicine, is the best representation of early Greek medical practices. The quotation from the *Iliad* stated at the beginning of this introduction reflects the importance that Homer ascribed to good, quality sleep. The god of sleep, Hypnos, from whom the terms *hypnotic* and *hypnotism* have developed, was first reported in the 14th book of the *Iliad* by Homer, and was mentioned again in the *Theogony* of Hesiod (ca. 700 B.C.) about two centuries later.

Also mentioned in Homer was the chieftain Asclepios and his two sons: Machanon, who in subsequent centuries became known as the father of surgery, and Podalirios, the father of internal medicine. In subsequent years, Asclepios became known as the god of healing, and temples were erected in his honor, the first being established about the sixth century B.C. in Thessaly or Ipidauros. The Asclepieian temples were a collection of several buildings that in many cases were very elaborate and ornate. They consisted of a tholos, a round building that contained water for purification, and a main temple, which were separated by a building called the abaton. The abaton was a most important structure as it was the site where ill patients were placed for a cure. The cure consisted of an "incubation" ceremony in which the cure took place in each worshipper's dreams. The medical ceremony began at dusk and the ill patient lay on a bed of skins to await a visit by Asclepios, the god for healing. During the night the priest would visit each patient and administer a treatment, which often consisted of medicines derived from such animals as snakes and geese. Upon awakening the next morning after dreaming of Asclepios, the patient was expected to have been cured. This treatment was clearly the forerunner of sleep therapy, which has been practiced through the ages until the present day, particularly in eastern countries. Although Asclepieian medicine was used to treat any type of illness, it was most effective for those of a psychological nature. Much of the healing was probably related to the impressive ceremony and the relaxation that occurred in conjunction with the setting. The priest-physicians instilled faith in the cures—not only in their patients but also in themselves. However, many attempted cures were in the realm of magic and fantasy.

A more rational style of medicine developed around the fifth century B.C. largely due to the influence of the Greek scientist-philosophers, such as Thales and Pythagoras.

Thales of Miletos (640–546 B.C.), who believed that water was an important basic element of all animal and plant life, made many contributions not only to medicine, but also to geometry, astronomy and mathematics. His direction in medicine was not inspired by mythological or religious beliefs but rather by observing natural processes of the environment. Around the same time, Pythagoras (ca. 530 B.C.) was born on an island off the coast of Asia Minor and developed a school of medicine at Crotona in Southern Italy. Pythagoras developed a philosophical approach to medicine that was based on the science of numbers and the spiritual universe, but the importance of diet, exercise, music and meditation was emphasized.

Alcmaeon (fifth century B.C.), of the Crotona school of medical thought, concentrated on man, and his basic belief was that health was harmony and disease was a disturbance of harmony. He considered the brain essential for memory and thought, a belief that Aristotle, who believed that the mind resided in the heart, would reject 100 years later. Alcmaeon proposed what was probably the first theory on the cause of sleep, when he postulated that sleep occurred when the blood vessels of the brain filled with blood; withdrawal of blood from the brain was associated with waking. However, his major contribution to medicine was the detailed description of the optic pathways at the base of the brain. His much more rational concepts of medicine have led some to consider him the first true medical scientist.

Around the time of Alcmaeon, a center of medicine was established in Sicily, and Empedocles (ca. 493–ca. 443 B.C.) was credited with the original concept that all things are comprised of four basic elements: water, air, fire and earth (the importance of these four elements had been established earlier). Empedocles believed that sleep occurs when the fire in the blood cools, thus separating one of the four elements from the others. He believed that illnesses were due either to separation of the four elements or alterations in their balance. The principle of the balance of body humors, known as humoralism, became established medical doctrine around this time. Humoralism considered health to be due to the balance of four body fluids: blood, phlegm, yellow bile and black bile. These fluids were usually seen during severe illnesses and disappeared when the crises were over.

Two other major schools of medicine were developed in the fifth century B.C., one at Cnidos and the other at Cos. At Cnidos an elaborate classification system for diseases resulted in each specific disease being ascribed to one symptom. The school at Cos did not develop elaborate diagnoses but depended largely upon the development of rational treatments and rational diagnostic principles.

> In whatever disease sleep is laborious,
> it is a deadly symptom.
>
> —Hippocrates, *Aphorisms,* II

Hippocrates (460–370 B.C.) was born on the island of Cos and was responsible for that school of medicine's direction. No individual in history has had more influence upon medicine than Hippocrates, who produced many of the basic tenets that underlie the practice of modern medicine. Hippocrates produced numerous works that are gathered under the title *Corpus Hippocraticum,* which comprises not only his own writings but also the writings of others of the time. His approximately 72 books covered all aspects of medicine, including medical ethics, and are most widely known for the Hippocratic oath. In his writings, Hippocrates discussed not only his theory of the cause of sleep, but he also made suggestions on the cause of dreams, which he considered to be of "medical" origin. Hippocrates stated that "sleep is due to blood going from the limbs to the inner regions of the body." This statement was based upon the recognition of the importance of the blood being warmed by the inner part of the body in order to produce sleep—a theory contrary to that proposed by Alcmaeon. Hippocrates believed that narcotics derived from the opium poppy could be useful in treatment; therefore, they were most likely applied to treat insomnia at that time.

Following Hippocrates, the philosophers Plato and Aristotle had an important influence upon medicine. Plato (ca. 429–347 B.C.), a teacher of Aristotle, developed many medical speculations. He influenced the practice of medicine to the extent that medical practice became more dogma rather than patient evaluation. For this reason physicians who supported his doctrines were called "dogmatists" and their therapeutic endeavors largely included drastic purgings and bleedings. Aristotle (384–322 B.C.) believed that dreams were important predictors of the future but proposed a theory of sleep based upon the effect of food ingestion. He proposed that food once eaten induced fumes that were taken into the blood vessels and then transferred into the brain where they induced sleepiness. The fumes subsequently cooled and returned to the lower parts of the body taking heat away from the brain, thereby causing sleep onset. The sleep process continued as long as food was being digested. Following the Hippocratic era of medicine, Greek medicine began to develop in Rome, along with temples to Asclepios in 300 B.C.

Atomism, the concept that all physical objects are comprised of atoms in an infinite number that undergo random motion, was first developed by Democritus of Abdera (ca. 420 B.C.) and Leucippus of Miletus (ca. 430 B.C.). Leucippus regarded sleep as a state caused by the partial or complete splitting-off of atoms. Democritus considered insomnia the result of an unhealthy diet and daytime sleeping as being a sign of ill-health. Epicurus (ca. 300 B.C.) revived the theory of atomism and wrote extensively on sleep and dreams, although his own works have been lost. The Roman poet Titus Lucretius Carus (ca. 50 B.C.) wrote of the teachings of Epicurus on atomism, sleep and dreams, in a poem entitled "De rerum natura." In this poem, the loss of central control that leads to loss of peripheral muscle control and relaxation forms the foundation of a neural theory of sleep that took 2,000 years to be expanded upon:

> And so, when the motions are changed, sense withdraws deep within. And since there is nothing which can, as it were, support the limbs, the body

> grows feeble, and all the limbs are slackened; arms and eyelids droop, and the hams, even as you lie down, often give way, and relax their strength.

Asclepiades of Bithynia (ca. 120–ca. 70 B.C.), another figure in Roman medicine, believed that the physician was more important in curing disease than was nature. He used the term "phrenitis" for mental illness and invoked treatment that consisted of hygiene, opium and wine. He was also the first to popularize the tracheostomy as a treatment for upper airway obstruction.

Cornelius Celsus (ca. A.D. 20) and Caius Pliny the elder (A.D. 23–79) substantially documented medical practice of their time. *De Medicina,* the work of Celsus, covered a wide range of topics, including history, preventative medicine, surgery and anatomy. Pliny produced *Historia Naturalis,* a work that contained virtually every piece of medical information available.

Although Pliny's writings were regarded as the mainstay of medicine right through the Middle Ages, the Greek Galen (A.D. 129–ca. 200) had a greater impact on the subsequent development of medicine. Galen's detailed writings substantially contributed to the knowledge of anatomy and he outlined the important elements of diagnosis and treatment. He believed bloodletting was important in the treatment of many illnesses, but he also encouraged conservative treatments, such as diet, rest and exercise. He utilized many herbal medicines, often in complicated combinations. The anatomical works of Galen reigned supreme in medicine until the works of Vesalius in the 16th century.

Sleep in the Bible

The Bible contains numerous references to sleep and dreams, which were largely regarded as being predictors of the future (but less significant than in previous eras) The Bible emphasized the importance of sleep and rest: the essential elements for good sleep were regarded as being hard work, a clear conscience, freedom from anxiety and trust in Jehovah (Ecclesiastes 5:12; Psalms 3:5, 4:8; Proverbs 3:24–26). Sleep disturbance was less likely to occur if one was content with life's lot, and sleeplessness would result from excessive worry about material possessions (Ecclesiastes 5:12).

However, the Bible also indicated that wrongdoings made people unnecessarily content, "they do not sleep unless they do badness, and their sleep has been snatched away unless they cause someone to stumble" (Proverbs 4:16). Excessive sleeping was regarded as being unacceptable as it produced laziness and could subsequently lead to poverty. "Laziness causes a deep sleep to fall" (Proverbs 6:9–11, 10:5, 19:15, 20:13, 24:33–34). The apostle Paul emphasized (Romans 13:11–13) the importance of being active in order to spread the word of God:

> It is already the hour for you to awake from sleep, for now our salvation is nearer than at the time that we became believers. The night is well along; the day has drawn near. Let us therefore put off the works belonging to darkness and let us put on the weapons of the light: as in the daytime let us walk decently, not in revelries and drunken bouts, not in illicit intercourse and loose conduct, not in strife and jealousy.

Sleep was often used as a term in place of death. In ancient Rome and Greece the similarity between death and sleep was often emphasized. "Sleep and death, who are twin brothers," Homer said in the *Iliad* (ca. 850 B.C.); and Ovid (43 B.C.–A.D. 17) in the *Amores II,* "What else is sleep but the image of chill death?" In the Bible there were numerous references to death being similar to sleep in that it was God who caused people to awaken from sleep, otherwise they would never wake up (Psalms 76:6). However, death was contrasted with sleep in the example of a dead girl, where Jesus Christ said "the little girl did not die but she is sleeping" (Matthew 9:24; Mark 5:39; Luke 8:52). This reference may have referred to the fact that she could be resurrected from death as one is awakened from sleep.

Dreams played an important part in the Bible as a means of communicating between God and man. The first book of the Bible, Genesis (28:10–16), reports communication between Jacob and God:

> And Jacob went out from Beresheeba, and went toward Haran.
>
> And he lighted upon a certain place, and tarried there all night, because the sun was set; and he

> took one of the stones of that place and put them for his pillows, and laid down in that place to sleep.
>
> And he dreamed, and behold a ladder set up on the earth, and the top of it reached to heaven: and behold the angels of God ascending and descending on it.
>
> And, behold, the Lord stood above it, and said, I am the Lord God of Abraham thy father, and God of Isaac: the land whereon thou liest, to thee will I give it and to thy seed;
>
> and thy seed shall be as the dust of the earth, and thou shalt spread abroad to the west, and to the east, and to the north, and to the south: in thee and in thy seed shall all the families of the earth be blessed.
>
> And behold I am with thee, and will keep thee in all places whither thou goest, and will bring thee again into this land; for I will not leave thee, until I have done that which I have spoken to thee of.
>
> And Jacob awaked out of his sleep, and he said, surely the Lord is in this place; and I knew it not.

Many other examples of dreams are presented in the Bible, such as Joseph's dream to take Mary as his wife, his dream to flee to Egypt with his family, the dream that it was safe to return home, and the dream of the Magi.

Sleep in the Middle Ages and the Renaissance

> Long sleep at after-noones by stirring fumes
> Breeds Slouth, and Agues
> Aking heads and Rheumes.
>
> —School at Salerno, Regimen: Sanitatis Salernitanum (1095–1224)

The time from the fall of Rome in A.D. 476 until the fall of Constantinople in A.D. 1453 is often referred to as the Middle Ages, the first 500 years being the Dark Ages. Both Ages comprise the Medieval period, the Age of Faith, a time when medicine was greatly influenced by the rise of Christianity.

With the spread of the word of Christianity, man was convinced that the day of judgment was about to come, and disease was considered to be due to God's punishment. Prayer and good deeds were considered to be important for cures and to prevent illness. Concern for "thy neighbor" led to the establishment of facilities for the care of the ill, most of which were run with religious motives. Medicine involved strong religious mysticism, and there was a loss of the rational, clinical observation and management of disease that had begun to develop in earlier years. Monasteries that cared for the sick were developed but they scorned scientific, medical teaching. One of the first to be established was Monte Cassino in Italy by St. Benedict of Nursia (A.D. 480–554). It was in these times that the Temples of Asclepios were also popular for the treatment of illnesses by Incubatio. Although superstition and magic swept the western world, some physicians with skill in observation and deduction slowly advanced medical knowledge, such as Alexander of Tralles (A.D. 525–605).

In the Moslem world, a similar religious approach to medicine occurred. Although in Islam disease is regarded as a punishment by Allah, hospitals in Moslem countries were very much better than those in the West because of their improved sanitation and better and more spacious facilities. Although physicians were largely of the Christian and Jewish faiths, Moslem practitioners gradually helped spread medicine in the East. The Persian Razi (A.D. 850–ca. 923) (also known as Rhazes in the West) wrote more than 200 books on many topics, including medicine. Avicenna (A.D. 980–1037), who also contributed to medical understanding, was regarded both in Islam and Christendom as being of equal importance to Galen.

A little later, Moses ben Maimon (A.D. 1135–1204), also known as Maimonides, emerged as the most influential Jewish physician in Arabic medicine. He appeared to combine the thoughts of Hippocrates, Galen and Avicenna but his primary focus was on philosophy. Maimonides had his own view of how much and when a person should sleep:

> The day and night consist of 24 hours. It is sufficient for a person to sleep one third thereof which is eight hours. These should [preferably] be at the end of the night so that from the beginning of sleep

until the rising of the sun will be eight hours. Thus he will arise from his bed before the sun rises.

—Misheneh Torah, "Hilchoth De'oth" (Ch.IV, No. 4)

In the 10th century A.D., several medical schools came into prominence. Perhaps the oldest was that established at Salerno, not far from Monte Cassino. The school at Salerno developed a practical scientific approach to medicine, eschewing its neighbor's concentration on philosophy and religious mysticism. Several universities in France, including those at Montpellier and Paris, were also highly regarded. At Paris, the school had a medical rather than a surgical bias, being more influenced by the Church. At Montpellier, Greek practices were more in evidence.

By A.D. 1000, at the end of the Dark Ages, monastic medicine began to decline as the influence of the universities increased. Many hospitals developed that are well known today, such as St. Thomas's and St. Bartholomew's in England and the Hotel-Dieu in Paris. Here diet was regarded as an important form of treatment, as were medications, particularly those derived from plant materials. One of the most commonly used medications at this time was theriac, which had been developed in the first century A.D.; it consisted of many substances derived from plants and animals, including snake flesh. Theriac would have been used for the treatment of a variety of sleep disorders, particularly those thought to be caused by poisons. Mysticism and astrology were important elements of medicine in the Middle Ages. Often the most important treatment to be considered was exorcism; however, purgatives and bloodletting were treatments that were still commonly employed.

In the 15th and 16th centuries, the works of Hippocrates were revived. Paracelsus (1493–1541), known as the Father of Pharmacology, began using metals in treatment, often producing some outstanding cures. Although illnesses such as leprosy and the plague had largely disappeared, venereal diseases such as gonorrhea and syphilis were rampant. Art and medicine became allied, as evidenced in the anatomical drawings of Michelangelo Buonarroti (1475–1564) and Albrecht Dürer (1471–1528). Andreas Vesalius (1514–64) produced one of the greatest medical books in history, entitled *De Humani Corporis Fabrica.* The detailed anatomical drawings surpassed those of Galen, and *Fabrica* became the anatomical cornerstone in the development of scientific medicine in the centuries to come.

Sleep in the 17th and 18th Centuries

Methought I heard a voice cry, "Sleep no more!
Macbeth does murder sleep," the innocent sleep,
Sleep that knits up the ravell'd sleave of care,
The death of each day's life, sore labour's bath,
Balm of hurt minds, great nature's second course,
Chief nourisher in life's feast.

—Shakespeare: *Macbeth,* Act II (ca. 1605)

In the 17th century, medicine underwent a major change from the doctrines that had influenced it up to that time, such as Aristotelianism, Galenism and Paracelsianism, to more scientifically directed theories, with the underlying teleological desire to accumulate knowledge on the way things work. This time was known as the "Age of Scientific Revolution" and included the major medical developments of Francis Bacon, William Harvey and Marcello Malpighi.

The scientific revolution began with the theories of Rene Descartes (1596–1650), who rejected Aristotle's doctrines and developed theories based on mechanisms. In this regard he was similar to Francis Bacon (1561–1626), who espoused experimentation and utilitarianism. Descartes developed a hydraulic model of sleep, which considered that the pineal gland maintained fullness of the cerebral ventricles for the maintenance of alertness. The loss of "animal spirits" from the pineal causes the ventricles to collapse, thereby inducing sleep.

Even Shakespeare made innumerable references to sleep in his writings, and it has been considered that the playwright's clear descriptions of insomnia suggest that he himself suffered from this malady.

. . . O sleep, O gentle sleep,
Nature's soft nurse, how have I frighted thee,

> That thou no more wilt weight my eyelids down
> and steep my senses in forgetfulness . . .

Medicine was now being viewed as an advancement in man's control over nature and was more soundly based on scientific principles. However, it was still a time to be speculative and philosophical about medicine:

> He sleeps well who knows not that he
> sleeps ill.
>
> —Francis Bacon, *Ornamentata Rationalia*, IV
> (quote from Publilius Syrus, Sententiae)

The chemical principles of Paracelsus were advanced in the 17th century, and medicines, including the use of mercurials, began to take over from treatments such as purging and bloodletting. Illness was now considered to be something that attacked the body in a distinct manner, and the Galenic and earlier concepts that disease was a derangement of humors, the essential elements of the body, were starting to fade. Atomism, which had been proposed by Democritus, Leucippus and Epicurus several centuries before the time of Christ, underwent a revival in the 17th century and was supported by the findings of Jan Baptista Van Helmont (1577–1644), who coined the term "gas" and recognized that air was composed of a variety of gases. Robert Boyle (1627–91) demonstrated the importance of air for life and the effect of gases under pressure, which led to the discovery that the reddening of venous blood occurred because of exposure of blood to gases contained in the air. However, the major discovery of the 17th century was that of William Harvey (1578–1657), who was the first to demonstrate that blood was pumped around the body by the heart.

It was against this background that the great neurologists, Thomas Willis (1621–75) and Thomas Sydenham (1624–89), developed the principles and practice of clinical neurology. Willis made a number of contributions to the knowledge of various disorders in sleep, including restless legs syndrome, nightmares and insomnia. He recognized that a component contained in coffee could prevent sleep and that sleep was not a disease but primarily a symptom of underlying causes. His book *The Practice of Physick* (1692) devoted four chapters to disorders producing sleepiness and insomnia. As with Descartes, he considered that the animal spirits contained within the body undergo rest during sleep. However, he believed that those animal spirits residing in the cerebellum became active during sleep to maintain a control over physiology. He believed that some of the "animal spirits" became intermittently unrestrained, leading to the development of dreams. He also described restless legs syndrome, which he considered to be an escape of the animal humors into the nerves supplying the limbs:

> when being a bed, they betake themselves to sleep, presently in the arms and legs, leapings and contractions of the tendons, and so great a restlessness and tossings of their members ensue, that the diseased are no more able to sleep, than if they were in a place of the greatest torture.

Willis also discovered that laudanum, a solution of powdered opium, was effective in treating the restless legs syndrome.

Due to the generally unhygienic living conditions, epidemics—mainly the plague, measles, smallpox, scarlet fever and chicken pox—continued to rage through Europe at this time. Therapy was still largely based on practices of the past, such as purging, bloodletting, dietary restriction, exercise and the use of potions, such as theriac.

Although the 18th century is largely regarded as being a period when the scientific foundation of medicine was extended from the principles laid down in the 17th century, this was not entirely the situation. Some medical theorists played an influential role in maintaining concepts of vitalism. George Stahl (1660–1734) was a strong proponent of the "animal spirits" concept of earlier years and decried Descartes' theory of a machinistic approach to medicine. Stahl also expounded his enthusiasm for treatments such as bloodletting to get rid of the unwanted spirits.

Despite some setbacks, a scientific approach to medicine continued with the works of Linnaeus and Von Haller. Karl Von Linne (1707–78), called Linnaeus, made important contributions to the classifications of botany, zoology and medicine. He emphasized the important of cyclical changes in botany, which was nowhere more clearly presented than in his flower-clock. The flower-clock was developed upon the principle that different species of flowers open their leaves at various times of the day. Therefore, a garden of flowers arranged in a circular pattern could give an estimate of the time of day by the pattern of flower and leaf openings and closings. Linnaeus' finding was an important early milestone in the development of the science of biological rhythms in plants and animals. As far back as ancient Greece there had been some recognition of variation in the behavior of plants and animals, not only on a seasonal basis but also on a daily basis. Even the Bible makes mention of seasonal change in the following passage from Ecclesiastes (3:1): "To everything there is a season and a time to every purpose under the heavens."

One of the first chronobiological experiments was that of Sanctorious (ca. 1657), who measured the cyclical pattern of change in a number of his own physiological variables. His experimental apparatus has been regarded as the first "laboratory for chronobiology." Subsequently the intrinsic pattern of circadian activity was demonstrated in the experiment performed by Jacques De Mairan in 1729, which was reported by M. Marchant. De Mairan placed a heliotrope plant in a darkened closet and observed that the leaves continued to open in darkness, at the same time of day as they had in sunlight. This experiment illustrated the presence of an intrinsic circadian rhythm in the absence of environmental lighting conditions. De Mairan also recognized the importance of this observation for understanding the behavior of patients: "this seems to be related to the sensitivity of a great number of bed-ridden sick people, who, in their confinement, are aware of the differences of day and night."

During the 17th and 18th centuries, medical schools had rapidly expanded throughout Europe, with those north of the French-Italian Alps beginning to gain in prominence. The Swiss-born scientist Albrecht Von Haller (1708–77), a pupil of Boerhaave of the University of Leiden, an important medical center in Europe, made major contributions to many scientific topics, including medicine. Von Haller performed numerous experiments on the nervous system and demonstrated the sensitivity of nerve and the irritability of muscle; in doing so he dispelled much of the mysticism of previous eras. Von Haller produced a major work entitled *Elementa Physiologiae* in which he devoted 36 pages to the physiology of sleep and proposed a theory for its cause. In a vascular concept similar to that of Alcmaeon in the fifth century B.C. he believed that sleep was caused by the flow of blood to the head, which induced pressure on the brain, thereby inducing sleep. Von Haller's theory was expanded in the 19th century into the congestion theory of the causes of sleep, a theory that was still believed into the early part of the 20th century. He also considered dreams to be a symptom of disease, "a stimulating cause, by which the perfect tranquility of the sensorium is interrupted."

The late 17th century was also the time of the discovery of oxygen by Karl Scheele (1742–86) and Joseph Priestley (1733–1804), but it was Antoine-Laurent Lavoisier (1743–94) who coined the name "oxygen" and recognized its importance in the maintenance of living tissue. Despite the important advances in clinical medicine that occurred in the 17th century, there were very few therapeutic advances. Medications still consisted of potions developed from plant and animal tissues, and opium was still the main form of sedation, in a common formulation called "Hoffmann's Anodyne of Opium." However, the ancient practices of bleeding and purging continued to be widely prescribed throughout the 18th century. One medication that was particularly important was discovered as a herbal brew from the foxglove plant, *Digitalis purpurea*. This medication, found by William Withering in 1785, was most helpful in the treatment of dropsy (swelling of the limbs) caused by heart disease. This was also the time of the French Revolution, following which it was recognized that more humane care was necessary for people with psychiatric disease; Phillipe Pinel (1745–1826), who was a supporter of vitalism, has been considered to be the founder of modern psychiatry.

Despite the important advances in the science of medicine and in scientifically based principles of treatment, it was still a time of hoaxes and charlatanism. On the fringe of quackery was Franz Anton Mesmer (1734–1815), who utilized "animal magnetism" for a hypnotic treatment that lead to the term *mesmerism*. He attracted the gullible to undergo treatment in his darkened rooms, which were regarded as cradles of immorality. Mesmer was subsequently banished from Paris, despite producing some effective cures of hysteria by the use of hypnotic suggestion.

Perhaps the greatest advance made in the development of sleep medicine occurred in Bologna with Luigi Galvani's (1737–98) demonstration of electrical activity of the nervous system. His findings led to the subsequent development of the field of electrophysiology, and the gradual destruction of the humoralist theory of nervous activity.

With the development of the scientific approach to medicine, the discovery of atomism, animal electrophysiology, the advances in respiratory and cardiovascular physiology, as well as treatment advances, such as quinine for malaria and digitalis for heart disease, medicine was about to enter its modern era, the 19th century.

Sleep in the 19th Century

> "What probing deep
> Has ever solved the mystery of sleep?"
>
> —Thomas Aldrich (1836–1907),
> *Human Ignorance*

Medicine made rapid advances in the 19th century, largely due to the discovery of anesthesia, the practice of surgery and the finding that microorganisms were a major cause of disease. This was the time of the Industrial Revolution; people came from the depressed countryside to the abhorrent working conditions and slums of the cities to be employed in factories. Although sanitation, as well as preventive medicine, was important, epidemics continued to rage in both Europe and the United States. Cholera and typhoid fever were just two of several infective illnesses that claimed many victims.

There were major advances in understanding the cause of sleep, and in the latter half of the century a number of specific sleep disorders were recognized. The anatomy of sleep and wakefulness was partially revealed through the animal experiments of two outstanding neuroanatomists of the time, Luigi Rolando (1773–1831) and Marie Jan Pierre Flourens (1794–1867).

Rolando in 1809 demonstrated that a state of sleepiness occurred when the cerebral hemispheres of birds were removed, and his experiments were replicated by Flourens in 1822 with the ablation of the cerebral hemispheres of pigeons:

> Just imagine an animal which has been condemned to be permanently asleep, one that has been devoid even of the ability to dream during sleep; this is more or less the situation of the pigeon in which I had ablated the cerebral hemispheres.

The 19th century could be regarded as the "age of sleep theories" as some of the greatest physicians, psychologists and physiologists turned their attention to explanations of the cause of sleep. Advances were made in the clinical recognition of sleep disorders, particularly the causes of daytime sleepiness, and several comprehensive books were written entirely on the physiological and clinical aspects of sleep. Much of what was known about insomnia and its causes, however, was only a slight expansion of earlier knowledge.

The theories of the cause of sleep can be placed into four main groups: vascular (mechanical, anemic, congestive), chemical (humoral), neural (histological) and a fourth group, which explains the reason for sleep rather than the physiological cause of sleep, the behavioral (psychological, biological) theories.

The vascular theories of sleep were those most widely disputed in the early part of the 19th century. They were based upon the first rational theory for the cause of sleep, proposed by Alcmaeon in ancient Greece in the fifth century B.C. Alcmaeon believed that sleep was due to blood filling the brain, and waking associated with the return of blood to the rest of the body, a concept consistent with the notions of ancient times, when it was recognized that brain disorders such as apoplexy were associated with stupor (*karos*). Hippocrates had an alternative theory in that he believed that sleep was due to blood going in the opposite direction, from the limbs to the central part of the body. Von Haller in the 18th century agreed with Alcmaeon's concept and proposed that blood going to the head caused the brain to be pressed against the skull, thereby inducing sleep by cutting off the "animal spirits." Von Haller derived his beliefs from the views of his mentor Hermann Boerhaave (1667–1738), who had presented a similar theory a few years earlier. Johann Friedrich Blumenbach (1752–1840), professor at Göttingen, who is regarded as the founder of modern anthropology, was the first to observe the brain of a sleeping subject in 1795. He noted that the surface of the brain was pale during sleep compared with wakefulness; contrary to earlier theories, he proposed that sleep was caused by the lack of blood in the brain. It was against this background of early sleep theories that the 19th-century researchers looked for the cause of sleep.

The theory that sleep was due to congestion of the brain was the most accepted vascular theory in the first half of the 19th century. Robert MacNish in 1834 wrote a seminal volume on sleep and its disorders, entitled *The Philosophy of Sleep.* MacNish supported the previous concept that sleep was due to pressure on the brain by blood. In 1846 Johannes Evangelistica Purkinje (1787–1869), an outstanding neuroanatomist and professor of physiology and pathology at Breslau (Wroclaw, in modern Poland), proposed a slightly different theory for the cause of sleep that was consistent with the congestive concept. Purkinje proposed that the brain pathways (corona radiata) become compressed by blood congestion of the cell masses of the brain (basal ganglia), thereby severing neural transmission and inducing sleep. James Cappie in 1860 wrote in detail about the circulation of the brain and was one of the last supporters of the congestion theory, which was finally contradicted by the findings of the outstanding clinical neurologist John Hughlings Jackson (1835–1911). In 1863 Jackson observed the optic fundi during sleep and reported that the retinal arteries became pale during sleep, which was consistent with Blumenbach's earlier findings. He therefore reasoned that brain congestion was not a cause of sleep.

The main alternative to the congestion theory was that sleep was due to insufficient blood in the brain (anemia). William Alexander Hammond (1828–1900), the noted American physician, in 1854 was the first in the 19th century to direct attention to the anemia theory, after observing the brain of a patient who had a traumatic skull injury. In 1855, Alexander Fleming supported the anemia theory after he performed an experiment in which he occluded the carotid arteries and induced a sleep-like state. One of the strongest advocates for the anemia theory was Frans Cornelius Donders (1818–1889), a professor at Utrecht in Holland, who carefully observed the cerebral circulation in animals through windows placed in the skull. Donders and, subsequently, Angelo Mosso (1826–1910), who observed the cerebral circulation in humans with skull defects, believed that at sleep onset blood passed from the brain to the skin. Arthur Edward Durham (1833–1895), who wrote extensively on the topic in 1860, believed that the blood passed from the brain during sleep not only to supply the skin but also to supply the internal organs. The final advocates for the anemia theory of sleep were the physiologists William Henry Howell (1860–1945) and Sir Leonard Erskine Hill (1866–1952). Howell believed that the change in arterial blood pressure at the base of the brain was responsible for cerebral anemia. Hill extensively studied the cerebral circulation, and in 1896 he reported the absence of a change in cerebral blood pressure during sleep. He believed that the brain did not become anemic or congested during sleep, and he showed that intracranial pressure was normal during sleep compared with during wakefulness.

By the end of the 19th century the vascular sleep theories, based on congestion or anemia of the brain, were less enthusiastically supported. Subsequent research showed that changes during sleep of both cerebral blood flow and intracranial pressure do occur, but it was no longer believed that these changes were responsible for the cause of sleep.

The neural theories for the cause of sleep were based upon mid-19th-century developments in the histological understanding of the central nervous system. Camillo Golgi (1843–1926) demonstrated the first clear picture of the nerve cell and its processes. His studies were extended by Heinreich Waldeyer (1837–1921), who first named the nerve cell—the neuron—and demonstrated an afferent axon and efferent dendrites. In 1890, Rabl Ruckhardt developed a hypothesis, called "neurospongium," in which he believed that during sleep there was a partial paralysis of the neuron prolongations, which prevented communication with adjacent nerve cells. Subsequently, Raphael Jacques Lepine (1840–1919) of Paris in 1894 and Marie Mathias Duval (1844–1907) in 1895 proposed similar theories, agreeing that sleep was produced by retraction of amoeboid processes of the nerve cell. The outstanding histologist Santiago Ramon y Cajal (1852–1934) proposed that small cells termed neuroglia interacted between neurons and were able to promote or inhibit the transfer of information from one cell to another. Cajal, who in 1906 was awarded the Nobel prize along with Golgi for his work on neurohistology, suggested that the alteration in the transference of information by neuroglia could explain not only sleep but also the effect of hypnotic medications. Ernesto Lugaro in 1899 proposed an alternative histological theory that sleep was due to expansion of the neuron processes. He believed that neural impulses inducing sleep passed through expanded processes (gemmules) to allow transmission between cells. (In the early 20th century, the theories relating movements to parts of the neuron were largely discredited and theories based upon synaptic transmission of neurotransmitters became the prominent neural explanation for changes of sleep and wakefulness.)

The chemical theories of sleep originated with Aristotle who believed that sleep was due to the effects of "fumes" taken into the blood vessels following the ingestion of food. He believed that the fumes were transferred to the brain where they caused sleepiness. Wilhelm Sommer in 1868 proposed that sleep was due to the lack of oxygen. Sommer's theory was developed from the work of Carl Voit and Max Pettenkofer, who had shown in 1867 that the body absorbed more oxygen during sleep than during the day. Eduard Friedrich Wilhelm Pfluger (1829–1910) became the main advocate for the oxygen hypothesis in 1875. Thierry Wilhelm Preyer (1841–1897) in 1877 believed that the accumulation of lactic acid during daytime fatigue led to a deficiency of oxygen in the brain at night, thereby causing hypoxemia and subsequent sleep. This theory led to several others on the accumulation of toxic substances, which included cholesterol and other toxic waste products.

Perhaps the most widely disseminated theory was that of Leo Errera of Brussels. Errera believed that the accumulation of poisonous substances called "leucomaines" induced sleep by passing from the blood to the brain. The leucomaines were believed to be gradually broken down during sleep, thereby leading to subsequent wakefulness. Reymond Emil Du Bois (1818–1896) in 1895 proposed that sleep was a result of carbon dioxide toxicity, which in small amounts during wakefulness led to sleep, but large accumulations during sleep induced wakefulness. Abel Bouchard (1833–1899) in 1886 proposed that sleep was due to toxic agents, excreted in the urine during sleep, that he called "urotoxins"; he also believed that diurnally produced urine contained toxic agents that produced wakefulness. The chemical theories continued to be popular at the end of the 19th century.

The behavioral theories of sleep developed from those of ancient times when general explanations were given for sleep. Although many behavioral theories were proposed over the years, the inhibition theory was the most popular; it was first alluded to in 1889 by Charles Edouard Brown-Sequard (1817–94), an outstanding clinical neurologist and physiologist. Brown-Sequard, who believed that most glands had secretions that pass into the bloodstream, is also known as the father of endocrinology. Based upon the previous work of Rolando (1809) and Flourens (1822), who had demonstrated that the removal of the cerebral cortex was accompanied by a sleep-like state, Brown-Sequard proposed that sleep was due to an inhibitory reflex. The inhibitory theory of sleep was advanced with the experiment of Heubel, of Kiev University in Russia, who proposed that sleep was due to the loss of peripheral sensory stimulation, which was essential for the maintenance of alertness. Subsequently, the inhibitory theory of sleep was greatly expanded by the work of Ivan Pavlov in the early 20th century. Marie de Manceine in 1897, in his book entitled *Sleep: Physiology, Pathology, Hygiene and Psychology,* regarded sleep as being the "resting state of consciousness," which was an appealing truism, although it provided little information on the mechanism of sleep.

A few researchers believed that a specific site in the body was capable of inducing sleep. The thyroid had been considered to be a sleep-inducing gland, until it was recognized that removal of the thyroid was not associated with insomnia. Jonathon Osborne in 1849 proposed that the choroid plexus was the "organ of sleep." He reasoned that congestion of the choroid kept the ventricles distended to produce sleep, and that contraction of the choroid was associated with wakefulness.

In the latter part of the 19th century two neurologists, Maurice Edouard Marie Gayet and Ludwig Mauthner, reported clinical findings that eventually led to the discovery of the brain stem's role in sleep and wakefulness. In 1875 Gayet presented a patient with lethargy and associated eye movement paralysis who had upper brain stem pathology at autopsy, which led Gayet to believe that the lethargy was due to a thalamic defect that produced impaired transmission from the brain stem to the cerebral hemispheres. Mauthner in 1890 reported a similar association between an eye movement disorder and sleepiness but placed the site of the deficit at the brain stem level. These findings received little attention at the turn of the century because of the more popular vascular and chemical sleep theories.

The science of chronobiology made a few advances in the 19th century, largely through the studies of plant biologists such as Augustin Pyramus de Candolle (1778–1841), who demonstrated in 1832 that plants in constant conditions had a rhythm that differed slightly from 24 hours. Wilhelm Friedrich Phillip Pfeffer (1845–1920) in 1875 confirmed De Mairan's finding that plants had their own intrinsic rhythm when devoid of environmental influences. In 1845 James George Davy (1813–1895) reported circadian rhythms of his own core body temperature, and in 1866 William Ogle performed similar experiments:

> There is a rise in the early morning while we are still asleep, and a fall in the evening while we are still awake, which cannot be explained by reference to any of the hitherto mentioned influences. They are not due to variations in light; they are probably produced by periodic variations in the activity of the organic functions.

The 19th century was a time of rapid clinical advances in medicine. The mesmerism of the early part of the 19th century gave way to hypnotism, a term coined in 1843 by James Braid (1791–1860). Subsequently ether, nitrous oxide and chloroform were used to induce anesthesia for surgery. Although at this time the main focus of academic medicine was in Europe, medical practice in the United States developed rapidly, and the major American university medical centers were established by the end of the 19th century. Medical practice became specialized with the development of ophthalmology, otolaryngology and urology; neurology and psychiatry did not become separate specialties until the beginning of the 20th century. Bacteriology developed as a specialized area of medicine, and disease was no longer viewed as being due to supernatural causes but mainly as the result of infection. This was the time of Louis Pasteur (1822–95) who firmly established the association between disease and microorganisms.

Pharmacology was well established, although herbal cures were still given because pharmacology was not able to keep up with the rapid development of clinical medicine. The first medication introduced specifically as a hypnotic was bromide in 1853, and other hypnotic medications introduced before 1900 included paraldehyde, urethane and sulfonal.

Although the theories regarding the cause of sleep were the focus of attention in the second half of the 19th century, important contributions were made to sleep disorders medicine. Hammond, who was well known for his contributions to medicine during the Civil War, wrote a book entitled *Sleep and Its Derangements* in 1869, based on his series of publications on the topic of insomnia. Silas Weir Mitchell (1829–1914), a well-known and influential neurologist in America, wrote a number of clinical articles on sleep, including the recognition of abnormal respiration during sleep, night terrors, nocturnal epilepsy and the effect of stimulants on insomnia.

Perhaps the greatest clinical contribution in the field of sleep disorders medicine was the first description in 1880 of narcolepsy by Jean Baptiste Edouard Gelineau (1828–1906), who derived "narcolepsy" from the Greek words *narkosis* (a benumbing) and *lepsis* (to overtake). The term "cataplexy," for the emotionally-induced muscle weakness (a prominent symptom of narcolepsy), was subsequently coined in 1916 by Richard Henneberg. Although Gelineau was the first to clearly describe the clinical manifestations of narcolepsy, several patients had previously been described by Caffe in 1862, Carl Friedrich Otto Westphal (1833–90) in 1877 and Franz Fischer in 1878.

The leading sleep disorder of the 20th century, obstructive sleep apnea syndrome, was described in 1836, not by a clinician but by the novelist Charles Dickens (1812–70). Dickens published a series of papers entitled *The Posthumous Papers of the Pickwick Club* in which he described Joe, the fat boy, who was always excessively sleepy. Joe, a loud snorer, who was obese and somnolent, may have had right-sided heart failure that lead to his being called "young dropsy."

> Mr. Lowton hurried to the door . . . The object that presented itself to the eyes of the astonished clerk was a boy—a wonderfully fat boy— . . . standing upright on the mat, with his eyes closed as if in sleep. He had never seen such a fat boy, in or out of a traveling caravan; and this, coupled with the utter calmness and repose of his appearance, so very different from what was reasonably to have been expected of the inflicter of such knocks, smote him with wonder.
>
> "What's the matter?" inquired the clerk.
>
> The extraordinary boy replied not a word; but he nodded once, and seemed, to the clerk's imagination, to snore feebly.
>
> "Where do you come from?" inquired the clerk.
>
> The boy made no sign. He breathed heavily, but in all other respects was motionless.
>
> The clerk repeated the question thrice, and receiving no answer, prepared to shut the door, when the boy suddenly opened his eyes, winked several times, sneezed once, and raised his hand as if to repeat the knocking. Finding the door open, he stared about him with astonishment, and at length fixed his eyes on Mr. Lowton's face.
>
> "What the devil do you knock in that way for?" inquired the clerk, angrily.
>
> "Which way?" said the boy, in a slow, sleepy voice.
>
> "Why, like forty hackney-coachmen," replied the clerk.
>
> "Because master said I wasn't to leave off knocking till they opened the door, for fear I should go to sleep" said the boy.

More than 100 years followed Charles Dickens's description before the obstructive sleep apnea syndrome became a well recognized clinical entity. However, a number of writers in the 19th century did allude to some of the features of sleep apnea in their publications. William Wadd, surgeon to the king of England, in 1816 wrote about the relationship between obesity and sleepiness. George Catlin, a lawyer, in 1872 described the breathing habits of the American Indian in his book entitled *Breath of Life;* he graphically portrayed the effects of obstructed breathing during sleep. William Henry Broadbent (1835–1907) in 1877 was the first physician to report the clinical features of the obstructive sleep apnea syndrome, and William Hill in 1889 observed that upper airway obstruction contributed to "stupidity" in children. The most notable description was by William Hughes Wells (1854–1919) in 1878; he cured several patients of sleepiness by treatment of upper airway obstruction.

The 20th Century

> The interpretation of dreams is the royal road to a knowledge of the part the unconscious plays in the mental life.
>
> —Sigmund Freud,
> *The Interpretation of Dreams* (1905)

Medicine in the 20th century is radically different from that of previous eras. The major advances have been the development of new diagnostic means, the recognition of infectious disease, the development of antibiotic medications, the elimination of most global epidemics, the development of surgery and the treatment of cancer.

For the first time objective diagnostic procedures complemented the physician's skill. X-rays were discovered in 1895 by Wilhelm Konrad Roentgen (1845–1923) and the first clinical application was reported in 1896. Widespread routine use of X-ray procedures began in the early 20th century; sophisticated brain imaging techniques, such as computerized axial tomography (CAT scan) and nuclear magnetic resonance (NMR) scanning, began in the second half of the century.

The vascular theories of the cause of sleep were no longer popular, and although the chemical theories were briefly of interest due to the findings of Rene Legendre and Henri Pieron in 1907, they were overshadowed largely by the behavioral theory of Ivan Petrovitch Pavlov (1849–1936). Pavlov, who is regarded as one of the greatest physiologists of all time, published his initial lectures on conditional reflexes in 1927. There he believed that sleep was due to widespread cortical inhibition:

> Sleep . . . is an inhibition which has spread over the great section of the cerebrum, over the entire hemispheres and even into the lower lying midbrain.

Pavlov's studies on dogs showed that a continuous and monotonous stimulus would be followed by drowsiness and sleep. He reasoned that the continuous stimulus acts at a certain point of the central nervous system and leads to inhibition with resulting sleepiness. Although Pavlov's theories on conditioning were interesting, they held little information on physiological mechanisms. Vladimir Michailovitch Bekhterev (1857–1927) published his findings on human reflexology and sleep in 1894 (translated into English in 1932). Bekhterev also believed that sleep was a general inhibition due to a loss of higher-level reflexes:

> [Sleep is] a reflex which has been biologically evolved for the purpose of protecting the brain from further poisoning by the products of metabolism, and which may be evoked, as an association reflex, and the conditions of fatigue.

Bekhterev's theory, similar to that of Edouard Claparede, who in 1905 viewed sleep as an "instinct," was subsequently influenced by the work of Legendre and Pieron; it believed that the biochemical processes leading to the inhibition of the brain were the "hypnotoxins." Since that time electrophysiological studies have demonstrated that the passive, cortical inhibition proposed by Pavlov and Bekhterev does not occur; instead, the brain maintains its activity during sleep, particularly during REM sleep.

Since the days of ancient Greece, it had been recognized that sleep consisted of two different states, one associated with dreaming and the other with quiet sleep. Willis in the 17th century had noticed the difference and believed that dream sleep was associated with release of the "animal spirits" from the cerebellum. However, the physiological changes of dreaming sleep were not reported until 1868 when Wilhelm Griesinger (1816–1868) noted the associated eye movements. Sigmund Freud in 1895, before the publication of his first book on dreams in 1900, recognized that paralysis of skeletal muscles during dream sleep prevented the dreamer from acting out dreams.

Sleep research, both basic and clinical, had its greatest period of growth during the second half of the 20th century. The advances in neurochemistry, electrophysiology, neurophysiology, chronobiology, pathology of sleep, sleep disorders medicine and the development of sleep societies are too many to list but a summary is presented below.

NEUROCHEMISTRY

> Our studies have established that the accumulation of the hypnotoxin produces an increasing need for sleep.
>
> —Henri Pieron, *Le Probleme Physiologique du Sommeil* (1913)

The most significant advance in the chemical theories came in 1907 when Legendre and Pieron provided evidence for an agent, called "hypnotoxin," that was derived from the blood serum of sleep-deprived dogs. When introduced in dogs who were not sleep-deprived, hypnotoxin induced sleep. Although attempts to replicate Legendre's work were often unsuccessful, in 1967 John Pappenheimer and colleagues induced sleep with cerebrospinal fluid obtained from sleep-deprived goats. The transmissible chemical, called "Factor S," was subsequently identified as a muramyl peptide in 1982 and is thought to act via the leucocyte monokine Interleukin-1. Finding alternative sleep factors has met with mixed success; the number of putative sleep factors has grown enormously in the last 20 years. However, in 1988 Osamu Hayaishi discovered that prostaglandin PGD2, found in the preoptic nuclei, was capable of inducing sleep in rats, leading to the speculation that the preoptic nucleus is the site of the perennial and elusive "sleep center."

ELECTROPHYSIOLOGY

> Feeble currents of varying direction pass through the multiplier when electrodes are placed on two points of the external surface [of the brain] . . .
>
> —Richard Caton (1875)

The most useful objective diagnostic means for sleep disorders has proven to be electrophysiological techniques. Following Galvani's demonstration of the electrical activity of the nervous system in the late 18th century, Richard Caton (1842–1926) in 1875 demonstrated action potentials in the brains of animals, an important step in the development of the electroencephalograph. In 1929, Johannes [Hans] Berger (1873–1941), the first to record electrical activity of the human brain, demonstrated differences in activity between wakefulness and sleep. Berger's discovery led to the development of the electroencephalograph as a clinical tool for the diagnosis of brain disease. The electroencephalograph was applied to determine different sleep states in 1937, when Alfred L. Loomis, E. Newton Harvey (1887–1959) and Garret Hobart were able to classify sleep into five stages, from A to E.

Dreaming sleep was characterized in 1953 by Eugene Aserinsky and Nathaniel Kleitman, who demonstrated the occurrence of rapid eye movements during a stage of sleep that they called "rapid eye movement (REM) sleep." In 1957 Kleitman and William Dement discovered a recurring pattern of REM sleep and non-REM sleep during overnight electroencephalographic monitoring—a finding that made it clear that sleep no longer could be regarded as a homogeneous state. In 1968, Allan Rechtschaffen and Anthony Kales developed a scoring manual, *A Manual of Standardised Terminology, Techniques and Scoring System for Sleep Stages of Human Subjects,* which has become the standard in the field. The first report of an effective measure of daytime alertness was by Gary Richardson et al., in 1978. This study compared narcoleptics with normals by applying the Multiple Sleep Latency Test (MSLT) that had been conceived and developed by Mary Carskadon working with William Dement at Stanford University.

NEUROPHYSIOLOGY

> . . . analysis of hypnogenic mechanisms has thus underlined the paramount importance of inhibition and disinhibition in the determination of sleep onset and maintenance—a striking illustration of Sherrington's visionary concepts.
>
> —Frederic Bremer (1977)

In the early part of the 20th century, two schools of thought emerged regarding the neurophysiological basis of sleep and wakefulness. One characterized sleep as due to disinhibition with release of an active "sleep center," and the other as due to a passive event, the result of inhibition of a "waking center." The theories proposed at the end of the 19th century by Mauthner and others assumed an interruption of peripheral sensory stimulation, thereby allowing the cerebral cortex to produce sleep. This "deafferentation" theory had been suggested first by Purkinje in 1846. The notion of a specific sleep center did not receive much support, as illustrated by the comment of the prominent clinical neurologist Jacques Jean Lhermitte (1877–1959) in 1910:

> We absolutely object to the thought of the existence of a nerve center attributed to the function of sleep. The conception of a center for sleep is erroneous, as it disavows the most simple principles of physiology.

Lhermitte was supported in 1914 by a pioneer of brain localization, Joseph Jules Dejerine, who said, "Sleep cannot be localized." However, in 1929, Constantin Von Economo (1876–1931) proposed a "center for regulation of sleep" based on anatomical and clinical studies of "Encephalitis Lethargica" at the Psychiatric Clinic of Wagner Von Jauregg in Vienna. Viral encephalitis reached epidemic proportions between 1916 and 1920, and Von Economo had the opportunity to correlate the clinical features of sleep disturbance with the central nervous system pathology. His studies demonstrated inflammatory lesions in the posterior hypothalamus in patients with excessive sleepiness and lesions in the preoptic area and anterior hypothalamus in patients with insomnia. Von Economo, influenced by the studies by Pieron and Pavlov, suggested that the "sleep regulating center" was controlled by substances circulating in the blood. These substances caused the sleep center to exert an inhibitory influence on the cerebral cortex, thereby leading to sleep. The same year in Zurich, Walter Rudolph Hess (1881–1973), who was awarded the Nobel prize with Egas Moniz for his work in neuroanatomy, confirmed Von Economo's findings by demonstrating that stimulation of the central gray matter in the region of the thalamus induced sleep.

Kleitman in 1929 regarded the cerebral cortex as being the source of wakefulness and believed that sleep due to inactivity of the central nervous system was brought about by a reduction in peripheral stimulation because of fatigue. His hypothesis conformed to the "deafferentation" theory. Steven Walter Ranson (1880–1942) in 1932 demonstrated that lesions placed at the top of the brain stem produced sleepiness; experimentally, this was consistent with Von Economo's findings.

In 1935, Frederic Bremer, of the University of Brussels, experimentally gave support to the deafferentation theory. Bremer completely transected the midbrain, producing the "cerveau isole" preparation—an isolation of the cerebrum—and was able to show characteristic sleep patterns on the electroencephalogram. The studies up until this time were consistent with the concept that a lesion that prevented transmission of peripheral stimulation was important in the production of sleep. However, Ranson in 1939 showed that lesions of the lateral hypothalamus, in the absence of upper brain stem lesions, were associated with sleep due to a loss of the "waking center." A few years later, Walle Jetz Harinx Nauta demonstrated that posterior hypothalamic lesions produced sleepiness whereas anterior hypothalamic lesions produced insomnia, thereby supporting the concept of a waking center in the posterior hypothalamus and a sleep center in the anterior hypothalamus. According to Nauta:

> Whereas Ranson and his collaborators held that periods of sleep were caused by more or less intrinsic periodic decreases in activity of the waking center, we are inclined to attribute these decreases to the inhibitory influence of a sleep center.

Horace W. Magoun and Ruth Rhines, at the Northwestern University Medical School in Chicago, demonstrated in 1946 that the lower portion of the brain stem reticular formation was responsible for inhibiting skeletal muscle tone. This function of the lower brain stem had earlier been alluded to by the clinical studies of Jackson in 1897. That the lower reticular formation could have an inhibitory function through descending pathways led to Guiseppe Moruzzi and Magoun's finding in 1949 that the brain stem reticular formation also had ascending pathways. This resulted in the discovery of the "ascending reticular activating system," which led to a new emphasis in the physiological investigation of sleep. Stimulation of the ascending reticular acti_vating system produced electroencephalographic patterns of wakefulness. It was now recognized that the brain stem transection studies did not produce sleep because of "deafferentation" of peripheral sensory input, but because of the loss of the wakefulness stimulus from the ascending reticular activating system. As a result, sleep became regarded as a passive phenomenon.

At the beginning of the second half of the 20th century, research concentrated on determining the neurophysiological basis for non-REM and REM sleep. Following the electrophysiological documentation of REM sleep, Michel Jouvet in 1959 demonstrated REM sleep–related muscle atonia, and in 1967 he demonstrated that the brain stem, serotonin-containing neurons of the raphe nuclei were important in the maintenance of sleep. Subsequently, Jouvet demonstrated that the rostral raphe nucleus was important for non-REM sleep, whereas the caudal raphe nucleus was important in the maintenance of REM sleep. In 1975, Robert William McCarley and J. Allan Hobson proposed a reciprocal interaction model of REM and non-REM sleep, with rostral REM "on" cells and caudal REM "off" cells.

CHRONOBIOLOGY

> Despite the multiplicity of its constituents, the circadian system often behaves like one unit which is

> characterized by the durability of its oscillations and its internal temporal order.
>
> —Juergen Aschoff (1981)

Auguste Henri Forel (1848–1931), a Swiss physician, is credited with stimulating the investigation of circadian rhythms as important time measuring systems. His studies in 1910 on the accurate timing system of bees were consistent with those of Linnaeus in the 18th century on the opening of the flower petals at a given time of day. The circadian behavior of rodents was first reported by Curt P. Richter in his Ph.D. thesis in 1922; and Erwin Bunning in 1935 was able to demonstrate the genetic origin of circadian rhythms in plants and subsequently developed a concept of "biological clocks." In the early 1960s Richter searched for the biological clock in extensive studies that culminated with the report in 1965 that lesions placed in the anterior-ventral hypothalamus produced disruption of circadian rhythms. Two groups acting independently in 1972, Robert Y. Moore and Victor B. Eichler, and F.K. Stephan and Irving Zucker, discovered the "clock" to be two small, bilateral nuclei in the anterior hypothalamus, which were subsequently called the suprachiasmatic nuclei (SCN).

Human circadian rhythms were investigated in the absence of environmental time cues by Jules Aschoff and Kurt Wever in 1962 in an underground laboratory in Munich. They demonstrated a free-running pattern of sleep and wakefulness with a period length of greater than 24 hours. A similar free-running pattern was demonstrated in field experiments in 1974 by the speleologist Michel Siffre, who lived for three months in the absence of time cues on an ice glacier deep in the Franco-Italian mountains. Many human biological rhythms have recently been discovered, such as the 24-hour episodic secretory pattern of cortisol that was reported by Elliot David Weitzman (1929–1983) in 1966. In 1978, Weitzman and Charles Czeisler demonstrated the internal organization of temperature, neuroendocrine rhythms and the sleep-wake cycle, in subjects who were monitored in an environment free of time cues for periods of up to six months. Sutherland Simpson (1863–1926) and J.J. Galbraith in 1906 had demonstrated that the light-dark cycle could influence mammal behavior; however, it was not until the 1980s that Czeisler and colleagues demonstrated the importance of the light-dark cycle in the entrainment of human circadian rhythms.

PATHOLOGY OF SLEEP

> Five billion people go through the cycle of sleep and wakefulness every day, and relatively few of them know the joy of being fully rested and fully alert all day long.
>
> —William Dement (1988)

Sleep disorders were poorly described at the turn of the century, and, other than narcolepsy and sleeping sickness, few specific sleep disorders were recognized. In addition to general medical illness, environmental effects and anxiety were viewed as the main causes of sleep disturbance. However, a gradual recognition of the multiplicity of sleep diagnoses began to parallel progress in psychiatry. Freud's book *The Interpretation of Dreams* led to the development of psychoanalysis, which was applied to the treatment of insomnia until the evolution of a more "organic" or "biological" psychiatric approach.

Psychoactive medications became widely used with the introduction of the phenothiazines in the 1950s, but hypnotic medications, particularly the barbiturates, had been in common usage since barbital was introduced in 1903. The 1960s saw the introduction of the benzodiazepine hypnotics, which largely replaced the barbiturates in the late 1970s. However, the 1980s saw a decline in the use of hypnotics with increased physician and public awareness of the disadvantages of chronic hypnotic use. Insomnia became recognized as a symptom rather than a diagnosis, and treatment was directed to the underlying physical or psychological causes.

Several books on sleep had a major influence on the development of sleep disorders medicine. Pieron's *Le Probleme Physiologique du Sommeil* in 1913 summarized the scientific sleep literature at that time. A similar approach was taken by Nathaniel Kleitman, who produced his monumental treatise *Sleep and Wakefulness* in 1939 (updated in 1963 to contain 4,337 references). The Association of Sleep Disorder Centers classification committee chaired by Howard Roffwarg produced the *Diagnostic Classification of Sleep and Arousal Disorders* in 1979; it ushered in the modern era of sleep diagnoses and became the first classification to be widely used. The *Principles and Practices of Sleep Disorders Medicine,* edited by Meir Kryger, William Dement and Thomas Roth in 1989, was the first comprehensive textbook on basic sleep research and clinical sleep medicine.

Increased knowledge about sleep and sleep disorders in general has resulted from the research of a few core sleep disorders, which include narcolepsy, obstructive sleep apnea syndrome and the insomnias.

Following Gelineau's description in the late 19th century, narcolepsy was brought to general recognition in 1926 by the Australian-born neurologist William John Adie (1886–1935), and stimulants were first used for treatment by Otakar Janota in 1931. In 1941 John Burton Dynes and Knox H. Findley applied the electroencephalograph to the diagnosis of narcolepsy, and the characteristic sleep-onset REM period of night sleep was discovered in 1960 by Gerald Vogel. Dement and colleagues at Stanford University developed a narcoleptic dog colony in the 1970s, which advanced the understanding of the biochemical and neuroanatomical bases of the disorder. The Multiple Sleep Latency Test was applied to the diagnosis by Richardson in 1978, and the documentation of a strong association between the histocompatability antigen HLA-DR2 and narcolepsy was made by Yutaka Honda and colleagues in 1984.

Following the reports of snoring, sleepiness and obesity in the 19th century, Sir William Osler (1849–1919) in 1907 referred to Dickens' description of Joe: "An extraordinary phenomenon in excessively fat young persons is an uncontrollable tendency to sleep—like the fat boy in Pickwick."

Charles Sidney Burwell in 1956 brought general recognition to obstructive sleep apnea syndrome, which he called the "Pickwickian Syndrome"; and the first objective documentation of polysomnographic features was reported by Henri Gastaut in 1965. Although the tracheotomy had been performed since the time of Asclepiades (first century B.C.), Wolfgang Kuhlo and Erich Doll in 1972 reported that it provided an effective treatment of the obstructive sleep apnea syndrome. Tanenosuke Ikematsu in 1964 popularized uvulopalatopharyngoplasty (UPP) surgery for the treatment of snoring, which was subsequently applied to the obstructive sleep apnea syndrome by Shiro Fujita in 1981. The same year, nasal continuous positive airway pressure (CPAP) treatment was described by Colin Sullivan and subsequently became the treatment of choice.

Another sleep-related breathing disorder called "Ondine's Curse" was first reported by John W. Severinghaus and Robert A. Mitchell in 1962. Named after the water nymph in Jean Giraudoux's play *Ondine* (1939), this disorder was characterized by the failure of automatic ventilation that could lead to fatal apnea during sleep.

> Live! It's easy to say. If at least I could work up a little interest in living—but I'm too tired to make the effort. Since you left me, Ondine, all the things my body once did by itself, it now only does by special order . . . I have to supervise five senses, two hundred bones, a thousand muscles. A single moment of inattention, and I forget to breathe. He died, they will say, because it was a nuisance to breathe.
>
> —Jean Giraudoux, *Ondine,* Act III (1939)

Insomnia received more interest in earlier centuries than in the first half of the 20th century, probably because of the availability of effective hypnotic medications. Frederick Snyder in the 1960s recognized and promoted the importance of psychiatric disorders in sleep medicine, especially depression: "Troubled minds have troubled sleep, and troubled sleep causes troubled minds." The polysomnograph was applied to the investigation of patients with insomnia following the discovery of obstructive sleep apnea in 1965, and objective measures of hypnotic effectiveness were developed by Kales in 1969. The concept of a conditioned insomnia (psychophysiological insomnia) was first presented in *Diagnostic Classification of Sleep and Arousal Disorders* in 1979 and subsequently became recognized as a common form of insomnia. The behavioral technique "stimulus control" developed by Richard Bootzin in 1972 was an effective treatment of insomnia, as was "sleep restriction therapy," developed by Arthur Spielman in 1987.

Circadian rhythm sleep disorders were recognized in the late 1970s, partly due to recognition of the chronobiological features of "jet lag" and "shift work." Thomas A. Edison, who was responsible for the development of the electric light bulb, which allowed shift work to occur, had his own views on sleep:

> In my opinion sleep is a habit, acquired by the environment. Like all habits it is generally carried to extremes. The man that sleeps four hours soundly is better off than a dreamy sleeper of eight hours.

The atypical, sleep-onset insomnia called the "delayed sleep phase syndrome," discovered by Elliot Weitzman and colleagues in 1981, led to a radically different form of treatment called "chronotherapy," which was based on chronological principles.

Many other sleep disorders have been discovered in the 20th century, including REM sleep behavior disorder by Carlos Schenk in 1986; paroxysmal nocturnal dystonia in 1981 and fatal familial insomnia in 1986, by Elio Lugaresi; and food allergy insomnia by Andre Kahn in 1984.

General and medical awareness of sleep disorders has dramatically increased since the 1970s through the contributions of sleep disorders clinicians and the sleep societies. In addition to those mentioned, a few of the many who have contributed to this recognition include: Roger Broughton, Michel Billiard, Christian Guilleminault, Peter Hauri, J. David Parkes, the late Pierre Passouant and Bedrich Roth.

SLEEP DISORDERS MEDICINE

> . . . we have created a new clinical specialty, sleep disorders medicine, whose task is to watch over all of us while we are asleep.
>
> —William Dement (1985)

Organized sleep disorders medicine in the United States began with the founding of the Association for the Psychophysiological Study of Sleep (APSS) in 1961, an association comprised of sleep researchers, many with clinical interests. Sleep research led to the investigation of sleep disorders, which resulted in the establishment in the early 1970s of clinical sleep disorder centers for the diagnosis and treatment of patients. In 1976, the Association of Sleep Disorder Centers (ASDC) was founded. The first sleep disorder center to be engaged in active patient evaluations and treatment was that established at Stanford University in California by William Dement. An accreditation process for sleep disorders centers was established by the ASDC, and the first to be accredited in 1977 was the Sleep-Wake Disorders Unit, headed by Elliot Weitzman, at Montefiore Medical Center in New York. In 1978, the medical journal *Sleep* was created to present research and clinical articles on sleep, and in 1979 a complete issue was devoted to the *Diagnostic Classification of Sleep and Arousal Disorders*. In 1978, the Association of Polysomnographic Technologists, founded by Peter Anderson McGregor, set standards of practice for polysomnographic technologists. In 1983 the Association for the Psychophysiological Study of Sleep was renamed the Sleep Research Society (SRS) and in 1984 the Clinical Sleep Society (CSS) was founded as the membership branch of the Association of Sleep Disorder Centers. In 1986, the Association of Sleep Disorder Centers, the Clinical Sleep Society, the Sleep Research Society and the Association of Polysomnographic Technologists formed a federation called the Association of Professional Sleep Societies (APSS). The Association of Sleep Disorder Centers changed its name to the American Sleep Disorders Association in 1987 and to the American Academy of Sleep Medicine (AASM) in 1999.

With the increased recognition of the importance of sleep disorders medicine many international sleep societies have been founded, beginning with the European Sleep Research Society (ESRS) in 1971, the Japanese Society for Sleep Research (JSSR) in 1978, the Belgian Association for the study of Sleep (BASS) in 1982, the Scandinavian Sleep Research Society (SSRS) in 1985, the Latin American Sleep Society (LASS) in 1986, the Sleep Society of Canada (SSC) in 1986 and the British Sleep Society (BSS) in 1989.

(Selected references for the introduction are included in the bibliography at the end of this volume.)

PSYCHOLOGY AND SLEEP: THE INTERDEPENDENCE OF SLEEP AND WAKING STATES

Arthur J. Spielman, Ph.D., Paul D'Ambrosio, M.A., and Paul B. Glovinsky, Ph.D.
Department of Psychology, The City College of New York
Sleep Disorders Center,
New York Methodist Hospital, Brooklyn, NY

The focus of psychology is behavior, which at first glance might be thought to cease during sleep. Certainly most psychological investigations have focused on waking behavior, whether it be an easily observed action or mental activity inferred from behavior or verbal report. Of course, neither the mind nor the body truly ceases activity during sleep. Far from turning off, the brain in sleep generates a variety of states, accompanied by predictable physiological changes and typical forms of mentation. Moreover, this nocturnal activity is not totally separate from waking thought and action. Daytime experience has a direct effect on what transpires during sleep, and both the psychology and physiology of sleep in turn have profound influences on waking life.

If sleep and wakefulness are interdependent, this interdependence is embedded in the endogenous rhythmic alternation that governs both states. The clock that influences the appearance of sleep and wakefulness may itself be reset by psychological processes. Whether by the sleeplessness of distress or the prolonged wakefulness of creative output, the appearance and timing of an array of associated physiological rhythms can be affected by psychological states.

The Interaction of Sleep and Wakefulness

Events transpiring during sleep and wakefulness are interwoven, each serving as an antecedent and consequent condition. Wakefulness can take on a multitude of casts, from normal renderings through aberrant forms. As the night follows the day, so will sleep reflect this variation.

Psychopathology Influences Sleep

It is so common as to be a staple of clinical wisdom that emotional disturbance precedes and produces sleep disturbance. Practical and ethical considerations have precluded a systematic study of this causal relationship. However, few would disagree with the assumption.

The *Diagnostic and Statistical Manual of Mental Disorders* (4th ed.) contains 18 different disorders that are associated with insomnia or hypersomnia. Major diagnostic categories, such as major depression, mania, generalized anxiety and dysthymic disorder, employ insomnia as a possible diagnostic criterion. The nocturnal agitation of the manic state, the early morning awakening of the major depressive, and the sleeplessness of the prodrome of the schizophrenic reaction are common clinical examples of sleep disturbance associated with psychopathology.

It has been shown that the prevalence of sleep disturbance among psychiatric patients is three times higher than in a control population. Furthermore, a large survey of different medical specialties has discovered approximately twice the prevalence of insomnia in psychiatric practice compared to the average of other specialties.

The well documented evidence for a particular psychometric profile of depression and anxiety in insomniacs has generated a theory stating that individuals who deal with emotional distress by internal processes are more vulnerable to insomnia.

Investigations of the significant sleep disturbance associated with major depressive disorders has revealed a number of intrasleep anomalies. In addition to the nonspecific disturbance of the continuity of sleep, REM sleep abnormalities have been identified that may be biological markers of major depression. The group at Pittsburgh have been leaders in studies showing that a shortened latency from sleep onset to the first appearance of REM sleep and increased rapid eye movement activity is characteristic of primary depression. Reduced slow wave sleep preceding the first REM period, another sleep characteristic of depression, may be involved in the disinhibition of REM sleep. A recent population sample of ambulatory American adults has highlighted the increased prevalence of insomnia in individuals suffering emotional distress. The finding of elevated anxiety and depression is accompanied by a markedly increased prevalence of insomnia.

Psychological disturbance does not have to attain a magnitude warranting formal diagnosis before its effects on sleep become apparent. All individuals must cope with varying degrees of stress originating from a variety of sources. The physical environment may contain numerous stressors, such as noise and crowded conditions. One's body may present discomfort or pain to be endured. Social etiquette may make demands that are perceived as stressful. Any of these sources of stress has the potential of precipitating a sleep disturbance directly, without need of a mediating psychopathological process.

Physical Activity Influences Sleep

The recent Neurolab astronauts aboard the space shuttle who spent many days orbiting the Earth, with reduced postural muscle activity due to weightlessness, had significant difficulty falling asleep. While there may have been more than one reason for hyperalertness while orbiting the Earth, controlled studies at sea level have shown that vigorous exercise during the day will increase the amount of slow wave sleep that night. Furthermore, this increase in deep sleep is obtainable only when physically fit subjects exercise. It appears that fit people can exercise at a high rate for longer periods of time and as a result increase their body temperature for longer durations. The discovery that body temperature is one factor that mediates the effects of physical activity on sleep provides a vivid illustration of how behavior and physiology interact within the sleep-wake cycle.

Sleep Affects Psychological Well-Being

Numerous studies of sleep deprivation have consistently shown that sleep loss affects daytime performance, sleepiness and mood. Sleep loss does not have to be large-scale to produce demonstrable effects. Reductions in sleep duration, if suffered nightly, will accumulate and produce daytime decrements. One of the first capacities to be affected is the ability to produce creative solutions to problems. Sleep loss also leads to the inability to maintain vigilance. Individuals cannot attend to ongoing tasks and will exhibit lapses in performance. Sleepiness and brief sleep episodes, irritability, and dysphoric mood also impair functional capacity and quality of life.

Alertness and attention represent the gateway to cognitive processing, and thus a wide range of mental and emotional dysfunction is possible. Eventually the sleep-disturbed individual's self-image and self-esteem must deal with the fact of lowered effectiveness and achievement. Patients start to refer to themselves as insomniacs, avoiding challenges, explaining away mistakes, and generally taking refuge in the sick role. They are ever wary that insufficient sleep will erode their capacities.

The self-attribution of "I'm an insomniac" may serve as a focus for self-deprecatory ideas. A widening circle of thoughts surrounds the belief that "I cannot sleep well." Examples of these might include, "I'm not up to hosting Thanksgiving" or "I'd better maintain a low profile because I'm not capable of as much work as my colleagues." Eventually, these ideas may produce a degree of helplessness and hopelessness that, according to cognitive theorists, forms the basis of a mood disturbance.

The Vicious Cycle of Insomnia and Anticipatory Anxiety

The interaction of disturbances in sleep and wakefulness is clearly seen in the mutually reinforcing experiences of sleepless nights and anxious days. Transient insomnia is nearly a universal experience. The tossing and turning, the racing mind and half-completed thoughts, the frustration at being unable to bring oneself relief, all of these experiences are extremely unpleasant and avoided if possible. During the day, insomniacs will wonder whether these experiences are again in store. A dread of the night to come may appear as evening approaches. This anticipation of a sleepless night produces anxiety and physiological arousal. Thus, fear of insomnia has itself produced sufficient arousal to perpetuate the sleep disturbance.

This vicious cycle persists despite occasional nights of good sleep. Variability of sleep from night to night is characteristic of insomnia. This renders the sleep of insomnia unpredictable and provides the basis for the insomniac's worry.

Insomnia as a Pathology of Sleep and Wakefulness

The problem of insomnia has been alluded to many times in the foregoing discussion, since the interaction of sleep and wakefulness is perhaps most clearly illustrated when the smooth transition between these states is disrupted. In narrowing the focus to the evaluation and treatment of insomnia, the practical application of this psychological viewpoint in clinical practice will be illustrated.

Let us take, for example, the case of a mid-level manager who has been denied promotion. He is seething with resentment, yet, in order to preserve his chances for the next review, he must maintain a "team player" attitude at work and carefully restrict any expression of hostility there. His wife notices growing irritability in the evening; rather than being a respite from work pressures, the evening hours at home become tainted from these pressures. A sleep-onset insomnia develops. Our manager becomes preoccupied with perceived or actual slights endured during the day; only after two or more hours of such obsessing is he exhausted enough to drop off to sleep. He cannot afford to come into the office late, so he diligently sets two alarm clocks and begins to build up a significant sleep loss. Daytime irritability mounts until one day a snide comment from a recently promoted colleague triggers an explosive outburst.

This scenario could be subjected to several straightforward analyses. One formulation would take as its context the pressures of the workplace and see the insult as sufficient to produce the outburst. A somewhat wider scope would include the development of the insomnia in its purview. This formulation would hold both the insomnia and the outburst to be secondary to emotional turmoil. The denial of promotion has stirred up feelings of inadequacy and dependency that produce an extensive disturbance, with both daytime and nocturnal manifestations.

Our analysis would underscore the mutual interaction between mood and sleep: The insomnia both reflects the underlying emotional state and influences this state. Heightened cognitive and physiological activation during the evening hours interferes with sleep onset at our patient's usual bedtime. He is less cognizant of this change in evening demeanor but acutely aware of the experience, a few hours later, of lying wide-eyed in bed, restless and angry. He reaches back to the last salient cue of change—slights at the workplace—in order to fix blame for his sleeplessness.

During the day our patient has to contend with increased irritability, diminished powers of concentration, and other mood and performance deficits resulting directly from sleep loss. In addition, the experience of insomnia has added an overlay: a sense of lost control, feelings of incompetence and concerns regarding health consequences. Against this backdrop, our patient's tolerance for assault on his self-esteem is especially low, and his successful colleague's comment especially stinging.

The course of insomnia is determined by the interacting sequence of daytime and nocturnal experiences. Either an understandably bad day or inexplicably bad night may serve as the first link in a chain of experiences and compensatory adaptations that result in chronic insomnia. Examining and categorizing these individual links in the chain of insomnia results in a clearer formulation and more directed treatment plan.

Predisposing, Precipitating and Perpetuating Factors in Insomnia

The nosological scheme of the International Classification of Sleep Disorders has produced a clear and consistent description of the sleep disorder's clinical phenomena. In the sense that this classification is descriptive rather than etiologically formulated, appropriate intervention strategies are not automatically derived from diagnosis. With regards to the insomnias we have urged the use of a simple categorization of case material that helps focus on the roles of different factors in the pathogenesis of the disorder, thereby assisting in a rational approach to treatment.

In the development of insomnia, characteristics of the person may serve as predisposing factors by increasing the vulnerability to develop a sleep disturbance. These characteristics might include susceptibility to anxious worrying or activation at night. Environmental features, such as noise and morning light exposure, may also predispose to insomnia. By definition, these characteristics are not sufficient to produce an insomnia, but they may set the stage for the development of a particular form of insomnia. Interventions that address these factors will help ameliorate the current insomnia and forestall the development of insomnia in the future.

The factors that trigger an insomnia are at the center of the initial clinical evaluation. An understanding of the factors that precipitate a sleep disturbance is often sufficient for developing a successful treatment plan. For example, a scientist may become increasingly keyed up and alter her bedtime hours as the deadline for submission of a grant application approaches. When writing is going well, she will stay up late; when it is going poorly, in the middle of the day she will take a nap: These changes weaken the synchronization of circadian rhythms that is sustained by a regular sleep-wake cycle. While she may believe that nothing can be done about her sleeplessness until after the deadline, strict structuring of her bedtime may substantially improve the sleep problem.

Table 1
COMMON PRACTICES AND RESPONSES TO INSOMNIA THAT PERPETUATE SLEEPLESSNESS

- Irregular timing of retiring and arising
- Excessive time in bed
- Napping at irregular times
- Worry that insomnia will produce daytime deficits
- Expectation of a bad night's sleep
- Increased caffeine consumption
- Use of hypnotic medication and alcohol
- Maladaptive conditioning
- "Sleeping in" on weekends

Insomnia may last for decades. When it persists beyond a transient period, the clinician may have to go beyond the uncovering of predisposing and precipitating factors. As insomnia becomes a chronic experience the individual may instigate compensatory practices to deal with the problem. Returning to the frantic grant writer, if a habit of napping at irregular hours continues after the deadline is long past, this may maintain her insomnia. Or if she increases her caffeine consumption to buttress her flagging alertness and then continues this habit, her insomnia may persist. In these cases, the precipitating circumstance has long subsided yet the secondary factors are sufficient to maintain the insomnia. Perpetuating factors may go unnoticed, especially when clear predisposing and precipitating aspects are still present. Therefore, one must thoroughly evaluate the common practices and experiences (see Table 1) that may accrue onto any insomnia so that a comprehensive treatment plan may be designed.

Behavioral Treatment of Insomnia

TREATMENT BASED ON CONDITIONING

The role of conditioning in sleep was extensively discussed by Pavlov. More recent demonstrations of the classical conditioning of sleep onset in cats have been conducted by Sterman and Clemente and colleagues. These investigators paired a neutral tone with electrical stimulation of the pre-optic basal forebrain. The electrical stimulation of the pre-optic basal forebrain was capable of rapidly producing high voltage slow waves and sleep. After a number of pairings, the formerly neutral tone was capable of independency eliciting high voltage slow waves and sleep. In "A Behavioral Perspective on Insomnia Treatment," we present preliminary data in humans suggesting that pairing contextual cues with the sleep-promoting properties of a hypnotic medication produces a conditioned response of rapid sleep onset.

One of the most widely tested and efficacious behavioral treatments of insomnia is based on the rationale that associative mechanisms can exert control over the sleep onset process. In normal conditions cues such as darkness, sleep rituals, the bed, quiet and recumbency are regularly associated with rapid sleep onset. Repeated experiences render these cues as discriminative stimuli for sleep. In other words, these cues signal that sleep is the appropriate response given the situation. If an individual engages in behaviors other than sleep in association with these cues, then these stimuli will lose their discriminative properties. This is what happens, for example, when an individual uses the bed as a dining table, TV viewing platform, telephone booth and so on. In this case the bed, bedroom environment and rituals have lost their control over the sleep process; they no longer signal that sleep is the appropriate and expected behavior.

Stimulus control instructions were developed by Richard Bootzin and consist of a short set of rules to reestablish the connection between bedroom cues and sleep. Excerpted, these rules are as follows:

1. Use the bed only for sleep (sex is exempt from this rule).
2. Go to bed only when sleepy.
3. If you do not fall asleep within about 15 minutes of getting into bed, then get out of bed. Do not return to bed until you are sleepy or feel you can fall asleep.
4. When you return to bed abide by rule number 3. The following additional rules keep sleep in line with principles of good sleep hygiene:
5. Get up at the same time every morning.
6. Do not nap.

Following these instructions leads to repeated experiences of rapidly falling asleep after getting into bed. Sleep improves, according to the theory, because the bedroom cues regain their discriminative properties and exert control over the sleep process.

TREATMENT BASED ON INCREASING THE DRIVE TO SLEEP

Analogous to the idea that there are individual differences in nocturnal sleep duration, differences in basal sleep propensity may reflect a trait. A range of habitual sleep times, approximating a bell-shaped curve with a mean of about 7.5 hours, has been reported by Daniel F. Kripke et al. This trait characteristic is distinct from state evoked changes (e.g., increasing or decreasing the amount of time spent in bed yields commensurate changes in sleep duration). Applying this familiar example of coexisting state and trait aspects of sleep duration, let us assume that daytime sleep latency also distributes normally, with a mean of about 12 to 14 minutes. In this view, the fact that, more or less, sleep affects sleepiness does not negate the possibility that sleepiness or activation may have a relatively stable trait influence.

If we have two traits of nocturnal sleep time and diurnal sleep propensity, the question arises as to how these traits might be related. Although a positive correlation between nocturnal sleep time and diurnal sleep latency is tacitly assumed to exist in individuals, there is surprisingly little evidence to this effect. Mary A. Carskadon and colleagues, for example, in elderly noncomplaining individuals obtained a nonsignificant positive correlation between night sleep and day sleepiness. However, recent evidence suggests that individuals with insomnia may exhibit an inverse relationship between nocturnal sleep and daytime sleep latency. Seidel and the Stanford group have shown that despite sleeping less than normal at night, insomniacs are no sleepier by day. Stepanski and colleagues at Henry Ford Hospital have shown a strong association ($r = -.67$) between sleep and daytime sleep latency. Therefore, a reduced drive for sleep, during both the night and day, appears to contribute to the difficulties facing insomniacs.

Sleep restriction therapy (see Spielman et al.) aims to increase sleep drive in insomniac patients. An initial sleep loss is produced by curtailing time in bed to an amount approximating the patient's subjective report of sleep time. The sleep loss heightens sleep propensity and increases the likelihood that most of the short time allotted for sleep will be spent actually sleeping. Anticipatory anxiety is reduced, sleep onset is rapid, sleep is less interrupted and sleep duration is more consistent across nights. As sleep improves, the patient is allowed to spend progressively more time in bed. Some insomniacs who may be deficient in sleep drive will require continued mild sleep restriction to maintain this improvement. Others can be returned to a schedule that does not impose sleep loss because the treatment has addressed factors other than a deficient sleep drive, such as anticipatory anxiety or irregular sleep-wake scheduling.

RELAXATION AND BIOFEEDBACK TRAINING

The clinical impression of increased autonomic activity and muscle tension has been documented in such studies of insomniacs as Monroe's. The goal of progressive muscle relaxation is to increase the patient's awareness of high and low muscle tension. The patient practices contracting a particular muscle group and holding the tension in order to heighten awareness. Next, the patient relaxes the muscle and focuses on the tension waning. These two steps—tensing and relaxing—are repeated for all the major muscle groups. This training helps patients avoid and counteract the tonic muscular tension that is a barrier to sleep. To assist with the fine discrimination of behavioral states that relaxation training requires, biofeedback devices are used, such as those that produce an auditory signal corresponding to the level of frontalis muscle tone.

COGNITIVE TREATMENTS

The mind can be its own worst enemy when it comes to sleep. The same ability to solve problems, plan ahead and generate options, which is so adaptive for waking life, becomes maladaptive when it is exercised at the expense of sleep. Cognitive therapies have been devised that train patients to exert more control over the content and timing of thought processes. Specific time can be set aside for worry, the mind can be guided through a sequence of relaxing images, or thoughts can be restructured so as to minimize the importance of distressing experiences. These and other similar techniques aim at ensuring a reasonably calm state for the relatively short time it takes to fall asleep, when all else is in place.

The Rhythm of Sleep and Wakefulness

Daytime functioning is affected not only by the amount of sleep attained the night before, but also by the time at which parameters such as mood, alertness and performance capacity are assessed. This distinction points to the importance of a new regulatory principle, that of circadian organization, which has taken its place alongside the classic homeostatic view (the system by which the body maintains a steady-state or balanced internal milieu). The homeostatic view is that optimal functioning occurs within a circumscribed range of physiological values; deviations from this range are aberrant and will mobilize mechanisms to reestablish the basal levels. For example, a body temperature of 98.6 degrees Fahrenheit is the normal value that is maintained by a variety of thermoregulatory mechanisms.

The biological rhythm perspective holds that certain deviations from normal values are endogenously generated and periodic. An important group of biological rhythms have period lengths (the duration of a complete cycle) of about one day, and hence are called circadian rhythms. For example, body temperature has a regular endogenous variation of about one and a half degrees Fahrenheit and a period length of about 24.2 hours. This regular fluctuation about a mean value of 98.6 degrees Fahrenheit does not represent error in the biological system but is, rather, a key structural factor.

Rhythmic systems are characterized by the amplitude of variation and period length of a given parameter and the phase relationship between different parameters. In the context of sleep and wakefulness, amplitude might refer to the range of arousal experienced. Ideally, there should be a great range between peak alertness during the daytime and minimal alertness at night. This range appears restricted in some chronic insomniacs. Arousal in this group is heightened both day and night.

With regard to phase relationship, the coordinated sequence of increasing sleepiness, fall in body temperature, and sleep onset regularly recurs at approximately the same time of night under normal conditions. In contrast to this synchrony, the timing of rhythmic processes may be displaced, so that there is an inappropriate interval between the fall of the temperature cycle and sleep onset. This is commonly experienced, for example, when eastbound airline passengers who have crossed five time zones try to go to sleep at a time that matches the nighttime in their new surroundings. Under these new conditions, bedtime is before the fall in body temperature, and falling asleep will likely be difficult.

We have seen how the vicissitudes of sleep and wakefulness can be conceptualized within a framework that emphasizes their mutual interdependence. Both of these states are comprised of a myriad of behaviors, each capable of reflecting the past and influencing the future. These behaviors are in turn influenced by the timing of their occurrence with respect to the sleep-wake cycle. Conceptualization of insomnia along these lines is particularly instructive, in that waking life, sleep behavior, circadian timing, physiological and psychological predispositions, maladaptive learning and environmental influences are all relevant to the genesis, course and treatment of this prevalent health problem.

(Selected references for this chapter are included in the Bibliography.)

A

abnormal movements Some sleep disorders can be characterized by atypical movements of limbs. For example, movement occurs in response to the creepy, crawly feeling in the legs due to the disorder known as RESTLESS LEGS SYNDROME (RLS). The relief that these movements bring, however, is only temporary. The disorder is mainly of unknown cause although (rarely) it may be associated with metabolic disorders such as anemia or renal failure. However, once correctly diagnosed, medication can effectively treat RLS and bring relief. Repetitive, abnormal movements of the legs or arms during sleep, occurring as frequently as every 10 seconds, are typical of PERIODIC LIMB MOVEMENT DISORDER (PLMD). These leg or arm movements are often powerful enough to cause an awakening as well as to disturb a bed partner because of the shaking of the bed or accidentally being kicked. Those suffering from REM SLEEP BEHAVIOR DISORDER, in which dream content is acted out during the REM (dreaming) stage of sleep, display movements such as punching, kicking or running, sometimes inadvertently causing injury.

The presence of abnormal movements during sleep that cause INSOMNIA or lead to EXCESSIVE SLEEPINESS during the day should be discussed with a physician to see if tests need to be performed, such as POLYSOMNOGRAPHY (sleep test).

abnormal swallowing syndrome, sleep-related See SLEEP-RELATED ABNORMAL SWALLOWING SYNDROME.

accidents Common in persons with sleep disorders, especially those who suffer from EXCESSIVE SLEEPINESS. Sleepiness produces impaired ALERTNESS and awareness, and this can be a problem for those who operate dangerous machinery or drive cars.

Motor vehicle driving is particularly hazardous in persons who are sleepy, since riding in a motor vehicle has a soporific effect and will bring out underlying sleepiness. Excessive sleepiness as a cause of crashes is often unrecognized either because the individual is wide awake once an accident occurs or does not survive to report the sleepiness. It is not uncommon to find that people who suffer from sleepiness while driving (DROWSY DRIVING) will open the window to get fresh air, turn the radio on loud or employ other techniques, such as moving around in the seat, to increase alertness. There may be frequent stops to get a cup of coffee or to walk around to get refreshed. Some may also use OVER-THE-COUNTER MEDICATIONS containing CAFFEINE, such as NoDoz, to increase alertness while driving. Naps taken in the car at the side of the road are also common for persons who have moderate to severe daytime sleepiness. However, the driver does not always appreciate the degree of sleepiness while driving and therefore motor vehicle accidents often result. Falling asleep while waiting for a red light or in traffic jams, veering to the side of the road and driving onto the road shoulder commonly occur.

Sleepiness, and accidents caused by sleepiness, can be exacerbated by the ingestion of alcohol, particularly if the amount of sleep the night before was less than required. Alcohol can also increase the severity of the OBSTRUCTIVE SLEEP APNEA SYNDROME, a common disorder in middle-aged males, thereby leading to increased sleepiness (and the greater possibility of accidents) the next day.

In addition to motor vehicle accidents due to sleepiness, people with sleep disorders are at risk of injuring themselves, even when sleeping in bed at home. Some sleep disorders, especially those associated with abnormal movement, such as the obstructive sleep apnea syndrome or REM SLEEP BEHAVIOR DISORDER, can cause an individual to fall out of bed or hit a nightstand. The violent movements during sleep may also injure a bed partner, and excessive movement during sleep is a common cause of a couple moving to separate beds in order to prevent injuries.

Some disorders can be associated with very violent activity, such as SLEEP TERRORS, which are often characterized by a rush from the bed in a violent and uncontrolled panic. People with sleep terrors have occasionally gone through glass doors or fallen out of windows during their intense panic. Also, sleepwalkers can suffer from accidents during their nocturnal wanderings. A fall from a window is not uncommon as a result of sleepwalking, and walking into furniture or other objects can cause injuries (see SLEEPWALKING).

When sleep terror and sleepwalking coexist, even death can be the consequence of an individual running or walking out of the house and rushing in front of a passing car or falling from a window.

Sometimes accidental injury can be produced indirectly. Snorers have reported accidents related to their snoring. One woman broke her arm as a result of her husband's SNORING. Used to sleeping in a double bed where she could touch her husband to get him to change position whenever he was snoring, she fell out of bed when staying in a separate bed in a hotel; her husband commenced snoring, she stretched out to touch him and, not realizing she was in a separate bed, fell and broke her arm. Another loud snorer was almost suffocated by his army colleagues when they stuffed socks in his mouth in order to stop his snoring. Another patient with sleep-related epileptic SEIZURES so frightened his wife that she thought her life was in danger; she hit him over the head with a bedpost causing him to require numerous scalp sutures.

accreditation standards for sleep disorder centers
In 1975, the ASSOCIATION OF SLEEP DISORDER CENTERS (ASDC) began to develop guidelines and standards for the practice of SLEEP DISORDERS MEDICINE. These standards resulted in the accreditation of the first sleep disorder center in 1977. Since that time, the Association of Sleep Disorder Centers has merged with the CLINICAL SLEEP SOCIETY to form the American Sleep Disorders Association (now called the AMERICAN ACADEMY OF SLEEP MEDICINE), which is responsible for producing guidelines for sleep disorder centers. An accreditation committee visits sites and ensures that sleep disorder centers throughout the United States meet appropriate standards for the practice of sleep disorders medicine. The standards involve a review of the following areas: the relationship of the center to the host medical institution, to ensure that there is a stable relationship among the medical structure of the sleep disorder center, the physical environment and the personnel; the way in which patient referrals and evaluation procedures are handled; the polysomnographic and other monitoring procedures; the interpretation and documentation of the polysomnographic data; and the physical equipment of the recording laboratory.

In order to become accredited, a comprehensive application for accreditation must be completed by the applying sleep disorder center. If the information presented indicates that the center meets the standards for accreditation, a site visit is organized. Two official site visitors go to the sleep disorder center to observe a patient undergoing polysomnographic evaluation and to review with the center its procedures and the ability to diagnose and treat sleep disorders. Upon completion of a site visit, the visitors recommend to the national chairman of the accreditation committee whether or not to accredit the center. If favorable, the sleep disorder center is given full accreditation status for five years.

Accreditation status can be contingent upon the sleep disorder center meeting a number of provisions, if all aspects of the center's activity do not conform entirely to the standards and guidelines. Then, after a period of five years, the sleep disorder center must reapply for accreditation. (By 2000, more than 500 sleep disorder centers had been accredited by the American Academy of Sleep Medicine.) In this way, the development of sleep disorder centers in the United States has proceeded in an orderly and appropriate manner, with the highest standards of patient care being maintained. (See also ACCREDITED CLINICAL POLYSOMNOGRAPHER [ACP], ASSOCIATION OF POLYSOMNOGRAPHIC TECHNOLOGISTS, SLEEP DISORDER CENTERS.)

accredited clinical polysomnographer (ACP) Individual trained and tested to administer the polysomnograph, the test that measures sleep activity and other physiological variables by recording brain, eye and muscle activity in sleep (see POLYSOMNOGRAPHY). In order to become an ACP, candidates studied basic physiology of sleep and its clinical ramifications and passed a test administered by the American Sleep Disorders Association (now called the AMERICAN ACADEMY OF SLEEP MEDICINE). This examination is now administered by the AMERICAN BOARD OF SLEEP MEDICINE, and those who pass the exam are no longer called ACPs but are board certified in sleep medicine. There were more than 1,500 board certified sleep specialists in the United States in 2001. Clinicians who pass the examination become fellows of the American Academy of Sleep Medicine.

acetazolamide (Diamox) See RESPIRATORY STIMULANTS.

acetylcholine A neurotransmitter involved in the regulation of sleep and wakefulness. Acetylcholine is found in the central and peripheral nervous system and is synthesized from acetaldehyde and choline. The effect of the release of acetylcholine from the nerve endings is modified by the enzyme acetylcholinesterase. Inhibition of the acetylcholinesterase enzyme leads to prolonged wakefulness in animals; however, the same inhibitors administered during sleep will enhance the appearance of REM SLEEP. Agents that stimulate the production of acetylcholine, such as carbachol, can induce a state that resembles REM sleep, but the effect of such agents very much depends upon the part of the central nervous system where these agents are inserted.

Many medications that affect the central nervous system have anticholinergic properties, and the blockage of acetylcholine accounts for many of the adverse reactions that are seen. The medications that have most pronounced anticholinergic effects are the tricyclic ANTIDEPRESSANTS, such as imipramine, which are often used in sleep medicine for the treatment of sleep disturbance in patients with depression. The anticholinergic tricyclic antidepressants are also used for the treatment of CATAPLEXY in patients with NARCOLEPSY. The adverse reactions of the medications include dry mouth, constipation and urinary retention, and can produce restlessness, irritability, disorientation, hallucinations and even delirium. The tricyclic antidepressants are now largely being replaced by the serotonin reuptake inhibitors such as fluoxetine (Prozac).

Acetylcholine is also believed to be involved in the maintenance of muscle tone in REM sleep. Acetylcholine blockers, such as atropine, can produce a profound loss of muscle tone resembling that seen during REM sleep.

acromegaly A disorder characterized by an excessive production of growth hormone, which causes an enlargement of the skeletal and soft tissues of the body. This disorder is produced by a tumor of the hormone-secreting cells of the pituitary gland. Patients with acromegaly have an increased likelihood of developing sleep-related breathing disorders, such as OBSTRUCTIVE SLEEP APNEA SYNDROME.

Excessive growth hormone causes an increase in the size of soft tissues of the upper airway, particularly the tongue. Bony changes can also occur that, in combination with the soft tissue changes, cause a narrowing of the upper airway. Consequently, upper airway obstruction during sleep is more likely to occur. Some acromegalic patients, particularly female patients, suffer CENTRAL SLEEP APNEA which may be due to a central nervous system abnormality as a direct effect of the pituitary tumor. In addition to the soft tissue changes of the upper airway, tissues throughout the body enlarge, and this is most noticeable by an increase in hand and foot size. Internal organs, such as the liver and heart, can also increase in size.

The obstructive sleep apnea syndrome associated with acromegaly may be dealt with by reduction of soft tissue enlargement through treatment of the excessive growth hormone production. Acromegaly treatment may involve surgical removal of, or radiation of, the pituitary gland, or the use of medications, such as bromocriptine, that suppress the production of growth hormone. Despite optimal treatment of the excessive growth hormone production, the obstructive sleep apnea syndrome may continue and require treatment by standard means, such as the use of a CONTINUOUS POSITIVE AIR PRESSURE device or TRACHEOSTOMY. (See also UPPER AIRWAY OBSTRUCTION.)

acroparesthesia See CARPAL TUNNEL SYNDROME.

acrophase The peak of a BIOLOGICAL RHYTHM in contrast to the NADIR, the lowest point of a biological rhythm. (See also BIOLOGICAL CLOCKS, CHRONOBIOLOGY, CIRCADIAN RHYTHMS.

ACTH See ADRENOCORTICOTROPHIN HORMONE (ACTH).

actigraphy A biomedical instrument capable of monitoring motor activity in order to identify the presence or absence of body motion during sleep or wakefulness. Activity monitoring by means of an actigraph is useful in detecting sleep episodes and differentiating periods of sleep and rest from periods of wakefulness.

Actigraphy is commonly employed for long-term CIRCADIAN RHYTHM studies to document the pattern of sleep and wakefulness with little inconvenience to the patient. A typical actigraph has a simple-to-wear, easily programmable microprocessor device, which is usually attached to the non-dominant wrist, but can also be attached to one or both legs. The device works on the principle that movement of the non-dominant wrist is correlated with wakefulness, whereas long, quiescent periods are associated with rest or sleep. Studies have demonstrated an 88.9% correlation of accuracy with polysomnographically measured sleep. Special computer programs interpret the information recorded, and it can be displayed in many different formats.

New forms of actigraphs include light-detecting monitors for measuring light exposure and actigraphs that include radio frequency transmitters for relaying information cordlessly to a distant computer.

Wrist activity monitors have also been used to measure abnormal movements that can occur in patients suffering neurological disease, such as Parkinson's disease or other types of movement disorders. (See also SHIFT-WORK SLEEP DISORDER.)

activated sleep See ACTIVE SLEEP.

active sleep The low voltage, mixed frequency EEG and rapid eye movement (REM) activity. This term, a phylogenetic and ontogenetic term for REM SLEEP, is synonymous with the term "activated sleep."

activity monitors Devices used to detect motion as a way of differentiating periods of wakefulness or rest. (See also ACTIGRAPHY.)

activity-rest cycle Term used to describe the cyclical pattern of activity that alternates with rest in animals and humans; it is commonly considered to be the same as wakefulness and sleep. The activity-rest cycle is usually determined in animal research studies of CHRONOBIOLOGY and CIRCADIAN RHYTHMS; it is more easily measured than sleep and wakefulness. The activity-rest patterns of rodents alternate wheel running activity with rest periods.

In addition to the 24-hour pattern of activity and rest there is a BASIC REST ACTIVITY CYCLE (BRAC) that has a shorter PERIOD LENGTH, of approximately three hours, than the activity-rest cycle. BRAC is believed to be indicative of an underlying ultradian cycle that is manifest during sleep by the NREM-REM SLEEP CYCLE.

acute mountain sickness See ALTITUDE INSOMNIA.

adenoids Lymphoid tissue present in the posterior nasopharynx. Adenoids are similar to tonsils and are involved in the immune system during childhood. The adenoids are typically enlarged in the prepubertal age group and gradually decrease in size, with very little tissue present in most adults. In childhood, enlarged adenoidal tissue can cause

UPPER AIRWAY OBSTRUCTION, predisposing the child to upper respiratory tract infections and the OBSTRUCTIVE SLEEP APNEA SYNDROME. Enlarged adenoidal tissue in adults can also contribute to upper airway obstruction.

An assessment of the extent of adenoid and tonsillar tissue is required in patients who have the obstructive sleep apnea syndrome; if indicated, surgical removal may be necessary. (See also SURGERY AND SLEEP DISORDERS, TONSILLECTOMY AND ADENOIDECTOMY.)

adenosine A basic element of the nucleic acids, adenosine consists of a sugar attached to a purine base. There is evidence that suggests that adenosine is a sedative or otherwise induces sleep. Adenosine may have its effect directly on neurons or through the inhibition of the release of other neurotransmitters, such as ACETYLCHOLINE or NOREPINEPHRINE.

Interest in adenosine was stimulated when CAFFEINE was found to inhibit adenosine release rather than inhibiting the enzyme phosphodiesterase, the previously-held view. Caffeine, which is one of the methylxanthines (see RESPIRATORY STIMULANTS), has very pronounced stimulation effects and increases wakefulness.

Radulovacki, M., "Role of Adenosine in Sleep of Rats," *Review of Clinical and Basic Pharmacology* 5 (1985): 327–339.

adjustment sleep disorder INSOMNIA resulting from an acute emotional stress that can be related to conflict, loss or a perceived threat, for example, a death in the family, an upcoming examination, marital, financial or work stress. Typically, adjustment sleep disorder lasts for a few days, and always less than three weeks, after which the sleep pattern returns to normal.

Features of adjustment sleep disorder are prolonged sleep latency (see SLEEP LATENCY), frequent awakenings, or EARLY MORNING AROUSAL. There may also be a tendency for excessive SLEEPINESS during the day. In acute circumstances, there can be loss of the ability to maintain normal social activities or employment until the acute reaction is over. Intense anxiety or depression may be associated with the stress response and the sleep disturbance. The sleep pattern returns to normal with the resolution of these acute psychological symptoms.

Polysomnography or a multiple sleep latency test may help diagnose a condition either of hyperarousal or of excessive daytime sleepiness. Treatment is essential soon after the sleep disturbance begins to prevent its development into chronic PSYCHOPHYSIOLOGICAL INSOMNIA. Hypnotic medication therapy, lasting only several days, is recommended. Attention to good SLEEP HYGIENE is essential, not only during the time of the stress reaction, but also in the days immediately following.

Adjustment sleep disorder, synonymous with transient psychophysiological insomnia and situational insomnia, is the preferred term.

Kales, Anthony and Kales, J., *Evaluation and Treatment of Insomnia.* New York: Oxford University Press, 1984.

adrenocorticotrophin hormone (ACTH) Hormone secreted by the pituitary gland that controls the secretion of CORTISOL from the adrenal gland. ACTH secretion occurs throughout the day with about 10 secretory episodes and is mainly secreted at the end of the sleep period, at the time of awakening. The resulting large increase in cortisol at this time is important for the maintenance of metabolic integrity and therefore physical activity.

Reduction of ACTH release can occur due to pituitary tumors and leads to fatigue and weight loss. Excessive production of ACTH leads to weight gain and hypertension, producing a disorder called Cushing's syndrome (overactive adrenal glands). (See also GROWTH HORMONE, MELATONIN, PROLACTIN.)

advanced sleep phase syndrome A CIRCADIAN RHYTHM SLEEP DISORDER characterized by difficulty in remaining awake until the desired bedtime, and getting up too early, or early morning INSOMNIA. This disorder, which is seen typically in elderly persons, often causes embarrassment due to an inability to remain awake in social situations in the mid-evening hours. The patient may also be at risk of ACCIDENT, for instance, by falling asleep at the wheel of a car. After a late night out, the inability to delay the time of the final awakening often produces a tendency to daytime sleepiness. Inappropriate daytime napping may result.

Polysomnographic studies have demonstrated an early onset in the timing of the low point of the circadian body temperature rhythm. Sleep onset time occurs at a time earlier than desired, and a normal duration and quantity of sleep follows. The spontaneous awakening is typically earlier than desired.

The origin of advanced sleep phase syndrome is unknown, but, as it seems more common in the elderly, it has been suggested that it is due to degeneration of the nerve cells of the circadian pacemaker, so that the circadian pacemaker is unable to induce a delay of the sleep pattern. As with the delayed sleep phase syndrome, the advanced sleep phase syndrome may be due to an abnormality of the PHASE RESPONSE CURVE. The disorder is apparently rare.

Advanced sleep phase syndrome differs from other causes of early morning awakening. Mood disorders, particularly depression, are associated with early morning awakening but are also associated with sleep onset and sleep maintenance difficulties. The advanced sleep phase syndrome needs to be differentiated from INSUFFICIENT SLEEP SYNDROME, which typically can also produce evening sleepiness but is caused by a forced early morning awakening. Individuals who are classified as short sleepers may have an early morning awakening but do not have evening sleepiness.

The diagnosis of advanced sleep phase syndrome is usually made by the typical complaint of an inability to stay awake till the desired bedtime, and an inability to remain asleep till the desired time of the morning. The disorder must be present for at least a three-month period. When the person is not required to remain awake till the desired bedtime (that is, goes to bed early), then the sleep episode is of normal quality and duration. The final awakening is always earlier than desired.

Mild disturbances can be treated by close attention to maintaining a regular sleep onset and waketime. Incremental delays of sleep onset on a daily basis, by 15 to 30 minutes, may assist in delaying the sleep pattern. One patient has been reported to have been treated by CHRONOTHERAPY, which involved advancing the sleep pattern by three hours per day. The sleep pattern was rotated around the clock so that a more appropriate sleep onset time was reached. Exposure to bright light prior to sleep onset may assist in producing a more normal sleep onset time. (See also AGE, LIGHT THERAPY.)

Kamei, R., Hughes, L., Miles, L. and Dement, W., "Advanced-sleep Phase Syndrome Studied in a Time Isolation Facility," *Chronobiologia* 6 (1979): 115.

affective disorders Term describing mental disorders characterized by mood disturbances, typically DEPRESSION or mania. More recently, the terms MOOD DISORDERS and ANXIETY DISORDERS have been applied to this group of psychiatric disorders.

age CIRCADIAN RHYTHMS, sleep and sleep disorders undergo distinct changes from infancy through old age. Some hormones, such as GROWTH HORMONE, are produced in amounts that are essential for normal growth in childhood, but may be absent in the elderly. High amounts of stage three and stage four sleep (see SLEEP STAGES) are usually present in prepubertal children, and altogether absent in the elderly. Some sleep disorders, such as REM SLEEP BEHAVIOR DISORDER, are more commonly seen in persons over 60 years of age, whereas SLEEPWALKING and SLEEP TERRORS are more commonly seen in children.

Infant sleep is characterized by a long, total sleep time of up to 20 hours in the 24-hour day. REM sleep may account for as much as 50% of the total sleep time. Newborn sleep is characterized by frequent awakenings, and sleep episodes are often associated with a direct transition from wakefulness into REM. REM sleep in older children and adults is never associated with the immediate onset of REM sleep, unless a specific sleep disorder is present.

The infant's sleep pattern gradually becomes more consolidated during the nocturnal hours so that by six weeks of age the majority of sleep occurs during the nocturnal half of the day. However, daytime naps are frequent.

Sleep disorders that can occur in infancy are most commonly related to sleep-disordered breathing, such as INFANT SLEEP APNEA. A central nervous system lesion or upper airway obstruction are causes in this age group. Other medical illnesses, such as infection, cardiorespiratory disease, metabolic changes or neurological disorders, can cause respiratory disturbance in infancy. Sleep-related epilepsy can occur, although usually epileptic SEIZURES in this age group occur during wakefulness as well as during sleep. Of particular concern in the first year of life is the possibility of SUDDEN INFANT DEATH SYNDROME (SIDS).

Because an infant's respiratory system is immature and small, infants are predisposed to lung collapse and airway obstruction. The muscles are relatively weak and are more susceptible to fatigue. The high percentage of REM sleep may also predispose the infant to more sleep-related breathing disorders because of the associated ATONIA that affects the accessory muscles of respiration.

BENIGN NEONATAL SLEEP MYOCLONUS, a disorder that occurs during non-REM sleep, causes muscle jerking that usually spontaneously resolves itself within the first few weeks of life. Irregular sleep patterns, characterized by frequent awakenings, are common around six months of age. This is an important time for the establishment of a stable sleep-wake pattern and the development of good SLEEP HYGIENE in the child. Limits need to be instituted so that the majority of sleep occurs during the nocturnal hours and not during the daytime; LIMIT-SETTING SLEEP DISORDER is a common problem in this age group and can be corrected by behavioral means.

The older child has typically established a sleep pattern at night consisting of 10 to 12 hours of nocturnal sleep and a short nap, in the mid-afternoon, of one to two hours. Circadian patterns of growth hormone, CORTISOL and PROLACTIN, start to establish a fixed pattern with the sleep-wake cycle. Between the ages of four and six years, the amount of REM sleep diminishes, and the percentage of SLOW WAVE SLEEP increases to maximum levels.

The most common sleep disorders in the prepubertal child include CONFUSIONAL AROUSALS (brief arousals or awakenings that occur during slow wave sleep), sleepwalking and sleep terrors. SLEEP ONSET ASSOCIATION DISORDER may occur from infancy to prepubertal ages so that a child may be unable to fall asleep without the presence of a particular behavior or object, such as a teddy bear. OBSTRUCTIVE SLEEP APNEA is a common occurrence in the prepubertal child due to enlarged tonsils and ADENOIDS and may be an indication for tonsillectomy or adenoidectomy (see TONSILLECTOMY AND ADENOIDECTOMY). Other sleep disorders, such as NARCOLEPSY and PERIODIC LIMB MOVEMENT DISORDER, rarely occur before puberty.

Around the time of puberty, growth hormone production and gonadotrophin reach high levels. Sleep is very efficient, with few awakenings occurring during nocturnal sleep and maximal alertness during the daytime. During adolescence there is a tendency for a later sleep onset time and difficulty in awakening in the morning.

Obstructive sleep apnea syndrome, due to enlarged tonsils, continues to be a major cause of sleep-related breathing disorders in adolescents. DELAYED SLEEP PHASE SYNDROME, causing difficulty in falling asleep at an early hour and trouble awakening in the morning for school, also becomes a common problem. Psychological or psychiatric disorders, characterized by ANXIETY and DEPRESSION, are also seen in this age group and may cause disturbed sleep.

Sleep often becomes less efficient in young adults, with an increased number of awakenings and a greater tendency for EXCESSIVE SLEEPINESS. SLEEP DEPRIVATION is a common cause. Obstructive sleep apnea and narcolepsy are other common causes of pathological sleepiness in this age group. Sleep disturbance related to the transition from school to college, or an employment situation, are typical, with psychiatric disorders, such as anxiety and depression, as contributing factors.

In middle age, sleep reduces even further in efficiency so that a shorter total sleep time with more frequent awakenings is common. In males between the ages of 40 and 60, obstructive sleep apnea syndrome is likely to occur. INSOMNIA is the main cause of sleep disturbance of females in middle age. Patterns of growth hormone secretion are reduced in this age group, as is the amount of slow wave sleep. With the development of other medical disorders or psychiatric disturbances, sleep disorders are commonly encountered in middle age and are more typical in the elderly.

The elderly have less efficient sleep with a short total sleep time during the nocturnal hours, a great tendency for daytime napping, less deep sleep with more light stage one and stage two sleep, and often the complete absence of slow wave sleep. Growth hormone secretion may be absent in the elderly. Other circadian rhythm patterns, such as body temperature or cortisol secretion, may be flatter than those seen in middle age. However, prolactin secretion seems to be fairly well established into old age. Gonadotrophin hormone secretion is reduced, and sexual difficulties, such as impotence, are more often encountered in this age group. Among the middle-aged to the elderly, SLEEP-RELATED PENILE ERECTIONS become less frequent and organic causes of impotence are commonly encountered.

Sleep-related breathing disorders are common causes of disturbed sleep in the elderly, particularly CENTRAL SLEEP APNEA due to a central nervous system or cardiovascular cause. Obstructive sleep apnea syndrome is also present in this age group and is more typically associated with the complaint of insomnia than it is in younger age groups. Periodic limb movement disorder and general nonspecific sleep disruption is also frequent in the middle-aged and elderly.

In the elderly, medical and psychiatric disorders, including depression, are also very common, and may be the cause of insomnia. DEMENTIA is more typically seen and is often associated with a breakdown of the sleep-wake pattern, leading to nocturnal confusion and wandering that is sometimes called the sundown syndrome. Sleep disturbance in the geriatric group is a common cause of institutionalization. Death is more likely to occur during sleep. (See also SLEEP EFFICIENCY, SLEEP NEED, TOTAL SLEEP TIME.)

Asplund, R., "Sleep Disorders in the Elderly," *Drugs and Aging* 14, no. 2 (1999): 91–103.

Weitzman, E.D., "Sleep and Aging," in Katzman, R. and Terry, R.D., eds., *The Neurology of Aging*. Philadelphia: F.A. Davis, 1983. pp. 167–188.

airway obstruction The predominant cause of OBSTRUCTIVE SLEEP APNEA SYNDROME. This disorder is associated with obstruction at any site from the nose to the larynx. Upper airway obstruction is assessed by means of CEPHALOMETRIC RADIOGRAPHS and FIBEROPTIC-ENDOSCOPY; treatment may be by surgical or mechanical means. (See also CONTINUOUS POSITIVE AIR PRESSURE, HYOID MYOTOMY, MANDIBULAR ADVANCEMENT SURGERY, SURGERY AND SLEEP DISORDERS, TONSILLECTOMY AND ADENOIDECTOMY, TRACHEOSTOMY; UPPER AIRWAY OBSTRUCTION, UVULOPALATOPHARYNGOPLASTY.

alcohol Commonly used to help insomnia sufferers get to sleep at night—with very deleterious effects on sleep. Drinking alcohol in the evening may help sleep onset, but headaches upon awakening the next morning are typical, particularly with excessive alcohol use. The routine use of alcohol as a sedative produces an improved sleep onset time, often with a deeper sleep in the first third of the night, but then sleep becomes lighter and more fragmented.

ALCOHOL-DEPENDENT SLEEP DISORDER occurs in people who chronically use alcohol for its sleep-inducing effects. This disorder is *not* associated with heavy alcohol ingestion during the daytime and is not a symptom of alcoholism; as tolerance develops, the amount of alcohol ingested increases, but persons with alcohol-dependent sleep disorder usually do not go on to become alcoholics. Alcohol will shorten the SLEEP LATENCY and increase the amount of stage three and four SLEEP (see SLEEP STAGES), but REM SLEEP is reduced and becomes fragmented. Awakenings frequently intrude into the second half of the nocturnal sleep episode.

It is commonly recognized that alcohol will increase the amount and loudness of SNORING, but it can also exacerbate OBSTRUCTIVE SLEEP APNEA SYNDROME. ALCOHOLISM is associated with an increased number of sleep-related disturbances, such as NOCTURNAL ENURESIS, NIGHT TERRORS, SLEEPWALKING.

Alcohol has detrimental effects on daytime alertness. The sleep fragmentation and disruption at night can lead to excessive sleepiness and diminished alertness during the daytime. The effects of alcohol upon performance, particularly driving, may be greatly influenced by the amount of the prior night's sleep so that ACCIDENTS due to alcohol abuse are often, in part, related to the soporific effects of alcohol.

The effects of alcohol are exacerbated by the ingestion of other drugs, particularly sedatives. This combination may be dangerous and lead to stupor and even coma or death.

Alcohol will impair the arousal and ventilatory response to the apneic episodes in obstructive sleep apnea syndrome, causing the apneas to be longer and the oxygen desaturation to be more severe. The association of alcohol with exacerbation of obstructive sleep apnea may lead to serious cardiovascular consequences that could prove fatal.

Treatment of obstructive sleep apnea syndrome often involves use of a CONTINUOUS POSITIVE AIRWAY PRESSURE device (CPAP), and alcohol ingestion can be a common cause of failure of an adequate CPAP response. A patient who consumes alcohol on a nightly basis may fail to do so in a sleep laboratory and therefore the adjustment phase of CPAP may lead to an inadequate pressure setting. Following alcohol ingestion, a higher than usual pressure may be required in order to overcome the apneic events. There is also evidence that alcohol can produce obstructive sleep apnea syndrome in persons who otherwise would not have apneic events.

Alcohol can exacerbate other sleep disorders, such as JET LAG and SLEEP-RELATED EPILEPSY. Epilepsy may also be exacerbated by the disruptive sleep pattern caused by alcohol, which leads to sleep deprivation and possibly the precipitation of epileptic seizures.

alcohol-dependent sleep disorder Disorder characterized by the chronic drinking of alcohol for its soporific effect. The self-prescribed use of ethanol (ALCOHOL) as a sedative is the cause of this disorder that often results from an underlying insomnia, such as an ADJUSTMENT SLEEP DISORDER or INADEQUATE SLEEP HYGIENE. Typically, alcohol is drunk late in the evening, a few hours before bedtime, usually in quantities of up to eight drinks. However, in this disorder, the alcohol ingestion is rarely associated with excessive alcohol intake during the daytime, or the development of chronic ALCOHOLISM.

The sedative properties of the alcohol are greatest at the onset of the pattern of alcohol ingestion. However, with chronic usage, tolerance develops and there is a loss of the sleep-inducing effect. In addition, withdrawal effects occur in the second half of the nocturnal sleep episode, so that a pattern of frequent awakenings and difficulty in maintaining sleep often results. Other symptoms of alcohol withdrawal, such as headaches, dry mouth, fatigue and tiredness upon awakening, may also occur.

In addition to the ingestion of alcohol, other sedative agents may be taken, although more typically the alcohol is the sole sedative ingested. The use of alcohol is generally longstanding and most often occurs in individuals after the age of 40 years.

Polysomnographic monitoring shows an increase in stage three and four sleep (see SLEEP STAGES) and a short SLEEP ONSET latency; however, REM SLEEP fragmentation is present with frequent awakenings, sometimes with early morning awakening.

Treatment of the alcohol dependency is the same as for any other drug dependency. A gradual drug withdrawal, with the institution of SLEEP HYGIENE measures, is essential to prevent further sleep disruption. In some situations, it may be necessary to supplant the alcohol with a more effective hypnotic agent during the alcohol withdrawal phase, and then the prescribed hypnotic can be gradually withdrawn.

Williams, H.L. and Salamy, A., "Alcohol and Sleep," in Kissin, B. and Begleiter, H., eds., *The Biology of Alcoholism*. New York: Plenum Press, 1972. pp. 435–483.

alcoholism Chronic alcohol intake with alcohol abuse and dependency. Sleep disturbances are a common feature of alcoholism, particularly INSOMNIA as well as EXCESSIVE SLEEPINESS during the day.

Alcohol produces an increased tendency for sleepiness that lasts for approximately four hours after drinking (depending upon the amount actually consumed). When taken before bedtime, it will reduce the SLEEP LATENCY and reduce wakefulness in the first third of the night, but as the alcohol is metabolized, there can be withdrawal effects, with increased sleep fragmentation. Individuals who drink chronically and excessively find that sleep disruption occurs with abstinence from alcohol, and very often alcohol is used to improve sleep. The chronic alcohol abuser may also suffer from NIGHTMARES and other REM phenomena as a result of REM SLEEP fragmentation during chronic ingestion of alcohol as well as abstinence. Alcoholics are susceptible to other sleep disrupting factors, such as environmental stimuli. Alcohol in alcoholics will often induce increased amounts of slow wave sleep in the first half of the night, and REM fragmentation and decrease is typically seen in the second half of the night. Sleep becomes so fragmented that STAGE TWO SLEEP SPINDLES and increased muscle tone can occur during REM sleep.

Associated features of alcoholism include an increased incidence of BED-WETTING, SLEEP TERRORS, SLEEPWALKING, nightmares and exacerbation of SNORING and OBSTRUCTIVE SLEEP APNEA SYNDROME. Alcoholic liver disease and encephalopathy with the development of a Korsakoff psychosis are common results of chronic alcohol ingestion. The direct effect of these disorders can also contribute to sleep disturbances. (See also ALCOHOL for other effects of chronic drinking.)

The alcoholic, when withdrawing from alcohol, can develop delirium tremors within a week of stopping the alcohol intake. This state is marked by severe autonomic hyperactivity, with tachycardia, sweating and tremulousness. Withdrawal seizures, called "rum fits," can occur within the first few days of alcohol withdrawal and always precede the development of delirium. During the time of delirium and hallucinosis, sleep is severely disrupted.

There may be an excessive amount of REM sleep that occurs in the first few days after alcohol withdrawal, although it may be fragmented. Slow wave sleep can be reduced and may recover very gradually following abstinence from alcohol, often never returning to pre-alcohol levels. Disturbed sleep may continue to be present for up to two years following complete abstinence.

Treatment of the alcohol-induced sleep disturbance is usually restricted to managing alcohol abstinence and may involve the use of short-term HYPNOTICS to reduce the severe sleep disruption. Attention to good SLEEP HYGIENE is essential. (See also ALCOHOL-DEPENDENT SLEEP DISORDER.)

Wagman, A. and Allen, R., "Effects of Alcohol Ingestion and Abstinence on Slow Wave Sleep of Alcoholics," in Gross, M.M., ed., *Alcohol Intoxication and Withdrawal* 2. New York: Plenum Press, 1975. pp. 453–466.

alertness Opposite of SLEEPINESS. Ideally, alertness should be full for the approximately two-thirds of the day when we are awake. Persons who have sleep disorders often notice an increased tendency for sleepiness in the midafternoon, an exaggerated form of a natural dip in alertness that occurs at that time. This midafternoon dip is part of the biphasic CIRCADIAN RHYTHM of sleep, which is reflected in the major sleep episode at night and the increased tendency for sleepiness that occurs 12 hours later, in the midafternoon. Some cultures take advantage of this decreased alertness by scheduling a SIESTA for several hours. The decrease in alertness also can be exacerbated by a large lunch or the ingestion of ALCOHOL.

Subjective measures of alertness include the STANFORD SLEEPINESS SCALE (SSS), which rates the degree of alertness and sleepiness on a scale from one to seven, and the EPWORTH SLEEPINESS SCALE. Objective alertness measures include PUPILLOMETRY, a measure of fluctuations in pupil diameter size that reflects changes in alertness. Decreased pupil size and oscillations of the pupil indicate decreased alertness. The most widely used objective measure of alertness, however, is the MULTIPLE SLEEP LATENCY TEST, which measures at two-hour intervals the tendency to fall asleep throughout the day. Five nap tests are scheduled from 10 A.M. to 6 P.M. and the electrophysiological measures of sleep are monitored for SLEEP STAGES. A short SLEEP LATENCY to the first epoch of sleep indicates decreased alertness and the presence of sleepiness, particularly if the mean sleep latency over the five naps is 10 minutes or less.

Daytime alertness can be influenced by a number of factors, including the quality and quantity of the prior night's sleep as well as medications or drugs taken during the daytime. Caffeine found in coffee and many sodas is a commonly-used central nervous system stimulant that will increase daytime alertness. STIMULANT MEDICATIONS, often used to improve alertness in persons with excessive sleepiness due to disorders such as NARCOLEPSY, include amphetamines, methylphenidate hydrochloride and pemoline. These agents improve alertness but have less of an effect on multiple sleep latency measures of sleepiness. Methylphenidate and amphetamines have been objectively shown to produce a reduction in sleepiness.

The cycle of daily alertness appears to be independent of the cycle of daytime sleepiness. This is most evident in a person's ability to maintain alertness unless placed in an environment conductive to sleep, where severe sleepiness may readily become apparent. The findings on the multiple sleep latency test for the effects of stimulant medications tend to support this notion of two independent processes.

For this reason, the MAINTENANCE OF WAKEFULNESS TEST was developed. This test measures the ability to remain awake and is performed in a manner similar to the multiple sleep latency test.

Measurement of alertness following treatment of some sleep disorders can be valuable in establishing whether or not an individual is sufficiently alert to drive a motor vehicle or operate dangerous machinery, for instance. (See also EXCESSIVE SLEEPINESS, VIGILANCE.)

Roth, T., Roehrs, T., Carskadon, M. and Dement, W., "Daytime Sleepiness and Alertness," in Kryger, M.H., Roth, T. and Dement, W.C., eds., *The Principles and Practices of Sleep Disorders Medicine*. Philadelphia: Saunders, 1989. pp. 14–23.

alpha activity A sequence of alpha waves of 8 to 13 hertz (cycles per second) seen in recordings on an electroencephalogram. Alpha activity is an indication of lightening of sleep and becomes more prevalent as wakefulness approaches. This activity is a faster rhythm than that seen during SLEEP STAGES, which most typically consist of theta and delta activity. (See also ALPHA RHYTHM.)

alpha-delta activity Term describing the presence of the alpha EEG rhythm, which occurs simultaneously with the slower delta EEG pattern of sleep. Alpha-delta activity is typically seen in disorders that disrupt nocturnal sleep, such as INSOMNIA, and is also a characteristic feature of the FIBROSITIS SYNDROME. (See also ALPHA RHYTHM.)

alpha infiltration See ALPHA INTRUSION.

alpha insertion See ALPHA INTRUSION.

alpha interruption See ALPHA INTRUSION.

alpha intrusion Also known as alpha infiltration, alpha insertion or alpha interruption. This is a brief superimposition of ALPHA ACTIVITY upon sleep activities during SLEEP STAGES. Alpha intrusion is characteristic of sleep disorders where the sleep-wake pattern is disrupted and is also a characteristic feature of FIBROSITIS SYNDROME.

alpha rhythm ELECTROENCEPHALOGRAM (EEG) wave activity that occurs with a frequency of 8 to 13 hertz (cycles per second) in adults. This activity occurs in the central to posterior portions of the head and is indicative of the awake state in humans. ALPHA ACTIVITY is usually present during relaxed wakefulness when visual input is reduced (for instance, when the eyes are closed). The activity tends to be slower in children and the elderly compared to young and middle-aged adults. It may occur during SLEEP STAGES if sleep is disrupted, as is seen in the many disorders of INSOMNIA. Alpha activity during slow wave sleep is a particular characteristic of the FIBROSITIS SYNDROME. (See also ALPHA INTRUSION.)

alprazolam See BENZODIAZEPINES.

altitude insomnia An acute INSOMNIA that occurs with the ascent to high altitudes; also known as acute mountain sickness. Altitude insomnia typically occurs in individuals, such as mountain climbers, who ascend to levels higher than 4,000 meters (13,200 feet) above sea level. Some symptoms may be evident at levels above 2,500 meters (8,250 feet), although the most predominant symptoms occur within 72 hours of exposure to higher altitudes. The disorder is characterized by difficulty in initiating and maintaining sleep, as well as other symptoms, such as headaches and fatigue.

This disturbance appears to be related to the low level of atmospheric oxygen that produces HYPOXEMIA and associated APNEA. The apnea is due to a post-hypoxemic period of hyperventilation that lowers the carbon dioxide to produce the central apneic episode.

People with lung disorders, anemia or impaired cardiac function are more likely to develop altitude insomnia.

The disorder may be treated by means of RESPIRATORY STIMULANTS, such as acetazolamide, and may be improved by breathing a high level of inspired oxygen. After a few days at altitude, changes in body chemistry occur that lead initially to alkalosis, but the condition gradually corrects itself. Severe hypoxemia at altitude may lead to the development of cardiac complications, with acute pulmonary edema, and lead to compensatory changes such as a stimulation of red blood cell production.

Altitude insomnia can be differentiated from other sleep or respiratory disorders by means of polysomnographic investigations. The usual pattern consists of 10 to 20 seconds of apnea followed by three to five breaths of hyperventilation, with associated arousals or awakenings. Arterial blood gases will demonstrate hypoxemia and reduced carbon dioxide levels.

The syndrome rapidly resolves itself upon return to lower altitudes. (See also CENTRAL ALVEOLAR HYPOVENTILATION SYNDROME, CENTRAL SLEEP APNEA SYNDROME, OBSTRUCTIVE SLEEP APNEA SYNDROME.

Krieger, B.P. et al., "Altitude-Related Pulmonary Disorders," *Critical Care Clinics* 15, no. 2 (1999): 265–280.

Weil, J.V., "Sleep at High Altitudes," Kryger, M., Roth, T., and Dement, W., eds., *The Principles and Practices of Sleep Disorders Medicine.* Philadelphia: Saunders, 1989. pp. 269–275.

alveolar hypoventilation Inadequate VENTILATION of the terminal units of the lungs, the alveoli. Patients who suffer from alveolar hypoventilation have inadequate gas transfer across the lungs to and from the blood and therefore have elevated carbon dioxide and lowered oxygen levels in their blood.

Alveolar hypoventilation can be produced by disorders that affect the lung directly or harm ventilation because of impaired respiratory drive. Typically, patients with alveolar hypoventilation have deterioration of ventilation during sleep. Daytime alveolar hypoventilation may be due entirely to SLEEP-RELATED BREATHING DISORDERS, such as OBSTRUCTIVE SLEEP APNEA SYNDROME, CENTRAL SLEEP APNEA SYNDROME, or CENTRAL ALVEOLAR HYPOVENTILATION SYNDROME.

Ambien See HYPNOTICS.

ambulatory monitoring The continuous measurement of physiological variables in a patient who is not confined to bed or a specific room. Typically, ambulatory monitoring employs a portable recording device that records data while attached to the patient.

Ambulatory monitoring techniques have been used for many years for the continuous measurement of heart rhythm by Holter monitoring. More recently, ambulatory techniques have been developed for the continuous recording of ELECTROENCEPHALOGRAM activity to detect seizures. Ambulatory monitoring devices have also been developed for the measurement of a variety of other physiological variables and the assessment of sleep disorders.

Twenty-four-hour ambulatory sleep-wake monitoring can determine the presence of the sleep pattern in patients who have INSOMNIA or patients who complain of EXCESSIVE SLEEPINESS. Continuous monitoring may also be helpful for the daytime assessment of unintended sleep episodes in patients with NARCOLEPSY or IDIOPATHIC HYPERSOMNIA. Continuous monitoring throughout the 24-hour period has some advantages over the usual intermittent nap testing by means of a MULTIPLE SLEEP LATENCY TEST, as it detects sleepiness that might be missed between naps. However, it is less standardized and therefore less useful for comparison purposes among patients or for comparing a patient's status at different times. Ambulatory monitoring is particularly useful for the documentation of abnormal events and can be used for screening of such disturbances as episodes of APNEA or PERIODIC LEG MOVEMENTS during sleep. This form of monitoring can be helpful in detecting events that occur infrequently, as patients can wear the monitoring device for several days or even weeks. Activities such as SLEEPWALKING, SLEEP TERRORS or abnormal SEIZURE episodes may be detected on ambulatory recorders.

Ambulatory monitoring is also useful for determining disturbed patterns of sleep and wakefulness, such as are seen in the CIRCADIAN RHYTHM SLEEP DISORDERS. It is particularly useful for the detection of the rest-activity cycle of shift workers and individuals who undergo frequent time zone changes (see JET LAG).

Several ambulatory monitoring systems are currently available in the United States. Typically they consist of a microcomputer digital system that monitors respiration, oxygen saturation, electrocardiography, and body temperature, position and movement. Some monitors are capable of detecting electroencephalographic activity for the measurement of sleep.

Ambulatory monitoring has the potential to become the ideal means of recording physiological information from a patient in his usual environment. However, present systems are unable to measure a number of physiological variables accurately, especially given the risk of sensors malfunctioning when the patient is not under constant supervision. Another factor limiting its usefulness is that the number of physiological variables that can be measured is necessarily limited. When more channels of information are recorded, there is a greater chance of either obtaining erroneous information or losing information. While the device is recording there may be an error (artifact) in the signal being monitored, which may not be recognized until the study is completed and the information is played back.

Because of the major disadvantages of current ambulatory monitoring, it cannot be applied to the routine clinical evaluation of patients with most sleep disorders. Its usage currently is primarily for screening purposes, follow-up evaluations after treatment has been initiated, research experimentation or for determining patterns of rest and activity. (See also ACTIVITY MONITORS, POLYSOMNOGRAPHY.)

American Academy of Sleep Medicine (AASM)

A multidisciplinary organization formed in 1983 by the union of the CLINICAL SLEEP SOCIETY and the ASSOCIATION OF SLEEP DISORDER CENTERS. Previously called the American Sleep Disorders Association, in 1999 it was renamed the American Academy of Sleep Medicine. The individual member branches include: clinicians involved in the diagnosis and treatment of patients with disorders of sleep and alertness; scientists involved in basic research of sleep as well as clinical research; and other professionals who are interested in learning more about the field of SLEEP DISORDERS MEDICINE. The association, through its two branches, is active in professional education, concerns itself over standards of practice, encourages the certification of SLEEP DISORDER SPECIALISTS and is an accrediting body for SLEEP DISORDERS CENTERS.

The primary goals of the American Academy of Sleep Medicine are to facilitate information exchange, educate new professionals and train new practitioners in the area of sleep and its disorders. It establishes, updates and maintains standards for the evaluation and treatment of human sleep disorders. It also promotes the role of sleep disorders medicine to health professional organizations, federal and local regulatory bodies, as well as to federal and private health insurers.

Members of the American Academy of Sleep Medicine are eligible for: reduced rates on the INTERNATIONAL CLASSIFICATION OF SLEEP DISORDERS; an annual subscription to the professional journal *SLEEP*, an authoritative international peer review journal of the field of sleep disorders medicine and research; an AASM newsletter; a membership certificate; a membership directory; updated information on governmental agency and insurance reimbursement policies that affect sleep disorders medicine; and reduced fees for the annual APSS scientific meeting, and for courses, seminars and workshops related to the practice of sleep medicine.

Membership in the AASM was more than 3,800 at the end of 2000. Categories include regular membership, affiliate membership, fellowship, and honorary fellowship. Regular membership is open to all individuals who hold an M.D., Ph.D., D.D.S. or other academic degree in the health care field and who are active in sleep disorders medicine. An affiliate membership (student) is offered to individuals enrolled in formal training programs that upon completion would make them eligible for regular membership. Fellowship in the American Academy of Sleep Medicine is open only to individuals who have successfully completed the AMERICAN BOARD OF SLEEP MEDICINE examination, which demonstrates their competency in sleep disorders medicine and POLYSOMNOGRAPHY. Honorary fellowship in the association is reserved for exceptional individuals who have shown a lifetime contribution to the field of sleep disorders medicine or research. This award is held by NATHANIEL KLEITMAN, Ph.D., and ELIO LUGARESI, M.D.

The AASM confers several awards each year at its annual meeting, including the William C. Dement Academic Achievement Award and the NATHANIEL KLEITMAN DISTINGUISHED SERVICE AWARD.

The American Academy of Sleep Medicine is located at 6301 Bandel Road, Suite 101, Rochester, Minnesota 55901. E-mail: aasm@aasmnet.org; Web: www.aasmnet.org.

American Board of Sleep Medicine In 1978 the ASSOCIATION OF SLEEP DISORDER CENTERS formed a committee to produce an examination for the purpose of establishing and maintaining standards of individual proficiency in clinical POLYSOMNOGRAPHY. This committee, which became the Examination Committee of the American Sleep Disorders Association, directed by Helmut S. Schmidt, M.D., had certified 432 physicians and Ph.D.s as ACCREDITED CLINICAL POLYSOMNOGRAPHERS (ACPs) by the middle of 1991. By the end of 2000, some 1,500 sleep specialists had been board certified in sleep medicine.

Culminating many years of planning, the American Board of Sleep Medicine was incorporated by WILLIAM C. DEMENT, M.D., Ph.D., as an independent, nonprofit, self-designated board on January 28, 1991. The 11 directors of the board are nominated by the AMERICAN ACADEMY OF SLEEP MEDICINE (formerly called the American Sleep Disorders Association) and other professional associations that have a significant role in sleep medicine. In order to reflect the fact that sleep medicine is based on a broad medical field, the board has discontinued the term ACP and, instead, refers to its diplomates—those individuals certified both before and after its establishment as an independent board—as board certified sleep specialists.

The board directs all aspects of the certifying process. Committees of the board review applicants' credentials and produce and evaluate the two-part examination. Part I is a multiple-choice written exam which tests general knowledge of sleep medicine and polysomnography. It is divided into three sections: the basic science of sleep, clinical sleep disorders and polysomnogram recognition. Applicants can take Part II when Part I has been successfully completed. Part II consists of clinical and polysomnographic data interpretation and patient management skills. It consists of record review, questions and essays. Successful completion of both Part I and Part II leads to certification in the specialty of sleep medicine.

To be eligible to apply for board certification in sleep medicine, applicants must have the following qualifications:

1. A medical degree (M.D. or D.O.) and an unlimited license to practice medicine in a state, commonwealth or territory of the U.S. or Canada.
2. Successful completion of a residency program accredited by the Accreditation Council for Graduate Medical Education, or its equivalent.
3. Certification by a primary board that is recognized by the American Board of Medical Specialties (ABMS), the Royal College of Physicians and Surgeons of Canada, the Certificate College of Family Physicians of Canada, or the equivalent board for osteopathic medicine.
4. One year of training (PGY 3 or later) in sleep medicine under the supervision of a diplomate of the American Board of Sleep Medicine or in an accredited fellowship training program. (Waivers may apply.) Graduates of fellowship programs in pulmonary medicine or clinical neurophysiology can satisfy this requirement with six full-time months (or the equivalent part-time) of training in a sleep medicine within their subspecialty fellowship, plus six months of full-time training in sleep medicine.
5. Knowledge of the fundamentals in interpretation and quality assurance of procedures related to sleep medicine. As a guideline, a minimum experience of interpretation and review of the raw data of 200 POLYSOMNOGRAMS and 25 MULTIPLE SLEEP LATENCY TESTS is suggested. The applicant should have seen a broad range of patients with different sleep disorders encompassing a minimum of 200 new patients and 200 follow-up patients.
6. A fully completed application, including a satisfactory evaluation from a board-certified sleep specialist, and three letters of reference.

For up-to-date and more specific details on examination requirements or for applications, contact: American Board of Sleep Medicine, 6301 Bandel Road, Suite 101, Rochester, Minnesota 55901. E-mail: absm@absm.org; Web: www.absm.org.

American Narcolepsy Association (ANA) An independent, not-for-profit organization established in 1975 in the San Francisco Bay Area by nine people who suffered from NARCOLEPSY. Its purpose was to "improve the quality of living of persons who have narcolepsy." By 1989 the association member/donor base numbered more than 4,000 persons, and ANA maintained contact with more than 10,000 persons suffering from narcolepsy. The ANA provided information and referral services nationwide and provided funds for narcolepsy-related sleep research. Volunteers were recruited for research projects; it provided direct mail assistance for narcolepsy survey research. Its governing board consisted of patients, scientists and industry representatives.

The executive director of ANA was WILLIAM BAIRD. The ANA ceased to function in the early 1990s and no longer exists. (See also NARCOLEPSY NETWORK, NARCOLEPSY-CATAPLEXY FOUNDATION.)

American Sleep Disorders Association (ASDA) See AMERICAN ACADEMY OF SLEEP MEDICINE (AASM).

amitriptyline See ANTIDEPRESSANTS.

amphetamines See STIMULANT MEDICATIONS.

ANA See AMERICAN NARCOLEPSY ASSOCIATION (ANA).

Anafranil See ANTIDEPRESSANTS.

analeptic medications A group of medications that stimulate the central nervous system. The term was derived from the Greek word *analepsis* meaning "to repair." But the term "analeptics" most commonly applies to those medications that stimulate arousal, in particular CAFFEINE and the amphetamines, and other stimulants such as pemoline and strychnine, and the respiratory stimulants doxapram and nikethimide. The central nervous system stimulants that produce arousal are usually used for the treatment of disorders of excessive sleepiness, such as NARCOLEPSY and IDIOPATHIC HYPERSOMNIA, whereas the respiratory stimulants are used for disorders such as INFANT SLEEP APNEA. (See also STIMULANT MEDICATIONS.)

angina decubitus See NOCTURNAL CARDIAC ISCHEMIA.

anorectics See STIMULANT MEDICATIONS.

antidepressants Medications used for the treatment of the psychiatric disorders associated with DEPRESSION. These disorders, previously called affective disorders and currently called mood disorders, can have pronounced effects upon sleep. INSOMNIA is a typical feature of mood disorders, as are altered sleep-wake patterns. The antidepressant medications can be useful for treating not only the predominant mood disorders but also the underlying sleep disturbance. The group of antidepressant medications most commonly used are the SEROTONIN reuptake inhibitors; however, other medications, including the tricyclic antidepressants and the monoamine oxidase (MAO) inhibitors, are frequently recommended. In addition to their role in treating sleep disturbance related to depression, the antidepressant medications are commonly used for the treatment of CATAPLEXY in patients who have NARCOLEPSY.

Selective serotonin reuptake inhibitors (SSRIs) are a group of medications used for the treatment of depression. These antidepressant medications are classified on the basis of their selective blockade or neuronal reuptake of serotonin (5HT). The SSRIs include agents such as fluoxetine, sertraline and paroxetine. These newer antidepressants generally have fewer side effects than the older antidepressants. The side effects, if they occur, happen at the start of treatment or after dosage increases.

The SSRIs have little effect upon monoamine uptake systems other than serotonin, and they cause only minimal inhibition of muscarinic cholinergic, histaminergic or adrenergic receptors.

Blocking the reuptake of 5HT increases the time that 5HT molecules remain in the synapse and therefore increases the chance that they will bind with 5HT receptors.

The SSRIs are as effective as the tricyclic antidepressants but have a better benefit-to-risk ratio because they are relatively safe if overdosed and are not cardiotoxic. The most common side effects of the SSRIs are nausea, loose stools, tremor, dry mouth and sexual dysfunction, including reduced libido, delayed ejaculation in men and anorgasmia in women. Several adverse effects are dose-related, such as anxiety, agitation, akathisia, tremor and nausea.

The tricyclic antidepressants are medications with a three-ringed biochemical structure. Their primary use is in improving depression, but they are also used for other psychiatric illnesses, such as panic attacks. The main tricyclic antidepressants used are amitriptyline, clomipramine, imipramine, and protriptyline. Anticholinergic side effects, such as dry mouth, anorexia, sweating, hypotension, tachycardia, urinary retention, constipation, blurred vision and sexual dysfunction are common. These side effects limit the usefulness of the tricyclic antidepressants in many patients.

The tricyclics are also commonly used for the treatment of insomnia. Sedating tricyclic medications can be used to improve the quality of nighttime sleep by reducing awakenings. The stimulating tricyclic medications, such as protriptyline, can be used during the daytime to reduce the psychomotor retardation that often occurs in patients with depression. They may also reduce the tendency for daytime lethargy and napping in such patients.

The tricyclic antidepressants have a pronounced REM sleep suppressant effect. Once the medication is stopped, there can be a rebound of REM sleep with enhancement of REM sleep-related phenomena, such as NIGHTMARES, SLEEP PARALYSIS or HYPNAGOGIC HALLUCINATIONS.

Amitriptyline (Elavil)

A tricyclic antidepressant with sedating effects that is commonly used in the treatment of insomnia due to DEPRESSION. This medication has been shown to decrease the number of awakenings, increase the amount of stage four sleep (see SLEEP STAGES) and markedly reduce the amount of REM SLEEP. Amitriptyline typically will suppress the sleep onset REM period that is commonly seen in patients with depression.

Amitriptyline is given in doses from 10 milligrams to 150 milligrams per day, higher doses being preferred for the treatment of endogenous depression, whereas the lower dosages are often effective in treating insomnia that is unrelated to primary depression.

Side effects of daytime sedation, and anticholinergic effects that are typical of all the tricyclic antidepressants, include dry mouth, anorexia, sweating, hypotension, tachycardia, urinary retention, constipation, blurred vision and sexual dysfunction; such side effects can commonly occur. As with the other tricyclic antidepressants, amitriptyline can be cardiotoxic and can induce cardiac arrhythmias in patients with cardiac disease.

This drug is not used for the treatment of cataplexy because of its tendency for side effects and its sedation. Other tricyclic antidepressants, such as protriptyline and clomipramine, that have little sedating effects, are more useful for the treatment of cataplexy. However, the serotonin reuptake inhibitors such as Prozac are commonly used.

Amitriptyline also suppresses ALPHA ACTIVITY in the electroencephalogram. Consequently, the drug has been used in the treatment of patients with nonrestorative sleep due to FIBROSITIS SYNDROME.

Clomipramine

Trade name Anafranil, a tricyclic antidepressant and a potent serotonin uptake blocker used for the treatment of depression and the cataplexy caused by narcolepsy.

Clomipramine is given in divided doses during the day, with dosages ranging from 10 to 20 milligrams per day. It is limited by its side effects, which include sedation, dry mouth, anorexia (loss of appetite), hypertension, sweating, tachycardia, urinary retention, constipation, blurred vision and sexual dysfunction.

Clomipramine is commonly used outside of the United States for the treatment for cataplexy in patients with narcolepsy. As this agent has powerful REM-suppressant effects, it is an effective agent for treatment of REM-sleep phenomena. Its effect on cataplexy appears to be greater than that of most other tricyclic antidepressants.

Imipramine

Trade name Tofranil, it was one of the first tricyclic antidepressants to be used. It appears to act by stimulation of the central nervous system and blocks the uptake of norepinephrine at nerve endings. This medication is primarily used for the relief of the symptoms of depression, especially endogenous depression; however, it is also used for the treatment of childhood ENURESIS and narcolepsy.

Imipramine is available in tablets of 10, 25 and 50 milligrams. Doses of up to 100 milligrams per day are usually required in adults. As the potential for cardiac toxicity is greater in children, it should be used in childhood only with caution. Overdosage in childhood has been reported to cause death.

The medication produces mild sedation and therefore can be given prior to sleep at night, where it can help the quality of sleep by improving deep stage three/four sleep (see SLEEP STAGES). But there is a marked reduction in REM sleep. Sudden withdrawal of the medication is frequently accompanied by an increase in REM sleep, with the development of nightmares and other REM sleep phenomena, such as sleep paralysis and hypnagogic hallucinations.

The main adverse reactions of imipramine are related to its cardiotoxicity and anticholinergic effects, such as dry mouth, blurred vision, constipation and urinary retention. In addition, central nervous system effects, such as confusion, disorientation and nightmares with exacerbation of insomnia, can occur.

When used for the treatment of cataplexy, the medication is usually given in divided doses during the daytime. However, the side effect of sedation limits its usefulness in treating narcolepsy. Other more stimulating tricyclic antidepressants, such as protriptyline or the serotonin reuptake inhibitors, are more useful. Also, because methylphenidate (Ritalin) can inhibit the metabolism of imipramine, the dose of imipramine may have to be reduced in patients receiving both medications.

A nighttime dose of 25 to 50 milligrams has been effective in suppressing nocturnal enuresis in childhood. This effect is believed to be produced by delaying the time of urinating till the final morning awakening and is not thought to be produced by its effect on either sleep stages or by its anticholinergic effects.

Protriptyline

Trade name Vivactil, a tricyclic antidepressant medication used for the treatment of depression and cataplexy in patients with narcolepsy. Protriptyline is commonly given in divided doses during the daytime in a dose from 15 to 30 milligrams per day. It is often used for treating cataplexy because of its effectiveness and its advantageous stimulant effects. Although patients report an alerting effect of protriptyline, this has not been confirmed by objective testing.

As with the other tricyclic antidepressants, the predominant side effects include the typical anticholinergic effects; the tendency to these side effects limits its usefulness in some patients with cataplexy.

Protriptyline reduces REM sleep at night but also, because of the stimulant effect, can produce an increased number of awakenings and lead to insomnia if given before nocturnal sleep. It can induce cardiac arrhythmias and should be given with caution to patients with cardiac disease.

Femoxetine

Has been shown to be useful in the treatment of cataplexy in patients with narcolepsy. This agent is less effective than the tricyclic antidepressants but has the advantage of lacking anticholinergic side effects, such as dry mouth, anorexia, hypertension and sweating. This medication is not yet available in the United States but is available for use in Europe, although it is believed that it has only a small role to play in the treatment of cataplexy, because more effective agents are available, such as protriptyline.

Fluoxetine

Trade name Prozac, a reuptake blocker. Sixty milligrams given in a single morning dose has been shown to be effective in reducing cataplexy in some patients. However, there have been rare reports of an increase in cataplexy on this medication, and its use may be limited by the side effect of nausea. Fluoxetine is limited in its usefulness of the treatment of cataplexy because other more effective agents, such as protriptyline, are available. Fluoxetine is an effective antidepressant.

Fluvoxamine

A potent serotonin uptake blocker that is used for the treatment of cataplexy in patients with narcolepsy. It is an antidepressant medication with slight sedative effects, but little anticholinergic effect. It is less effective in treating cataplexy than the tricyclic medication protriptyline.

Sertraline

Trade name Zoloft. A serotonin reuptake inhibitor that can disturb sleep. It also can produce REM-sleep suppression and BRUXISM.

Paroxetine

Trade name Paxil. A serotonin reuptake inhibitor that can induce rapid eye movements in NREM sleep. It is useful for daytime anxiety disorders.

Nefazodone

Trade name Serzone. This medication is sedative and can be useful for treating insomnia. It can increase REM sleep.

Mirtazapine

Trade name Remeron. It produces mild sedation and can suppress REM sleep.

Venlafaxine

Trade name Effexor. It can induce sedation or insomnia.

Thase, M.E., "Antidepressant Treatment of the Depressed Patient with Insomnia," *Journal of Clinical Psychiatry* 60, Suppl. 1 (1999): 28–31.

antihistamines Medications that block the effect of HISTAMINE, an irritant agent released in response to trauma or an allergic reaction. Antihistamines, particularly diphenhydramine, have sedative properties and are sometimes used as HYPNOTICS. However, their primary use is as blockers of acute allergic reactions, such as allergic skin reactions, nasal allergies, gastrointestinal allergies or for the treatment of severe whole body allergic reactions, such as anaphylaxis or angioedema. Other antihistamine agents do not have sedative properties, and are effective in inhibiting gastric acid secretion. They are commonly used for the treatment of peptic ulcers.

Diphenhydramine

Antihistamine primarily used for allergic reactions. Its pronounced tendency to induce sedation and sleepiness leads to its use by parents for the treatment of childhood INSOMNIA, as a sedative agent. However, diphenhydramine has pronounced anticholinergic effects (constipation, dry mouth, urine retention and hypotension), and its sedative effect is a side effect of the histamine blocker. It is not recommended for routine use as a hypnotic agent. Other, more specific hypnotics, the BENZODIAZEPINES, are preferable for patients who have sleep disturbance. Benadryl is the pharmaceutical name for diphenhydramine.

antipsychotic medication See NEUROLEPTICS.

anxiety A feeling of dread and apprehension regarding one or more life circumstances. A common cause of sleep disturbance, anxiety may be a short-lived, acute stress, such as that related to an examination or a marital, financial or work problem. Acute anxiety in these situations can lead to an ADJUSTMENT SLEEP DISORDER, which typically resolves itself within a few days of the acute anxiety, but it may persist for several weeks. Chronic anxiety often indicates an ANXIETY DISORDER and may lead to an enduring and pervasive sleep disorder.

Individuals with chronic sleep disorders, such as PSYCHOPHYSIOLOGICAL INSOMNIA, may become anxious as a secondary feature of the sleep disorder. Treatment of the underlying sleep disorder in these situations usually leads to resolution of the anxiety. (See also PANIC DISORDER.)

anxiety disorders Psychiatric disorders characterized by symptoms of anxiety and dread, and avoidance behavior. Sleep disturbance commonly occurs in association with anxiety disorders. Anxiety disorders include PANIC DISORDER, with or without agoraphobia, phobias, obsessive-compulsive disorder, post-traumatic stress disorder and general anxiety disorder.

Patients with general anxiety disorder typically have a sleep onset or maintenance INSOMNIA, with frequent awakenings that may be associated with anxiety dreams. Typically there is ruminative thinking that occurs at sleep onset or during the awakenings. Individuals often complain of being unable to "turn off their minds" because of the flood of thoughts and concerns, many of which are trivial in nature. Following the disturbed night of sleep, there may be feelings of unrest, tiredness, fatigue and sleepiness. Often during the daytime there is intense anxiety over the thought of another impending night of inadequate sleep. Associated with the daytime anxiety is evidence of increased muscle tension, restlessness, shortness of breath, palpitations, dry mouth, dizziness, trembling and difficulty in concentration. Most patients with anxiety disorders have little ability to take daytime naps, as the difficulty in being able to fall asleep persists around the clock.

The anxiety disorders characteristic of early adulthood are more common in females than in males. There appears to be a familial tendency for general anxiety disorder. Polysomnographic studies demonstrate a prolonged sleep latency, with frequent awakenings during the night, reduced sleep efficiency and increased amount of lighter stages one and two sleep, with reduced slow wave sleep. REM SLEEP latencies are normal although REM sleep may be reduced in percentage (see SLEEP STAGES).

The chronic nature of anxiety differentiates patients with anxiety disorders from those who are experiencing an ADJUSTMENT SLEEP DISORDER, which is typically seen in association with acute stress. Sleep disturbance associated with anxiety disorders should be distinguished from that seen in patients who have PSYCHOPHYSIOLOGICAL INSOMNIA; the anxiety in psychophysiological insomnia is less generalized and is more focused on the sleep disturbance, which, when effectively treated, leads to resolution of the anxiety. Patients with generalized anxiety disorders have more pervasive anxiety that may persist even though the sleep disturbance is otherwise resolved.

Anxiety disorders are treated either by pharmacological means or through counseling and psychotherapy. Pharmacological agents used to treat anxiety disorders include HYPNOTICS and BENZODIAZEPINES; the use of ANTIDEPRESSANTS may be required if elements of depression coexist. Good SLEEP HYGIENE and treatment of the sleep disturbance by behavioral means, such as STIMULUS CONTROL THERAPY or SLEEP RESTRICTION THERAPY, are usually necessary in patients with sleep disturbance because of anxiety disorders.

Case History

A 39-year-old male high school teacher had a long history of sleep disturbance, a condition that had deteriorated in the prior three years. In addition to teaching, he also had a part-time job as a landlord, which contributed a number of anxieties and rather complicated his life. His sleep pattern was disrupted by a constant feeling that he couldn't turn off his mind. He became very annoyed and angry at his inability to fall asleep. Occasionally, he would perform RELAXATION EXERCISES before getting into bed at night and would avoid any activities that might be stimulating or disruptive to his sleep. He usually was unable to sleep for more than an hour at a time before awakening, and then he would be in and out of sleep for the rest of the night. Occasionally he tried drinking a small amount of ALCOHOL to improve his sleep but stopped this when he found it did not produce any benefit. Upon awakening in the morning, he would be tired and had difficulty in maintaining concentration, which affected his conversations. He found that he would often have to repeat himself. He became slightly depressed and irritable because of the sleep disturbance.

His problem with initiating and maintaining sleep was finally diagnosed as secondary to chronic anxiety and depression. There was no evidence of major depression; the anxiety features were more prominent. Treatment was initiated by scheduling his time for sleep within the limits of 10:45 at night with an awakening at 6:45 in the morning. With 0.5 milligrams of alprazolam (Xanax; see BENZODIAPENES) the sleep disturbances abated but were not resolved. After several weeks of treatment, combined with close attention to his hours, a small dose of sedating antidepressant medication was added to his treatment. He commenced 50 milligrams of amitryptiline (see ANTIDEPRESSANTS) taken one hour before sleep.

On the new treatment regime, he dramatically improved and the quality of sleep was the best he had had in years. In addition, the intermittent feelings of daytime depression were eliminated and he did not suffer from fatigue and tiredness. He was maintained on the medications with strict adherence to a regular sleeping-waking schedule.

Gillin, J.C., "Are Sleep Disturbances Risk Factors for Anxiety, Depressive and Addictive Disorders?" *Acta Psychiatrica Scandinavica* Suppl. 393 (1998): 39–43.

Rosa, R.R., Bonnett, M.M. and Kramer, M., "The Relationship of Sleep and Anxiety in Anxious Subjects," *Biological Psychology* 16 (1983): 119–126.

Sussman, N., "Anxiety Disorders," *Psychiatric Annals* 18 (1988): 134–189.

apnea Derived from the Greek word that means "want of breath," apnea has occurred if breathing stops for at least 10 seconds, as detected by airflow at the nostrils and mouth. Respiratory movement may or may not be present during an apneic episode. Typically there are three forms of apnea, depending upon the degree of respiratory movement activity: obstructive, central and mixed.

Obstructive apnea is associated with upper airway obstruction and is characterized by loss of airflow while respiratory movements remain normal. Airflow is usually measured by means of a nasal THERMISTOR (a temperature-sensitive metal strip) that records changes in air temperature with inspiration and expiration, whereas respiratory muscle movement activity can be measured by means of the electromyogram, strain gauges or by a bellows pneumograph. Obstructive apnea is usually accompanied by sounds of snoring.

Central apnea is cessation of airflow associated with complete cessation of all respiratory movements. The diaphragm and chest muscles are immobile. This type of apnea can occur among those who have diseases such as poliomyelitis or spinal-cord injuries.

Mixed apnea typically has an initial central apnea component for about 10 seconds followed by an obstructive component.

Apnea during sleep can produce a lowering of the blood oxygen level, increased blood carbon dioxide levels, cardiac arrhythmias, and sleep disruption with resulting excessive sleepiness. If the number of apneas becomes frequent enough to produce clinical symptoms and signs, then the patient may have either an OBSTRUCTIVE SLEEP APNEA SYNDROME or CENTRAL SLEEP APNEA SYNDROME.

apnea-hypopnea index The number of obstructive, central and mixed APNEA episodes, plus the number of episodes of shallow breathing (HYPOPNEA), expressed per hour of total sleep time, as determined by all-night polysomnographic recording. Most clinicians believe that the apnea-hypopnea index is a more reliable measure of apnea severity than the APNEA INDEX because it monitors all three types of respiratory irregularity during sleep. The apnea-hypopnea index is sometimes referred to as the RESPIRATORY DISTURBANCE INDEX (RDI).

apnea index A measure of APNEA frequency most commonly used in determining the severity of respiratory impairment during sleep. The number of obstructive, central and mixed apneic episodes is expressed per hour of total sleep time as measured by all-night polysomnographic recording. Occasionally an obstructive apnea index, which is a measure of the obstructive apneas per hour of total sleep time, or a central apnea index, is stated. Typically an apnea index of 20 or less is regarded as mild apnea, an index of 20 to 50 as moderate and above 50 as a severe degree of apnea. The term "apnea index" is only one index of apnea severity because the duration of apneic episodes and severity of associated features, such as oxygen saturation and the presence of electrocardiographic abnormalities, are also important in determining apnea severity.

If the number of episodes of shallow breathing during sleep (HYPOPNEA) are added to the apneas in calculating the index, then an APNEA-HYPOPNEA INDEX is produced, an index preferred by many clinicians.

apnea monitor A biomedical device developed primarily for detection of episodes of cessation of breathing that occur in infants and young children.

An apnea monitor detects respiratory movement and heart rhythm. Typically, an apnea monitor is set to signal a breathing pause of 20 seconds or greater, or an episode of slowing of the heart rhythm, a rate that is determined according to the age of the child.

Apnea monitors are usually recommended for use on children who have been known to stop breathing in their sleep. Any subsequent events can be detected and will set off an alarm so that the parent can check the condition of the child. With infants, it often occurs that the alarm will sound and by the time the parents get to the infant, the child has recommenced breathing. However, in some situations the child may need to be stimulated to start respiration, particularly those children with sleep-related breathing disorders, such as the CENTRAL SLEEP APNEA SYNDROME. Apnea monitors are not useful for detecting upper airway obstruction in association with the OBSTRUCTIVE SLEEP APNEA SYNDROME.

Apnea monitors do not replace the use of more extensive polysomnographic evaluation when sleep-related breathing disorders are suspected. Polysomnographic monitoring has the advantage of being able to detect upper airway obstructive events as well as determining whether alterations in ventilation occur during sleep or specific sleep stages. In addition, polysomnographic monitoring is able to detect other physiological variables that may be associated with a respiratory pause, for example, the electroencephalographic pattern in a child who has epileptic seizures as a cause of respiratory cessation.

apnea of prematurity (AOP) Episodes of interrupted breathing present in otherwise healthy, prematurely born infants. The breathing pauses are typically greater than 20 seconds in duration; however, shorter pauses may be associated with cyanosis, abrupt pallor or hypotonia. The majority of the apneic episodes occur during sleep; however, some are associated with movement when the infant is awake. Up to 10% of the apneic episodes are purely obstructive, with the site of obstruction being in the pharynx. The episodes always terminate spontaneously and, if necessary, stimulation can assist in promoting ventilation.

Immaturity of the respiratory system is believed to be the primary cause of apnea of prematurity. However, this form of apnea can be precipitated by general anesthesia or the use of other central nervous system depressant medications.

Normal healthy infants can have brief apneic pauses, typically between five and 10 seconds in duration; however, these episodes are not of clinical significance and it is the longer apneas associated with cyanosis and reduction of cerebral blood flow that are of particular concern.

The majority of infants born before 31 weeks of gestation will have this form of apnea; the prevalence falls to less than 15% of infants born after 32 weeks of gestation and older.

Episodes of apnea may occur infrequently (once a week) or can occur several times per hour. The course of the disordered breathing is shorter the older the child is at birth, and typically the course is less than four weeks for infants older than 31 weeks gestation.

Apnea of prematurity can be demonstrated by polysomnographic monitoring, which shows apneic episodes occurring during both QUIET SLEEP and inactive sleep. However, the most severe episodes occur during ACTIVE SLEEP, often in association with cardiac arrhythmias, such as bradycardia.

The disorder may produce severe HYPOXEMIA and require ventilatory support. There is some suggestion that infants with apnea of prematurity may be at high risk of developing SUDDEN INFANT DEATH SYNDROME (SIDS).

Treatment is mainly supportive. Assisted ventilation and constant respiratory monitoring in a neonatal intensive care unit may be necessary. (See also CENTRAL ALVEOLAR HYPOVENTILATION SYNDROME, CENTRAL SLEEP APNEA SYNDROME, INFANT SLEEP, INFANT SLEEP APNEA, OBSTRUCTIVE SLEEP APNEA SYNDROME.)

Durand, M., Cabal, L., Gonzalez, F., Georgia, S., Barberis, C., Hoppenbrouwers, T. and Hodgman, J.E., "Ventilatory Control and Carbon Dioxide Response in Preterm Infants with Idiopathic Apnea," *American Diseases of Childhood* 139 (1985): 717–720.

Thach, B., "Sleep Apnea in Infancy and Childhood," *Medical Clinics of North America* 69 (1985): 1289–1315.

arginine vasotocin (AVT) A peptide that was initially discovered in the pineal gland. This agent has a variety of effects, including modification of conditioned behavior, inhibition of gonadotrophin hormone (sex gland stimulating hormone) release and the stimulation of SLOW WAVE SLEEP. Very low doses of AVT are reported to be effective in increasing slow wave sleep in animals. (It is thought that the effects may be mediated through the gamma-aminobutyric acid pathways to serotonergic neurons.)

There is evidence in humans to suggest that AVT is released during sleep into the cerebrospinal fluid. Recent evidence in patients with NARCOLEPSY and other disorders of excessive sleepiness has shown that sleep, and particularly sleep onset REM periods, can be increased by the administration of AVT. These studies suggest that AVT may be involved primarily in the regulation of REM SLEEP. (See also GAMMA-AMINOBUTYRIC ACID, SEROTONIN, SLEEP-INDUCING FACTORS.)

Argonne anti-jet-lag diet Developed by Dr. Charles Ehret of Argonne's Division of Biological and Medical Research as part of his studies of biological rhythms. (The Argonne National Laboratory is a center of research in energy and fundamental sciences of the United States Department of Energy and is located in Argonne, Illinois.) The Argonne anti-jet-lag diet is based upon the finding that high carbohydrate food, such as pasta, fruit and some desserts, will produce an increased level of energy for about one hour, and subsequently will produce tiredness and sleepiness. Conversely, high protein foods, such as fish, eggs, dairy products and meat, will give a sustained increased level of energy, possibly by its metabolism to catecholamines such as adrenaline. In addition, caffeine-containing drinks, such as coffee, can advance or delay the sleep pattern, depending upon the time they are taken.

The Argonne anti-jet-lag diet consists of a pattern of feasting and fasting for four days prior to departure. The first day, breakfast and lunch consist of high protein meals and the evening meal consists largely of carbohydrates. This pattern of food intake is repeated on the third day. On the second and fourth days of the diet, fasting occurs so that only light meals of fruits, soups and selected solids are taken. Caffeinated beverages are allowed only between 3 and 5 P.M. Upon the day of departure, if the traveler is westbound, he is advised to drink caffeine beverages in the morning before departure. When traveling eastbound, caffeine beverages are taken between 6 and 12 P.M.

The first day in the new environment is one of fasting.

The Argonne anti-jet-lag diet may be useful for some people; however, many find its pattern of feasting and fasting impractical and it has not been effective for everyone who has rigidly adhered to the plan. (See also DIET AND SLEEP, TIME ZONE CHANGE [JET LAG] SYNDROME.)

arise time Time on the clock after final wake up, at which an individual gets out of bed.

arousal A change in the sleep state to a lighter stage of sleep. Typically, arousal will occur from a deep stage of non-REM sleep to a lighter non-REM sleep stage, or from REM sleep to stage one or wakefulness (see SLEEP STAGES). Arousals sometimes result in a full awakening and are often accompanied by body movement and an increase in heart rate.

Arousals occurring from stage three and four sleep may be accompanied by the characteristic features of AROUSAL DISORDERS, namely, SLEEPWALKING, SLEEP TERRORS and CONFUSIONAL AROUSALS. In these disorders, arousal is followed by an incomplete waking and the persistence of electroencephalographic patterns of sleep.

arousal disorders Disorders of normal AROUSAL. In 1968, ROGER BROUGHTON described four important common sleep disorders as abnormalities of the arousal process: SLEEP ENURESIS (bedwetting), somnambulism (SLEEPWALKING), SLEEP TERRORS and NIGHTMARES. At that time, it was believed that all four of these disorders shared common electrophysiological and clinical features.

Two of the disorders, somnambulism and sleep terror, most consistently demonstrate the classical feature of the arousal disorders. They occur during an arousal from slow wave sleep, rather than REM sleep. Since Broughton's original description, a third disorder, the nightmare, has been shown to occur more typically from REM sleep; and sleep enuresis, although occurring from slow wave sleep, can also occur out of other sleep stages.

In addition to the sleep stage association, the other major features of the four arousal disorders are: (1) the presence of mental confusion and disorientation during the episode; (2) automatic and repetitive motor behavior; (3) reduced reaction and insensitivity to external stimulation; (4) difficulty in coming to full wakefulness despite vigorous attempts to awaken the individual; (5) inability to recall the event the next morning (retrograde amnesia); and (6) very little dream recall associated with the event.

Although mentioned by Broughton in his original article, the disorder of CONFUSIONAL AROUSALS has recently been established as another arousal disorder.

Broughton, R., "Sleep Disorders: Disorders of Arousal?" *Science* 159 (1968): 1070–1078.

arrhythmias Heart rhythm irregularities. The most common cause of sleep-related arrhythmias is OBSTRUCTIVE SLEEP APNEA SYNDROME, which produces a pattern of slowing and speeding up of the heart (brady-tachycardia). This pattern may be picked up on a 24-hour electrocardiographic recording (for instance, during Holter monitoring). The presence of brady-tachycardia during sleep, and its absence during wakefulness, is a characteristic feature of obstructive sleep apnea syndrome. Other cardiac arrhythmias that can occur in association with the obstructive sleep apnea syndrome include episodes of sinus arrest, lasting up to 15 seconds in duration, and tachyarrhythmias, such as ventricular tachycardia (see VENTRICULAR ARRHYTHMIAS). Cardiac arrhythmias due to obstructive sleep apnea are believed to be a cause of sudden death during sleep.

Other disorders that can produce cardiac irregularity during sleep include REM SLEEP-RELATED SINUS ARREST. This disorder is characterized by episodes of cardiac pause, lasting several seconds, that occur during REM sleep in otherwise healthy individuals. This disorder may require the implantation of a cardiac pacemaker in order to prevent complete cardiac arrest.

Another disorder that may be associated with cardiac irregularity is SUDDEN UNEXPLAINED NOCTURNAL DEATH SYNDROME (SUND) which is seen in Southeast Asian refugees. In this disorder, sudden death occurs during sleep and a cardiac cause is suspected. Ventricular tachycardia has been detected in the few patients who have been resuscitated.

Patients who have cardiac arrhythmias due solely to heart disease often have an improvement in the cardiac irregularity during sleep, particularly during non-REM sleep, when the heart rate slows and the rhythm becomes more stable. During REM sleep there can be an exacerbation of cardiac irregularity, particularly during the episode of phasic rapid eye movement activity. (See also SLEEP-RELATED BREATHING DISORDERS.)

artifact Interfering electrical signals that occur during the recording of sleep. They may be caused by the person being studied or by environmental interference, sometimes from the sleep lab itself, and can obscure the information being recorded.

Too much artifact may make a sleep recording impossible to score and analyze and therefore render it useless.

Sixty hertz activity, often due to nearby electrical appliances or cables, is a common cause of artifact during sleep recordings.

Ascending Reticular Activating System (ARAS) A portion of the brain stem and cerebrum involved in the maintenance of wakefulness. The cells in this area consist of a loose network that forms the central gray matter of the brain stem.

In the 1940s, Morruzi and Magoun discovered that electrical stimulation of the brain stem reticular formation produced an increase in cortical activation indicative of wakefulness. The ascending reticular formation interacts with the brain stem regions for the induction and maintenance of sleep, as well as the cerebral regions involved in the production of sleep, thereby producing the sleep-wake cycle. The Ascending Reticular Activating System anatomically consists of the brain stem reticular formation, including that of the medullary, pontine and midbrain levels, as well as the subhypothalamic and thalamic regions. Excitation of these areas leads to cortical activity by means of a diffuse thalamic projection system that covers the entire cerebral cortex.

In addition to the sleep-related functions, the reticular formation of the brain stem contains those neurons involved in the respiratory, cardiovascular and other autonomic systems.

Moruzzi, G. and Magoun, H.W., "Brain Stem Reticular Formation and Activation of the EEG," *Electroencephalography and Clinical Neurophysiology* 1 (1949): 455–473.

ASDA sleep code A number used in the American Sleep Disorders Association (ASDA) diagnostic and coding manual that allows information, such as associated symptoms, and the severity and duration of particular disorders, to be coded for research purposes. (See also AMERICAN ACADEMY OF SLEEP MEDICINE, INTERNATIONAL CLASSIFICATION OF SLEEP DISORDERS.)

Aserinsky, Eugene Considered one of the pioneers of modern sleep research, Dr. Aserinsky (1921–98), in 1952, while a graduate student at the University of Chicago working in the laboratory of NATHANIEL KLEITMAN in the Department of Physiology, discovered the presence of the RAPID EYE MOVEMENT (REM) phase of sleep.

Association for the Psychophysiological Study of Sleep Founded in Chicago in 1961, at which time it consisted of only a few interested sleep researchers. The first meeting outside of Chicago was held in 1963 at the Downstate Medical Center in Brooklyn, New York. By 1964, Association for the Psychophysiological Study of Sleep had become the official name of the organization.

In 1983, the Association for the Psychophysiological Study of Sleep changed its name to the SLEEP RESEARCH SOCIETY.

Association of Polysomnographic Technologists (APT) Founded in 1978 by Peter A. McGregor, chief polysomnographic technologist at the Sleep-Wake Disorders Center of Montefiore Medical Center in New York. An organizational meeting of polysomnographic technologists was held in April 1978 at the annual convention of the ASSOCIATION FOR THE PSYCHOPHYSIOLOGICAL STUDY OF SLEEP and the ASSOCIATION OF SLEEP DISORDER CENTERS.

The main aims of the APT are to develop standards of professional competence within the area of polysomnographic technology, to provide and administer a registration process for polysomnographic technologists, to help technologists develop the finest possible patient care and safety and produce the highest quality of polysomnographic data, to provide a means of communication among technicians and others working in the field of SLEEP DISORDERS MEDICINE and sleep research, to support and advance the professional identities of technologists in health care and to standardize polysomnographic procedures.

The Association of Polysomnographic Technologists started with about 50 members in 1978 and by 1999 had increased its membership to almost 2,000. Nearly 3,000 technicians have passed the association's registration examination and are registered polysomnographic technologists (R.P.S.G.T.).

Association of Professional Sleep Societies (APSS) Founded in 1985, a federation of two professional sleep societies: the SLEEP RESEARCH SOCIETY (SRS) and the AMERICAN ACADEMY OF SLEEP MEDICINE. Although it was an original member of the APSS, the ASSOCIATION OF POLYSOMNOGRAPHIC TECHNOLOGISTS (APT) is no longer a member.

APSS organizes and implements an annual national scientific and clinical meeting. The association was specifically created to represent the common interests of sleep researchers and sleep disorders medicine, and to provide a single body for representation to the general public and the government. Dr. WILLIAM C. DEMENT of Stanford University was the first chairman of APSS.

Association of Sleep Disorder Centers (ASDC) Founded in 1975 and accredited its first centers in 1977. The first sleep disorder center to be accredited by the ASDC was the Sleep-Wake Disorders Unit of Montefiore Medical Center in New York. The two other disorder centers accredited in the first year of the association were at Stanford University in Palo Alto and at Ohio University in Columbus.

The primary function of the ASDC was to develop accreditation standards and guidelines to ensure that the highest level of care would be provided by the sleep disorder centers. In 1987, the Association of Sleep Disorder Centers was merged with the CLINICAL SLEEP SOCIETY into one organization, the AMERICAN ACADEMY OF SLEEP MEDICINE (AASM). There were 400 sleep disorder centers accredited by ASDA as of 2000. The American Sleep Disorders Association is one of several members of the federation known as the ASSOCIATION OF PROFESSIONAL SLEEP SOCIETIES. (See also ACCREDITATION STANDARDS FOR SLEEP DISORDER CENTERS.)

asthma See SLEEP-RELATED ASTHMA, SLEEP-RELATED BREATHING DISORDERS.

asymptomatic polysomnographic finding Any asymptomatic abnormality detected by polysomnography that when present in other patients can be symptomatic. For example, PERIODIC LEG MOVEMENT can produce symptoms associated with INSOMNIA or EXCESSIVE SLEEPINESS; however, in many otherwise healthy individuals, periodic leg movements may be asymptomatic. These asymptomatic features may be detected during polysomnographic monitoring performed for other reasons, for example, for impotence or for unrelated sleep disorders, such as nocturnal epilepsy or SLEEPWALKING. Other asymptomatic polysomnographic findings include infrequent episodes of obstructive or CENTRAL SLEEP APNEA and FRAGMENTARY MYOCLONUS.

atonia The absence of muscle activity. Skeletal muscle, even in the resting state, has a degree of muscle activity that maintains the tension in muscles (muscle tone). A reduction in muscle tone causes the muscle to relax and become weak and unable to maintain tension. Atonia is typically seen in a muscle that is removed from its neurological input, such as when a nerve is severed; it is also seen as a characteristic feature of REM SLEEP when all skeletal muscles, except for the inner ear muscles, the eye muscles and the respiratory muscles, have absent tone. In general, muscle tone is highest in wakefulness, reduces as sleep becomes deeper and is typically absent during REM sleep.

autogenic training A behavioral technique used in the treatment of INSOMNIA. A form of self-hypnosis, autogenic training conditions patients to concentrate on sensations of heaviness and warmth in the limbs, thus inducing sleepiness. Although some studies have questioned how effective this technique is for all patients, it seems that at least some are helped by it. (See also BEHAVIORAL TREATMENT OF INSOMNIA, DISORDERS OF INITIATING AND MAINTAINING SLEEP, HYPNOSIS, PSYCHOPHYSIOLOGICAL INSOMNIA.)

automatic behavior Unconscious psychological and physical actions. Such behavior includes repetitive movements typical of some forms of SLEEP-RELATED EPILEPSY. Automatic behavior can also occur with normal activities, such as driving, and is seen in patients with NARCOLEPSY and other forms of severe sleepiness. In automatic behavior, an individual may perform complex normal activities, yet have amnesia for these acts.

awakening A change from non-REM or REM SLEEP to the awake state or WAKEFULNESS. Wakefulness is characterized by fast, low-voltage EEG activity with both alpha waves and beta waves. There is an increase in tonic EMG activity and rapid eye movements, and eye blinks occur. An awakening is always accompanied by a change in the level of consciousness to the alert state. (See also NREM-REM SLEEP CYCLE.)

awakening epilepsies Term referring to epileptic seizures that occur during WAKEFULNESS as compared to epilepsies that occur during sleep. The most common form of awakening epilepsies are generalized epilepsies, such as tonic-clonic epilepsy or petit mal epilepsy. In addition, some forms of juvenile myoclonic epilepsy occur upon awakening.

The awakening epilepsies are contrasted with the sleep epilepsies, which primarily consist of generalized tonic-clonic SEIZURES or complex partial seizures. (See also SLEEP-RELATED EPILEPSY.)

B

background activity See BASELINE.

barbiturates Medications used as hypnotic agents since the turn of the century; about 50 are available commercially. Since the 1960s, barbiturates have largely been replaced by the BENZODIAZEPINES because the latter have less potential for drug addiction and a reduced risk of death from overdose. Yet, despite disadvantages of barbiturates, they are effective hypnotic agents although rarely prescribed now. The most commonly prescribed barbiturates include amyobarbital (Amytal), pentobarbital (Nembutal) and secobarbital (Seconal).

Barbiturates depress the central nervous system and therefore can be very toxic in high doses, producing coma and even death. Clinically they produce a range of effects from mild sedation through sleep induction. Phenobarbital is commonly used as an effective anticonvulsive agent. Short-acting, intravenous barbiturates are used for general anesthesia.

Hypnotic barbiturates have profound effects upon sleep. They decrease SLEEP LATENCY, reduce the number of sleep stage shifts to WAKEFULNESS, and reduce stage one sleep (see SLEEP STAGES). The drug also increases the amount of fast EEG beta activity throughout the sleep recording. SLOW WAVE SLEEP is generally reduced in amount; however, phenobarbital sometimes increases stage four sleep in healthy individuals. The REM SLEEP latency is increased, and there is reduction in the total amount of REM sleep, the number of REM sleep cycles and the density of rapid eye movements during REM sleep.

Tolerance to the beneficial hypnotic effect of the medication generally occurs within two weeks of continuous use. There are variable effects of the rebound in slow wave and REM sleep after termination of barbiturate use.

The development of a cycle of tolerance, abuse and dependence is the main cause for the withdrawal of barbiturates from common prescription use. Barbiturates can also depress respiration and may exacerbate SLEEP-RELATED BREATHING DISORDERS. Another effect of barbiturates is the induction of microsomal enzymes, which degrade or otherwise alter other medications a patient may be taking.

Typical side effects of barbiturates include: the sedative effects, which may impair performance for up to 24 hours after their administration; excitement, with an intoxicated or euphoric feeling; and irritability and temper changes. These effects are paradoxical in that barbiturates can induce excitement rather than sedation; they are a more common problem in the geriatric age group (see ELDERLY AND SLEEP). (See also HYPNOTICS.)

baseline Term describing the usual or normal state of an investigative variable. The baseline state implies that there is a change in amplitude in the variable, typically due to an experimental manipulation. The term is often used for the first night of POLYSOMNOGRAPHY prior to the application of a CONTINUOUS POSITIVE AIRWAY PRESSURE device (CPAP).

basic rest-activity cycle (BRAC) In 1960, NATHANIEL KLEITMAN first suggested that a cycle of activity and rest occurs throughout a 24-hour period. His original suggestion was based upon recognizing a periodicity in the feeding intervals of infants. Kleitman had noticed that there were four cycles of feeding and rest during the day, and five at night. Similar cycles of behavior have been demonstrated in adults for many activities, such as eating, drinking and smoking. The NREM-REM SLEEP CYCLE of approximately 90 minutes in nocturnal sleep and the cycle of alertness as determined by pupillary measures are other examples.

The periodicity of the basic rest-activity cycle may vary among species and appears to be 23 minutes in cats, which correlates with the self-feeding cycle as well as the non-REM-REM sleep cycle. The longer cycle of 72 minutes has been determined in monkeys. The human basic rest-activity cycle is approximately 96 minutes in adults.

This basic rest-activity cycle is believed to be determined by a central nervous system mechanism. Studies in cats have shown that lesions in the basal forebrain of cats will alter the period of the sleep-wake cycle but do not alter the basic rest-activity cycle, suggesting that the underlying basic rest-activity cycle is independent of sleep and wakefulness.

beds There was probably a time in the early Neolithic period when a transition occurred from sleeping on the ground to sleeping in a bed. The change to sleeping in a bedroom occurred around the time of the Sun King of France, Louis XIV, who developed a separate room for sleeping, which was in a very prominent position in his palace. Prior to that time, most people would sleep in a communal room.

The kings and queens of ancient days often had varied types of beds, ranging from flat tables with wooden headrests to cushions on the floor or beds encrusted with gold and jewels. In the Middle Ages, the typical bed consisted of pallets of straw; however, the wealthy developed ornate canopied beds with thick hangings to prevent drafts in otherwise austere castles.

Louis XIV would hold court while lying in his bed, which was placed in a key position in his palace so it was more like a public room. At that time, beds became more elaborate and were often regarded as prized items to be passed down through the family.

Nowadays, beds are used for a variety of activities, including writing, reading, watching television and sexual intimacy, as well as sleeping. Charles Darwin is reported to have written his *Origin of Species* while lying in bed, and Benjamin Franklin is reported to have had four beds in his bedroom so he could move to a fresh bed whenever he felt the need. Lawrence of Arabia is reported to have slept usually in a sleeping bag, and Charles Dickens rearranged the bed so that the head was always pointing to the north.

In recent years, the bed has undergone some modern changes. Mattresses have been improved with the use of inner springs. The more typical single-sized bed has given way to queen- or king-size beds. Water beds have been popular, particularly with young adults, and various forms are available, some with a single water-filled bag and others with numerous tubes of water contained within a padded mattress covering.

The accessories to the bed have also developed, with some beds having built-in electronic equipment so that a person can lie in bed and watch television, or listen to stereophonic music that can be adjusted by remote control.

It is evident that if someone needs to sleep, he or she can sleep on any surface. During wartime, soldiers have slept under the most arduous conditions in trenches, exposed to the weather and the noise of gunfire. In many primitive cultures, the bed consists of a matting placed on the floor of a room inside a dwelling or even on the ground exposed to the environment.

For most westerners, selecting a bed or a pillow is a matter of personal preference. However, certain physical concerns, such as height, should be taken into consideration; very tall or heavyset persons may need larger beds to comfortably accommodate their body size. The firmness or softness of a mattress is also a matter of taste. (See SLEEP SURFACE.)

Whether or not sheets are used on a bed, as well as the type of material (cotton, satin, combination fabrics), is another matter of personal taste, as well as whether both a bottom and top, or just a bottom, sheet are used.

Since persons adapt to their typical bed, a change in a bed may require a period of adjustment. Hence vacationers will complain they failed to get a good night's sleep, even in the most comfortable bed in the finest hotel, simply because the bed is unfamiliar. Similarly, infants changing from a crib to a bed for the first time may require a period of time to adjust to the new bed and mattress.

If someone has difficulties initiating sleep, it may be better to restrict the number of non-sleep-related activities that are associated with the bed. For example, children who have difficulty falling asleep may need to have distracting toys or books removed from their beds, or from the area immediately surrounding the bed.

Finding a comfortable position in bed for sleeping can be influenced by such factors as pregnancy or back problems. During pregnancy, it may be necessary to use pillows under the stomach and between the knees and thighs to enable a woman to sleep on her side, a more comfortable position for some than sleeping on the back. A larger bed may also help the pregnant woman to spread out more as her increasing size makes a smaller bed uncomfortable. Those with back problems might be in less agony if they avoid sleeping on their stomachs and sleep on a firm surface, and those with breathing problems might find their breathing is improved if they sleep on their sides. (See also SLEEP HYGIENE.)

Hales, Diane, *The Complete Book of Sleep*. Reading, Mass.: Addison-Wesley, 1981.

bedtime The time when an individual attempts to fall asleep, *not* the time when an individual gets into bed, which may not be the same. Typically, bedtime is associated with the time that the bedroom light is turned off in anticipation of sleep.

Especially for young children, bedtime rituals are thought to ease the transition from wakefulness to sleep. Activities to help the child wind down from wakefulness to sleep include soft music, such as lullabies, either prerecorded and played on a tape recorder, or sung by a parent, or reading or telling a story. Children or adults may find that taking a bath immediately before bedtime can produce relaxation and assist the ability to fall asleep.

The ideal bedtime is tied to the anticipated wake up time the next morning. Thus, on a weekday bedtime may be earlier than over the weekend. Consistency in the precise bedtime, however, helps to regulate sleep and wakefulness. Too wide a variation in bedtime hours—say, from 11 P.M. for adults on a workday night to 1 or 2 A.M. on weekend nights, or for children from 8 P.M. on a school night to 11 P.M. on a weekend night—may make adjusting to the weekday bedtime hour difficult on Sunday night. The resulting difficulty in falling asleep on Sunday night is often called SUNDAY NIGHT INSOMNIA, and the difficulty awakening on Monday morning is called the MONDAY MORNING BLUES. Too much variation in bedtime or waketime may cause a form of insomnia called INADEQUATE SLEEP HYGIENE, if mild, or IRREGULAR SLEEP-WAKE PATTERN, if severe.

Bedtimes for a young child have to be set by the parent or caretaker, as these children are too young to understand the need to ensure an adequate duration of sleep. If the parent does not establish appropriate bedtimes and waketimes, LIMIT-SETTING SLEEP DISORDER may result.

If a child finds a particular bedtime ritual helpful in getting to sleep, such as clutching a special stuffed animal or a blanket, using a night-light in the room or listening to a particular kind of music, it may be helpful to bring those props along when sleeping away from home for any period of time. But if a particular bedtime ritual becomes a major endeavor and sleep is markedly disturbed without it, then a form of insomnia called SLEEP ONSET ASSOCIATION DISORDER may result.

bed-wetting See SLEEP ENURESIS.

behavioral treatment of insomnia The use of nonpharmacological techniques to improve nighttime sleep. Behavioral treatments can be useful for most patients who have INSOMNIA, even if it is due to a physical or organic cause. However, these treatments are most useful for the psychophysiological forms of insomnia or insomnia related to psychiatric disorders, particularly ANXIETY DISORDERS.

Behavioral treatments include SLEEP HYGIENE, specific sleep behavior programs, RELAXATION EXERCISES to reduce arousal, and techniques to reduce excessive rumination during sleep, including COGNITIVE FOCUSING, SYSTEMIC DESENSITIZATION, PARADOXICAL TECHNIQUES and SLEEP RESTRICTION THERAPY.

There is an increase in the use of behavioral techniques in the management of chronic insomnia as physicians become warier of hypnotic medications. In fact, hypnotic medications are now recommended only for transient use, particularly in patients who have situational or transient insomnia. Behavioral techniques get to the source of the sleep disturbance and prevent the continuation of poor practices that maintain the insomnia. Typically these techniques are utilized along with other treatments, particularly in patients with PSYCHIATRIC DISORDERS who may need specific medications, to treat the psychiatric disorders. (See also AUTOGENIC TRAINING, BIOFEEDBACK.)

Spielman, A.J., Caruso, L.S. and Glovinsky, P.B., "A Behavioral Perspective on Insomnia Treatment," *Psychiatric Clinics of North America* 10 (1987): 541–554.

Belgian Association for the Study of Sleep (BASS) Founded in 1982, the Belgian Association for the Study of Sleep is one of a number of sleep societies that has been founded around the world to promote sleep research and the development of clinical sleep disorders medicine. The first society to be founded outside the United States was the EUROPEAN SLEEP RESEARCH SOCIETY, in 1971. (See also INTERNATIONAL SLEEP SOCIETIES.)

Benadryl See ANTIHISTAMINES.

benign epilepsy with Rolandic spikes (BERS) An unusual form of epilepsy that occurs primarily during non-REM sleep (see SLEEP STAGES). This disorder, which is more common in children, has an onset between four and 13 years of age, and produces clinically-obvious SEIZURES in about 60% of children with the abnormal encephalographic pattern. A typical pattern consists of focal spikes that occur at a rate of five to 10 per minute, which can be present during WAKEFULNESS and REM SLEEP but increase in frequency during non-REM sleep. In non-REM sleep, the manifestations can become generalized, causing the clinical seizures. In addition to the focal spikes, there can be spike activity, with slow waves, that appears like the more typical spike and slow wave pattern characteristic of absence or petit mal epilepsy.

Benign epilepsy with Rolandic spikes may have a hereditary predisposition and usually is a benign form of epilepsy, lasting only about four years. Its course appears to be independent of whether the disorder is treated or not.

The clinical features of the epilepsy include generalized tonic-clonic seizures that occur in about 25% of patients; more commonly, focal seizures involve the face, with twitching on one side and sometimes jerking movements of a limb.

If a treatment is required, phenytion is regarded as the most effective anticonvulsant and is preferred over the use of barbiturates. (See also SLEEP-RELATED EPILEPSY.)

benign neonatal sleep myoclonus An abnormal form of jerking that occurs in newborn infants. This asynchronous jerking (MYOCLONUS) occurs primarily during quiet or SLOW WAVE SLEEP, in clusters of four or five at a time, and recurs approximately once every second throughout sleep. Each myoclonic episode lasts between 40 and 300 milliseconds and causes jerking of the arms or legs, particularly the distal muscle groups. More major movements can cause the whole body to move. Usually the jerks occur asynchronously in a pattern that varies among infants.

This jerking usually lasts for only a few days or, at the most, a few months. It always has a benign course, and its cause is unknown. No treatment is necessary as this disorder always spontaneously resolves. It can affect both male and female infants and usually occurs within the first week of life.

There is no evidence of any underlying biochemical or neurological abnormality.

Benign neonatal sleep myoclonus needs to be differentiated from neonatal epileptic SEIZURES that most commonly occur in association with biochemical or infective causes. Drug withdrawal can also be a cause of similar movements.

Other forms of jerking, such as infantile spasms, commonly occur after the first month of life and therefore can be easily differentiated from benign neonatal sleep myoclonus. Infantile spasms also have a specific electroencephalographic pattern termed hypsarrhythmia, which does not occur in benign neonatal sleep myoclonus.

Other movement disorders that occur during sleep include the benign infantile myoclonus of Lombroso and Fejerman, which usually appears after the third month of life and during wakefulness, not during sleep. PERIODIC LIMB MOVEMENT DISORDER is typically seen in older children and adults; the movements are of longer duration and are not true myoclonic episodes. The FRAGMENTARY MYOCLONUS of non-REM sleep produces a similar twitch-like muscle jerk; however, this disorder persists during non-REM sleep and is not typically associated with observable movements such as is seen in benign neonatal sleep myoclonus.

Coulter, D.L. and Allen, R.J., "Benign Neonatal Sleep Myoclonus," *Archives of Neurology* 39 (1982): 191–192.

benign snoring See PRIMARY SNORING.

benzodiazepine receptors Specific receptors for the benzodiazepine medications appear to exist in different areas of the central nervous system, primarily in the cerebral cortex. These receptors are associated with GAMMA-AMINOBUTYRIC ACID (GABA) receptors, and it appears that the BENZODIAZEPINES modulate GABAergic transmission. It is believed that there may be two types of benzodiazepine receptor, although this is unclear. However, it appears that the interaction between benzodiazepines and GABA is mediated through the benzodiazepine receptors, and that this interaction is important in the induction and maintenance of sleep.

benzodiazepines Benzodiazepines were first introduced in the 1960s, primarily for their anti-anxiety effect. The first agent to be introduced was chlordiazepoxide, which had little hypnotic effect but appeared to be an effective anti-anxiety agent. The benzodiazepines were preferred over the previously-used barbiturate sedative medications because of a decreased tendency to produce fatal central nervous system depression, drug abuse and toxic side effects. The term "benzodiazepine" refers to the group structure, which is composed of a benzene ring fused to a seven-membered diazepine ring. Approximately 25 benzodiazepines that are slight variations of this basic structure are currently in clinical use.

The first primarily hypnotic benzodiazepine, introduced in 1970, was flurazepam. The three major benzodiazepine hypnotic agents currently in use in the United States are the long-acting flurazepam (Dalmane), the intermediate-acting temazepam (Restoril) and the short-acting triazolam (Halcion).

In addition to their hypnotic effect, benzodiazepines are also effective muscle relaxants and anti-epileptic medications and can be used to induce general anesthesia. Other benzodiazepine hypnotics commonly used outside of the United States include flunitrazepam, nitrazepam, brotizolam, midazolam and quazepam.

The benzodiazepine effect on the waking EEG is characterized by a decrease in ALPHA ACTIVITY with an increase in the low-voltage, fast beta activity. The increase in beta activity appears to correlate with the anti-anxiety effects of the benzodiazepines.

In general, the benzodiazepines tend to decrease SLEEP LATENCY and reduce the number of awakenings and the amount of wakefulness that occurs during the major sleep episode. The amount of stage one sleep is usually decreased and the time spent in non-REM stage two sleep is increased. The amount of stage three and four (slow wave) sleep is reduced as is the total amount of REM sleep. REM sleep latency is usually increased and the frequency of the rapid eye movements during REM sleep is reduced.

The effect of benzodiazepines on sleep gradually diminishes over a few nights of consecutive use. If the medication is abruptly stopped after several weeks of chronic use there may be a REBOUND INSOMNIA that typically lasts one or two nights. This effect can be minimized by instituting a gradual withdrawal of medication.

The benzodiazepines appear to have their central nervous system effect by increasing neural inhibition that is mediated by gamma-aminobutyric acid (GABA). The safety of the benzodiazepine hypnotics over the barbiturates may be because of this effect upon the GABA inhibitory neurotransmitters, whereas the barbiturates have their effect by inhibiting excitatory neurotransmitter action.

The benzodiazepines have a slight effect on suppression of respiration and are particularly contraindicated in the treatment of patients with SLEEP-RELATED BREATHING DISORDERS. There are only minor cardiovascular effects of the benzodiazepines, such as reduction of blood pressure and increase in heart rate.

The effectiveness of the benzodiazepine hypnotics depends upon their rapidity of onset of action, which is effected by absorption and passage through the blood brain barrier. Ideally the benzodiazepine hypnotics should be eliminated by the next morning; however, a slow rate of elimination and metabolism of long-acting metabolites may be a disadvantage of some benzodiazepine hypnotics, such as flurazepam. Untoward effects of the benzodiazepines include light-headedness, fatigue, reduced reaction time, motor incoordination, ataxia and impaired mental and psychomotor functions. There can be confusion, dysarthria, retrograde amnesia, dry mouth and a bitter taste. Benzodiazepines may interact with alcohol to produce more severe sedation and this effect of the benzodiazepines may be most prominent in the elderly.

Benzodiazepines have a low incidence of abuse and dependency; however, increasing dosages and the development of a HYPNOTIC-DEPENDENT SLEEP DISORDER can occur.

The benzodiazepines are most commonly used for the treatment of either insomnia related to anxiety or PSYCHOPHYSIOLOGICAL INSOMNIA. The medications are preferably used for transient or short-term insomnia and are best avoided in the management of long-term chronic insomnia. Transient forms of insomnia, such as those due to JET LAG or SHIFT-WORK SLEEP DISORDER, and sleep disturbance associated with acute situational stress or anxiety, for example an ADJUSTMENT SLEEP DISORDER, can also be helped by a short course of a hypnotic benzodiazepine.

Flurazepam

A long-acting benzodiazepine hypnotic agent. The pharmaceutical name is Dalmane. The medication is available in 15 and 30 milligrams, and a typical dose is 15 or 30 milligrams before bedtime. Flurazepam reduces sleep latency, increases total sleep time and reduces intermittent wakefulness. Subjective reports indicate that flurazepam can improve sleep quality, depth and duration. The most pronounced effects of flurazepam can be demonstrated for the first one or two nights, and longer term studies have shown improved sleep for at least four weeks.

Flurazepam has a long-acting metabolite, desalkylflurazepam, which has a half-life of between 40 and 103 hours. The hypnotic effects of flurazepam are partly related to the activity of this metabolite and therefore residual effects are likely; accumulation of the metabolite can occur with continuous ingestion. Accumulation is of particular concern in the elderly in whom excretion of the drug may be slowed. Conversely, the long-acting effect may be useful in some patients, who have a high degree of anxiety, where mild daytime sedation is useful. However, the adverse effects of flurazepam are primarily related to the excessive daytime sedation.

Temazepam

An intermediate-acting benzodiazepine hypnotic medication used primarily for the treatment of insomnia. The majority of patients who take temazepam find that they initially have a good or very good response; however, there is not a consistently beneficial response. This drug is processed in two forms, one with a soft gelatin capsule, which enhances the onset of action and therefore is of most benefit for sleep onset insomnia, and a hard gelatin capsule form, which has a slower rate of absorption and therefore daytime sedative effects can occur. The soft capsule form is currently available only in Europe; the hard capsule form is available in the United States. Temazepam is available in 15 or 30 milligram capsules, and the usual dose is either 15 or 30 milligrams taken before bedtime. Restoril is the brand name for temazepam.

Polysomnographic studies have demonstrated that temazepam produces a reduced sleep latency and increased total sleep time. The number of waking episodes is decreased. The hypnotic effects of temazepam appear to be reduced after several nights of continuous usage; however, benefits have been demonstrated up to at least five weeks.

The most common side effects of temazepam are due to the residual effects of the medication at or soon after the time of awakening in the morning. These effects are the usual sedative effects of the benzodiazepine hypnotics.

Triazolam

A short-acting benzodiazepine hypnotic medication used for the treatment of insomnia. Triazolam, with the brand name of Halcion, is available in tablets of 0.0625, 0.125 and 0.25 milligram. The rapid onset of action is particularly useful for sleep-onset insomniacs, and its short half-life of 2.6 hours is beneficial in preventing daytime sedation. Patient studies have generally shown a benefit on sleep latency and the quality of nighttime sleep; however, early morning awakening may show little improvement with triazolam.

Polysomnographic studies have demonstrated a reduction in sleep latency, an increase in total sleep time, and reduced wake time during the night. Sleep efficiency is increased.

Triazolam can improve alertness during the day following the night of administration, as demonstrated by MULTIPLE SLEEP LATENCY TESTING. However, there are also reports of triazolam increasing anxiety, and retrograde amnesia can occur, but typically with the 0.5 milligram dosage. The recommended dosage for geriatric patients is 0.125 milligram or less per night.

Triazolam has also been shown to be effective in a variety of sleep disorders other than insomnia, such as suppression of the parasomnia activity, SLEEP TERRORS and somnambulism (SLEEPWALKING), for instance. It also appears to be an effective agent for treatment of PERIODIC LIMB MOVEMENT DISORDER, particularly when it is associated with EXCESSIVE SLEEPINESS.

Clonazepam

A long-lasting benzodiazepine commonly used for the treatment of epilepsy. However, clonazepam is also used for the treatment of some sleep disorders, such as periodic limb movement disorder and REM SLEEP BEHAVIOR DISORDER. The brand name of clonazepam is Klonopin.

The main side effects of clonazepam are drowsiness, sleepiness, fatigue and lethargy. Incoordination, ataxia, dizziness and behavioral disturbances have also been described.

Clonazepam is available in 0.5, 1 and 2 milligram tablets. The usual starting dose is 0.5 milligram and the usual maintenance dose is 1 milligram.

Alprazolam

A benzodiazepine that has been used for the treatment of anxiety and is effective in suppressing panic attacks. The trade name for alprazolam is Xanax.

Diazepam

A benzodiazepine that is utilized as a sedative agent. It has little hypnotic properties, although it has been demonstrated to be effective in the treatment of insomnia due to anxiety disorders. Diazepam has a long half-life, and in the elderly it may accumulate and produce daytime effects, such as lethargy and sleepiness. Diazepam is used primarily for sleep disturbances associated with anxiety disorders and is rarely used today for its hypnotic properties. The pharmaceutical name for diazepam is Valium.

Nitrazepam

A benzodiazepine hypnotic medication used for the treatment of INSOMNIA. It is not available in the United States but is commonly used in Europe. The brand name of nitrazepam is Mogodon.

Nitrazepam has been shown to increase total sleep time and reduce the number of nocturnal awakenings. There is also a reduction in body movement during sleep. The sleep stages are altered by nitrazepam, with an increase in SPINDLE sleep and spindle rate, and electroencephalographic beta activity. Total REM sleep is initially decreased by nitrazepam with an increase in the REM sleep latency and a reduction in REM density. There is also an increase in electroencephalographic beta activity during REM sleep.

Nicholson, A.N., "Hypnotics: Clinical Pharmacology and Therapeutics," Kryger, M.H., Roth, T. and Dement, W.C., eds., *The Principles and Practice of Sleep Disorders Medicine.* Philadelphia: Saunders, 1989. pp. 219–227.

bereavement It is not unusual for the death of a loved one to be the precipitating cause of SHORT-

TERM INSOMNIA. If a spouse with whom one has shared a bed or a bedroom has died, a person may find it hard to fall asleep alone. This type of short-term insomnia, an ADJUSTMENT SLEEP DISORDER, usually resolves itself within a few weeks. Continued insomnia may produce conditioned associations and lead to a PSYCHOPHYSIOLOGICAL INSOMNIA. Bereavement is one indication for the use of short-term HYPNOTICS to prevent such a conditioned insomnia from developing. The bereavement may be helped by consulting a bereavement counseling center or a therapist.

Berger, Hans The first person to measure and record brain electrical activity, Hans Berger (1873–1941) reported the first human ELECTROENCEPHALOGRAM in 1929. Berger began to study electrical activity in animals in 1910 at a hospital in Germany. In 1924, he first studied electrical activity in the brains of humans, particularly of those who had skull defects where the needles could be placed directly on the surface of the brain. His first report of alpha waves, recorded with the patient's eyes closed, was presented in 1929. The presence of alpha waves did not find general recognition until 1933, when Berger's work was publicized by the physiologist Lord Adrian, who called the ALPHA RHYTHM the Berger rhythm.

Berger's discovery led to the subsequent recognition of differences in the electroencephalogram during wakefulness and sleep, and this forms the basis of the electroencephalographic determination of SLEEP STAGES.

Berger rhythm See ALPHA RHYTHM.

BERS See BENIGN EPILEPSY WITH ROLANDIC SPIKES.

beta rhythm Electroencephalographic frequency of 13 to 35 hertz that is typically seen during alert wakefulness. This activity may be associated with the ingestion of a variety of different medications, such as BARBITURATES and BENZODIAZEPINES. Beta activity, when seen in association with high ELECTROMYOGRAM (EMG) activity and a low voltage mixed frequency ELECTROENCEPHALOGRAM (EEG), is indicative of wakefulness. With relaxed wakefulness, the EEG frequency slows, and if the eyes are closed, alpha activity of 13 hertz or lower is typically seen. (See also ALPHA RHYTHM.)

Billiard, Michel Dr. Michel Billiard is a professor of neurology in the School of Medicine of Montpellier University (France) as well as director of the Sleep Disorders Center of Gui De Chauliac Medical Center, Montpellier. He was secretary of the European Sleep Research Society (1978–1984).

Dr. Billiard's main sleep research contributions are in the areas of narcolepsy, periodic hypersomnia and epilepsy and sleep.

Billiard, M., Quera Salva, M., DeKoninck, J., Besset, A., Touchon, J. and Cadilhac, J., "Daytime Sleep Characteristics and Their Relationships with Night Sleep in the Narcoleptic Patient," *Sleep* 9 (1986): 167–174.

biofeedback Biofeedback technique can assist in recognizing when muscle tension is high, which may reflect impaired ability to fall asleep. Biofeedback involves sensors that detect changes in muscle activity and convey this information by means of different sounds. The individual can use the sounds to assist in relaxing the muscles as a change in the muscle tension is detected by the alteration in the sound produced by the muscles. After biofeedback training, a person can relax the muscles without the need for feedback sound information from the sensors. The relaxation technique can then be performed in bed, prior to SLEEP ONSET to assist sleep. (See also SLEEP EXERCISES, STRESS.)

biological clocks The periodic oscillation that occurs in a wide variety of biological systems; the frequency of the oscillations serves an internal timing system. Virtually all plants and animals have an internal timing system, or biological clock, and there may be several of these processes that control different aspects of the physiology of the biological systems. The biological clocks measure time and synchronize an organism's internal processes with daily environmental events. The site of the major biological clock in humans is believed to be the SUPRACHIASMATIC NUCLEUS. (See also CIRCADIAN RHYTHMS; CHRONOBIOLOGY.)

biorhythm A recurrent pattern of change in a physiological variable, such as a CIRCADIAN RHYTHM. However, the term *biorhythm* more commonly has become associated with the astrological prediction of life events and is not scientifically based. Biorhythm is rarely used in CHRONOBIOLOGY; the term *biological rhythm* is preferred.

Block, A. Jay Born in Baltimore, Maryland, Dr. Block (1938–) received his B.A. in 1958 and his M.D. in 1962 from Johns Hopkins University. He is currently professor of medicine and anesthesiology and chief, Division of Pulmonary Medicine, University of Florida College of Medicine.

Dr. Block's research activities have been in the areas of respiratory failure and disease, including the relationship of these disorders to sleep and obesity. From 1987 to 1988, Dr. Block was president of the American College of Chest Physicians.

Block, A.J., "Disorders of Breathing Control During Sleep," *Respiratory Care* 24 (1979): 715–721.

Block, A.J., Wynne, J.W. and Boysen, P.G., "Sleep-disordered Breathing and Nocturnal Oxygen Desaturation in Postmenopausal Women," *American Journal of Medicine* 69 (1980): 75–79.

body clock Another term for BIOLOGICAL CLOCKS and CIRCADIAN RHYTHMS, it is related to CHRONOBIOLOGY, the scientific study of biological rhythms. The everyday cycle of sleep and wakefulness is systematized by the biological or body clock. Practically all plants and animals have an internal timing system, or biological clock. The plant experiment conducted by JEAN-JACQUES D'ORTOUS DE MAIRAN in 1729 was significant because it demonstrated the presence of biological rhythms even when the ENVIRONMENTAL TIME CUES of light and dark were missing.

body movements Those movements detected during polysomnographic recording that indicate a specific physiological event, as indicated by an increase in amplitude of the ELECTROMYOGRAM that lasts one second or longer. Body movements are associated with muscle artifact that can be seen obscuring the ELECTROENCEPHALOGRAM or ELECTRO-OCULOGRAM recording. Brief body movements are a normal accompaniment of healthy sleep but are increased in number in disorders that cause lighter sleep, such as INSOMNIA. (See also MOVEMENT AROUSAL, MOVEMENT TIME.)

bodyrocking One of three disorders—bodyrocking, HEADBANGING and HEAD ROLLING—that involve repetitive movement of the head and occasionally of the whole body. These disorders are now known under the collective name rhythmic movement disorder.

Bodyrocking may occur during times of rest, drowsiness or sleep, as well as during full wakefulness. It is usually performed on the hands and knees with the whole body rocking in an anterior/posterior direction, with the head being pushed into the pillow.

The disorder most commonly occurs in children below the age of four years, with the highest incidence at six months of age. Treatment is usually unnecessary when the condition occurs in infancy as it typically disappears within 18 months. Bodyrocking can persist into older childhood, adolescence and, rarely, adulthood. Behavioral or pharmacological treatment may then be required. (See also INFANT SLEEP DISORDERS.)

body temperature See TEMPERATURE.

brachialgia parasthetica nocturna See CARPAL TUNNEL SYNDROME.

brain-wave rhythms A lay term that is often used to describe electroencephalographic patterns. *EEG wave* is the preferred term. (See also ELECTROENCEPHALOGRAM.)

British Sleep Research Society (BSRS) Founded in 1989, the British Sleep Research Society is the most recent of the numerous international sleep associations founded to aid the growth of clinical sleep disorders medicine. (See also ASSOCIATION OF PROFESSIONAL SLEEP SOCIETIES and EUROPEAN SLEEP RESEARCH SOCIETY.)

bromocriptine A medication that is used to suppress the production of GROWTH HORMONE in the treatment of ACROMEGALY, a disorder characterized by an enlargement of the skeletal and soft tissues of the body. Individuals with acromegaly have an increased incidence of SLEEP-RELATED BREATHING DISORDERS, particularly OBSTRUCTIVE SLEEP APNEA SYNDROME.

Broughton, Roger J. Dr. Broughton (1936–) graduated in medicine at Queen's University in Kingston, Ontario, Canada, in 1960. From 1962 to 1964, he trained in clinical neurophysiology, epileptology and sleep disorders with Henri Gastaut in Marseilles, France. Broughton received his Ph.D. in neurology and neurosurgery at McGill University in 1967. Since 1968, he has been in the Department of Medicine at the University of Ottawa where he is professor of medicine with cross appointments in the Departments of Pharmacology and Experimental Psychology. From 1972 to 1975, he was president of the ASSOCIATION FOR THE PSYCHOPHYSIOLOGICAL STUDY OF SLEEP. Founder and president of the Canadian Sleep Society (1986–88), Dr. Broughton has written or edited five books and over 200 articles on parasomnias, hypersomnias, vigilance, chronobiology and epilepsy. For lifetime achievement in the field, he received the 1997 William C. Dement Academic Achievement Award of the American Sleep Disorders Association (now the AMERICAN ACADEMY OF SLEEP MEDICINE).

Broughton, Roger, "Sleep Disorders: Disorders of Arousal?" *Science* 159 (1968): 1070–1078.

Dinges, D.F. and Broughton, R.J., eds., *Sleep and Alertness: Chronobiological, Behavioral, and Medical Aspects of Napping*. New York: Raven Press, 1989.

bruxism A stereotyped movement disorder characterized by grinding or clenching of teeth that can occur during sleep or wakefulness. When bruxism occurs predominantly during sleep, it is termed SLEEP BRUXISM. Bruxism can be associated with discomfort of the jaw and may produce abnormal destruction of the cusps of the teeth.

C

caffeine Probably one of the first medications used for the treatment of EXCESSIVE SLEEPINESS. Caffeine is used to increase the level of alertness and is taken in the form of drinks, most commonly tea, coffee or cola. A typical cup of coffee contains about 100 milligrams caffeine, a bottle of cola drink about 50 milligrams. Also, OVER-THE-COUNTER MEDICATIONS containing caffeine are available (Vivarin, 200 milligrams caffeine; No Doz, 100 milligrams caffeine).

Caffeine can disturb the quality of nighttime sleep if ingested prior to bedtime. Sleep onset and sleep maintenance difficulties are not uncommon due to the effects of caffeine; even some individuals who believe that they sleep well after a cup of coffee have been shown to have increased sleep disturbance with frequent awakenings and reduced total sleep time.

Caffeine is not recommended for the treatment of daytime tiredness or sleepiness. It has a general stimulant effect that can produce cardiac stimulation with palpitations and hypertension as well as increased nervousness, irritability and tremulousness. Other more effective STIMULANT MEDICATIONS, such as methylphenidate, pemoline or amphetamines, are available for the treatment of sleepiness in patients who have disorders of excessive sleepiness.

Withdrawal of caffeine may produce an increased feeling of tiredness and lethargy during the first few days, which may lead to resumption of the caffeine intake. Therefore, excessive caffeine intake may be the cause of symptoms of excessive sleepiness.

Curatolo, P.W. and Robertson, D., "The Health Consequences of Caffeine," *Annals of Internal Medicine* 98 (1983): 641–653.

Canadian Sleep Society Founded in 1986, the sleep society is one of several sleep societies around the world founded to promote sleep research and clinical sleep disorders medicine. (See also ASSOCIATION OF PROFESSIONAL SLEEP SOCIETIES, ASSOCIATION FOR THE PSYCHOPHYSIOLOGICAL STUDY OF SLEEP, INTERNATIONAL SLEEP SOCIETIES.)

canthus The corner of the eye. Typically, the electrodes associated with measuring eye movement are placed just lateral to the outer canthus of each eye. When electrodes are placed at each outer canthus, one electrode is placed slightly above the outer canthus, and the other electrode slightly below the outer canthus, in order to most accurately document eye movement activity. (See also ELECTROOCULOGRAM.)

carbamazepine Trade name Tegretol; chemically related to the tricyclic antidepressants. It was first employed as an antiepileptic agent but has had a variety of uses since that time. It is still a major drug for the treatment of epilepsy, particularly partial complex and generalized tonic-clonic epilepsy. Carbamazepine is also used for the treatment of some sleep disorders.

Its primary toxicity is hematological, with the potential for producing aplastic anemia and agranulocytosis. Initial reports of the common occurrence of these hematological effects have largely been displaced and such adverse reactions are now considered to be rare. Carbamazepine has been used for the treatment of pain disorders and is occasionally used for the management of RESTLESS LEGS SYNDROME. It is also used as a treatment of NOCTURNAL PAROXYSMAL DYSTONIA, which is not thought to have an epileptic basis even though it is responsive to this anticonvulsive medication.

Carbamazepine is available in 100 milligram and 200 milligram tablets, as well as a 100 milligram/5 milliliter suspension. The usual adult dose is 600 milligrams per day.

carbon dioxide Gas produced as a result of body metabolism. This metabolic product is eliminated from the body through the lungs during a process of exchange with oxygen from the atmosphere. Alterations of ventilation can cause a retention of carbon dioxide in the body and a reduction of blood oxygen.

Carbon dioxide and oxygen are the two most important blood gases in the regulation of respiration. The SLEEP-RELATED BREATHING DISORDERS commonly will affect lung ventilation, thereby producing an increased carbon dioxide level (HYPERCAPNIA) and a lowering of oxygen (HYPOXEMIA). Some patients with OBSTRUCTIVE SLEEP APNEA SYNDROME may have an increased level of carbon dioxide detectable during wakefulness, which is in part due to a resetting of the regulation of ventilation. Most patients with obstructive sleep apnea syndrome have only a transient elevation of carbon dioxide in association with the apneic episodes.

Increased levels of carbon dioxide produce a body acidosis that may be irritating to the heart, producing cardiac ARRHYTHMIAS. An elevated carbon dioxide level also stimulates ventilation through its chemoreceptors, thereby causing a lowering of the level by means of a feedback mechanism.

cardiovascular symptoms, sleep-related See SLEEP-RELATED CARDIOVASCULAR SYMPTOMS.

carpal tunnel syndrome Disorder, also known as acroparesthesia, characterized by compression of the median nerve at the wrist, which typically causes pain and discomfort in the hands upon awakening. The discomfort in the hands is exacerbated by the lack of movement of the hands during sleep, allowing fluid to accumulate in the sheaves of the tendons in the carpal tunnel. Typically, individuals with carpal tunnel syndrome will shake or rub their hands together in order to restore normal sensation, which occurs within a few minutes of awakening. Pressure in the carpal tunnel presses on the median nerve at the wrist. Eventually sensation is lost in the median nerve distribution of the hand, and weakness and atrophy of the muscles occur. The hand often feels swollen, stiff, clumsy and numb, even throughout the day. The disorder is more commonly seen in people who are overweight and those who have hypothyroidism. In mild cases, weight loss or intermittent steroid injections into the tendon sheaves in the carpal tunnel can relieve the symptoms. However, the most effective treatment is surgical decompression of the carpal tunnel. The lining of the fluid-filled sac around the tendons becomes inflamed, swollen and thickened and is surgically removed.

Carskadon, Mary A. First woman president of the North American Sleep Research Society (SRS) and cofounder of the Northeastern Sleep Society (NESS), Dr. Carskadon (1947–) is director of chronobiology and sleep research at E.P. Bradley Hospital in Providence and an associate professor of psychiatry and human behavior at Brown University School of Medicine.

Dr. Carskadon obtained her Ph.D. with distinction in neuro- and biobehavioral sciences from Stanford University in 1979. Her dissertation topic was "Determinants of Daytime Sleepiness: Adolescent Development, Extended and Restricted Nocturnal Sleep." A major focus of Dr. Carskadon's subsequent research has been the development and application of a standardized measure of daytime sleep tendency, the MULTIPLE SLEEP LATENCY TEST. Her primary areas of interest continue to be patterns of daytime sleepiness and adolescent sleep behavior, as well as the exploration of olfactory sensitivity during sleep. Dr. Carskadon is a Fellow of the AMERICAN ACADEMY OF SLEEP MEDICINE (formerly the American Sleep Disorders Association), which honored her with the NATHANIEL KLEITMAN DISTINGUISHED SERVICE AWARD in 1991.

Carskadon, M.A. and Dement, W.C., "Daytime Sleepiness: Quantification of a Behavioral State," *Neuroscience & Biobehavioral Reviews* 11 (1987): 307–317.

Carskadon, M.A., Harvey, K., Duke, P., Anders, T.F., Litt, I.F. and Dement, W.C., "Pubertal Changes in Daytime Sleepiness," *Sleep* 2 (1980): 453–460.

Carskadon, M.A., Labyak, S.E., Acebo, C., and Seifer, R., "Intrinsic Circadian Period of Adolescent Humans Measured in Conditions of Forced Desynchrony," *Neuroscience Letters* 260 (1999): 129–132.

Carskadon, M.A., Wolfson, A.R., Acebo, C., Tzischinsky, O., and Seifer, R., "Adolescent Sleep Patterns, Circadian Timing, and Sleepiness at a Transition to Early School Days," *Sleep* 21 (1998): 871–881.

catalepsy Synonymous with catatonia. Catalepsy refers to a rigidity of the limbs so that when they are placed in a particular position, that position is maintained for a long period of time. This is most commonly associated with hysteria or schizophrenia. Catalepsy is sometimes confused with CATAPLEXY, which refers to the sudden reduction in muscle tone associated with NARCOLEPSY. However, catalepsy and cataplexy are distinctive from each other. (See also PSYCHIATRIC DISORDERS.)

cataplexy A sudden loss of muscle power in response to an emotional stimulus. Cataplexy is typically seen in persons suffering from NARCOLEPSY, which is characterized by EXCESSIVE SLEEPINESS during the day. Cataplexy will usually cause a reduction in muscle power, leading either to complete collapse or, more typically, a drooping of the head, weakness of the facial muscles, weakness of the arms or sagging at the knees. Cataplexy is most often induced by laughter, but anger, surprise, startle, pride, elation or sadness can also induce episodes.

Cataplexy is an ATONIA (loss of muscle tone) that is normal of REM sleep. However, cataplexy is produced by an emotional change and not due to sleepiness. If episodes of cataplexy are long in duration, typical REM sleep occurs, with the usual change of the EEG activity and associated rapid eye movements.

Individuals who have pronounced episodes of cataplexy may suffer injuries due to a sudden collapse to the ground. Episodes of cataplexy usually last a few seconds. If the emotional stimulus continues, a state of continuous cataplexy can occur, termed STATUS CATAPLECTICUS. Cataplexy can be effectively treated by the use of tricyclic ANTIDEPRESSANTS, such as imipramine or protriptyline or the SEROTONIN reuptake inhibitors such as fluoxetine.

catatonia See CATALEPSY.

central alveolar hypoventilation syndrome (CAHS) A breathing disorder that results in arterial oxygen desaturation during sleep. CAHS occurs in persons with normal mechanical properties of the lungs, such as intact ribs, muscles, and lung fields. During sleep in healthy individuals there is a normal slight reduction in TIDAL VOLUME (the amount of air usually taken into the lungs during a normal breath at rest); however, in patients with CAHS the tidal volume greatly decreases. The reduction in tidal volume leads to an increase in the carbon dioxide level in the blood as well as reduced blood oxygen saturation. This change in the arterial blood gases (carbon dioxide and oxygen) can produce arousals that increase respiratory drive. The arousals disturb sleep quality and therefore sleep may be characterized by a complaint of insomnia. If the arousals and awakenings are frequent enough, excessive sleepiness may develop. CAHS is due to an abnormality of the central nervous system control of lung ventilation.

Other features of sleep-related hypoventilation include morning headaches caused by the change in blood gases during sleep. The sleep-related breathing disturbance is typically exacerbated during REM SLEEP when ventilation is entirely dependent upon diaphragmatic function. Cardiac ARRHYTHMIAS commonly occur, particularly slowing of the cardiac rhythm. There may be tachycardia at the time of the awakening, leading to premature ventricular contractions. Typically the episodes of sleep-related hypoventilation are long, sometimes several minutes or several hours in duration. The long episodes of low oxygen saturation are liable to induce the development of pulmonary hypertension and heart failure, which is more commonly seen in this disorder than in the OBSTRUCTIVE SLEEP APNEA SYNDROME or CENTRAL SLEEP APNEA SYNDROME.

The respiratory disturbance in central alveolar hypoventilation syndrome is exacerbated by obesity, which impairs diaphragmatic function.

This disorder also occurs in infants and is known by the name "congenital central alveolar hypoventilation syndrome." These children are also liable to develop pulmonary hypertension and right-sided heart failure, as well as brain damage due to the low oxygen saturation. Central nervous system insults at birth can contribute to the development of acquired central alveolar hypoventilation syndrome, such as infection, brain stem trauma, hemorrhage or the presence of brain tumors.

Patients with central alveolar hypoventilation syndrome may also have central or obstructive sleep apneas; however, these are not the primary cause of the clinical features. The disorder in infants and children may improve as the respiratory system matures; however, some children require artificial ventilation.

The incidence of this disorder is not known but it appears to be quite rare. There is some evidence to suggest that it is more common in males.

Studies of ventilation during wakefulness have demonstrated a nonresponsiveness to elevated carbon dioxide levels or hypoxia. The idiopathic form of central alveolar hypoventilation syndrome is believed to be due to a defect of the medullary chemoreceptors controlling ventilation.

The nature of this disorder can best be demonstrated by means of POLYSOMNOGRAPHY. Episodes of reduced tidal volume lasting several minutes in duration are commonly associated with sustained oxygen desaturation or elevation of carbon dioxide levels. The disorder is exacerbated during REM sleep; however, in infants it may be at its worst during slow wave sleep. Frequent awakenings and arousals may be associated with the oxygen desaturation, and multiple sleep latency testing may demonstrate excessive sleepiness.

Patients with this disorder require investigative testing of respiratory and central nervous system function. Brain CT scanning, MRI scanning, nerve conduction testing, electromyography, muscle biopsy, pulmonary function tests and cardiac function tests may be required. Blood tests may demonstrate an elevated hemocrit and hemoglobin level reflecting POLYCYTHEMIA as a result of the severe hypoxemia.

Central alveolar hypoventilation syndrome is treated with RESPIRATORY STIMULANTS, for instance, doxapram or almitrine in children and medroxyprogesterone, acetazolamide or protriptyline in adults. Many patients require the use of assisted ventilation either by means of CONTINUOUS POSITIVE AIRWAY PRESSURE, a negative pressure ventilator such as a cuirass ventilator or, if the disorder is severe enough, a positive pressure ventilator applied through either a tracheostomy or a nasal mask. Weight reduction is essential for any overweight patient who has central alveolar hypoventilation syndrome.

Oren, J., Kelly, D.H. and Shannon, D.C., "Long-term Follow-up of Children with Congenital Hypoventilation Syndrome," *Pediatrics* 80 (1987): 375–380.

Rochester, D.F. and Enson, Y., "Current Concepts in the Pathogenesis of the Obesity-Hypoventilation Syndrome," *American Journal of Medicine* 57 (1974): 402–420.

central sleep apnea syndrome Disorder marked by a cessation of ventilation during sleep, usually associated with oxygen desaturation with an absence of airflow that lasts 10 seconds or more in adults, 20 seconds or more in infants.

This syndrome is typically associated with the complaint of INSOMNIA, particularly in older adults, or a complaint of EXCESSIVE SLEEPINESS during the day. Typically, patients will awaken several times at night, often with the sensation of gasping or choking during sleep. Not uncommonly, episodes of apnea will be asymptomatic, and if the episodes are frequent enough to cause disruption of much of the sleep episode, then daytime sleepiness will result. In children, central apneas are usually accompanied by a change in their facial color, such as cyanosis or pallor, and there may also be marked changes of the muscle tone with generalized body limpness.

Central sleep apnea syndrome is most commonly seen in patients with neurological disorders that affect the control of respiration. Spinal cord lesions or lesions of the brain stem commonly will produce central sleep apnea. Ventilation can be normal during wakefulness; however, complete cessation of breathing can occur during sleep and the patient may be able to breathe only during arousals or wakefulness. This inability to breathe during sleep has been called ONDINE'S CURSE and, if left untreated, may have a fatal outcome.

If the brain stem and lower neurological control of respiration is intact, patients may have central apneas that occur in conjunction with CHEYNE-

STOKES RESPIRATION, which is characterized by a crescendo, decrescendo respiratory pattern. Central apneas usually occur during non-REM sleep, and regular rhythmical ventilation occurs during REM sleep. Disorders affecting the cerebral hemispheres, such as cerebrovascular disease or cardiovascular disorders that produce an increased circulation time, are typically associated with the Cheyne-Stokes pattern of ventilation. Such patients may have complaints of insomnia due to the arousals that are associated with the crescendo ventilatory pattern.

Central apnea is apt to occur in infants who are prematurely born, or for unexplained reasons in the neonatal period. Such central sleep apnea generally subsides spontaneously in the first six months of age; however, there is an increased risk for SUDDEN INFANT DEATH SYNDROME in infants who suffer central sleep apnea syndrome.

The prevalence of central sleep apnea syndrome in the general population is unknown; however, certain patient groups have a higher predisposition, such as those with neuromuscular disorders, and there is also an increased prevalence in the elderly.

The presence of central sleep apnea syndrome is usually determined by all-night POLYSOMNOGRAPHY, and typically most apneic events last from 10 to 30 seconds. However, episodes as long as several minutes in duration can sometimes be seen. Associated with the apneic episodes is a reduction of the oxygen saturation value and an increase in CARBON DIOXIDE levels. There may be cardiac ARRHYTHMIAS that are characterized by bradycardia during the apneic episodes. Bradycardia is a particular feature of central apnea in infants.

A MULTIPLE SLEEP LATENCY TEST may demonstrate excessive daytime sleepiness if the central apneas are frequent enough to cause severe sleep disruption.

Obesity will exacerbate central sleep apnea syndrome by impairing the ventilation-perfusion because of underperfused basal portions of the lung. Occasionally patients with severe central sleep apnea syndrome will have abnormal daytime blood gases that are improved by treatment of the SLEEP-RELATED BREATHING DISORDER. As a result of the oxygen desaturation during sleep, pulmonary hypertension and right-sided heart failure may develop, which further impairs circulation time, thereby exacerbating the apnea.

Patients with central sleep apnea syndrome need to be differentiated from those with other sleep-related disorders, such as OBSTRUCTIVE SLEEP APNEA SYNDROME. In some patients, it may be necessary to insert an intraesophageal balloon in order to measure pressure changes so that obstructive apneic events can be differentiated from central apneas, because standard polysomnography may not clearly differentiate the two disorders.

Other causes of insomnia must be distinguished from insomnia due to the central sleep apnea syndrome, particularly in elderly patients. As patients with NARCOLEPSY have an increased incidence of central sleep apnea, consideration must be given to this diagnosis in patients presenting with the complaint of excessive sleepiness.

Treatment of central sleep apnea syndrome is primarily by pharmacological or mechanical means. Recent reports have indicated that some patients with central sleep apnea syndrome may respond favorably to the nasal CONTINUOUS POSITIVE AIRWAY PRESSURE (CPAP) device that typically is used for patients with obstructive sleep apnea syndrome. As CPAP is a relatively easily applied treatment, it is worthwhile attempting treatment with this device before trying other treatment modalities.

Pharmacological treatments include the use of RESPIRATORY STIMULANTS such as medroxyprogesterone or acetazolamide. These drugs may be partially effective but rarely will totally eliminate moderate to severe central sleep apnea syndrome. The tricyclic ANTIDEPRESSANT medication protriptyline may be helpful in some patients, particularly those who have mainly ventilatory impairment during REM sleep.

Assisted ventilation devices—such as a negative pressure ventilator, the cuirass—are usually required for patients who have severe central sleep apnea syndrome. This ventilator may induce obstructive sleep apnea episodes in some patients and therefore should be used with caution. Some patients may require the use of a positive pressure ventilator applied either through a TRACHEOSTOMY or a nasal mask.

Treatment of any underlying exacerbating disorders should also be encouraged. For example, the treatment of cardiac failure may greatly improve central sleep apnea syndrome that is due to neurological disorders. Weight reduction is also an essential part of management for any obese patient who has a sleep-related breathing disorder.

Guilleminault, C. and Kowall, J., "Central Sleep Apnea in Adults," in Thorpy, Michael J. (ed.), *Handbook of Sleep Disorders*. New York: Marcel Dekker, 1990.

Thalfofer, S., et al, "Central Sleep Apnea," *Respiration* 64, no. 1 (1997): 2–9.

cephalometric radiograph An X ray of the head performed in a standardized manner so that comparative skeletal measurements can be made. The patient is usually placed in a sitting position with the head in a natural position, the teeth together, the lips relaxed and the X-ray film placed next to the left side of the face, with the X-ray beam exactly five feet from the film. These X rays are used for analysis of cranial and mandibular changes, for the assessment of skeletal abnormalities and for other medical and dental evaluations.

Cephalometric radiographs are also performed in sleep medicine, primarily for determining skeletal and soft tissue features in patients who have the OBSTRUCTIVE SLEEP APNEA SYNDROME. Specific abnormalities that have been seen in obstructive sleep apnea syndrome patients include an increased mandibular plane to hyoid bone distance (MP-H); also, the posterior airway space (PAS) is often narrowed. The position of the maxillary bone and mandible can be determined by two angles (the SNA and SNB angles), which, if less than 80 degrees, suggest a maxillary or mandibular deficiency. Such deficiencies are commonly seen in patients with obstructive sleep apnea syndrome who are not obese.

Many SLEEP DISORDER CENTERS use cephalometric radiographs in the routine evaluations of patients with obstructive sleep apnea syndrome. This information is often used to determine whether corrective surgical treatment, such as UVULOPALATOPHARYNGOPLASTY or MANDIBULAR ADVANCEMENT SURGERY, is indicated.

Riley, R., Guilleminault, C., Heron, J. and Powell, N., "Cephalometric and Flow-Volume Loops in Obstructive Sleep Apnea Patients," *Sleep* 6 (1983): 303–311.

cerebral degenerative disorders Slowly progressive disorders of the central nervous system that are often associated with abnormal movements and behaviors. These disorders include Huntington's disease, the dystonias, olivopontocerebellar degeneration, hereditary ataxias, PARKINSONISM, dementias and Rett's syndrome. Sleep disturbances—characterized both by difficulty in maintaining sleep and by EXCESSIVE SLEEPINESS—are typical of cerebral degenerative disorders. There may be concurrent abnormal movement activity that occurs during sleep as well as CIRCADIAN RHYTHM SLEEP DISORDERS.

The sleep disturbance can be severe and is often associated with increasing severity of the underlying disorder. As some of these disorders, such as torsion dystonia, occur in childhood, the sleep disturbance can be present from an early age. Typically the movement disorders are present only in light, non-REM sleep and are suppressed by the deeper stages of sleep. In the early stages of some cerebral degenerative disorders, abnormal movements may be difficult to differentiate from movements due to hysteria. However, the occurrence of abnormal movements during the lighter stages of sleep is often a diagnostic feature of the movement disorders because voluntary motor activity usually decreases with the onset of sleep.

Other sleep disorders that are characterized by abnormal movements are frequently present in patients with cerebral degenerative disorders, such as FRAGMENTARY MYOCLONUS, PERIODIC LEG MOVEMENTS, and increased muscle activity during REM sleep, which is seen in the REM SLEEP BEHAVIOR DISORDER. There may also be abnormalities of the upper airway muscles leading to sleep-related breathing disorders, such as the OBSTRUCTIVE SLEEP APNEA SYNDROME.

Typically, POLYSOMNOGRAPHY will demonstrate the abnormal movement activity, reduced amounts of slow wave and REM sleep, and abnormal eye movements, particularly in those degenerative disorders that effect eye movements. In addition, there may be reduced SLEEP SPINDLE activity, which is commonly seen in patients with Rett syndrome, or there may be increased sleep spindle activity as has been reported in the dystonias. The spinocerebellar degenerations are often associated with central or obstructive sleep apnea syndrome. Rett syndrome may demonstrate an electroencephalographic pattern that is similar to the changes seen in some forms of epilepsy.

The cerebral degenerative disorders are diagnosed by investigations, such as brain imaging or an ELECTROENCEPHALOGRAM.

The cerebral degenerative disorders need to be differentiated from PSYCHIATRIC DISORDERS or the effects of central nervous system depressant medications. The abnormal limb activity during sleep has to be distinguished from other sleep disorders characterized by limb movement, such as the periodic limb movement disorder or REM sleep behavior disorder.

The treatment of the sleep disorder depends on the underlying cause of the movement disorder, but very often the sleep disturbance is pervasive and therefore SLEEP HYGIENE measures, plus the use of NEUROLEPTICS, are necessary in order to produce a state of restfulness at night.

Chase, Michael H., Ph.D. Has a B.A. in zoology and sociology from the University of California at Berkeley and a Ph.D. in physiology from the University of California at Los Angeles. Currently a professor in the Department of Physiology of the School of Medicine of the University of California in Los Angeles, Dr. Chase (1937–) has conducted extensive sleep research.

Dr. Chase's term as president of the World Federation of Sleep Research Societies was from 1988 to 1992. His term as president of the Sleep Research Society ended in 1990. Dr. Chase was active in the Association of Professional Sleep Societies and, from 1987 to 1990, served as a member of the Board of Directors and on the Finance and Governmental Affairs Committees. He is editor of *SLEEP RESEARCH ONLINE*.

Chase, Michael H. and Morales, F.R., "The Control of Motoneurons During Sleep," Kryger, M.H., Roth, Thomas and Dement, William C., eds, *The Principles and Practices of Sleep Disorders Medicine.* Philadelphia: W.B. Saunders, 1989. pp. 74–85.

Chase, Michael H., Soja, P.J. and Morales, F.R., "Evidence that Glycine Mediates the Postsynaptic Potentials that Inhibit Lumbar Motoneurons During the Atonia of Active Sleep," *Journal of Neuroscience* 9 (1989): 743–751.

Cheyne-Stokes respiration A pattern of breathing described by John Cheyne and William Stokes in 1818 that is characterized by a regular crescendo and decrescendo fluctuation in respiratory rate and volume. This breathing pattern can occur during wakefulness, but it is most commonly is seen in drowsiness and can persist into non-REM sleep (see SLEEP STAGES). Cheyne-Stokes breathing usually does not occur during REM SLEEP.

Cheyne-Stokes respiration has been associated with a change in circulation time that may be induced by cardiovascular disease. It also has been associated with intracerebral disease, such as might occur as a result of strokes. The periodic pattern of breathing produces wide fluctuations in blood oxygen and CARBON DIOXIDE levels, which can induce an arousal at the peak of the crescendo respiratory pattern. INSOMNIA, characterized by arousals and awakening, may occur due to Cheyne-Stokes respiration, and treatment may involve the administration of a continuous flow of oxygen or the use of RESPIRATORY STIMULANTS, such as acetazolamide.

childhood onset insomnia See IDIOPATHIC INSOMNIA.

chloral hydrate See HYPNOTICS.

cholecystokinin (CCK) A group of peptides, of approximately 33 amino acid residues long, that originally was found in the gastrointestinal tract but more recently has been discovered to be present in the central nervous system. Cholecystokinin (CCK) is primarily found in the cerebral cortex, hypothalamus and the basal ganglia. It has been shown to reduce SLEEP LATENCY but has very little effect on SLEEP STAGES. The soporific effect of a big meal may be mediated through the large increase of cholecystokinin that occurs following meals. Cholecystokinin may have its greatest effect as a behavioral sedative that allows sleep to occur, rather than by any direct effect on inducing sleep. (See also DELTA SLEEP INDUCING PEPTIDE, DIET AND SLEEP, FACTOR S, MURAMYL DIPEPTIDE, SLEEP-INDUCING FACTORS.)

...a See LONG-TERM INSOMNIA.

...ostructive pulmonary disease Also ...onic obstructive respiratory disease; this ...piratory disorder characterized by a chronic impairment of airflow through the respiratory tract. This disorder can disrupt sleep due to the altered cardiorespiratory physiology. Persons with chronic obstructive pulmonary disease frequently will complain of disturbed sleep and INSOMNIA.

The sleep disturbance that occurs is typically one of difficulty in initiating sleep, and there are frequent awakenings at night, often with the sensation of shortness of breath and difficulty in breathing. There may be excessive coughing during sleep and the need to get out of bed in order to breathe more easily. Some of the sleep disturbance may be due to MEDICATIONS that are required to improve breathing, which often have a stimulant effect, thereby adding to the complaint of insomnia.

Typically during sleep, patients with chronic obstructive pulmonary disease will demonstrate a reduction in TIDAL VOLUME, with increasing HYPOXEMIA or elevation of the carbon dioxide level in the bloodstream. This particular pattern is more common in patients called "blue bloaters," who have evidence of right-sided heart failure due to pulmonary hypertension and an increase in the blood hemocrit level. Patients who are blue bloaters usually suffer severe oxygen desaturation during sleep.

A second group called "pink puffers" characteristically has shortness of breath associated with increased lung volumes. The hypoxemia and elevation of carbon dioxide levels during sleep is not as severe as that seen in blue bloaters.

Chronic obstructive pulmonary disease can be due to a variety of disorders, such as respiratory infections or bronchopulmonary dysplasia; however, the most common cause in adults is chronic SMOKING.

POLYSOMNOGRAPHY demonstrates a prolonged SLEEP LATENCY and frequent awakenings during the major sleep episode. Some patients may be unable to lie flat during sleep because of severe shortness of breath and therefore polysomnography may need to be performed with the patient in a semi-recumbent position. There is typically a reduction of SLOW WAVE SLEEP as well as REM SLEEP with fragmentation of the sleep stages—particularly REM sleep, due to oxygen desaturation. Obstructive and central apneic events may occur concurrently with the sleep-related hypoxemia. Cardiac ARRYTHMIAS may be associated with the hypoxemia or may occur independently. A MULTIPLE SLEEP LATENCY TEST may demonstrate a reduced mean sleep latency, particularly in patients with frequent nocturnal sleep disruption or a complaint of EXCESSIVE SLEEPINESS during the day.

The sleep disturbance of a patient with chronic obstructive pulmonary disease needs to be differentiated from other causes of complaints of insomnia. Anxiety and DEPRESSION, or PSYCHOPHYSIOLOGICAL INSOMNIA, may coexist with the chronic obstructive pulmonary disease. Acute anxiety due to an exacerbation of lung disease may produce an ADJUSTMENT SLEEP DISORDER.

The blue bloater form of chronic obstructive pulmonary disease is similar to CENTRAL ALVEOLAR HYPOVENTILATION SYNDROME. It may be difficult to differentiate the two disorders if the history of development of chronic obstructive pulmonary disease is unknown.

Treatment involves ensuring optimum treatment of the chronic obstructive pulmonary disease. Stimulant bronchodilator medications, used for the treatment of the lung disease, should be reduced to effective but not excessive doses. If OBSTRUCTIVE SLEEP APNEA SYNDROME or CENTRAL SLEEP APNEA SYNDROME is present, or even alveolar hypoventilation, the use of a CONTINUOUS POSITIVE AIRWAY PRESSURE device (CPAP), with or without the addition of low oxygen therapy, may be helpful. Such treatment is best performed under polysomnographic monitoring. Attention should be given to SLEEP HYGIENE measures, and other lifestyle changes should be strongly recommended, such as weight reduction and avoidance of smoking.

Flenly, C., "Chronic Obstructive Pulmonary Disease," in Kryger, M., Roth., T. and Dement, W.C., eds., *The Principles and Practices of Sleep Disorders Medicine.* Philadelphia: Saunders, 1989. pp. 601–610.

Guilleminault, C., Kaminsky, J. and Motta, J., "Chronic Obstructive Air Flow Disease in Sleep Studies," *American Review of Respiratory Disease* 112 (1987): 397–406.

chronic obstructive respiratory disease See CHRONIC OBSTRUCTIVE PULMONARY DISEASE.

chronic paroxysmal hemicrania A headache consisting of one-sided repetitive head pains. These headaches appear to have a very close relationship with REM SLEEP and they can be so tightly linked with REM sleep that they are often called REM SLEEP-LOCKED. Whereas CLUSTER HEADACHES are much more common in males, chronic paroxysmal hemicrania is more common in females. (See also SLEEP-RELATED HEADACHES.)

chronobiology The scientific study of biological rhythms. Biological rhythms can have markedly varying period lengths, from less than a second for heart rate to as long as a year for hibernational cycles in animals. In humans, the biological rhythms of approximately one day are those that are commonly referred to under the term CIRCADIAN RHYTHMS.

chronotherapy Treatment developed by CHARLES CZEISLER in 1981 to correct the displaced sleep period of patients with the circadian rhythm sleep disorder of DELAYED SLEEP PHASE SYNDROME. The treatment involves a progressive delay of a sleep period so the major sleep period is rotated around the clock to an improved SLEEP ONSET time. For example, prior to shifting the sleep period an individual who is unable to fall asleep before 3 A.M. would be instructed to maintain a regular sleep onset time at 3 A.M., sleeping for eight hours until 11 A.M., for a period of five days. After the five-day stabilization period, the patient would be instructed to go to bed three hours later, and arise three hours later each day until the sleep onset time reaches a more appropriate time at night. Depending upon the amount of time that the sleep period is displaced, the process of shifting the sleep periods takes about six to seven days. Once having reached a more desirable sleep onset time, the patient is instructed to maintain a regular bedtime and arise eight hours later so that the sleep period can become stabilized at the new sleep onset and awake times.

Some patients find they are able to maintain the improved timing of the sleep episode; however, others will find that they drift to a later period of time and may require a repeat course of chronotherapy in order to reestablish more appropriate sleep onset and wake times.

The same process of shifting the sleep by three hours has been applied successfully to one patient with ADVANCED SLEEP PHASE SYNDROME, who rotated the sleep period in an anticlockwise direction.

circadian rhythms Franz Halberg in 1959 proposed this term to describe endogenous rhythms that had a period length of about 24 hours. The term was coined from the Latin *circa,* meaning "about," and *dies,* meaning "a day." Although most circadian rhythms are 24 hours in duration, the term was originally applied to the endogenous rhythms that run in humans at a slightly longer period of approximately 25 hours. ENVIRONMENTAL TIME CUES prevent the true period length of the underlying circadian rhythm from becoming manifest, so the circadian rhythm length is maintained at 24 hours. Without environmental time cues sleep onset would occur on average one hour later and we would awaken one hour later. Therefore, we would live on a 25-hour-long day. (See also ENDOGENOUS CIRCADIAN PACEMAKER, FREE RUNNING, TEMPORAL ISOLATION.)

Kennaway, D.J., "Generation and Entrainment of Circadian Rhythms," *Clinical Experiments in Pharmacology and Physiology* 25, no. 10 (1998): 862–865.

circadian rhythm sleep disorders Previously called sleep-wake schedule disorders, these are disorders of the timing of sleep within the 24-hour day. These disorders were originally grouped together in the first edition of the "Diagnostic Classification of Sleep and Arousal Disorders," published in 1979 in the journal *SLEEP*. The disorders were divided into two groups—transient and persistent.

The main disorders in the transient group include TIME ZONE CHANGE (JET LAG) SYNDROME and SHIFT-WORK SLEEP DISORDER. The five persistent circadian rhythm sleep disorders are: FREQUENTLY CHANGING SLEEP-WAKE SCHEDULE, DELAYED SLEEP PHASE SYNDROME, ADVANCED SLEEP PHASE SYNDROME, NON-24-HOUR SLEEP-WAKE SYNDROME and IRREGULAR

SLEEP-WAKE PATTERN. In all of these disorders, there is an alteration in the timing of sleep in that it is either advanced, delayed or occurs irregularly during a 24-hour period. Some of these disorders are related to an irregularity or disruption of the normal ENVIRONMENTAL TIME CUES and are thereby thought to be of socio-environmental cause. Other circadian rhythm sleep disorders suggest a defect in the intrinsic mechanism of the circadian pacemaker or its mechanism of entrainment (ability to keep to a set pattern) and hence are thought to be of endogenous or organic cause. Recently, new types of chronobiological tests have become available, such as the CONSTANT ROUTINE, that can determine whether the abnormality in the circadian pacemaker is of endogenous etiology.

Some of the circadian rhythm sleep disorders, such as delayed sleep phase syndrome, have been subtyped into an intrinsic type, in which the circadian pacemaker or its mechanism is believed to be abnormal, and an extrinsic type, in which socio-environmental factors appear to be responsible.

Sedgwick, P.M., "Disorders of the Sleep-Wake Cycle in Adults," *Postgraduate Medical Journal* 74, no. 869 (1998): 134–138.

circadian timing system The physiological system responsible for measuring time and synchronizing an organism's internal physiological processes with its environmental daily events. (See also BIOLOGICAL CLOCKS, CHRONOBIOLOGY, CIRCADIAN RHYTHMS.)

circasmedian rhythm A chronobiological term applied to a rhythm that has a PERIOD LENGTH of about half a day, as opposed to a CIRCADIAN RHYTHM, which has a period length of one full day. An example of a circasmedian rhythm is seen in the tendency for sleepiness that peaks not only at night but also in the mid-afternoon. (See also CHRONOBIOLOGY.)

clinical polysomnographer Specialist trained in the clinical interpretation of the results of the POLYSOMNOGRAMS of patients with a wide variety of sleep disorders. This term has now been superseded by the term "sleep specialist" (see SLEEP DISORDER SPECIALIST). Most clinical polysomnographers work in full-service SLEEP DISORDER CENTERS. Certification in clinical polysomnography was a requirement for the accreditation of sleep disorder centers by the American Sleep Disorders Association (now the AMERICAN ACADEMY OF SLEEP MEDICINE). The new examination for sleep specialists is run by the AMERICAN BOARD OF SLEEP MEDICINE.

A clinical polysomnographer usually had clinical training in one of the medical sciences, most commonly medicine, but also in psychology or other clinical specialties. The American Sleep Disorders Association held a CLINICAL POLYSOMNOGRAPHER EXAMINATION to certify competence in clinical polysomnography. An applicant who successfully passed the examination was certified in clinical polysomnography and received an ACCREDITED CLINICAL POLYSOMNOGRAPHER (ACP) degree. (See also ACCREDITATION STANDARDS FOR SLEEP DISORDER CENTERS, ASSOCIATION OF POLYSOMNOGRAPHIC TECHNOLOGISTS, ASSOCIATION OF PROFESSIONAL SLEEP SOCIETIES, POLYSOMNOGRAPHY.)

clinical polysomnographer examination A test given by the AMERICAN ACADEMY OF SLEEP MEDICINE (formerly the American Sleep Disorders Association) in order to assure competence and knowledge of the basic and clinical science of sleep disorders medicine. The first examination for clinical polysomnographers was held in 1978 and tests are held yearly. Applicants who passed the clinical polysomnographer examination became ACCREDITED CLINICAL POLYSOMNOGRAPHERS (ACP). The examination is now called the board examination in sleep medicine and is administered by the AMERICAN BOARD OF SLEEP MEDICINE. There are approximately 1,000 accredited clinical polysomnographers in the United States today.

The clinical polysomnographer examination consisted of two parts held four months apart. One part of the examination tested competence in the basic sciences of sleep, disorders of sleep, biological rhythms and chronobiology, and other medical disorders that affect sleep. The other part was a practical examination that tested the ability to interpret sleep studies and score sleep recordings. (See also POLYSOMNOGRAPHY, SLEEP DISORDER CENTERS, SLEEP DISORDERS MEDICINE.)

Clinical Sleep Society (CSS) This organization was founded in 1984 as the clinical branch of the ASSOCIATION OF SLEEP DISORDER CENTERS (ASDC). The individual members of the Clinical Sleep Society were clinicians involved in the diagnosis and treatment of patients with sleep and alertness disorders, scientists involved in basic or clinical sleep research, and other professionals interested in learning more about the field of SLEEP DISORDERS MEDICINE. In 1988, the Clinical Sleep Society and the Association of Sleep Disorder Centers (formerly known as ASDC-CSS) changed the name of its combined form to the American Sleep Disorders Association (ASDA), now known as the AMERICAN ACADEMY OF SLEEP MEDICINE (AASM). (See also SLEEP RESEARCH SOCIETY, ASSOCIATION OF PROFESSIONAL SLEEP SOCIETIES.)

clomipramine See ANTIDEPRESSANTS.

clonazepam See BENZODIAZEPINES.

cluster headaches Severe unilateral headaches felt behind the eye. The headaches produce autonomic dysfunction in the region around the eye. Cluster headaches predominantly occur in association with REM SLEEP at night. Other symptoms include nasal stuffiness, rhinorrhea and unilateral forehead sweating. (See also SLEEP-RELATED HEADACHES.)

cocaine Drug derived from the leaves of the coca; commonly used by drug abusers for its euphoric effects. This drug is an amino-alcohol base closely related to tropine, the amino alcohol in atropine. It has been used in medicine for many years as a local anesthetic, particularly for ophthalmological procedures. Cocaine can have pronounced effects upon sleep due to its stimulation of the central nervous system; it produces restlessness and INSOMNIA. There is also some evidence to suggest that the chronic nasal ingestion of cocaine induces a nasal congestion that can exacerbate the OBSTRUCTIVE SLEEP APNEA SYNDROME.

O'Brien, Robert and Cohen, Sidney, M.D., *The Encyclopedia of Drug Abuse.* New York: Facts On File, 1984. pp. 63–65.

codeine Drug shown to improve alertness in patients with EXCESSIVE SLEEPINESS. It can achieve this without the side effects of central nervous system or peripheral stimulation. However, side effects such as constipation, and the potential for drug abuse, may occur.

In doses of 30 to 180 milligrams per day, codeine phosphate is effective in the treatment of NARCOLEPSY but is rarely used because other STIMULANT MEDICATIONS, such as pemoline, methylphenidate, dextroamphetamine, and MODAFINIL, are more effective. However, codeine may be useful for patients who are unable to tolerate these other central nervous system stimulants.

cognitive effects of sleep states Recall of information presented during an awakening from slow wave sleep is not as good as when the information is presented following an awakening from REM sleep. Learned material is better remembered after a sleep episode than following a similar duration of wakefulness. This ability to retain information better following sleep has been seen as support for the interference theory of forgetting (ITF). Some studies have suggested that there is better retention for the first half of the night compared with the second half. However, the difference in the ability to recall learned information following sleep compared with wakefulness is very small and does not appear to be long-lasting.

Brain activity is high during the REM stage of sleep and hence DREAM recall is often very vivid and complex. Some mental activity does occur during slow wave sleep but dream recall is greatly reduced compared with REM sleep. (See also LEARNING DURING SLEEP, SLEEP STAGES.)

cognitive focusing A technique used in the management of INSOMNIA that involves focusing on reassuring thoughts. Patients with insomnia typically awaken at night and are unable to return to sleep because they are haunted by recurring, unwanted and unpleasant thoughts. Cognitive focusing involves learning to focus on reassuring thoughts and pleasant images so that sleep is more likely to occur. (See also BEHAVIORAL TREATMENT OF INSOMNIA, DISORDERS OF INITIATING AND

MAINTAINING SLEEP, HYPNOSIS, PSYCHOPHYSIOLOGICAL INSOMNIA.)

coma A state of psychological unresponsiveness that can be differentiated from sleep and wakefulness. The primary difference from sleep is that there is no psychologically understandable response to an external stimulus, or to an inner need. Patients in acute coma may look as if they are asleep; however, this state never lasts more than two or four weeks, no matter how severe the brain injury. Patients in sleeplike coma then pass into a chronic state of unresponsiveness in which they appear to be awake but lack cognitive mental ability. This state has variously been termed *vegetative state, akinetic mutism, coma vigil* or the *apallic syndrome*. Coma can be the result of chemical toxicity that affects the whole central nervous system, or it may result from extensive damage to the cerebral hemispheres or the brain stem.

Normal sleep-wake patterns and cycling of REM and NREM sleep usually do not occur in patients with acute coma until they pass into the chronic vegetative state where the pattern of sleep and wakefulness usually returns. There are several forms of coma in which the electroencephalographic pattern differs. The more typical form of acute coma and coma due to metabolic or pharmacological causes has a 1-to-5-hertz slow wave EEG pattern. A form of coma termed *alpha coma* has a pattern of nonreactive alpha activity that is not blocked by eye opening or other sensory stimuli. This particular form of coma is most often due to brain stem lesions at the level of the pons or to post-anoxic encephalopathy.

A form of coma called spindle coma occurs in approximately 6% of all comatose patients; it is characterized by the presence of 14 hertz SLEEP SPINDLES with vertex sharp waves and K complexes superimposed on a background of slower delta and theta activity. The sleep spindle activity resembles that seen in stage two sleep. This form of coma appears to result from interruption of the ascending reticulo-thalamo-cortical pathways.

Another coma pattern is called theta coma and is characterized by typical 4-to-7-hertz theta activity that is superimposed on a low voltage delta pattern of activity. This particular pattern is often indicative of a disruption of brain stem reticular pathways to the thalamus and is highly predictive of a poor outcome—typically, death.

With all forms of coma, the occurrence of a normal sleep-wake pattern, or presence of non-REM/REM cycling, is typically associated with an improved prognosis. (See also NON-REM-STAGE SLEEP, REM SLEEP, STAGE TWO SLEEP, UNCONSCIOUSNESS.)

Plum, F. and Posner, J.B., *The Diagnosis of Stupor and Coma*, 3rd ed. Philadelphia: F.A. Davis, 1982, p. 377.

conditioned insomnia An essential part of PSYCHOPHYSIOLOGICAL INSOMNIA that develops through a process of negative associations between the usual sleep environment and sleep patterns. A prior episode of poor quality sleep leads to the development of the negative associations, which produce the conditioned insomnia, a learned pattern of poor quality sleep. For instance, if a person has difficulty falling asleep in his or her bedroom, the person may come to believe sleep is difficult or impossible there. Also, a person who frequently reads or works in bed may have difficulty in accepting the bed as a sleeping place.

confusional arousals Episodes of mental confusion that typically occur during arousals from sleep. These episodes most often occur with arousals from DEEP SLEEP in the first third of the night. The individual usually sits forward in bed and feels disoriented in time and space, with behavior that may be inappropriate, such as picking up a phone to speak into it in response to a ringing alarm clock. There may also be slowness in speech and thought. Responses to commands and questions are often slow and inappropriate. Episodes may last from several minutes to several hours.

Confusional arousals were first mentioned by Roger J. Broughton in 1968 in his classic article on the arousal disorders. Other terms that have been applied to confusional arousals are *sleep drunkenness, excessive sleep inertia* and *Schlaftrunkenheit* (in the German literature) and *l'ivresse du sommeil* (in the French literature).

The confusional arousals are thought to be related to an abnormality of the normal arousal mechanism during sleep. The abnormality may be a defect of the ASCENDING RETICULAR ACTIVATING SYSTEM (ARAS).

Confusional arousals are most typical in childhood, often before puberty, less common in older children or adolescents and even rarer in adults.

Episodes may be precipitated by conditions that predispose the individual to excessive fatigue, such as SLEEP DEPRIVATION or an altered sleep-wake pattern. MEDICATIONS, particularly depressants of the central nervous system, can also induce episodes. Sometimes confusional arousals are seen in association with other sleep disorders, such as IDIOPATHIC HYPERSOMNIA or SLEEP APNEA. More typically, episodes of confusional arousal occur in individuals who are predisposed to have SLEEPWALKING or SLEEP TERRORS, with a strong familial tendency marking all three behaviors.

Polysomnographic recordings of confusional arousals generally show an arousal occurring from the slow wave non-REM sleep (see SLEEP STAGES) in the first third of the night; the recordings are characterized by delta activity with mixes of theta and poorly-reactive ALPHA RHYTHMS.

Confusional arousals are a generally benign phenomenon, although injuries may occur if the individual accidentally knocks into furniture or other objects near the bedside. Confusional arousals may be considered to be a minor manifestation of sleepwalking or sleep terrors. Sleep terrors are characterized by an intensely loud scream that heralds the episode, whereas sleepwalking is characterized by walking during the event. Other behaviors that may have some similarities with confusional arousals are sleep-related epileptic SEIZURES, particularly those of the partial complex type.

Treatment of confusional arousals is rarely necessary unless the episodes occur in conjunction with other arousal disorders, such as sleepwalking or sleep terrors. In certain circumstances, it may be helpful to use either BENZODIAZEPINES or tricyclic ANTIDEPRESSANTS, such as imipramine, in order to suppress episodes. However, more commonly the only action that need be taken for confusional arousals is to secure the bedroom and prevent injuries from objects or furniture near the bedside. (See also AROUSAL DISORDERS.)

Ferber, Richard, "Sleep Disorders in Infants and Children," in Riley, T.L., ed., *Clinical Aspects of Sleep and Sleep Disturbance.* Boston: Butterworth, 1985.

Broughton, R., "Sleep Disorders: Disorders of Arousal?" *Science* 159 (1968): 1070–1078.

congenital central alveolar hypoventilation syndrome (CCHS) See CENTRAL ALVEOLAR HYPOVENTILATION SYNDROME.

congestive heart failure The inability of the heart to pump blood, with resulting elevation of systemic, venous and capillary pressure and the transudation of fluid into the tissues. Congestive heart failure can occur as a result of disorders that affect cardiac function.

OBSTRUCTIVE SLEEP APNEA SYNDROME can produce pulmonary hypertension and result in right-sided heart failure, with the development of liver congestion and ankle edema. Treatment of obstructive sleep apnea syndrome usually results in improved cardiac function, with correction of the congestion and edema.

Congestive heart failure can produce CHEYNE-STOKES RESPIRATION which is a crescendo-decrescendo pattern of ventilation that can produce awakenings due to fluctuations in blood gases. This pattern of breathing can lead to LONG-TERM INSOMNIA.

Patients who have impaired cardiac function that results in lung congestion can present symptoms such as ORTHOPNEA or PAROXYSMAL NOCTURNAL DYSPNEA when in a recumbent or reclining position during sleep. (See also SLEEP-RELATED BREATHING DISORDERS, SLEEP-RELATED CARDIOVASCULAR SYMPTOMS.)

constant routine A biological test of the ENDOGENOUS CIRCADIAN PACEMAKER that involves a 36-hour episode of BASELINE monitoring, followed by a 40-hour episode of monitoring, with the individual on a constant routine of food intake, position, activity and light exposure. During this time, the sleep pattern is monitored as well as the core body TEMPERATURE. The cycle of the core body temperature allows a determination of the natural period length of the pacemaker control in body temperature and allows a comparison of the phase position of body temperature to other individuals so as to determine whether the pattern is advanced or delayed. This test may be useful in determining the timing of the circadian pacemaker in individuals who suffer from CIRCADIAN RHYTHM SLEEP DISORDERS, such as DELAYED SLEEP PHASE SYNDROME or ADVANCED SLEEP PHASE SYNDROME. (See also ENDOGENOUS CIRCADIAN PHASE ASSESSMENT; PERIOD LENGTH.)

continuous positive airway pressure (CPAP) An effective and commonly used treatment for OBSTRUCTIVE SLEEP APNEA SYNDROME. The system was first devised in 1981 by Colin Sullivan of Australia; today a number of commercially-developed systems are available for home use.

The CPAP device consists of an air pump housed in a small box about one cubic foot in size, which is placed at the patient's bedside. Tubing of approximately one inch in diameter conveys the air to a mask, which is placed over the patient's nose so that the mouth is free. The mask is attached to the head with elasticized straps. The patient puts on the CPAP mask, turns on the machine and sleeps with the mask in place during the night until awakening, when the mask is removed. This system has been demonstrated to relieve severe obstructive sleep apnea syndrome, with resumption of normal quality sleep at night and resolution of the cardiac features, as well as complete resolution of the associated daytime sleepiness.

The CPAP system provides an air splint to the upper airway thereby preventing its collapse. During the inspiratory phase of an obstructive apnea, the upper airway tissues collapse because of a negative inspiratory pressure, thereby producing upper airway obstruction. The continuous positive air pressure device provides a low flow of air with a pressure of between 2 and 20 centimeters of water, which prevents the negative suction effect on the tissues of the upper airway, thus preventing their collapse.

Most patients with obstructive sleep apnea syndrome are capable of using a CPAP system; however, some patients find the mask makes them feel claustrophobic, preventing its regular use. The development of chronic nasal irritation due to the air flow is also a major complication of the device. This irritation can be partially relieved by the use of extra humidification of the inspired air; however, occasionally nasal decongestant inhalers may be necessary. Despite optimum treatment of the nasal irritation, some patients will find relief only by discontinuing use of the CPAP system.

One of the major concerns regarding the use of nasal CPAP is that it is very dependent upon patient compliance with the treatment recommendations. Although for most patients the benefits are very apparent and reinforce the desire to use the system, some patients may not be motivated to utilize the system. This is of particular concern for patients with severe daytime sleepiness, who are employed in positions where sleepiness may put them or others at risk, such as bus drivers. Alternative treatments for obstructive sleep apnea may not be readily available, as the UVULOPALATOPHARYNGOPLASTY surgical procedure is not effective in approximately 50% of patients who have obstructive sleep apnea syndrome. The only effective surgical alternative is TRACHEOSTOMY, which is often rejected by the patient for cosmetic, social or medical reasons.

Despite the limitations of nasal CPAP treatment, this device has dramatically changed the management of obstructive sleep apnea syndrome and is a major advance in its treatment. (See also CEPHALOMETRIC RADIOGRAPH, FIBEROPTIC ENDOSCOPY.)

Sullivan, C.E., Issa, F.D., Berthon-Jones, M. and Eves, L., "Reversal of Obstructive Sleep Apnea by Continuous Positive Airway Pressure Applied Through the Nares," *Lancet* 1 (1981): 862–865.

convulsions Generalized whole body movements that occur in association with epileptic activity. SLEEP-RELATED EPILEPSY is a primary cause of convulsions during sleep.

cortisol A hormone released from the adrenal gland in response to stimulation by ACTH (ADRENOCORTICOTROPHIN HORMONE), which is released from the pituitary gland. The secretion of cortisol is reduced during sleep but is greatly increased around the time of awakening. It is important for the maintenance of body metabolism, and its absence leads to reduced energy and weight loss.

Cortisol is often measured in the blood to detect the specific phase of the CIRCADIAN RHYTHM. Shifts of the sleep pattern by 12 hours are usually not accompanied by acute shifts of the cortisol circadian rhythm, which takes up to two weeks to realign with the new time of sleep. The cortisol rhythm appears to be linked to the body temperature rhythm, which takes a similar amount of time to shift to coincide with the new time of sleep. (See also GROWTH HORMONE, MELATONIN, PROLACTIN, REVERSAL OF SLEEP.)

cot death A term used, mainly in Britain, for SUDDEN INFANT DEATH SYNDROME (SIDS).

coughing Coughing during sleep is due to an irritation of the upper airway and typically is associated with abrupt awakening, and difficulty in breathing. Patients with sleep-related breathing disorders are liable to have episodes of choking and coughing during sleep, particularly those with CHRONIC OBSTRUCTIVE PULMONARY DISEASE or SLEEP-RELATED ASTHMA.

Coughing can have many causes, such as inflammatory reactions to inhaled allergens, mechanical irritation due to dust particles, chemical irritation due to smoke or gas, and thermal irritation due to very hot or cold air. Treatment depends upon the cause of the coughing. Specific therapy should be directed to any underlying medical disorder, such as sleep-related asthma. A cough suppressant (antitussive) medication such as CODEINE can be of help. If secretions are thick and are the cause of coughing, an ultrasonic nebulizer will allow the secretions to be expectorated. Ipratropium, a bronchodilator with anticholinergic effects, is helpful for coughs due to asthma. (See also SLEEP-RELATED BREATHING DISORDERS.)

CPAP See CONTINUOUS POSITIVE AIRWAY PRESSURE (CPAP).

"C" process See ENDOGENOUS CIRCADIAN PACEMAKER.

CPS See HERTZ.

cramps Contractions of muscles that typically result in a painful sensation. The most common site for cramps during sleep is in the calf muscles. Cramps may be induced by metabolic changes, such as an alteration in the serum electrolytes.

Acute cramps can be partially relieved by stretching the muscle involved. Quinine sulfate is an effective medication for the prevention of muscle cramps. (See also NOCTURNAL LEG CRAMPS.)

craniofacial disorders A number of genetically-determined disorders that affect head and face growth. They typically produce abnormalities of the upper airway so that there is obstruction to air flow, which is worsened during sleep. These disorders can produce OBSTRUCTIVE SLEEP APNEA SYNDROME.

Achondroplasia, a hereditary disorder that is characterized by abnormal growth of endochondral bone, results in dwarfism. Patients with this disorder have abnormalities at the base of the skull and deficient growth of the mid-facial region. Achondroplastics can also suffer compression of the brain stem and upper spinal cord, which can contribute to impaired control of the pharyngeal muscles. Patients with achondroplasia have a higher incidence of obstructive sleep apnea syndrome than the general population, and this may cause reduced growth as well as the development of EXCESSIVE SLEEPINESS. Treatment of the obstructive sleep apnea syndrome can improve growth and eliminate the clinical features of obstructive sleep apnea syndrome.

Pierre-Robin Syndrome, also known as the Robin Sequence, is characterized by head and jaw abnormalities. There may be microcephaly and a small and retroplaced jaw. The tongue can fall back and obstruct the airway, leading to the development of obstructive sleep apnea syndrome with features of inability to thrive and the development of right-sided heart failure. Treatment may be necessary by either TRACHEOSTOMY or MANDIBULAR ADVANCEMENT SURGERY.

An autosomal dominant condition, termed Treacher Collins syndrome, is characterized by mandibular and mid-face growth abnormalities as well as mental retardation. Patients are also liable to suffer obstructive sleep apnea syndrome and may require tracheostomy or mandibular advancement surgery.

The velo-cardio-facial syndrome, which is also known as Shprintzen's syndrome, was first described in 1978 in individuals with learning disabilities, small stature, hearing loss and a retruded mandible. These patients also have cardiac defects. The craniofacial abnormalities in velo-cardio-facial syndrome children may produce obstructive sleep apnea syndrome, which can be worsened by repair of cleft palate, which is commonly seen in this syndrome. Tonsillectomy, or mandibular advancement surgery, may be indicated to treat the obstructive sleep apnea syndrome.

Goldenhars syndrome, also known as oculo-auriculo-vertebral dysplasia, is a disorder characterized by eye, ear and vertebral anomalies. There is an associated small lower jaw and reduced growth of the bony tissues of the face. These patients are also liable to develop obstructive sleep apnea syndrome.

crib death Term that has been used, largely in the United States, for the SUDDEN INFANT DEATH SYNDROME.

cycles per second (CPS) See HERTZ.

Cylert See STIMULANT MEDICATIONS.

Czeisler, Charles A. Dr. Czeisler (1952–) received his A.B. degree in 1974 in biochemistry and molecular biology from Harvard College, his Ph.D. in 1978 in neuro- and biobehavioral sciences from Stanford University and his M.D. in 1981 from the Stanford University School of Medicine. He has been on the faculty of Harvard Medical School since 1983 and has been a professor of medicine since 1998.

Working with the late Professor ELLIOT D. WEITZMAN at the Albert Einstein College of Medicine/Montefiore Medical Center in New York, Dr. Czeisler established one of the first TEMPORAL ISOLATION facilities, where the relationship between the episodic secretory pattern of hormones and the output of the ENDOGENOUS CIRCADIAN PACEMAKER was studied. They demonstrated the influence of that pacemaker on the duration and internal organization of sleep, and in 1981 Czeisler developed CHRONOTHERAPY for delayed sleep phase syndrome.

Dr. Czeisler is chief of the Division of Sleep Medicine in the Department of Medicine at the Brigham and Women's Hospital and Harvard Medical School in Boston, Massachusetts. Czeisler carried out one of the first studies to show that shift-work schedules that disrupt sleep could be improved by applying circadian principles.

Dr. Czeisler was the first to demonstrate that light exposure could reset the human circadian clock independent of the timing of the sleep-wake cycle. He then went on to demonstrate that properly timed light exposure to light and darkness could effectively treat maladaptation to night shift work. He has applied this research to the scheduling of NASA astronauts and conducted a sleep experiment on Senator John Glenn during his 1998 return to space flight.

In his 1999 article in *Science*, cited below, Dr. Czeisler and his associates demonstrated that the intrinsic period of the human circadian pacemaker is very close to 24 hours, rather than 25 hours as had been previously believed.

Czeisler, C.A., Duffy, J.F., Shanahan, T.L., et al., "Stability, Precision, and Near-24-Hour Period of the Human Circadian Pacemaker." *Science* 284 (1999): 2177–2181.

D

D sleep Term sometimes used to describe dreaming sleep or desynchronized sleep. D sleep is synonymous with REM SLEEP and should not be confused with the original STAGE D SLEEP.

Dalmane See BENZODIAZEPINES.

dauerschlaf See SLEEP THERAPY.

daydreaming The state of mind associated with withdrawal from environmental influences. Sleep does not occur but there may be DROWSINESS. Full alertness to the environment is reduced. Sleepiness can erroneously be mistaken for daydreaming, particularly in adolescents who tend to be sleep deprived and may not concentrate on schoolwork (see EXCESSIVE SLEEPINESS, SLEEP DEPRIVATION). If other features of sleepiness occur, such as eye closure, head drooping or even snoring, then there should be a consideration of a sleep disorder as a cause.

True dream phenomenon (see DREAMS) is a state associated with pronounced physiological changes, such as rapid eye movements and loss of muscle tone. Daydreaming does not represent daytime dreams and therefore should be differentiated from true dreaming sleep.

daytime sleepiness See EXCESSIVE SLEEPINESS.

deaths during sleep Several extensive epidemiological studies have demonstrated that death is most likely to occur over the usual nocturnal hours, with the greatest likelihood of death occurring between 4 A.M. and 7 A.M. The reason for this circadian variation in deaths is unknown; however, there are several disorders that are believed to increase the likelihood of death during sleep. SLEEP-RELATED BREATHING DISORDERS, including OBSTRUCTIVE SLEEP APNEA SYNDROME, have been reported to be associated with sudden death during sleep, and in patients with asthma there is a higher rate of death during the nocturnal hours compared to the daytime. (See SLEEP-RELATED ASTHMA.)

Patients with the obstructive sleep apnea syndrome have a high rate of sleep-related hypoxemia and cardiac arrhythmias related to the apneic episodes. The cardiac arrhythmias are believed to be the primary cause for the sudden unexpected death during sleep.

An American Cancer Society study conducted in 1964 (data was analyzed in 1979) of more than 1 million people found that men who slept four hours or less, or more than 10 hours, had a higher mortality rate than those who slept a normal six to eight hours. This association between sleep length and death may be related either to underlying medical illness, which produces sleep disturbance at night, or to disorders, such as sleep apnea, that usually produce a prolonged nighttime sleep episode.

There is also some evidence that people who take sleeping pills (HYPNOTICS) are more likely to have a nocturnal death. (See also MYOCARDIAL INFARCTION.)

Mitler, M.M., Carskadon, M.A., Czeisler, C.A., Dement, W.C., Dinges, D.F. and Graeber, R.C., "Catastrophes, Sleep, and Public Policy: Consensus Report," *Sleep* 11 (1988): 100–109.

Kripke, D.F., Simmons, R.M., Garfinkel, L. and Hammond, E.C., "Short and Long Sleep and Sleeping Pills," *Archives of General Psychiatry* 36 (1979): 103–116.

deep sleep Term describing STAGE THREE and STAGE FOUR non-REM (NREM) sleep. This term was developed because of the increased threshold to awakening by various stimuli that occurs during these SLEEP STAGES. Rarely, in the older literature, the term was applied to REM sleep, but the term is most appropriately applied to stages three and four sleep.

delayed sleep phase Term applied to a delay in falling asleep in relation to the usual time of sleep, according to the 24-hour clock; the sleep episode is consequently delayed in relation to underlying circadian patterns of other physiological variables (see CIRCADIAN RHYTHMS). The delay of the sleep phase can be temporary, such as typically seen with TIME ZONE CHANGE (JET LAG) SYNDROME, or can be a chronic state, such as seen in DELAYED SLEEP PHASE SYNDROME.

delayed sleep phase syndrome One of the CIRCADIAN RHYTHM SLEEP DISORDERS. It is characterized by SLEEP ONSET and WAKE TIMES that are usually later than desired, with difficulty in initiating sleep onset. Once sleep onset does occur, sleep is of good quality, with few awakenings until the time of final awakening. This sleep pattern is mainly a difficulty in falling asleep at night, or a difficulty in awakening in the morning, which prevents fulfilling social or occupational obligations.

Delayed sleep phase syndrome was first described by ELLIOT D. WEITZMAN and CHARLES CZEISLER in 1981. Their analysis of 450 patients who complained of INSOMNIA showed that 7% fulfilled the criteria for having delayed sleep phase syndrome.

Persons with delayed sleep phase syndrome have great difficulty falling asleep at a desired time. Attempts to fall asleep earlier are accompanied by prolonged periods of lying in bed awake until the time that they usually fall asleep. These patients are often prescribed MEDICATIONS to aid sleep, but sleeping medications are ineffective and only add to both the difficulty of awakening and the daytime sleepiness.

In typical cases of delayed sleep phase syndrome, the individual will be unable to initiate sleep onset until 2 A.M. or even as late as 6 A.M. In younger children, the sleep onset time may be earlier, but typically occurs two or more hours after the desired time to go to bed. Because there are attempts to get up at the desired time in the morning, which are only partially successful, the individual with delayed sleep phase syndrome is often sleep deprived and therefore suffers from symptoms of excessive daytime sleepiness, such as fatigue and tiredness. Episodes of sleep can occur inappropriately during the day whenever the individual is in a quiet situation, and this can cause school or work difficulties. Children are typically late to school, and adults are frequently late to their jobs.

On weekends, because there is usually no need to arise early in the morning, these individuals will sleep into the day, often sleeping till midday or even later. These long sleep episodes on the weekend help to make up for the chronic sleep deprivation that accumulates during the week.

The diagnosis of delayed sleep phase syndrome is made on the complaint of either an inability to fall asleep at the desired time, or the inability to awaken at the desired time in the morning. Sometimes the complaint of EXCESSIVE SLEEPINESS during the day will be given. The symptoms will be present for at least three months, and when not required to maintain a strict schedule, such as on weekends and while on vacations, individuals will have a normal sleep pattern in duration and quality, and will awaken spontaneously at a later time than desired.

Investigative studies have shown that the circadian pattern of body temperature is shifted to a later time so that the nadir (low point) does not occur at the more typical time of 5 A.M. but occurs after 8 or 9 A.M. (see CIRCADIAN RHYTHMS). Polysomnographic studies have shown that the sleep period is of short duration when the individual arises at the desired time and is characterized by reduced REM sleep. When the sleep period is allowed to proceed without interruption, such as is seen on the weekend, the sleep period is of normal duration, with normal amounts of each sleep stage.

Although alcohol and hypnotic abuse are commonly used in an attempt to correct the problem, true psychopathology is not typical. An atypical form of depression may be present in adolescents with this syndrome. The depression may be directly related to the social and functional difficulties induced by the abnormal sleep pattern.

In childhood, other disorders, such as LIMIT-SETTING SLEEP DISORDER, SLEEP-ONSET ASSOCIATION DISORDER or IDIOPATHIC HYPERSOMNIA, need to be differentiated from delayed sleep phase syndrome.

The prevalence of the disorder is unknown, but may be as common as 10% in the adolescent population. Adolescents seem particularly predisposed toward developing a delayed sleep pattern because of the natural tendency to delay sleep onset. The onset of the disorder is in late puberty or early adolescence, although major difficulties are not encountered until late adolescence or until the commencement of employment.

Although a male predominance of the delayed sleep phase syndrome is reported in the literature, this may be because of a referral pattern bias. This disorder does not appear to be inherited.

In many cases of delayed sleep phase syndrome, social and environmental factors in inducing the delay of the sleep pattern appear to be the predominant causes. However, some individuals have a circadian pacemaker system that is abnormal and unresponsive to the usual environmental time cues. The time cues are weak stabilizers of the natural physiological tendency to delay sleep onset. An abnormality of the pacemaker's PHASE RESPONSE CURVE has been suggested as a cause.

Individuals who have delayed sleep phase syndrome should be differentiated from those who have a pattern of sequential delays of a sleep phase that occur continuously, the disorder known as the NON-24-HOUR SLEEP-WAKE SYNDROME. The delayed sleep phase syndrome may be a less severe alteration in the phase response curve than the non-24-hour sleep-wake syndrome, in which individuals will rotate the sleep pattern around the clock.

Individuals who have irregularity of the sleep onset time, with the ability to advance the sleep onset time some days each week, are characterized as having INADEQUATE SLEEP HYGIENE rather than delayed sleep phase syndrome.

For the diagnosis, the sleep disturbance should be illustrated on a SLEEP LOG for a period of at least two weeks, and if there is any doubt about the diagnosis, appropriate polysomnographic monitoring should be performed.

Treatment depends on the severity of the disorder. Mild delayed sleep phase syndrome may be improved by strict attention to regular sleep onset and awake times. More severe disturbances may require incremental advances by 15 or 30 minutes per day until a more appropriate sleep onset time is reached. The most severe form of the disorder may require making advancements of the sleep pattern by enforcing a night of sleep deprivation to assist in the sleep advance process, or, more effectively, by the use of a technique termed CHRONOTHERAPY, which involves a three-hour delay in the sleep period on a daily basis until the sleep pattern is rotated around the clock and sleep onset occurs at a more appropriate time.

Weitzman, E.D., Czeisler, C.A., Coleman, R.M. et al., "Delayed Sleep Phase Syndrome," *Archives of General Psychiatry* 38 (1981): 731–746.

Thorpy, Michael J., Korman, E., Spielman, Arthur J. and Glovinsky, P.B., "Delayed Sleep Phase Syndrome in Adolescents," *Journal of Adolescent Health Care* 9 (1988): 22–27.

delirium A clouded state of consciousness characterized by disorientation, fear, irritability, a misperception of sensory stimuli, and often hallucinations. Patients with delirium may alternate between being relatively unresponsive and being mentally very clear. Usually, delirious patients are unaware of environmental influences and do not act appropriately; very often such patients are uninhibited and talk in a loud and defensive manner, often with paranoid ideation and agitation.

The state of delirium is often of rapid onset, lasting a week in duration, although some manifestations may last for several weeks or longer. This disorder is often associated with a metabolic toxic encephalopathy, as with patients with ALCOHOLISM, or can be due to more diffuse intracerebral diseases, as with autoimmune vascular disease. (See also ALCOHOL, COMA, DEMENTIA, OBTUNDATION, STUPOR.)

delta sleep Term used to describe the stage of sleep when the ELECTROENCEPHALOGRAM (EEG) shows a high voltage, slow wave activity in the delta (up to four hertz) frequency. The term is synonymous with stage three and stage four sleep. Because of the slow frequency of activity seen on the EEG, this stage of sleep is also called SLOW WAVE SLEEP. (See also SLEEP STAGES.)

delta sleep inducing peptide (DSIP) First discovered in 1964 in the blood of rabbits in whom electrical stimulation of the thalamic nuclei of the brain induced a sleep-like state. Studies with the infusion of DSIP into rabbits have confirmed the slow wave sleep-inducing properties of this agent. Some studies have been performed in humans with INSOMNIA and the total amount of sleep appears to be increased; however, this peptide can be given only by an intravenous infusion. When administered during the day to patients with NARCOLEPSY, there is some evidence that it has an alerting effect with improvement of performance, as tested by different evaluative tests. (See also FACTOR S, MURAMYL DIPEPTIDE, SLEEP-INDUCING FACTORS.)

Schneider-Helmert, D., "Clinical Evaluation of DSIP," in Wauquier, A., Gaillard, J.M., Monti, J.M. and Radulovacki, M., eds., *Sleep: Neurotransmitters and Neuromodulators.* New York: Raven Press, 1985. pp. 279–290.

delta waves A cycle of electroencephalographic activity with a frequency of less than four hertz (see ELECTROENCEPHALOGRAM [EEG]). For sleep stage scoring the minimum requirements for delta waves are that the amplitude of the waves must be greater than 75 microvolts, and the frequency must be less than two hertz in duration. Delta waves are seen during stages three and four sleep, and occasionally in stage two sleep. (The stage three/four sleep, also known as delta sleep, is regarded as the most important stage of sleep.) (See also DELTA SLEEP, SLEEP STAGES.)

de Mairan, Jean Jacques d'Ortous Astronomer (1678–1771) who conducted an experiment in 1729 that led to an improved understanding of the internal control of CIRCADIAN RHYTHMS. De Mairan's experiment was reported in a communication written by M. Marchant to L'Academie Royale des Sciences de Paris. De Mairan had studied the leaf movements of the heliotrope plant, which opens its leaves during the day and closes them at night. De Mairan removed the plant from daylight and placed it in a dark cabinet; he found that the plant continued to open its leaves during the day, even in the absence of light in the cabinet, and to close them at night. This led de Mairan to conclude that there was an internal biological circadian rhythmicity that occurred despite the absence of ENVIRONMENTAL TIME CUES, and he related these rhythms to the sleep patterns of bedridden patients.

This experiment by de Mairan is heralded as one of the earliest scientific experiments to demonstrate the persistence of biological rhythms in the absence of environmental time cues, in this case, of light and dark.

de Mairan, Jean Jacques, "Observation Botanique," in *Histoire de L'Academie Royale des Sciences* (1729). pp. 35–36.

Dement, William C. Received both his M.D. with honors and a Ph.D. in neurophysiology from the University of Chicago. Dr. Dement (1928–) started the Sleep Laboratory at Stanford University in 1963, and he later founded, and now directs, the Sleep Disorders Center at Stanford University Medical Center in California and is professor of psychiatry at its medical school.

From 1952 to 1957, Dement, while in medical school, joined Eugene Aserinsky and Professor Nathaniel Kleitman; together they discovered and described rapid eye movement (REM) sleep.

Dement also conducted a series of experiments known as dream deprivation studies. The first experiments were done in conjunction with Charles Fisher at New York's Mount Sinai Hospital. Dement continued his experiments a few years later at Stanford University, first depriving volunteers of all REM sleep for 16 nights, then, along with MICHEL JOUVET, depriving cats of REM sleep. Dement's additional sleep research has included a study, along with Dr. CHRISTIAN GUILLEMINAULT, of 235 hypersomnias.

Dr. Dement was a cofounder of the ASSOCIATION FOR THE PSYCHOPHYSIOLOGICAL STUDY OF SLEEP, now the SLEEP RESEARCH SOCIETY. He was also the founding president of the ASSOCIATION OF SLEEP DISORDER CENTERS, now the AMERICAN ACADEMY OF SLEEP MED-

ICINE from 1985 to 1987, and a past president of the ASSOCIATION OF PROFESSIONAL SLEEP SOCIETIES. A member of the National Academy of Sciences, Dr. Dement has twice been the recipient of the NATHANIEL KLEITMAN DISTINGUISHED SERVICE AWARD and in 1991 he was awarded the Distinguished Service Award of the Sleep Research Society.

Dement, William C., *Some Must Watch While Some Must Sleep: Exploring the World of Sleep.* New York: W.W. Norton, 1976.

Dement, William C., and Christopher Vaughn, *The Promise of Sleep.* New York: Dell, 1999.

Kryger, M., Roth, T. and Dement, W.C., eds., *The Principles and Practices of Sleep Disorders Medicine.* Philadelphia: Saunders, 1989.

dementia A progressive and degenerative neurological disease that is associated with loss of memory and other intellectual functions. Patients with dementia commonly suffer sleep disturbances, typically due to behavioral disturbances during the sleep period; DELIRIUM, agitation, wandering and inappropriate talking often occur during nighttime hours. These disturbances in behavior begin in the evening, and therefore the term "sundown syndrome" has been used to describe patients with this form of sleep disturbance.

Patients suffering dementia commonly become major management problems for their families and often require institutionalization in a nursing home or hospital. The need for sedative medications (see HYPNOTICS) to suppress the behavior often contributes to the disturbance of sleep and wakefulness and can lead to further impairment of intellectual function. Patients may also suffer exaggerated NOCTURNAL CONFUSION, with the onset of acute medical illnesses, such as infections. The confusion can also be worsened by medications that are given for the infective illness.

The disturbance in sleep and wakefulness may be due to a loss of the brain center controlling the circadian pattern of sleep and wakefulness; disorders such as Alzheimer's disease and multiple cerebral infarction are typical causes of dementia. Polysomnographic studies have tended to show nonspecific sleep disruption with reduced sleep efficiency, and reduced stages of deep sleep (see SLEEP STAGES). Some patients can have respiratory disturbance during sleep, although this is not a typical feature of patients with dementia.

The diagnosis of dementia is made clinically and by tests such as brain imaging and electroencephalography. Reversible forms of dementia, for example, metabolic abnormalities and drug effects, must be considered. The treatment of sleep disturbance associated with dementia depends upon initiating good SLEEP HYGIENE and assuring that the dementia patient is fully active during the period of desired wakefulness and allowed to sleep in a quiet environment during the time of desired sleep. Hypnotic medications may have a paradoxical effect and increase activity in some patients. The longer-acting hypnotics may cause decreased behavior and alertness during the daytime, which will exacerbate the breakdown of the nighttime sleep pattern and therefore should be avoided. NEUROLEPTICS, such as haloperidol, and phenothiazines may be useful in some patients. (See also CEREBRAL DEGENERATIVE DISORDERS, IRREGULAR SLEEP-WAKE PATTERN.)

Mamelak, M., "Neurodegeneration, Sleep, and Cerebral Energy Metabolism: A Testable Hypothesis," *Journal of Geriatric Psychiatry and Neurology* 10, no. 1 (1997): 29–32.

Weitzman, E.D., "Sleep and Aging," in Katzman, R. and Terry, R.D., *The Neurology of Aging.* Philadelphia: F.A. Davis, 1983. pp. 167–188.

Vitiello, M.V. and Prinz, P.N., "Aging and Sleep Disorders," Williams, R.L., Karacan, I., Moore, C.A., eds., *Sleep Disorders: Diagnosis and Treatment.* New York: John Wiley, 1988. pp. 293–314.

depression Emotional condition characterized by an episode of loss of interest or pleasure in most daytime activities that lasts two weeks or longer. Most patients with depression have sleep disturbance that is accompanied by INSOMNIA or, less commonly, by EXCESSIVE SLEEPINESS. Other associated symptoms include appetite disturbance, weight change, decreased energy, feelings of worthlessness and helplessness, excessive and inappropriate feelings of guilt, difficulty in concentrating and recurrent thoughts of death, with suicidal ideation or attempts.

The characteristic sleep disturbance seen in patients with depression is one of EARLY MORNING AROUSAL, although this does not invariably occur, and particularly not in adolescents, where a prolonged nocturnal sleep period is commonly seen. Other features of depression include a short REM sleep latency on all-night polysomnography as well as an increased REM density.

Depression is one feature of the MOOD DISORDERS. One form of depression recurs at intervals depending upon the seasons of the year and is termed SEASONAL AFFECTIVE DISORDER (SAD). Recently light therapy has been demonstrated to be an effective treatment for this disorder. Depression can also be treated by psychotherapy or ANTIDEPRESSANT medications that include the tricyclic antidepressants, serotonin reuptake inhibitors and MONOAMINE OXIDASE INHIBITORS.

Thase, M.E., "Depression, Sleep, and Antidepressants," *Journal of Clinical Psychiatry* 59, no. 4 (1998): 55–65.

depth encephalography A form of electroencephalography that involves the implantation of electrodes into the brain. This type of EEG is typically performed prior to seizure surgery. By implanting electrodes into the brain, a more precise anatomical site of epilepsy can be obtained. This procedure is reserved for patients who have severe epilepsy and in whom surgical treatment of the epilepsy is indicated. (See also ELECTROENCEPHALOGRAM (EEG), SLEEP-RELATED EPILEPSY.)

desynchronization of circadian rhythms Refers to the loss of synchronized phase relationships between two or more biological rhythms so that, instead, they have their own period lengths. Desynchronization of human CIRCADIAN RHYTHMS occurs when individuals are in TEMPORAL ISOLATION and devoid of any ENVIRONMENTAL TIME CUES. The underlying body temperature rhythm and the sleep-wake cycle initially free run, then reach a point where desynchronization occurs, and each rhythm runs at its own frequency. Typically, the body temperature rhythm will have its own period length of about 24.5 hours, whereas the sleep-wake cycle may have a period length of 33 hours. (See also FREE RUNNING, PERIOD LENGTH.)

desynchronized sleep The sleep stage in which there is little evidence of synchronized ELECTROENCEPHALOGRAM (EEG) patterns so that slow or high amplitude waves are not seen. Typically, desynchronized sleep refers to RAPID EYE MOVEMENT (REM) SLEEP and not NON-REM-STAGE SLEEP. A desynchronized pattern suggests that the coordination of neuronal firing does not occur and that neuronal activity occurs independently throughout the central nervous system. The term *desynchronized sleep* is more often used in ontogenetic or phylogenetic sleep research when other features indicative of REM sleep are not clearly seen, such as rapid eye movements, sawtooth waves or loss of muscle tone. The term *REM sleep* is preferred when applicable. (See also REM PARASOMNIAS, SAWTOOTH WAVES.)

dextroamphetamine See STIMULANT MEDICATIONS.

Diagnostic Classification of Sleep and Arousal Disorders Classification system first published in the journal *Sleep* in 1979 that is the most widely used system in classifying sleep disorders. It was produced by the Diagnostic Classification Committee of the ASSOCIATION OF SLEEP DISORDER CENTERS, chaired by HOWARD ROFFWARG, M.D.

The *Diagnostic Classification of Sleep and Arousal Disorders* divides the sleep and arousal disorders into four major sections: the DISORDERS OF INITIATING AND MAINTAINING SLEEP, the DISORDERS OF EXCESSIVE SOMNOLENCE, the SLEEP-WAKE SCHEDULE DISORDERS, and the PARASOMNIAS.

The phrase "difficulty in initiating and maintaining sleep" was preferred over the term *insomnia* as it indicated that some disorders could produce difficulty in initiating sleep, whereas others might produce a disorder of maintaining sleep. However, it was recognized that some disorders not listed in the "disorders in initiating and maintaining sleep" section could also produce sleep onset insomnia, for example the CIRCADIAN RHYTHM SLEEP DISORDERS. DELAYED SLEEP PHASE SYNDROME typically has a complaint of difficulty in initiating sleep. In addition, some of the parasomnias could occur frequently enough to disrupt sleep at night. However, despite this deficiency, the classification system was felt to be extremely useful in helping physicians understand the differential diagnosis of the causes of insomnia.

The "disorders of excessive somnolence" section of classification includes disorders that produce excessive sleepiness, such as NARCOLEPSY or OBSTRUCTIVE SLEEP APNEA SYNDROME. Disorders in other sections could also contribute to excessive sleepiness, such as delayed sleep phase syndrome or ADVANCED SLEEP PHASE SYNDROME. However, despite the overlap with the sleep-wake schedule disorders, this section was found to be very useful in providing a diagnostic differential listing for consideration of a complaint of excessive sleepiness.

The "circadian rhythm sleep disorders" were listed as a third section because of their common, underlying, pathophysiological mechanisms. This group of disorders was broken down into transient and persistent subgroups. The transient forms include TIME ZONE CHANGE (JET LAG) SYNDROME and SHIFT-WORK SLEEP DISORDER due to their episodic and transient nature. The persistent subgroup included delayed sleep phase syndrome, advanced sleep phase syndrome, and NON-24-HOUR SLEEP-WAKE SYNDROME.

The final section of disorders consists of the "parasomnias"—dysfunctions associated with sleep, sleep stages or partial arousals. This grouping included such disorders as SLEEPWALKING or SLEEP TERRORS, which in themselves do not primarily cause a complaint of insomnia or of excessive daytime sleepiness but rather disrupt or intrude into the sleep-wake process.

The *Diagnostic Classification of Sleep and Arousal Disorders* has been extensively used in the United States and also internationally and has been translated into many different languages. It is highly regarded as a most useful classification system. (The *Diagnostic Classification of Sleep and Arousal Disorders* is reprinted in Appendix IV of this book.)

In 1985, the Association of Sleep Disorder Centers initiated a process for the revision of the *Diagnostic Classification of Sleep and Arousal Disorders* that was produced in early 1990. The newly developed classification is the INTERNATIONAL CLASSIFICATION OF SLEEP DISORDERS (ICSD); it includes not only a revision of the original diagnostic entries but adds those disorders that have been recognized since the first edition, such as the REM SLEEP BEHAVIOR DISORDER. The classification includes more detailed diagnostic and coding information. A minor revision of the ICSD was carried out in 1998.

Diamox See RESPIRATORY STIMULANTS.

diazepam See BENZODIAZEPINES.

diet and sleep Diet can have an important effect on the sleep-wake cycle; however, very few research studies have been performed in this area.

It is well recognized that stimulant drinks or foods, such as coffee or chocolate, can increase daytime alertness and reduce the ease of falling asleep at night. Patients with insomnia find that these agents typically cause them to have greater sleep difficulties and are usually advised to avoid the ingestion of CAFFEINE in any form.

The nighttime snack is believed to aid in sleep onset although the exact mechanism for this effect is unknown. It has been suggested that L-tryptophan (see HYPNOTICS), an important constitute of proteins, is useful in promoting sleep as it is known to be a precursor of SEROTONIN, a neurotransmitter believed to be involved in initiating and maintaining sleep. However, research studies on L-tryptophan have shown a mild effect, if any at all, in persons with insomnia. Furthermore, because of 30 cases in 1989 (including a few deaths) of eosinophilia-myalgia, a rare blood disorder possibly linked to supplements of L-tryptophan, the United States Center for Disease Control (CDC) requested that physicians temporarily stop prescribing L-tryptophan. The effect of the nighttime snack may not be due to its chemical constituents but through stimulation of the gastrointestinal neural pathways, producing a sensation of satiety and relaxation. Food drinks—containing milk products and cereal, such as Ovaltine and Horlicks—are useful in promoting sleep at night.

There is some evidence that the gastrointestinal effects of food ingestion may be mediated through a hormone called CHOLECYSTOKININ (CCK), which is found in both the gastrointestinal tract and the brain. This hormone is released in response to food ingestion, and some studies have shown that the administration of CCK will promote sleep onset.

The effect of carbohydrates compared to proteins in sleep initiation has been disputed. Carbohydrates will allow L-tryptophan to be taken up more readily by the central nervous system and therefore may potentiate L-tryptophan's sleep-inducing effects. Proteins, through their breakdown into amino acids, are believed to increase the catecholamines, which are agents that increase energy. Therefore, based on this biochemical evidence, the suggestion has been that carbohydrates, which initially may induce energy, subsequently have an effect on promoting sleep, whereas proteins will be more liable to increase alertness. The effect of carbohydrates and proteins on alertness and sleepiness appears to vary from person to person. However, a pattern of carbohydrate and protein ingestion is reported to be useful for the treatment of jet lag and has been outlined in the ARGONNE ANTI-JET-LAG DIET, publicized by the Argonne National Laboratory. This diet involves an alternating pattern of feast and fast, and utilizes the stimulating effect of caffeine-containing drinks to alter the timing of sleep.

Large meals are best avoided immediately before sleep as they can produce increased gastrointestinal activity that may lead to disrupted nocturnal sleep. In addition, big meals just before sleep can exacerbate OBSTRUCTIVE SLEEP APNEA SYNDROME by preventing diaphragm action, and are often associated with SLEEP-RELATED GASTROESOPHAGEAL REFLUX. Meals containing spicy foods are also best avoided before sleep because of their stimulating effects.

Several sleep disorders are associated with the excessive ingestion of food or fluid during sleep at night. The NOCTURNAL EATING (DRINKING) SYNDROME is associated with awakenings at night in order to eat food. The desire to eat food becomes overwhelming and the person often cannot stop the behavior. For some people with this syndrome, the majority of the caloric intake is taken in the nighttime hours. Excessive drinking at night is more common in children who are given fluids during the nighttime hours, particularly infants who have frequent nighttime feedings. Sleep enuresis may occur in children, especially infants.

Patients with the Kleine-Levin form of RECURRENT HYPERSOMNIA often eat excessively (megaphagia) during the cyclical periods of excessive sleepiness. This syndrome is characterized by recurrent episodes of sleepiness that last for about two weeks and occur several times each year in association with behavioral disorders, such as hypersexuality and excessive eating.

diffuse activity A term frequently used in electroencephalographic (EEG) recordings to indicate that EEG activity is being recorded from multiple sites on the scalp. The term "nonfocal" is often used synonymously with diffuse activity.

DIMS See DISORDERS OF INITIATING AND MAINTAINING SLEEP (DIMS).

diphenhydramine See ANTIHISTAMINES.

disorders of excessive somnolence (DOES) A category of the DIAGNOSTIC CLASSIFICATION OF SLEEP AND AROUSAL DISORDERS published in the journal *Sleep* in 1979. This group consists of disorders that primarily produce the complaint of inappropriate and undesirable sleepiness during waking hours. The sleepiness may produce impaired mental or work performance, induce a need for daytime NAPS, increase the total amount of sleep in a 24-hour day, increase the length of the major sleep episode or produce a difficulty in achieving full arousal upon awakening. The disorders of excessive somnolence should be differentiated from those disorders that produce tiredness and fatigue without an increased physiological drive for sleep, such as dysthymia, DEPRESSION or chronic illness.

There are 10 major groups among disorders of excessive somnolence that are induced by behavioral, psychological or medical causes, or may be induced by drugs or MEDICATIONS.

The most common cause of EXCESSIVE SLEEPINESS in the general population is insufficient sleep at night; however, other frequent causes of excessive somnolence include the effects of medications, which either disrupt nighttime sleep or induce sleepiness during the day, and psychiatric disorders, such as depression. However, the majority of patients that go to SLEEP DISORDER CENTERS with the complaint of excessive sleepiness have the OBSTRUCTIVE SLEEP APNEA SYNDROME. Respiratory impairment during sleep due to the obstructive sleep apnea syndrome, CENTRAL SLEEP APNEA SYNDROME or CENTRAL ALVEOLAR HYPOVENTILATION SYNDROME are major causes to be considered in any patient presenting with the complaint of excessive sleepiness. PERIODIC LIMB MOVEMENT DISORDER and, rarely, RESTLESS LEGS SYNDROME can also produce daytime sleepiness.

NARCOLEPSY is the most well-known pathological disorder inducing daytime sleepiness. This disorder can be differentiated from IDIOPATHIC HYPERSOMNIA, which has different clinical and polysomnographic features.

Recurrent episodes of sleepiness are seen in RECURRENT HYPERSOMNIA, such as the KLEINE-LEVIN SYNDROME, which is most typically seen in young adults in association with gluttony and hypersexuality. Another disorder that can produce intermittent excessive sleepiness is that related to the MENSTRUAL CYCLE.

Treatment of the disorders of excessive somnolence depends upon the underlying causes and can vary from behavioral techniques, such as extending the amount of time spent in bed at night, to the use of STIMULANT MEDICATIONS in the treatment of narcolepsy. Mechanical devices, such as CONTINUOUS POSITIVE AIRWAY PRESSURE devices, may be used in the treatment of obstructive sleep apnea syndrome.

disorders of initiating and maintaining sleep (DIMS) A group of disorders characterized by the symptom of INSOMNIA. These sleep disorders may result in difficulty getting to sleep, frequent awakenings or arousals during the night, EARLY MORNING AROUSAL or a complaint of NONRESTORATIVE SLEEP.

The term "disorders of initiating and maintaining sleep" was first publicized in the DIAGNOSTIC CLASSIFICATION OF SLEEP AND AROUSAL DISORDERS, published in the journal *Sleep* in 1979. This is one of four categories of sleep disorder in the classification system, and it consists of a list of nine major groups of disorders. The cause of these sleep disorders varies greatly and may be due to behavioral, psychological, psychiatric, or medical factors or may be due to medication and drug effects.

In the population as a whole, the most common disorder among the disorders of initiating and maintaining sleep is that due to an acute stressful event, such as a family, marital, work or other stress. Because this form of insomnia is usually self-limited and lasts only a few days, patients with this type of insomnia usually do not consult sleep disorder specialists or sleep disorder centers.

The most common insomnia disorders that are seen in most sleep disorder centers are either PSYCHOPHYSIOLOGICAL INSOMNIA caused by negative conditioning factors or insomnia due to psychiatric disorders, such as ANXIETY or DEPRESSION. Respiratory impairment can contribute to insomnia by means of CENTRAL SLEEP APNEA SYNDROME or OBSTRUCTIVE SLEEP APNEA SYNDROME. Abnormal limb activities, such as those seen in the PERIODIC LIMB MOVEMENT DISORDER or RESTLESS LEGS SYNDROME, are also causes of difficulty in initiating and maintaining sleep.

One form of insomnia, IDIOPATHIC INSOMNIA, appears to have a primary central nervous system cause, possibly on a genetic basis or due to an acquired subtle abnormality, perhaps in neurotransmitter function.

The treatment of DIMS depends upon the underlying cause of the disorder. For all patients good SLEEP HYGIENE is an essential part of treatment. Specific treatments can range from behavioral treatments of insomnia such as STIMULUS CONTROL THERAPY or SLEEP RESTRICTION THERAPY, to the use of HYPNOTICS or ANTIDEPRESSANTS. Mechanical treatments, such as the use of continuous positive airway pressure devices, may be required for the treatment of obstructive sleep apnea syndrome.

Kales, Anthony and Kales, J.D., *Evaluation and Treatment of Insomnia*. New York: Oxford University Press, 1984.

disorders of the sleep-wake schedule See CIRCADIAN RHYTHM SLEEP DISORDERS.

diurnal Occurring during the day. Opposite of NOCTURNAL.

DOES See DISORDERS OF EXCESSIVE SOMNOLENCE.

dopamine A central nervous system neurotransmitter that has very important effects upon both the cardiovascular and central nervous systems. Dopamine is the immediate metabolic precursor of NOREPINEPHRINE and epinephrine. It has stimulant effects upon the heart, causing an increase in heart rate and blood pressure. Dopamine appears to be involved in the maintenance of wakefulness; however, it may also have a role in REM SLEEP, possibly in its suppression.

Dopamine at low doses promotes sleep; but high doses delay sleep onset and increase wakefulness.

An alteration in dopamine metabolism appears to be present in patients with NARCOLEPSY; consequently, medications that stimulate the production of dopamine may be useful in the treatment of narcolepsy. The central nervous stimulants such as pemoline, methylphenidate and amphetamine have their effect upon narcolepsy through dopamine. L-Tyrosine (see STIMULANT MEDICATIONS), a precursor of dopamine, has been shown to have a beneficial effect on the clinical symptoms of narcolepsy.

Wauquier, A., Clincke, G.H.C., Van Den Broeck, W.A.E. and DePrins, E., "Active and Permissive Roles of Dopamine in Sleep-Wakefulness Regulation," in Wauquier, A., et al., eds., *Sleep Neurotransmittors and Neuromodulators.* New York: Raven Press, 1985. pp. 107–120.

dream anxiety attacks Synonymous with NIGHTMARES, the term was first proposed in the DIAGNOSTIC CLASSIFICATION OF SLEEP AND AROUSAL DISORDERS, published in the journal *Sleep* in 1979, as a means of indicating dreams that occurred in relationship to anxiety at night.

dream content Since classical Greece, DREAMS have been used to gain a better understanding, at first of the world and in the last century, of each individual. SIGMUND FREUD used dreams to try to better understand the conflicts of the patients in his psychoanalytic practice. His monumental work *The Interpretation of Dreams* (1900) spells out his complex ideas on the manifest and latent content of dreams.

Psychologist Carl Gustav Jung in his essay "Approaching the Unconscious" delves into the importance of dreams and dream symbolism. For Jung, dreams were a way to achieve psychological health and to work through daytime conflicts. Jung found Freud's use of free association with dreams too confining and instead he suggested ". . . to concentrate rather on the associations to the dream itself, believing that the latter expressed something specific that the unconscious was trying to say."

Dreams have contained the idea, or the entirety, of some literary works, composed partly or totally during a dream (see DREAMS AND CREATIVITY).

Researchers have discovered that the sex of the dreamer influences dream content. Women tend to have dreams with indoor settings, with less aggression than in male dreams. However, these differences may reflect the learned cultural traits of males and females rather than true gender differences.

Daytime experiences can influence dream content; disturbing dreams are often associated with daytime stress. (See also NIGHTMARES.)

Dement, William C., *Some Must Watch While Some Must Sleep.* New York: W.W. Norton, 1976.

Freud, Sigmund, *The Interpretation of Dreams* (1900), tr. J. Strachey; *The Standard Edition of the Complete Psychological Works of Sigmund Freud,* vols. 4 & 5. London: Hogarth Press, 1953.

Jung, Carl G., "Approaching the Unconscious," in *Man and His Symbols.* New York: Dell, 1968.

dreams Dreams have fascinated mankind since antiquity. For instance, the Bible contains many references to dreams, both in the Old and the New Testament. Aristotle, one of the first to observe that the brain can be very active during sleep, placed little importance upon the role of dreams and suggested that they were a means of eliminating excessive mental activity.

The scientific investigation of dreams began toward the end of the last century. The study by Mary Calkins of Wellesley College in 1893 accurately documented 205 dreams and confirmed the impression that most dreams were recalled from sleep that occurred in the latter third of the night.

The most significant advance in the interpretation of dreams occurred with SIGMUND FREUD's psychodynamic writings on dreams in his initial publication *The Interpretation of Dreams* in 1900.

Wrote Freud: "*The Interpretation of Dreams* is the royal road to a knowledge of the part the unconscious plays in the mental life."

The first major development in the scientific investigation of dreams occurred in 1953 when specific physiological changes were documented during dreaming sleep and REM (rapid eye movement) sleep. This discovery, made by Eugene Aserinsky and NATHANIEL KLEITMAN at the University of Chicago, led to an intense investigation, by electrophysiological means, of the nature of dreams. It became clear that dreams were more vivid and more easily recalled from awakenings out of REM sleep than out of non-REM. Although dreams occur in non-REM sleep, they contain less clarity and tend to be short sequences of vaguely recalled thoughts. The rapid eye movements that occur during REM sleep were initially believed to be related to the dream content and led to the development of the scanning hypothesis. Observations of eye movements under closed or partially opened eyelids were recorded and the subject awoken and interrogated as to the possible eye movements that would have occurred during the dream. By this means, the sequence of eye movements was traced and in some cases was correlated with the actual eye movements observed in the sleeper. This hypothesis has been viewed with skepticism by many researchers in recent years.

The function of dreams has been explored by many researchers. The importance of dreams in the development of a mature central nervous system was originally proposed by HOWARD PHILLIP ROFFWARG. The importance of REM sleep in consolidating learned material was emphasized by Edmond M. Dewan and Ramon Greenberg, and a similar theory has proposed that REM sleep is important in increasing protein synthesis in the central nervous system for the development of learning and memory. Some researchers have taken the opposite approach to explaining dreams in that they believe that dreams eliminate unwanted information from the central nervous system. Dreaming may be important in uncluttering the brain so that new information can be more easily retained in memory.

Many famous people have reported that dreaming was important in their development of great works of art (see DREAMS AND CREATIVITY).

Visual input is important for the development of typical dreaming. People who have been blind from birth do dream but their dreams contain less visual and more auditory content. People who have been rendered blind from an early age after the development of visual input tend to retain the ability to have visual dreams. The question of whether people dream in black and white or color was explored by Calvin Hall, and he determined that approximately 30% of dreams were reported to have vivid color content. The content of dreams is also influenced by the sex of the dreamer. Females tend to have dreams that are more likely to be set indoors and are less aggressive than the dreams of males. However, these differences may be related more to personality differences than to true sex difference.

Dream activity within the cerebral hemispheres is believed by some to occur primarily in the right hemisphere because of the association with the storage of visual memory. Right-hemisphere function in dreaming is supported by reports of patients with right-hemisphere lesions who have a loss of dream recall. However, lesions of the posterior region of the brain affecting either hemisphere are also associated with dream loss.

The ability to dream appears to be present from infancy, and some researchers, such as Howard Roffwarg, have hypothesized that REM sleep is important for normal brain development. Children as young as three years of age report dream content, although it is often difficult to assess whether the reported dream activity is elaborated upon. Young children tend to dream of unpleasant events, such as being chased, and by age four the dream content appears to include more animal dreams. By age five or six, the dreams include ghosts, physical injury and even death.

The content of dreams can be influenced by daytime experiences. Unpleasant dreams are usually associated with daytime psychological stress. Research has attempted to incorporate material into dreams, including using auditory, tactile or visual stimuli. Incorporation of auditory stimuli into dream content is rather poor, occurring in approximately 10% of attempts. If water is sprayed on the face of the dreamer, some content regarding water is found in about 40% of recalled dreams.

Exposure to light flashes can be incorporated into dream content, but only about 20% of the time is it recalled. Experimentation by having patients wear colored glasses throughout the day so that they experience only the color red have led to an increase in the recall of red content in the dreams. Mental activity that occurs immediately prior to the onset of sleep is often incorporated into the dream content.

REM sleep is associated with a number of phasic events of which the eye movement is the most prominent. In animals, ponto-geniculate-occipital (PGO) spikes can be detected by electrodes placed over the cortex. These spikes occur at the onset of REM sleep and are thought to be important in the initiation of the REM sleep state. Various theories have been reported as to the importance of PGO spikes. Some researchers think they may be related to hallucinatory behavior whereas others believe that they may improve brain function by the elimination of unwanted memories.

It has been hypothesized that the human equivalent of PGO spikes is more common in patients with psychiatric disorders characterized by hallucinations, such as schizophrenia. The PGO spikes are generated in the pons of the brain stem, which is believed to be the site of origin for REM sleep. During REM sleep, activity is relayed from the brain stem to the cortex where it is associated with the dreaming. Simultaneously, REM activity passes down the brain stem to the medullary region where stimulation causes an inhibition of the spinal cord motoneurons, leading to the loss of muscle tone during REM sleep. Additional information on the neurophysiology of REM sleep was discovered with the recognition of the syndrome of REM sleep without atonia, which occurs in cats following pontine lesions. In this syndrome, the output from the pons to the medullary inhibitory centers is prevented so that the atonia associated with REM sleep does not occur. Cats with such lesions tend to "act out" their dreams. This suggests that the muscle atonia of REM sleep is a protective mechanism to prevent excessive motor activity during that sleep stage.

In recent years there has been an increased interest in a phenomenon known as LUCID DREAMS where the dreamer is aware of being asleep and of dreaming. It seems almost as if the dreamer is awake and asleep at the same time. Various techniques, such as posthypnotic suggestions and somatic sensory stimulation during REM sleep, have been reported to increase the likelihood of lucid dreaming. It has been suggested that the increased ability to have lucid dreams might be useful in stimulating creativity and might even be useful in controlling NIGHTMARES.

Nightmares are unpleasant dreams that occur in connection with the REM sleep stage. These episodes can be confused with SLEEP TERRORS, in which panic occurs out of slow wave sleep. The nightmare, also known as a dream anxiety attack, produces an abrupt awakening from sleep with recall of frightening dream content. The nightmare sufferer can usually recall in detail the dream content—typically, a threat to the dreamer's safety. Nightmares are more common in the latter third of the night because of the increased likelihood of REM sleep at that time.

NARCOLEPSY, a disorder of excessive sleepiness and characterized by sleep onset REM periods, is also associated with frequent and vivid dreaming, and there may be a slight increase in a tendency for nightmares. The sleep onset dreams of the narcoleptic are often unpleasant. A more extreme form of nightmare activity can occur at sleep onset—TERRIFYING HYPNAGOGIC HALLUCINATIONS; however, these can also occur in people without any obvious precipitating disorder.

The dreaming stage of sleep is associated with penile erections in males. Although sexual dream content is not usually associated with REM SLEEP-RELATED PENILE ERECTIONS, sexual dreams are common in adolescence. Sexual dreams increase the likelihood of a NOCTURNAL EMISSION (wet dream) in which ejaculation occurs in association with the penile erection. Nocturnal emissions are more likely to occur in males who have abstained from sexual activity for a long period of time and are also more common in adolescence.

The dream stage of sleep is a very important sleep stage because of its association with dramatic changes in physiology and the association with nightmares, erectile ability during sleep, REM sleep behavior disorder, narcolepsy, and because of its psychoanalytical significance. Investigation into dreams and their associated pathophysiology is a fertile area of investigation. (See also ALCOHOLISM, DREAM ANXIETY ATTACKS.)

Dement, William C., *Some Must Watch While Some Must Sleep.* New York: W.W. Norton, 1976.

Freud, Sigmund, *The Interpretation of Dreams.* London: Allen & Unwin, 1954.

Hartmann, Ernest, *The Nightmare.* New York: Basic Books, 1984.

Hirshkowitz, M. and Howell, J.W., "Advances and Methodology in the Study of Dreaming," in Williams, R.L., Karacan, I. and Moore, C.A., eds., *Sleep Disorders: Diagnosis and Treatment.* New York: Wiley, 1988. pp. 215–244.

dreams and creativity History includes several examples of artists who have created works while dreaming, or have dreamed the solution to a creative problem they were coping with during the day. For instance, the English artist and poet William Blake stated that, while searching for a less expensive way to do engraving, he dreamed that his deceased brother came to him and suggested that Blake use copper engraving, a method he immediately began to explore. English poet Samuel Taylor Coleridge is reported to have dreamed part of his poem "Kubla Khan."

Other examples, cited in Patricia Garfield's book, *Creative Dreaming,* include Guiseppe Tartini, Italian violinist and composer; anthropologist Hermann V. Hilprecht; German chemist Friedrich A. Kekule, who discovered the molecular structure of benzene in a dream; and English author Robert Louis Stevenson (1850–1894), who wrote that he dreamed the essence of the Dr. Jekyll and Mr. Hyde story. Garfield includes a list of "what we can learn from creative dreamers," including the suggestion that if you have a creative dream, you should ". . . clearly visualize it and record it in some form as soon as possible: write it, paint it, play it, make it. Visualize it while you translate it into a concrete form." (See also DAYDREAMING, DREAM CONTENT and DREAMS.)

Garfield, Patricia, *Creative Dreaming.* New York: Ballantine, 1974.

drowsiness A state of wakefulness characterized by brief episodes of sleep, typically lasting only seconds. The individual is often not aware that sleep is actually occurring and perceives the state as one of tiredness and a strong desire for sleep.

During drowsiness, the ELECTROENCEPHALOGRAM (EEG) records an "alpha dropout" with reduced ALPHA ACTIVITY giving way to low-voltage, mixed slow and fast activity. Slow waves in the range of 2 to 7 hertz occur, often mixed with fast activity of 15 to 25 hertz. As the drowsiness deepens, the electroencephalogram rhythm slows, with more frequent episodes of two to three hertz activity intermixed with brief episodes of return to alpha activity in response to arousing stimuli.

Occasionally, when a person experiences drowsiness, the EEG will show the presence of positive occipital sharp transients of sleep (POSTS) that occur in the occipital regions and are most commonly seen in adolescents and young adults. In addition, transient sharp waves, termed benign epileptiform transients of sleep (BETS), can also be seen.

Drowsiness is a relaxed state that can be considered an intermediary stage between wakefulness and light sleep. During drowsiness, the individual is able to comprehend environmental stimuli and will deny being asleep. Not uncommonly, individuals who are in stage one sleep, which is characterized by loss of alpha activity and reduced appreciation of environmental stimuli, will report that they were in a state of drowsiness and deny being asleep.

Drowsiness occurs naturally prior to sleep onset, but it can also be brought on by medications prescribed specifically for that purpose or as a side effect of a medication prescribed for another purpose, such as for motion sickness, hay fever or colds (see ANTIHISTAMINES). Certain illicit substances, such as heroin or marijuana, may also induce drowsiness.

drowsy driving Term applied to driving a car or truck when not fully alert. The danger of drowsy driving, also referred to as driver fatigue, is that it may lead to falling asleep at the wheel with resultant injuries or even fatalities to the driver, passengers and any other individuals who come into contact with the vehicle which would be out of control due to the sleeping driver. Causes of drowsy driving include sleep deprivation, shift work, certain medications that have sleepiness as a side effect, drinking alcoholic beverages, eating a large meal, especially one that has an excess of carbohydrates, and the soporific effect of highway driving, especially at night. Fifty-one percent of the 1,154 adults surveyed by telephone for the National Sleep Foundation's 2000 poll said that they had actually dozed off while driving drowsy during the previous year. Men were more likely than women to drive drowsy (63% versus 43%) and younger adults were more likely than older adults to drive drowsy (60% of 18-year olds versus 21% of those 65 years and older).

The most common way to deal with drowsy driving, according to the National Sleep Foundation 2000 poll, was to use caffeine (63%). Roughly one of five drivers (22%) said they pulled over to take a nap when they feared their exhaustion might cause them to fall asleep at the wheel.

In recent years, consumer and driver education and public awareness campaigns from the Automobile Association of America as well as sleep associations like the National Sleep Foundation have emerged to get the word out about the hazards of drowsy driving.

drugs See ANTIDEPRESSANTS, ANTIHISTAMINES, BARBITURATES, BENZODIAZEPINES, HYPNOTICS, MONOAMINE OXIDASE INHIBITORS, NARCOTICS, RESPIRATORY STIMULANTS, STIMULANT MEDICATIONS.

dustman See SANDMAN.

dyssomnia A disorder of sleep or wakefulness that is associated with a complaint of difficulty of initiating or maintaining sleep or EXCESSIVE SLEEPINESS. Dyssomnia is used, as opposed to the term PARASOMNIA, which refers to a sleep disorder that occurs during sleep but does not primarily produce a complaint of insomnia or excessive sleepiness.

In the older literature, Nathaniel Kleitman used the term *dyssomnia* to refer to all disorders of sleep and wakefulness, including parasomnias. The term dyssomnia is also used as a major heading in the sleep disorders section of the American Psychiatric Association's section on sleep disorders in the *Diagnostic and Statistical Manual* (DSM-IV). In DSM-IV, dyssomnias refer to any disturbance of sleep and wakefulness other than the parasomnias. In the INTERNATIONAL CLASSIFICATION OF SLEEP DISORDERS, the term dyssomnia refers only to the major (primary) sleep disorders that are associated with insomnia or excessive sleepiness and excludes the secondary (other medical and psychiatric) causes.

E

early morning arousal Term used to denote final awakening that occurs following the major sleep episode at a time earlier than desired. The term is commonly used as synonymous with "premature morning awakening" and is usually associated with underlying DEPRESSION, although it may be caused by other medical or psychiatric disorders, such as DEMENTIA or mania. Early morning arousal may also be due to a CIRCADIAN RHYTHM SLEEP DISORDER, such as ADVANCED SLEEP PHASE SYNDROME, in which the sleep onset time is early and hence the wake time is also early. The early morning arousal is often preceded by numerous brief awakenings before the final awakening. (See also INSOMNIA.)

early morning awakening See EARLY MORNING AROUSAL.

ECOG See ELECTROCORTICOGRAM (ECOG).

EDS See EXCESSIVE SLEEPINESS.

EEG See ELECTROENCEPHALOGRAM (EEG).

Elavil See ANTIDEPRESSANTS.

elderly and sleep Sleep complaints are common in the elderly, usually the inability to fall asleep or to remain asleep; but there can also be complaints of excessive sleepiness during the daytime. Abnormal activity during sleep (particularly movements of the limbs), nightmares and other fears are also common. Old age is a time that is associated with light and unrefreshing sleep.

Sleep in the elderly is characterized by electroencephalographic changes in sleep stages, as well as an increase in the number of awakenings and wakefulness during the major sleep periods.

The amount and percentage of stage one sleep increases. The spindle activity of stage two sleep is reduced, and the total amount of stage three and four sleep is also reduced. The slow wave activity is reduced in amplitude. REM sleep becomes more fragmented and the density of rapid eye movements is reduced in the elderly.

Along with the changes in the polysomnographic features of sleep there is an increase in complaints regarding the quality of sleep, and sleep is bound to be less restful. The number of daytime naps increases and there is a general increase in sleepiness throughout the waking portion of the sleep-wake cycle.

The sleep-wake pattern can become so disrupted that there may be the loss of a definite main nocturnal sleep episode.

Certain sleep disorders become more prevalent in the elderly, particularly SLEEP-RELATED BREATHING DISORDERS and PERIODIC LEG MOVEMENTS. These physiological changes contribute to the sleep disruption and the tendency to increasing daytime sleepiness.

The elderly patient is more likely to request hypnotic medications than a younger patient. HYPNOTICS in the elderly may exacerbate sleep-related breathing disorders and, because of reduced metabolic clearance, there may be an accumulation of the hypnotic, which impairs mental performance. Elderly patients are also more likely to have medical illnesses, including psychiatric illness, factors that can disrupt nighttime sleep. The dementias are often associated with NOCTURNAL CONFUSION, which has been called the sundown syndrome. The sundown syndrome often leads to the elderly patient being placed in a nursing home where appropriate observation and control can be instituted at night.

Electroencephalogram

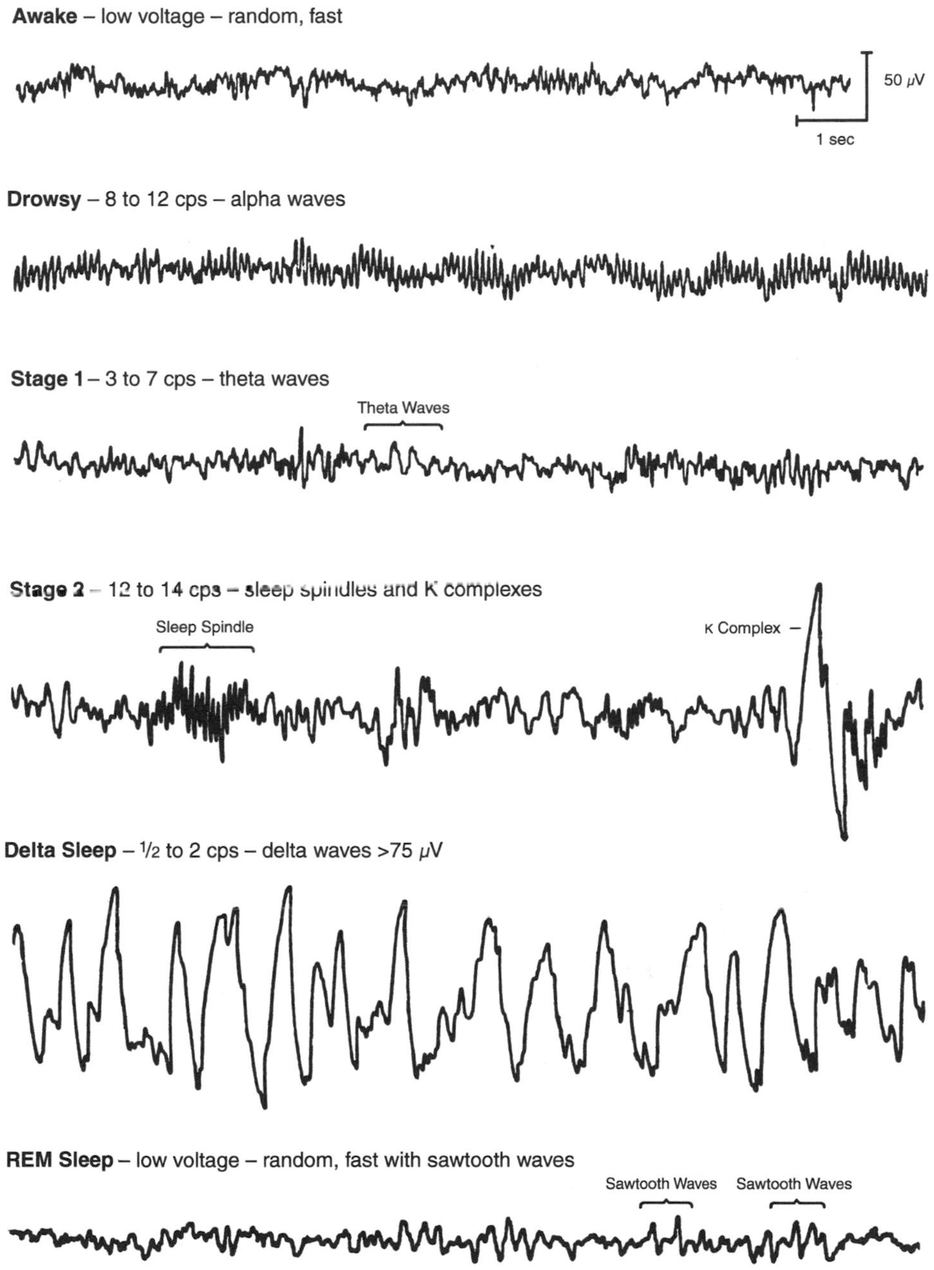

Electroencephalographic characteristics of the human sleep stages. (From Hauri, P.: *Current Concepts: The Sleep Disorders*: Kalamazoo, Michigan: The Upjohn Company, 1982; with permission.)

Medications and alcohol can contribute to this sleep disturbance in the elderly and can add to disruption of the sleep-wake pattern, which may exacerbate mental impairment.

Treatment of sleep disturbance in the elderly rests primarily upon the institution of good SLEEP HYGIENE measures and the institution of treatment for specific sleep disorders. In general, if possible, hypnotics are best avoided.

Case History

A 76-year-old retired insurance broker presented at a sleep disorder center because of excessive daytime sleepiness that appeared to be related to his very disturbed nighttime sleep. He weighed 215 pounds, which was about 45 pounds overweight, and was a loud snorer, although no apneic episodes were noticed during his sleep. He had a lot of activity during sleep, particularly brief twitching movements of his limbs.

He underwent all-night polysomnography, which showed a total sleep time of only 204 minutes with a sleep efficiency of 56%. He did not have any breathing disturbances during sleep but had 510 periodic leg movements, giving an index of 150 per hour of sleep (108 per hour were associated with arousals that were evident on the electroencephalogram during sleep).

In view of the findings, a diagnosis of insomnia due to periodic limb movement disorder was made and the patient was recommended to take the benzodiazepine triazolam, 0.25 milligram half an hour before sleep onset. This medication made a dramatic improvement in the quality of his nighttime sleep and his tendency for daytime sleepiness. In view of the severity of the periodic limb movement disorder, it is likely he will need to continue this medication indefinitely. The dosage can be reduced slightly if he remains free of significant sleep disturbance for about six months. (See also AGE, OBESITY, ONTOGENY OF SLEEP, SLEEP STAGES.)

Morin, E.M., et al., "Nonpharmacological Treatment of Late-Life Insomnia," *Journal of Psychosomatic Research* 42, no. 2(1999): 103–116.

Vitiello, M.V. and Prinz, P.N., "Aging and Sleep Disorders," in Williams, R.L., Karacan, I., and Moore, C.A., eds., *Sleep Disorders: Diagnosis and Treatment.* New York: John Wiley, 1988, pp. 293–314.

electrical status epilepticus of sleep (ESES) An abnormal ELECTROENCEPHALOGRAM pattern that occurs during NON-REM-STAGE SLEEP. This disorder is characterized by continuous, slow-spike-and-wave discharges that occur and persist throughout non-REM sleep. At least 85% of non-REM sleep is occupied by this abnormal pattern. Electrical status epilepticus of sleep does not produce direct clinical features of epilepsy and therefore its name is regarded as slightly inappropriate. It is really an electrical abnormality, rather than a true seizure disorder. However, children with electrical status epilepticus of sleep have significant cognitive and behavioral disorders that are believed to be directly related to the electroencephalographic pattern.

ESES is most often seen in childhood around eight years of age and affects males and females equally. It tends to disappear with increasing age and its duration, although difficult to know exactly, appears to be in terms of months or years. Some children who suffer from ESES also can have more typical epilepsy. Most often, the seizures are a generalized or focal seizure disorder that usually predates the discovery of the ESES.

This disorder appears to be rare although the exact prevalence is unknown. As it was first recognized in 1971 and has only been detected in childhood, it is not known whether a familial pattern exists. Pathological studies have failed to reveal any specific central nervous system abnormality to account for this disorder.

Children may have associated severe language impairment, with reduced mental ability, and impairment of memory and temporo-spatial orientation. There may be reduced attention span, hyperkinesis, aggressiveness and even psychotic states.

The disorder is diagnosed by demonstrating the characteristic electroencephalographic pattern that occurs for more than 85% of the non-REM sleep. This particular pattern does not occur during wakefulness. Sleep organization is generally preserved, with a normal proportion of non-REM and REM sleep. However, the electroencephalographic pattern tends to obscure the more typical features of slow wave sleep so that SPINDLES, K COMPLEXES and vertex transient waves (see VERTEX SHARP TRANSIENTS) are usually indistinguishable.

The abnormal slow wave activity needs to be distinguished from other epileptic disorders, such as BENIGN EPILEPSY WITH ROLANDIC SPIKES (BERS). The benign epilepsy of childhood has clinical seizures that are usually evident, and the electroencephalographic pattern is characterized by frequent spike activity. Although benign epilepsy of childhood commonly occurs during non-REM sleep, it never fills more than 85% of slow wave sleep.

Other seizure disorders, such as the Lennox-Gastaut syndrome, may need to be differentiated. However, this particular form of epilepsy has typical tonic seizures associated with the abnormal electroencephalographic pattern.

Another form of epilepsy associated with language difficulty is called the Landau-Kleffner syndrome. This form of epilepsy is associated with clinical features of epilepsy and a typical electroencephalographic pattern that is localized to one or both temporal lobes.

Electrical status epilepticus of sleep is treated by standard anticonvulsants that include phenytoin. SESE is an acronym for subclinical electrical status epilepticus of sleep, which is synonymous with electrical status epilepticus of sleep.

Patry, G., Lyagoubi, S. and Tassinari, C.A., "Sub-clinical 'Electrical Status Epilepticus' Induced by Sleep in Children," *Archives of Neurology* 24 (1971): 242–252.

electrocorticogram (ECoG) The recording of the electroencephalogram by means of electrodes that are applied on the cortex directly to the surface of the brain. This technique is most often used for detecting the site of intractable seizure activity prior to neurosurgical removal of a lesion.

electroencephalogram (EEG) Recording of the electrical activity of the brain. The term typically applies to measurements made by applying electrodes to the scalp. The electroencephalographic activity is composed of frequencies that are divided into four main groups: those that are below 3.5 per second (DELTA), 4 to 7.5 per second (THETA), 8 to 13 per second (ALPHA) and those above 13 per second (BETA). Sleep electroencephalographic frequencies are usually of the theta or delta range, except that of REM SLEEP which consists of mixed theta and alpha activities. The deepest stage of sleep, SLOW WAVE SLEEP, has EEG activity in the delta range.

EEG waves are also described in terms of their amplitudes. The amplitude of waves detected at the scalp is usually 10 to 100 microvolts (mv). Alpha activity is usually 10 to 20 mv. Beta activity is also low amplitude, rarely exceeding 30 mv. Theta waves can be higher, up to 50 mv, and delta waves are of the highest amplitude, up to 100 mv in children.

The recording is usually on paper, although it is now possible to record on magnetic tape and computer disk. Typically the electroencephalogram is measured along with the ELECTRO-OCULOGRAM and the ELECTROMYOGRAM for the recording of sleep stages and wakefulness. Electrodes for the measurement of the brain activity to document sleep are typically placed at the C3 or C4 positions according to the 10-20 system used throughout the world. Electroencephalograph electrodes can also record other electrical signals that come from the body, such as muscle activity or eye movements.

electromyogram (EMG) The recording of muscle electrical potentials in order to document the level of muscle activity. The electromyogram is usually recorded by a polysomnograph machine, along with the ELECTROENCEPHALOGRAM and ELECTRO-OCULOGRAM, in order to stage sleep. The electrodes for the measurement of the electromyogram are typically placed over the tip of the jaw to record activity in the mentalis muscle. Sometimes electromyographic activity is also recorded from other muscle groups to determine other abnormal activity during sleep. For example, measurements of the masseter muscle activity are useful for determining the presence of BRUXISM (tooth grinding), and activity recorded from the anterior tibialis muscles can document the presence of PERIODIC LEG MOVEMENTS during sleep.

Electromyographic activity recorded in the polysomnogram typically will show an increased level of activation during wakefulness; this decreases as the subject passes through the non-REM sleep stages (see NON-REM-STAGE SLEEP) to the deeper stages of sleep, when the chin muscle activity is very low. In REM SLEEP, electromyographic activity is characterized by a silent background, but with brief phasic muscle activity from most muscle groups. Rarely, background electromyographic activity can be increased in REM sleep in association with REM SLEEP BEHAVIOR DISORDER.

electronarcosis The alteration of the level of consciousness by electrical stimulation is called electronarcosis.

Electronarcotic experiments have been performed on animals since the early 1800s. A current is passed through electrodes that are placed on the neck of the animal. Starting at a rate of 100 pulses per second, a current of one to two milliamperes produces a loss of all motor activity and reflexes. This state can be maintained for several hours and upon termination of the electrical current, the animal immediately recovers.

The first electronarcosis performed on a human was in 1902 by Stephane Armand Nicolas Leduc (1853–1939). Leduc, experimenting on himself, maintained consciousness but speech and movement were lost. The sensation experienced was not unlike a feeling of paralysis that is experienced with dreams (see SLEEP PARALYSIS).

Electronarcosis was used in humans for the treatment of schizophrenia; it was felt to be more beneficial than treating patients with electroconvulsive therapy (ECT). However, electronarcosis can induce cerebral convulsions and ventricular arrhythmias and therefore is no longer regarded as an acceptable form of treatment. (See also ELECTROSLEEP.)

electro-oculogram (EOG) A recording of eye movements by means of changes in the electrical potentials between the retina and the cornea. There is a large potential difference, often over 200 microvolts, between the negatively-charged retina and the positively-charged cornea. Electrodes that are placed lateral to the outer CANTHUS of the eyes record changes in the dipole with movements of the eyes. Measurement of eye movement activity is essential for staging sleep.

In stage one sleep, there are slow rolling eye movements, and the eyes become quiescent (not moving) in deeper stages of non-REM sleep. REM SLEEP is characterized by rapid eye movement. Rapid eye movements similar to those seen in REM sleep can be seen during wakefulness, and the measurement of other physiological variables, such as the EEG and EMG, help in the differentiation of REM sleep from wakefulness. (See also SLEEP STAGES.)

electrosleep A form of SLEEP THERAPY that involves the induction of sleep by means of an electric current. A pulsating current lasting 0.2 to 0.3 millisecond, of voltage 0.5 to 2.5 and milliamperage of 0.2 to 1.5, has been recorded as being effective in inducing sleep in animals. When the current is terminated, sleep continues. It is believed that electrosleep is more effectively produced when low doses of hypnotics, such as the barbiturates or benzodiazepines, are given concurrently. Electrosleep has been used in the course of sleep therapy for treatment of a variety of medical disorders such as schizophrenia. This form of treatment is widely practiced in Eastern European countries, and there are differing opinions on its usefulness. (See also ELECTRONARCOSIS.)

EMG See ELECTROMYOGRAM (EMG).

encephalitis lethargica A disease suspected to be of viral cause, first reported in 1917. It affected thousands of people until 1927, when the disease gradually disappeared. Encephalitis lethargica produced inflammation of various portions of the brain, including the brain stem and hypothalamus. It was most prevalent in Vienna and France spreading to Western Europe and England.

The primary features of this disorder were stupor, excessive sleepiness, disturbed sleep at night and the development of features of Parkinsonism, with generalized rigidity and abnormal movements.

Constantin Von Economo (1876–1931) extensively studied patients with encephalitis lethargica and recognized three different sleep patterns: EXCESSIVE SLEEPINESS, INSOMNIA and REVERSAL OF SLEEP. He studied the pathology and determined that insomnia primarily occurred in those patients who had basal forebrain lesions whereas excessive sleepiness appeared to result from posterior hypothalamus lesions. Although features typical for NARCOLEPSY and CATAPLEXY have been reported in association with encephalitis lethargica, the development of true narcolepsy by encephalitis lethargica is questioned.

Other features of encephalitis lethargica included immobility of the eye muscles and oculogyric crises (bizarre, uncontrollable eye movements).

In recent years, encephalitis lethargica has rarely been reported, and polysomnographic testing has not been performed. However, the electroencephalogram has shown generalized slowing. There is no known treatment for the primary illness, and the features have to be treated symptomatically.

Von Economo, C., *Encephalitis Lethargica: Its Sequelae and Treatment.* London: Oxford University Press, 1931.

———, "Sleep as a Problem of Localization," *Journal of Nervous and Mental Disease* 71 (1930): 249–259.

endogenous circadian pacemaker An internal mechanism that triggers the periodic processes that are involved in the human circadian timing system, this structure controls the timing of various rhythmical processes in the body, such as the sleep-wake cycle, that have a cycle of approximately 24 hours. The site of the pacemaker appears to be the SUPRACHIASMATIC NUCLEUS at the base of the third ventricle in the hypothalamus of the brain. The endogenous circadian pacemaker is also known as the X-oscillator, the type-1 oscillator, the "C" process and the endogenous rhythm.

The endogenous circadian pacemaker appears to have a very stable periodicity that controls the timing of the CIRCADIAN RHYTHMS in the free-running condition. A number of physiological parameters, including the core-body temperature, cortisol release, REM sleep propensity, urinary potassium excretion, alertness, and cognitive and psychomotor performance, are all driven by the endogenous circadian pacemaker.

endogenous circadian phase assessment Term describing a means of determining the rhythm of the ENDOGENOUS CIRCADIAN PACEMAKER as illustrated by changes in the body TEMPERATURE. The CONSTANT ROUTINE method can be used for determining the circadian phase of the body temperature and allowing one to compare the circadian phase of one individual with the circadian phases of others. (See also CIRCADIAN RHYTHMS, PHASE SHIFT.)

endogenous rhythm See ENDOGENOUS CIRCADIAN PACEMAKER.

endoscopy A procedure whereby an observation can be made anywhere inside the body. In sleep disorders medicine, endoscopy commonly is performed in patients who have UPPER AIRWAY OBSTRUCTION in order to determine the site of that obstruction. A fiberoptic endoscope (see FIBEROPTIC ENDOSCOPY) is placed through the nose so that an observer can view the tissues of the nose and upper airway. This procedure can be performed not only on the awake patient but also on a patient who is asleep or under anesthesia. SOMNOENDOSCOPY is the term applied to the endoscopic evaluation of the upper airway in the sleeping patient. This procedure is rarely performed in patients with OBSTRUCTIVE SLEEP APNEA SYNDROME in order to determine the site of upper airway obstruction, because the presence of the endoscope is usually too uncomfortable to allow the patient to sleep. Endoscopy performed in the awake patient is a more common procedure.

end-tidal carbon dioxide Term referring to the measurement of the carbon dioxide value in expired air, which reflects the level of carbon dioxide in the lung alveoli. "End-tidal" refers to the end, or last portion, of the resting breath (TIDAL VOLUME). This value is normally detected by means of sampling air from the nostrils at the end of the expiration. The gas is analyzed by means of an infrared gas analyzer.

In addition to providing accurate measurements of alveolar carbon dioxide levels, the resultant tracing can also be used as an accurate measure of ventilation. The measurement of carbon dioxide values is most useful in determining impairment of gas exchange in the lungs, and this can give important information on lung function or ventilatory ability.

(See also SLEEP-RELATED BREATHING DISORDERS, SLEEP APNEA.)

enuresis, sleep-related See SLEEP ENURESIS.

environmental sleep disorder A sleep disorder that has its roots in a disturbing environmental condition that produces a complaint of INSOMNIA or EXCESSIVE SLEEPINESS. Light and environmental noise are typical causes. Usually the sleep disorder is resolved when the environmental disturbance is eliminated.

environmental time cues Environmental factors that influence a pattern of behavior, such as the sleep-wake cycle, and help to maintain regular 24-hour periodicity. Maintenance of a 24-hour sleep-wake cycle is dependent upon environmental time cues occurring prior to the onset of the major sleep episode and also at the time of awakening. Such time cues include alarm clocks, light stimuli, social interaction and noise stimulus. In an environment free of environmental time cues, an individual may free run with a sleep-wake cycle that is longer than 24 hours, typically 25 hours, causing the individual to fall asleep one hour later and arise one hour later on a daily basis. This FREE RUNNING pattern of sleep and wakefulness causes the sleep-wake pattern to occur out of synchrony with that of most other people. The German term *zeitgeber* is synonymous with environmental time cues. (See also CHRONOBIOLOGY, CIRCADIAN RHYTHM SLEEP DISORDERS, NON-24-HOUR SLEEP-WAKE SYNDROME, NREM-REM SLEEP CYCLE.)

EOG See ELECTRO-OCULOGRAM (EOG).

epilepsy Epileptic seizures may disturb sleep and, if they occur frequently enough, may be a cause of daytime sleepiness. Sometimes the medications used for epilepsy, such as phenobarbitol, can contribute to daytime sleepiness. SLEEP DEPRIVATION is a known precipitant of epileptic seizures. Most seizures, if they occur during sleep, occur during the non-REM sleep stages. Rarely do seizures occur during REM sleep. A particular type of epilepsy called benign focal epilepsy of childhood (Rolandic epilepsy) has a marked tendency to occur during sleep. In some patients, SLEEP TERRORS or SLEEPWALKING episodes may need to be distinguished from epileptic seizures. (See also RAPID EYE MOVEMENT SLEEP.)

epoch A measure of sleep activity used in order to stage sleep (see SLEEP STAGES); typically epochs are 20- to 30-second samples of sleep that have been recorded by POLYSOMNOGRAPHY. Epochs often reflect the recording speed of the polysomnograph, and refer to a single page of recording; polysomnograph recordings performed at 15 millimeters per second will typically produce a 20-second epoch on standard EEG paper, whereas recordings performed at 10 millimeters per second will produce 30-second epochs on standard EEG paper. A typical polysomnographic recording of sleep will produce approximately 1,000 epochs of sleep at the standard 10 millimeters per second recording rate.

Epworth Sleepiness Scale (ESS) A questionnaire that is used to assess whether someone is suffering from excessive daytime sleepiness. Eight questions are asked and you rank on a scale of 0 to 3 your chance of dozing in those situations (0+ would never doze; 1=slight chance of dozing; 2=moderate chance of dozing; and 3=high chance of dozing).

Situation	Chance of Dozing
1. Sitting and reading	________
2. Watching television	________
3. Sitting inactive in a public place such as a theater or a meeting	________
4. As a passenger in a car for an hour without a break	________
5. Lying down to read in the afternoon	________
6. Sitting and talking to someone	________
7. Sitting quietly after lunch (when you've had no alcohol)	________
8. In a car, when stopped for traffic	________

A score of less than 8 means you're not suffering from excessive daytime sleepiness. A score of 10 or more means that you are more sleepy than you should be and may need to think more about your sleep. A score of 15 or more means that you should discuss the results of this test and your sleep-related symptoms with your physician.

Murray W. Johns, M.D. developed the Epworth Sleepiness Scale at the Sleep Center at Epworth Hospital in Melbourne, Australia.

Equalizer A trade name for a dental appliance that is inserted in the mouth for the treatment of SNORING. This device consists of two fine tubes attached to the mouthpiece to allow air to be sucked through the mouth to the hypopharynx. The Equalizer prevents a negative suction effect from occurring in the upper airway, so obstruction does not occur. It is not particularly useful for the treatment of OBSTRUCTIVE SLEEP APNEA SYNDROME, but can be effective in some patients who have primary (benign) snoring.

erections during sleep Penile erections typically occur during sleep in all healthy males from infancy to old age. Erections are associated with REM SLEEP, not usually with sexual dreams. The erections occur during each of the episodes of REM sleep and can last up to 20 minutes. The presence of penile erections during sleep helps differentiate IMPOTENCE due to psychogenic causes from that due to physical causes, such as a neurological or vascular disorder. (See also IMPAIRED SLEEP-RELATED PENILE ERECTIONS, SLEEP-RELATED PAINFUL ERECTIONS.)

erratic hours Term applied to varied SLEEP ONSET and WAKE TIMES. Alterations in the time of going to bed at night, and of awakening in the morning, are common precipitating factors in the development of INSOMNIA. Regularity in going to bed and awakening is a key element of good SLEEP HYGIENE.

People who develop insomnia often find that their times of going to bed and awakening start to vary greatly. The insomniac will typically go to bed earlier some nights to catch up on sleep lost the night before, and typically will stay in bed later on some mornings, if there has been an inadequate amount of sleep, in the hope that more sleep will be obtained. However, some nights, because of the feeling of being wide awake, the insomniac may go to bed later than usual; and on some days, because of awakening early due to the insomnia, the patient may arise earlier than usual. Therefore the sleep episodes are spread out over at least a 10-hour period. There is a breakdown of the ENVIRONMENTAL TIME CUES that are essential for the maintenance of a stable sleep-wake pattern, in part because of the effect of disrupted sleep on underlying CIRCADIAN RHYTHMS. An essential element in treatment of patients with insomnia is to ensure that sleep does not occur before a set time at night, for example 11 P.M., or after a set time in the morning, such as 7 A.M. Ensuring that all sleep occurs between appropriate limits of no longer than eight hours helps develop a stable sleep-wake cycle.

Maintaining regular sleep onset and wake times is an important element of STIMULUS CONTROL THERAPY for insomnia, as well as SLEEP RESTRICTION THERAPY. (See also IRREGULAR SLEEP-WAKE PATTERN.)

ESES See ELECTRICAL STATUS EPILEPTICUS OF SLEEP (ESES).

esophageal pH monitoring Episodes of gastroesophageal reflux of acid can be detected by means of a stomach pH-sensitive electrode, which is passed by means of a polyurethane tube through the nose into the lower esophagus. The electrode is connected to a strip chart recorder so that continuous measurements of pH changes can be detected throughout sleep and often for a 24-hour period. (See also SLEEP-RELATED GASTROESOPHAGEAL REFLUX.)

esophageal reflux Term applied to the regurgitation of gastric contents into the esophagus. Esophageal reflux typically occurs in individuals who have some incompetence of the gastroesophageal sphincter between the esophagus and the stomach. This incompetence may be due to a hiatus hernia. Patients with OBSTRUCTIVE SLEEP APNEA SYNDROME are more likely to have esophageal reflux during the struggle to breathe that is associated with apneic events. This reflux may cause an awakening from sleep and produce gagging or COUGHING, sometimes associated with laryngospasm. (See SLEEP-RELATED GASTROESOPHAGEAL REFLUX, SLEEP-RELATED LARYNGOSPASM.)

ethchlorvynol (Placidyl) See HYPNOTICS.

European Sleep Research Society Founded in 1971, the European Sleep Research Society is the first international sleep society to be formed outside of the United States. Like the ASSOCIATION FOR THE PSYCHOPHYSIOLOGICAL STUDY OF SLEEP, founded in 1961 in the United States, the European Sleep Research Society is devoted to promoting sleep research and the development of clinical sleep disorders medicine. The European Sleep Research Society was one of four international societies that jointly sponsored the bimonthly journal *SLEEP*, published by Raven Press. The European Sleep Research Society now has its own journal, *The Journal of Sleep Research*, published by Blackwell Press in the United Kingdom. (See also ASSOCIATION OF PROFESSIONAL SLEEP SOCIETIES, LATIN AMERICAN SLEEP RESEARCH SOCIETY and JAPANESE SLEEP RESEARCH SOCIETY.)

evening person (night person) An individual who prefers to go to bed later, and arise later, than is typical for the general population. Such persons have a delay in their sleep phase, and the pattern of body TEMPERATURE and other circadian rhythms is delayed. An evening person is sometimes referred to as a "night owl." (See also ADVANCED SLEEP PHASE SYNDROME, DELAYED SLEEP PHASE SYNDROME, MORNING PERSON, OWL AND LARK QUESTIONNAIRE.)

evening shift Work shift from about 3 P.M. to 11 P.M. that is before the NIGHT SHIFT.

excessive daytime sleepiness See EXCESSIVE SLEEPINESS.

excessive sleepiness The inability to remain awake during the awake portion of an individual's sleep-wake cycle (see NREM-REM SLEEP CYCLE). Excessive sleepiness is synonymous with EXCESSIVE DAYTIME SLEEPINESS (or EDS) and somnolence but is the preferred term.

Excessive sleepiness may be present at night for an individual who has the major sleep period occurring during the day, for example, a shift worker. Excessive sleepiness may be reported subjectively or be quantified by means of electrophysiological measurements of sleep tendency. Tests that can quantify excessive sleepiness include the MULTIPLE SLEEP LATENCY TEST, the MAINTENANCE OF WAKEFULNESS TEST, PUPILLOMETRY and VIGILANCE TESTING. Subjective rating scales, such as the STANFORD SLEEPINESS SCALE (SSS) and the EPWORTH SLEEPINESS SCALE (ESS), are often used to determine a subject's level of sleepiness.

The causes of excessive sleepiness range from OBSTRUCTIVE SLEEP APNEA SYNDROME to NARCOLEPSY, TIME ZONE CHANGE (JET LAG) SYNDROME or INSOMNIA. The sleepiness can be caused by an ADJUSTMENT SLEEP DISORDER related to a temporary stressful event, such as illness or death in the family, midterm or final exams at school or anxiety about a particular crisis at work. The insomnia and the excessive sleepiness related to that insomnia clears up as soon as the interim situation is resolved.

Excessive sleepiness can also be chronic, such as that seen in children or adolescents suffering from DELAYED SLEEP PHASE SYNDROME so that every day, especially during the school week, they get too little sleep and are tired the next day.

Adults who suffer from INSUFFICIENT SLEEP SYNDROME may have a chronic problem with excessive sleepiness that has a negative impact on their health, career success or social relationships.

The consequences of excessive sleepiness may include mild to severe fatigue, crankiness, depression and reduced concentration, or even such catastrophic consequences as fatigue-related driving accidents (DROWSY DRIVING) as well as industrial or home ACCIDENTS.

El-Ad, B., et al., "Disorders of Excess in Daytime Sleepiness—An Update," *Journal of Neurological Science* 153, no. 2 (1998): 192–202.

exercise and sleep Exercise can increase or reduce the quality of sleep, or have no effect at all.

It is well recognized that intense exercise performed immediately before sleep will impair the ability to fall asleep. The increased autonomic system activation produced by the exercise increases AROUSAL and therefore sleep onset will be delayed. Good SLEEP HYGIENE includes avoiding intense exercise before going to bed at night.

However, a relaxing exercise, such as yoga, may be beneficial to sleep by reducing muscle tension. Mild relaxing exercises, such as those recommended by Edmund Jacobson, can be beneficial and are a well-recommended form of relaxation therapy (see JACOBSONIAN RELAXATION).

There are differing opinions on the role of daytime exercise in improving the quality of nighttime sleep. Initial reports have demonstrated that intense daytime exercise will increase the amount of SLOW WAVE SLEEP at night; however, this increase appears to occur only in trained athletes. Initially it was suggested that exercise by means of producing wear and tear on the tissues would lead to enhanced deep sleep as a restorative process. However, there is no evidence that deep sleep is restorative after exercise, and studies with invalids on complete bed rest show little difference in the amount of slow wave sleep present compared with more active populations.

The role of exercise in improving slow wave sleep in trained individuals is also controversial as there are some who believe that the increase is due to an increase in body TEMPERATURE. Trained athletes on sustained exercise are more liable to produce an increase in their core body temperature compared with unfit individuals. Other studies looking at the effects of body heating by artificial means have demonstrated that slow wave sleep can be increased in the absence of exercise. (See also SLEEP EXERCISES.)

Manfredini, R., et al., "Circadian Rhythms, Athletic Performance, and Jet Lag," *British Sports Medicine* 32, no. 2 (1998): 101–106.

exhaustion A state of extreme mental or physical fatigue. Exhaustion is not synonymous with EXCESSIVE SLEEPINESS. Persons can become exhausted from mental strain and feel a tiredness and weakness that has nothing to do with an increased physiological drive for sleep. Similarly, a form of exhaustion can occur following exercise where fatigue occurs; however, acute sudden exercise can lead to a state of relaxation that will allow an underlying drive for sleep to become manifest. For example, someone who is slightly sleepy, due to an insufficient quality or amount of sleep, may sleep during the day following exercise as the exercise causes him or her to become relaxed and sleep occurs.

exploding head syndrome Disorder in which an awakening is accompanied by a sensation of an explosion having gone off in the head. This disorder typically occurs in the elderly. The sensation causes intense fear but no pain. The syndrome mainly occurs in women with no neurological or psychiatric disorder. The moment the sufferer is awake, the sensation is gone, but the syndrome causes anxiety, rapid heart rate and sweating; there is usually a concern that one has had a stroke, or that it is a sign of an intracerebral tumor.

No known cause is evident for the disorder; however, disinhibition of the connection between the inner ear and the brain has been proposed as an explanation.

This syndrome does not require a specific treatment other than reassurance. (See also SLEEP-RELATED HEADACHES.)

Pearce, J.M.S., "Exploding Head Syndrome," *Lancet* 11 (1988): 270–271.

extrinsic sleep disorders Sleep disorders that originate, develop or arise from causes outside of the body. Examples of extrinsic sleep disorders include environmental sleep disorder, ADJUSTMENT SLEEP DISORDER and ALTITUDE INSOMNIA. Removal of the external factor usually resolves the sleep disturbance unless another sleep problem develops in the interim. For example, PSYCHOPHYSIOLOGICAL INSOMNIA may occur after the removal of the external factor, such as stress, that caused the development of an adjustment sleep disorder, so the person becomes conditioned to insomnia. This group of disorders is one of three subcategories of dyssomnias in the American Sleep Disorder Association's INTERNATIONAL CLASSIFICATION OF

SLEEP DISORDERS. (The other two subcategories are INTRINSIC SLEEP DISORDERS and CIRCADIAN RHYTHM SLEEP DISORDERS.)

eye movements Typically recorded for the detection of sleep stages. Usually, awake persons will have rapid eye movements; these slow during DROWSINESS so that slow eye movements are a common feature of STAGE ONE SLEEP. The eyes become quiescent during SLOW WAVE SLEEP. The REM stage of sleep (see REM SLEEP) is characterized by rapid eye movements that are similar to those seen during wakefulness.

The eye movement activity, in conjunction with the ELECTROENCEPHALOGRAM pattern and ELECTROMYOGRAM, is one of the three main physiological variables that are recorded during POLYSOMNOGRAPHY.

F

Factor S A substance discovered in the cerebrospinal fluid that appears to have a sleep-inducing effect. In 1913, Henri Pieron reported that substances accumulating in the spinal fluid have sleep-inducing properties. Pieron took spinal fluid from sleep-deprived dogs and injected it into the brain ventricles of normal dogs and found that it could induce sleep for up to 15 hours. Cerebrospinal fluid taken from non-sleep-deprived dogs did not have a similar effect. This sleep-inducing substance was subsequently isolated from huge amounts of human urine (4.5 tons). Factor S was found to consist of three amino acids—glutamic, alanine and diaminopimelic—and the sugar, muriac acid. Therefore, Factor S appears to be a small glucopeptide that has been identified as a muramylpeptide. Muramylpeptides are found in the cell walls of bacteria and plants, but are not substances that are present in human cells. It has been suggested that the production of muramylpeptide comes from bacteria that are taken in with food and then synthesized into Factor S (see MURAMYL DIPEPTIDES).

Factor S induces an increase in SLOW WAVE SLEEP when infused in rabbits. It also increases body TEMPERATURE, an effect that is thought to be due to the production of INTERLEUKIN-I. (See also DELTA SLEEP-INDUCING PEPTIDE, SLEEP-INDUCING FACTORS.)

Pappenheimer, J.L., Miller, T.B. and Goodrich, C.A., "Sleep-Promoting Effects of Cerebrospinal Fluid From Sleep-deprived Goats," *Proceedings of the National Academy of Science* 58 (1967): 513–517.

family bed The practice of having an infant or child sleep in bed with its mother, father or both parents. Advocates of the family bed emphasize that it helps promote bonding among child and parents as well as promoting an adult-type sleep-wake cycle. In the early months or years, if a mother is breast-feeding, it can minimize the disruption to her sleep if she just turns to the nearby infant for a feeding, rather than going into another room. However, infants have died because the sleeping parent has accidentally smothered the child.

The child sleep expert Richard Ferber advises against letting a child sleep with a parent, except for a night or two when a child is ill or temporarily upset. As a general rule, however, a separate bed offers the child the opportunity to develop independence. Children as young as two or three may find a family bed offers intimacy with their parents that is excessive and overstimulating. Ferber also cautions against allowing a child into a parent's bed because one parent is away, on a business trip out of town, for example.

Ferber suggests that if there are temporary or long-term circumstances that necessitate a child sleeping in a parent's room—there is only one bedroom, grandparents have taken over the child's room or the family is away and sharing a hotel room—the child should be given his or her own place to sleep, even if it is a mattress on the floor in the corner of the room. If possible, use curtains to close off that area.

If a child enters a parent's bed in the middle of the night, the parent should carry, or walk, the child back to his or her own room. If the child has difficulty falling asleep, the parent could comfort the child till sleep occurs, or just sit in a nearby chair, rather than allowing a return to the parent's bed. (See also BEDS, INFANT SLEEP, INFANT SLEEP DISORDERS.)

Ferber, Richard, *Solve Your Child's Sleep Problems*. New York: Simon & Schuster, 1985.

fast sleep See REM SLEEP.

fatal familial insomnia A rare disorder, primarily seen in people of Italian descent, characterized by a severe insomnia associated with degeneration of the central nervous system; it is ultimately fatal. This disorder is associated with abnormalities of the autonomic neurological system that produce symptoms of insomnia, temperature changes, excessive salivation, excessive sweating and rapid heart and breathing rates.

Fatal familial insomnia has insomnia persistent throughout the course of the disorder. As the autonomic symptoms develop, sleep becomes more disrupted and there is usually development of other neurological features; dysarthria, tremors, muscle jerks (myoclonus) and dystonic posturing can occur. The patient has a deteriorating level of mental alertness and frequently lapses from wakefulness into sleep. Often there can be an "acting out" of dreams during sleep. The disorder leads to coma and finally to death.

Fatal familial insomnia is a prion disease which primarily occurs in adults between the fifth and sixth decades of life, affecting males and females equally. It appears to have a familial transmission as several members of one family with the disease have been reported.

Polysomnographic investigations in the early stages of this disease generally show severely disrupted sleep patterns with wakefulness intervening between short episodes of sleep. There is very disrupted REM SLEEP with maintenance of muscle tone and abnormal movements associated with DREAMS. Slow wave sleep diminishes and becomes absent during the course of the disease. The electroencephalogram gradually becomes less reactive to environmental stimuli and progressively decreases in amplitude until death.

Fatal familial insomnia needs to be differentiated from other forms of degenerative neurological disease such as Creutzfeldt-Jakob disease, which is characterized by a progressive deteriorating dementia and myoclonic jerks. Other forms of dementia, such as Alzheimer's disease, are relatively easily distinguished from fatal familial insomnia. The abnormal movements that occur during REM sleep are similar to those seen in REM SLEEP BEHAVIOR DISORDER, which does not have a progressively deteriorating course. Other sleep stages are generally intact in the REM sleep behavior disorder, whereas in fatal familial insomnia, loss of stage three and four sleep, and a severely disrupted sleep pattern, are characteristic.

No treatment is known to affect the course of the underlying disorder. (See also CEREBRAL DEGENERATIVE DISORDERS, DEMENTIA, NOCTURNAL PAROXYSMAL DYSTONIA.)

Lugaresi, E., Midori, R., Montagna, P. et al., "Fatal Familial Insomnia and Dysautonomia with Selective Degeneration of Thalmic Nuclei," *New England Journal of Medicine* 315 (1986): 997–1003.

fatigue A state of reduced efficiency due to prolonged or excessive exertion. Fatigue needs to be differentiated from EXCESSIVE SLEEPINESS, which is a state of increased drive for sleep. The term "fatigue" is often erroneously interpreted as meaning sleepy; however, individuals can be severely fatigued without the ability to fall asleep during a day of usual wakefulness. The state of EXHAUSTION is similar to fatigue and indicates primarily a mental rather than a muscular form of fatigue.

femoxetine See ANTIDEPRESSANTS.

Ferber, Richard A graduate magna cum laude of Harvard College in chemistry and physics in 1965, and of Harvard Medical School in 1970. From 1970 to 1971 and 1973 to 1979, Dr. Ferber (1944–) trained at the Children's Hospital Medical Center in Boston as pediatric intern and resident, psychiatry research fellow, and pediatric fellow in psychosomatic medicine. In 1978, he cofounded the Center for Pediatric Sleep Disorders, where he has been director since 1979. Affiliated with Harvard Medical School since 1973, he is currently an associate professor of neurology. Since that time, he has helped to describe and characterize sleep disorders in children, and to develop new methods of evaluation and treatment. Dr. Ferber's major research interests include behavioral aspects of sleep disorders in children, sleep apnea in children, chronobiological sleep disorders in children and parasomnias in children.

Chesson, A.L. Jr., Ferber, R.A., Fry, J.M., Grigg-Damberger, M., Hartse, K.M., Hurwitz, T.D., Johnson, S., Kader, G.A., Littner, M., Rosen, G., Sangal, R.B., Schmidt-Nowara, W. and Sher, A., "The Indications for Polysomnography and Related Procedures," *Sleep* 20 (1997): 423–487.

Ferber, R., "Sleep Disorders of Childhood," in Chokroverty, S. and Daroff, B.B., eds., *Sleep Disorders Medicine.* Boston: Butterworth-Heinemann, 1999. pp. 683–696.

———. *Solve Your Child's Sleep Problems.* New York: Simon & Schuster, 1985.

Ferber, R. and Kryger, M., eds., *Principles and Practice of Sleep Medicine in the Child.* Philadelphia: W.B. Saunders, 1995.

fiberoptic endoscopy Otolaryngological procedure typically performed in sleep medicine for the evaluation of the upper airway. The procedure involves passing a fiberoptiscope through the nose and into the pharynx and hypopharynx for the visualization of lesions in the upper airway. The fiberoptic endoscope, which is a few millimeters in diameter, is a flexible tube that can allow an experienced individual to observe the pharynx by means of the light transmitted in the optical fibers of the device. This procedure is commonly performed in patients with OBSTRUCTIVE SLEEP APNEA SYNDROME in order to determine the site of upper airway obstruction.

Some examiners perform a test called a muller maneuver while the fiberoptiscope is in place in order to observe movement of the tissues of the upper airway. This maneuver is performed by closing the mouth and nares and having the patient inspire so that a negative pressure is exerted on the upper airway, thereby causing its collapse. This procedure has been reported to be helpful in the evaluation of the site of upper airway obstruction and in predicating a patient's response to UVULOPALATOPHARYNGOPLASTY. CEPHALOMETRIC RADIOGRAPHS are often employed along with fiberoptic endoscopy in the evaluation of the upper airway changes in patients with obstructive sleep apnea syndrome. (See also SURGERY AND SLEEP DISORDERS.)

Sher, A.E., Thorpy, Michael J., Shprintzen, R.J., Spielman, Arthur J., Burrack, B. and McGregor, P.A., "Predictive Value of Muller Maneuver in Selection of Patients for Uvulopalatopharyngoplasty," *Laryngoscope* 95 (1985): 1483–1487.

fibromyositis syndrome See FIBROSITIS SYNDROME.

fibrositis syndrome Syndrome characterized by diffuse, nonspecific muscle aches and pains that are typically associated with complaints of unrefreshing sleep at night. The musculoskeletal symptoms are not due to any articular, nonarticular or metabolic disease.

The sleep disturbance is one of frequent arousals and brief awakenings and a feeling upon awakening in the morning of being unrefreshed. There may be discomfort in the muscles and joints during the night and morning stiffness upon awakening. Tiredness, fatigue and, rarely, sleepiness may be present during the daytime. An increased prevalence of periodic limb movements has also been described.

There is a specific pattern to the muscular discomfort, which primarily affects the muscles of the neck and shoulders. The upper border of the trapezius, the muscles in the neck, the lumbar spine muscles and the mid-lateral thigh are particularly sensitive to pressure. The muscle discomfort is rapid in onset and becomes chronic. Usually the onset of the disorder occurs in early adulthood, although it may present for the first time in the elderly. It is more common in females.

Patients often go through intensive investigations for other forms of rheumatic disorders, such as rheumatoid arthritis, systemic lupus erythematosis or osteoarthritis, without diagnostic features of these disorders being found.

Polysomnographic investigations show a characteristic pattern of alpha sleep in which ALPHA ACTIVITY occurs superimposed on other sleep stages. When this pattern occurs during slow wave sleep it is often termed ALPHA-DELTA ACTIVITY. The sleep stages are otherwise normal in percentage; however, there may be an increased number of brief awakenings and arousals. Patients usually lack evidence of pathological daytime sleepiness.

There is no clear cause or pathology found to explain the discomfort.

Fibrositis syndrome must be differentiated from other rheumatic disorders. When the sleep disturbance is prominent, other causes of nonrestorative sleep need to be distinguished, such as psychophysiological insomnia or insomnia due to psychiatric disorders. Sleep disturbances due to dysthymic disorder or neuromyasthenia may be more difficult to differentiate from the fibrositis syndrome. However, such patients do not have the characteristic alpha sleep finding, and the specific areas of muscle tenderness are not found in these other disorders.

Treatment of the sleep disturbance is with the tricyclic ANTIDEPRESSANT medication amitriptyline. In addition, attention to good SLEEP HYGIENE is helpful. Typically the anti-inflammatory medications that are used for rheumatic disorders are not effective in the fibrositis syndrome.

Fibrositis syndrome has also been called rheumatic pain modulation disorder, fibromyositis syndrome or fibromyalgia.

Moldofsky, H., Saskin, P. and Lue, F.A., "Sleep and Symptoms in Fibrositis Syndrome after a Febrile Illness," *Journal of Rheumatology* 15 (1988): 1701–1704.

Moldofsky, H., Tullis, C. and Lue, F.A., "Sleep-related Myoclonus in Rheumatic Pain Modulation Disorder (fibrositis syndrome)," *Journal of Rheumatology* 13 (1986): 614–617.

final awakening See ARISE TIME.

final wake-up See ARISE TIME.

first night effect A pattern of increased SLEEP LATENCY, and reduced TOTAL SLEEP TIME on the first night of a polysomnographic recording in the laboratory. The first night effect is believed to be due to several factors, including the discomfort to the subject of the recording electrodes, the new sleep environment and psychological effects, including anxiety regarding a polysomnographic recording. However, the subject adjusts to the above factors, and the disruptive effects on sleep typically are present only on the first night of recording. (See also POLYSOMNOGRAPHY, SLEEP-WAKE DISORDERS CENTER.)

5-hydroxytryptamine The biochemical name for SEROTONIN, which is a component of blood that causes constriction of the blood vessels, allowing the blood to clot. This constricting agent has been found in neurons and is involved in the regulation of the sleep-wake cycle. Serotonin is derived from the amino acid L-tryptophan (see HYPNOTICS), which is present in normal dietary intake, usually up to two grams per day. Extra L-tryptophan is sometimes taken by sufferers of insomnia to elevate brain serotonin levels in the hope that this will improve the quality of nocturnal sleep. L-tryptophan is believed to have some sleep-inducing properties, although these are considered to be mild. A metabolic product of L-tryptophan, which is called 5-hydroxytryptophan, has been demonstrated to increase both REM SLEEP and SLOW WAVE SLEEP. However, this agent is not very useful in improving sleep in patients with INSOMNIA. (See DIET AND SLEEP for cautionary note about L-tryptophan because of 1989 report of 30 cases of eosinophilia-myalgia linked to dietary supplements of L-tryptophan.)

The serotonin reuptake inhibitors are a class of antidepressant medications that increase serotonin at the synapse. (See ANTIDEPRESSANTS.)

Parachlorphenylamine (PCPA) inhibits the production of 5-hydroxytryptamine, thereby leading to a reduction in brain serotonin levels and, typically, producing insomnia. But other medications that affect the synthesis, storage and release of 5-hydroxytryptamine have little effect on sleep or wakefulness.

fluoxetine See ANTIDEPRESSANTS.

flurazepam See BENZODIAZEPINES.

fluvoxamine See ANTIDEPRESSANTS.

food allergy insomnia A disorder of initiating and maintaining sleep that is caused by food allergy; typically occurring in infants and associated with irritability, frequent arousals, crying episodes and daytime lethargy. Other signs or features of an allergic response may be present, but they are usually not the predominant feature of the disorder. For example, skin irritation, gastrointestinal upset or respiratory difficulties may all occur.

Although this is a disorder that primarily affects children, it can also occur in adults who may develop an allergy to eggs or fish, with resultant insomnia. When the disorder occurs in children, it usually occurs in infancy and resolves spontaneously by the age of four years at the latest. There may well be a family history of allergic phenomena. The allergy most commonly is related to the ingestion of cow's milk and therefore may occur soon after the introduction of cow's milk to the diet.

Food allergy insomnia should be differentiated from infant colic in which sleep disturbance may be associated with acute crying spells that occur episodically (gastrointestinal symptoms may accompany the acute episodes). SLEEP-RELATED GASTROESOPHAGEAL REFLUX, INFANT SLEEP APNEA and infantile epileptic seizures need to be differentiated from food allergy insomnia.

Treatment involves removal of the offending allergen. Allergy tests may be necessary to determine the exact allergen, but once it is removed from the diet, the sleep disturbance usually resolves rapidly.

Kahn, A., Mozin, N.J., Casimir, G., Montauk, L. and Blum, D., "Insomnia in Cow's Milk Allergy in Infants," *Pediatrics* 76 (1985): 880–884.

fragmentary myoclonus Disorder characterized by clusters of brief muscle jerks that occur predominantly in NON-REM-STAGE SLEEP. These involuntary "twitch-like" contractions can occur in various skeletal muscles in an asynchronous and asymmetrical manner. Muscles of the limbs and face and trunk can all be involved. The brief muscle contractions can occur for prolonged periods throughout sleep. At times, the muscle jerks produce ELECTROENCEPHALOGRAM (EEG) evidence of an AROUSAL with a transient K-COMPLEX; however, there is usually no change in the EEG in association with the activity.

The muscle jerks are very brief, usually 75 to 150 milliseconds in duration, with an amplitude of about 50 to several hundred microvolts. The activity usually commences soon after sleep onset and continues throughout non-REM sleep, including SLOW WAVE SLEEP, and persists into REM SLEEP.

Fragmentary myoclonus is associated with EXCESSIVE SLEEPINESS. The activity has been described in other sleep disorders, including the SLEEP-RELATED BREATHING DISORDERS, NARCOLEPSY, PERIODIC LIMB MOVEMENT DISORDER and other causes of INSOMNIA.

This disorder should be differentiated from PERIODIC LEG MOVEMENTS, which are of longer duration and are more typically associated with an EEG arousal or awakening. It should also be differentiated from the physiological REM sleep myoclonus, which typically occurs throughout normal REM sleep and can be associated with the eye movements of REM sleep. Neurological disorders, such as the degenerative disorders, can produce myoclonus, which is typically present throughout wakefulness and usually decreases during sleep. More generalized synchronous movements due to sleep starts are easy to distinguish from the asynchronous and briefer muscle jerks of fragmentary myoclonus.

In most situations, fragmentary myoclonus does not require treatment. However, if frequent EEG arousals are associated with the activity and excessive sleepiness is a feature, then suppression of the arousals by means of BENZODIAZEPINES may be helpful.

Broughton, Roger, Tolentino, M.A. and Krelenia, M., "Excessive Fragmentary Myoclonus in Non-REM Sleep: A Report of 38 Cases," *Electroencephalography and Clinical Neurophysiology* 61 (1985): 123–309.

fragmentation See NREM-REM SLEEP CYCLE.

free running A chronobiological term that applies to a biological rhythm isolated from ENVIRONMENTAL TIME CUES such as light, food, temperature, social interactions and clock time. Under these conditions, the rhythm will continue with its own internal period length, which for CIRCADIAN RHYTHM is close to, but not exactly, 24 hours in duration.

frequently changing sleep-wake schedule One of the sleep-wake schedule disorders of the *Diagnostic Classification of Sleep and Arousal Disorders,* which was published in the journal *SLEEP* in 1979.

This term refers to sleep disorders that are due to persistent alteration of the sleep-wake schedule, such as those due to a changing work shift pattern or flight across time zones. The sleep-wake pattern is constantly disrupted. The terms SHIFT-WORK SLEEP DISORDER and TIME ZONE CHANGE (JET LAG) SYNDROME are preferred.

Freud, Sigmund "Father of Psychoanalysis" (1856–1939) who viewed DREAMS as doors to the unconscious, the keys to understanding and eventually unblocking repressed sexual and aggressive forces that motivate and perhaps unconsciously control a person's behavior. In 1900, Freud published his groundbreaking treatise, *The Interpretation of Dreams,* which explained dreams as the fulfillment of certain unconscious impulses considered unacceptable on a conscious level.

Freud believed repressed sexual and aggressive desires are disguised in dreams in three ways: through symbolism, such as by using objects to represent sexual organs; by condensation, where one dream image represents several aspects of a person's life; and by displacement, in which an unacceptable wish is focused on something other than the real object of the wish.

He also believed DREAM CONTENT took two forms: the manifest content, or that part of the dream we remember, and the latent content, the true underlying meaning of the dream.

In their treatment, Freudian psychoanalysts use dream interpretation to help patients gain insight, and eventual control, over the unconscious forces causing conflicts and emotional disturbances.

Freud, Sigmund, *The Interpretation of Dreams,* J. Strachey, *The Standard Edition of the Complete Psychological Works of Sigmund Freud,* vols. 4 and 5. London: Hogarth Press, 1953.

G

GABA See GAMMA-AMINOBUTYRIC ACID.

Gaillard, Jean-Michel Trained at the Medical School of the University of Lausanne (Switzerland) and Paris between 1957 and 1963, Dr. Gaillard (1939–) has been working since 1968 in the research department of the University Psychiatric Institute of Geneva, where he is presently chief of the Division of Biochemistry and Clinical Neurophysiology.

His contributions to sleep research have included development of an automatic sleep scoring system, which has been used continuously since 1971; the sleep pharmacology of benzodiazepines; pharmacological study of the involvement of brain catecholamine systems in the regulation of paradoxical sleep and waking; study of hemispheric activation during sleep; a detailed investigation of sleep onset; and a study of chronic insomnia and the use of short-term dynamic psychotherapy.

Gaillard, J.M., "Temporal Organization of Human Sleep: General Trends of Sleep Stages and their Ultradian Cyclic Components," *Encephale* 5 (1979): 71–93.

gamma-aminobutyric acid (GABA) An inhibitory amino acid neurotransmitter that is widely spread throughout the central nervous system. It is found in highest concentration in the hypothalamus and is believed to be involved in the induction of sleep. The BENZODIAZEPINES are known to have their sedative action through binding to the GABA receptor. In addition, the BARBITURATES bind with GABA in the brain. Drugs that increase GABA levels in the brain, such as those that inhibit the breakdown enzyme of GABA, can increase SLOW WAVE SLEEP. GABA is found in neurons that extend from the hypothalamus to the cortex, and the release of GABA from the cortex has been shown to be highest during natural sleep or in lesions that affect the midbrain reticular formation.

GABA will enhance sleep induced by benzodiazepines, and therefore it appears to have an affect on the affinity of benzodiazepines for their final receptor sites; however, the exact role in the induction of sleep is still undetermined.

gamma-hydroxybutyrate (GHB) The precursor of the naturally occurring agent gamma-aminobutyric acid. This agent has been found to be effective in controlling the auxiliary symptoms of NARCOLEPSY, primarily the symptom of CATAPLEXY. Gamma- hydroxybutyrate has been shown to have little effect in improving daytime sleepiness. It is known to increase SLOW WAVE SLEEP, with little effect upon REM SLEEP. The medication is given once or twice in two- or three-gram doses at night. As the medication has a short duration of action, it is necessary to give a second dose halfway through the sleep period. Gamma-hydroxybutyrate may be useful in the treatment of cataplexy in patients who are unable to use the tricyclic ANTIDEPRESSANTS because of anticholinergic side effects. Very few side effects have been recorded with gamma-hydroxybutyrate. However, the drug has been abused, and when combined with benzodiazepines has been called the "date rape" drug. One side effect reported is SLEEPWALKING, possibly due to the effect of gamma-hydroxybutyrate in increasing the amount of slow wave sleep. Gamma-hydroxybutyrate is available in Canada but unavailable in the United States except on a research basis for the treatment of narcolepsy.

Gardner, Randy San Diego high school senior who, in 1964, broke the *Guinness Book of World Records* record by staying awake the longest—264 hours, or 11 days. Sleep researcher WILLIAM C. DEMENT observed Gardner during his ordeal and concluded, "staying awake for 264 hours did not cause any psychiatric problems whatsoever." In his book *The Promise of Sleep* (1999), however, Dement wondered if Gardner may have been sleepwalking for some of the time since, back in 1965, the recording devices for monitoring sleep were much less sophisticated than today's devices.

Gelineau, J.B.E. Jean Baptiste Edouard Gelineau (1828–1906) was a French physician who is credited with first suggesting the term NARCOLEPSY for a mysterious syndrome characterized by sudden sleeping, especially at inappropriate times during the day. Gelineau, in his 1880 article published in the *Gazette des Hopitaux,* proposed the word "narcolepsy" along with a detailed description of a 38-year-old male wine barrel retailer who had sleep attacks and accompanying falls. The falls are now known as CATAPLEXY but Gelineau called them "astasia."

The next year, in his work "On Narcolepsy," Gelineau discussed 14 cases of narcolepsy, distinguishing two types of the syndrome, the first an idiopathic syndrome, and the second related to other illnesses.

Gelineau, J., "De La Narcolepsie," *Gazette des Hopitaux* 53 (1880): 626–628.

Passouant, Pierre, "Historical Note: Doctor Gelineau (1828–1906); Narcolepsy Centennial," *Sleep* 3 (1981): 241–246.

genetics The science of the biological unit of heredity that is transmitted from one cell to another during the process of reproduction. Although a number of sleep disorders, including SLEEPWALKING and SLEEP TERRORS, are believed to have a genetic origin, with a genetic predisposition passed on through the family, only NARCOLEPSY has been demonstrated to have a specific genetic factor, which is present in nearly every patient with the disease. The human leukocyte antigen DR2 is present in more than 90% of patients diagnosed with narcolepsy. The allele HLA DQB1-0602 is the most specific genetic factor also found in more than 90% of patients with narcolepsy. (See also HISTOCOMPATABILITY ANTIGEN TESTING, HLA-DR2.)

Faraco, J., et al., "Genetic Studies in Narcolepsy, a Disorder Affecting REM Sleep," *Journal of Heredity* 90, no. 1 (1999): 129–132.

GHB See GAMMA-HYDROXYBUTYRATE.

gigantocellular tegmental field One of three divisions of the reticular formation. (The other two divisions include the lateral tegmental field, FTL, and the magnocellular tegmental field, TM.) The gigantocellular tegmental field consists of large cells of the pontine and medullary reticular formation. The cholinergic cells of the pontine portion of the gigantocellular tegmental field have been demonstrated to increase their activity during the onset of REM SLEEP. The cells have been called the REM-ON CELLS in the reciprocal interaction model of sleep regulation that was proposed by J. Allan Hobson, ROBERT W. MCCARLEY and Peter W. Wyzinski in 1975. (See also ASCENDING RETICULAR ACTIVATING SYSTEM, INTERACTION MODEL OF SLEEP.)

Gillin, J. Christian Received his M.D. from Case-Western Reserve School of Medicine. Since 1982, Gillin (1938–) has been a professor of psychiatry at the University of California at San Diego (UCSD), and since 1986 he has been a director of the Mental Health Clinical Research Center at UCSD.

Dr. Gillin's areas of sleep research have included the effects of depression and alcoholism on sleep, pharmacologic studies of sleep, the use of hypnotics, and brain metabolism of sleep and sleep deprivation. He is past president of both the Sleep Research Society and the Society for Biological Rhythms and Light Therapy.

Drummond, S.P., Brown, G., Gillin, J.C., Stricker, J., Wong, E. and Buxton, R., "Altered Brain Response to Verbal Learning Following Sleep Deprivation," *Nature* (February 10, 2000): 655–657.

glottic spasm See LARYNGOSPASM.

growth hormone Secreted from the pituitary gland in relation to the onset of sleep, with maximal secretion occurring in the first third of the night. Although originally thought to be primarily related to the onset of stages three and four sleep, it is now believed to be more related to the time following the onset of sleep (see SLEEP STAGES). Growth hormone is tied to the sleep-wake cycle so that acute shifts of sleep by 12 hours will cause an acute shift of the growth hormone secretory pattern. There is minimal growth hormone secretion during the daytime, with small peaks of production that occur in relation to stress or exercise. A shift of the sleep pattern by several hours is immediately accompanied by a shift of growth hormone secretion. This shift is not accompanied by an immediate shift in some other hormone rhythms, such as cortisol. The cortisol circadian rhythm, although related to the sleep-wake cycle, can become disassociated from sleep following an acute shift of the timing of sleep. After one or two weeks, the cortisol pattern readjusts to the new time of sleep and therefore its relationship with growth hormone is reestablished.

Growth hormone is important for growth, particularly in childhood. Maximal levels are secreted around the time of puberty and are important in the maintenance of normal body size. Absence of growth hormone will lead to dwarfism and excessive production of growth hormone will lead to gigantism. However, the removal of the pituitary and loss of growth hormone secretion in adults appears to have few physical effects.

Although prolactin, which is inhibited by dopamine, is very much affected by medications, growth hormone secretion during sleep is largely unaffected. Medications that do influence the production of growth hormone during sleep include cholinergic inhibitory medications, such as methscopolamine, which causes a large increase in the sleep-related growth hormone release. (See also ADRENOCORTICOTROPHIN HORMONE, CORTISOL, DOPAMINE, PROLACTIN.)

Guilleminault, Christian Born in Marseilles, France, Dr. Guilleminault (1938–) received his medical degree from the University of Paris in 1956 and his doctorate in biology from the University of Grenoble. Since 1972, he has been affiliated with the Stanford Sleep Disorders Clinic and Research Center as associate director. Since 1985, Dr. Guilleminault has been professor of psychiatry and behavioral sciences, Stanford University. In 1986, he was the recipient of the NATHANIEL KLEITMAN DISTINGUISHED SERVICE AWARD. He was editor in chief of the journal *SLEEP* until 1998.

Dr. Guilleminault's hundreds of journal articles, books, monographs and chapters in books reflect his research in the areas of sleep apnea, narcolepsy, insomnia, parasomnia and sleep disorders of children.

Guilleminault, C., "Sleep Apnea Syndromes: Impact of Sleep and Sleep States," *Sleep* 3 (1980): 227–246.

Guilleminault, C. and Dement, W.C., eds., *Sleep Apnea Syndromes*. New York: Alan R. Liss, 1978.

H

Halberg, Franz Born in Bistritz, Romania, Dr. Halberg (1919–) received his medical degree in 1943. In 1959, Halberg coined the term "circadian rhythm" to describe physiologic rhythms with a frequency of one cycle in about 24 (20 to 28) hours. The term was created from the Latin words *circa,* meaning "about," and *dies* ("a day"). Halberg contributed the science (*logos*) of life's (*bios*) time (*chronos*) structure—CHRONOBIOLOGY.

Halberg, Franz, "Chronobiology," *Annual Review of Physiology* 31 (1969): 675–725.

Halcion See BENZODIAZEPINES.

Hall, Calvin S. Well-known dream theorist. In 1961, Hall (1909–1985) founded the Institute of Dream Research. Hall was best known for his cognitive theory of dreaming and his research into the content analysis of DREAMS. One of his surveys of DREAM CONTENT found that only one-third of those surveyed dreamed in color.

After early work in the field of behavioral genetics, Hall, while professor and chairman of the psychology department at Western Reserve University from 1937 to 1957, turned his attention to dreams. In 1947, his first article, "Diagnosing Personality by the Analysis of Dreams," was published in the *Journal of Abnormal and Social Psychology.* His cognitive theory of dreams was presented in his book *The Meaning of Dreams,* published in 1953; and in 1966, along with R. Van de Castle, he published *The Content Analysis of Dreams,* which surveyed 500 dreams of men and the same number for women, along with guidelines for scoring dreams according to scales that they devised.

In addition to numerous books on dreams as well as textbooks on introductory psychology, Jung and Freud, Hall, in collaboration with G.W. Domhoff, K. Blick and K. Weesner, wrote an article in *Sleep* in 1982 that reaffirmed the results of his research on dream content from 30 years before. "The Dreams of College Men and Women in 1950 and 1980: A Comparison of Dream Contents and Sex Differences" is a classic contribution in the field of dream research.

Hall, Calvin S., "What People Dream About," *Scientific American* 184 (1951): 60–63.
———, *The Meaning of Dreams.* New York: Harper, 1953.
Editors, "In Memoriam: Calvin S. Hall," *Sleep* 8 (1985): 298.

Hartmann, Ernest Born in Vienna, Austria, Dr. Hartmann (1934–) received his M.D. from Yale University in 1958. Since 1962, Dr. Hartmann has been involved in sleep research. He has contributed basic studies on the chemistry and biology of REM and non-REM sleep as well as the role of serotonin in sleep states. He has also studied sleep need in terms of natural long, short and variable-length sleepers, leading to a theory on the functions of sleep. He has carried out extensive work on nightmares and nightmare sufferers. Dr. Hartmann is currently professor of psychiatry at the Tufts University School of Medicine, director of the Sleep Research Laboratory at Lemurel Shattuck Hospital, and director of the Sleep Disorders Center, Newton-Wellesley Hospital, in Boston.

Hartmann, Ernest, *The Nightmare.* New York: Basic Books, 1984.
———, *The Sleep Book.* Glenview, Illinois: Scott, Foresman–AARP, 1988.

Hauri, Peter J. Received his Ph.D. in clinical psychology at the University of Chicago in 1966. Since

1988, Dr. Hauri (1933–) has been consultant to the Sleep Disorders Center and Division of Psychology at the Mayo Clinic in Rochester, Minnesota, as well as professor of psychology at the Mayo Medical School. Prior to that, Dr. Hauri held teaching positions at Dartmouth Medical School and College in New Hampshire (1971–88).

His Ph.D. dissertation was on "The Influence of Evening Activity on Sleeping and Dreaming." Insomnia and the effect of depression on sleep and dreaming have been some of his major sleep research areas. Dr. Hauri is director of the Mayo Sleep Disorders Center. In 1989 he was the recipient of the NATHANIEL KLEITMAN DISTINGUISHED SERVICE AWARD presented by the Association of Professional Sleep Societies.

Hauri, Peter, "Primary Insomnia," in Kryger, M.H., Roth, T. and Dement, W.C., eds., *The Principles and Practices of Sleep Disorders Medicine.* Philadelphia: Saunders, 1989. pp. 14–23.

———, *The Sleep Disorders.* 2nd ed. Kalamazoo, Michigan: Upjohn Company, 1982.

Hauri, Peter J., and Shirley Lind. *No More Sleepless Nights.* New York: Wiley, 1991.

headaches Pain or discomfort in the head that is experienced during wakefulness; however, some headache forms can occur during sleep or may be present upon awakening from sleep. MIGRAINE and CHRONIC PAROXYSMAL HEMICRANIA have been demonstrated to have an association with REM SLEEP, and patients with the OBSTRUCTIVE SLEEP APNEA SYNDROME can have headaches upon awakening in the morning. (See also CLUSTER HEADACHES, SLEEP-RELATED HEADACHES.)

headbanging (jactatio capitis nocturna) Also known as rhythmic movement disorder. This behavior is included in a group of three disorders—headbanging, HEAD ROLLING and BODYROCKING—that have as their main characteristic a repetitive movement of the head and, occasionally, of the whole body. These disorders may occur during the time of rest, drowsiness, sleep or full wakefulness. The condition has been reported to occur during deep slow wave sleep, as well as in REM sleep. The episodes occur very frequently, on an almost nightly basis, and usually last for about 15 minutes. The frequency of the movement can vary, but it typically occurs at the rate of 45 episodes per minute and can be as fast as 120 episodes per minute.

The disorder was first described clinically in 1905, by Zappert, when he coined the Latin term *jactatio capitis nocturna,* which is still commonly used.

The head movements in the headbanging form of this disorder are in an anterior/posterior direction. Usually the head is banged into a pillow or a mattress. Occasionally the head movement can be into solid objects, such as a wall or the side of a crib.

When the head movements occur side to side, the condition is termed *head rolling.*

Bodyrocking is most often performed on the hands and knees. The whole body is rocked in an anterior/posterior direction, with the head being pushed into the pillow.

It has been reported that as many as 66% of children exhibit some sort of rhythmical activity at nine months of age, and the prevalence decreases to approximately 8% at four years of age. It is rare for the condition to occur for the first time after two years of age; however, it may persist through adolescence into adulthood.

Headbanging is reported to be more common in males than in females, and rarely has been reported to occur in families. The mentally retarded are more likely to exhibit the behavior. The disorder has to be distinguished from an epileptic disorder and from the fine head oscillations of spasmus nutans.

Polysomnograph studies of the activity usually demonstrate frequent episodes during sleep, most often in the lighter stages one and two sleep. Rarely has the condition been reported to occur only during REM sleep, which may indicate a variant of the disorder. Episodes can occur during deep slow wave sleep, although, again, this has rarely been reported. Daytime electroencephalography is usually normal between episodes.

The cause of the movements is unknown, but numerous theories have been proposed. There is little evidence to support a psychiatric or organic neurological disorder to account for the behavior. A neurophysiological basis for the activity is the most likely, related to normal development. It has been suggested that the activity may be a pleasurable sensation, and therefore a form of vestibular self-stimulation.

Treatment is usually unnecessary when the condition occurs in childhood, as it typically will disappear within 18 months, often at around four years of age. When the condition persists into adolescence or adulthood, behavioral or pharmacological approaches may be needed. Sedative medications have been beneficial, and some patients have had a favorable response to tricyclic ANTIDEPRESSANTS. Measures may have to be taken to prevent injury from the repetitive movements in young children.

head rolling Repetitive movement of the head from side to side, which may occur during rest, drowsiness, sleep or wakefulness; more typical in children below the age of four than in older children or adults. (See also HEADBANGING.)

heart attack See MYOCARDIAL INFARCTION.

heartburn Discomfort experienced in the middle of the chest; associated with reflux of acid from the stomach into the esophagus. Heartburn commonly accompanies gastroesophageal reflux and can occur during sleep as a symptom of SLEEP-RELATED GASTROESOPHAGEAL REFLUX. Heartburn during sleep may be due to the OBSTRUCTIVE SLEEP APNEA SYNDROME during which increased abdominal pressure produces a reflux of acid into the esophagus.

hemolysis, sleep-related See PAROXYSMAL NOCTURNAL HEMOGLOBINURIA.

hertz (Hz) Term synonymous with cycles per second (cps); it refers to a rhythm frequency most commonly applied to the ELECTROENCEPHALOGRAM (EEG).

hibernation A state produced in animals as a response to seasonal environmental changes. During winter, animals are at risk in the environment due to the cold and the lack of food. Hibernating animals are typically those who are unable to travel long distances to make a major environmental change.

During hibernation, a sleep-like state exists with a reduction of metabolic activity and respiratory and circulatory rates. Body temperature can gradually drop to near freezing point; this is associated with a change in the electroencephalographic pattern, typically one of SLOW WAVE SLEEP with reduced or almost absent REM SLEEP. During the hibernation, the animal typically withdraws to its usual sleeping environment and reserves of stored fat are used to maintain the metabolic rate at only 10% to 15% of its normal rate. During the depth of the hibernation, the slow wave pattern of non-REM sleep gives way to a flattening of the electroencephalographic pattern, with no resemblance to sleep or wakefulness.

With the rising environmental temperatures at the end of hibernation, the electroencephalographic patterns revert back to normal as the body temperature slowly returns to a level typical during warmer seasons. (See also ELECTROENCEPHALOGRAM.)

histamine A naturally occurring substance that is released during injury to tissues. The word is derived from the Greek word for tissue, *histos*. Histamine appears to act via two distinct receptors, the H1 and H2 receptors. The antihistamines have their effects primarily through blocking the H1 receptors; medications that inhibit gastric secretion work through blocking the H2 receptors.

There is some evidence to suggest that histamine is involved in the control of arousal and wakefulness. Animal studies have demonstrated that histamine is increased in the brains of animals during darkness, and that inhibition of histamine synthesis reduces wakefulness.

histocompatability antigen testing A test of the genetic constituents that play a role in determining rejection of a tissue graft. The major histocompatability complex (MHC) is composed of a group of genes that are located on chromosome 6, and the products of these genes are present on cell surfaces. The MHC in humans is called the human leukocyte antigen (HLA). There are three classes of human leukocyte genes and products, which are called class I, II, III. The HLA class I and class II products are located on cell surfaces. HLA class I products are found on most cell surfaces and consist of the HLA types A, B, C and E. The HLA class II products are found on the surface of the immune cells, such as lymphocytes. The HLA class II products consist of DR, DQ and DP.

The HLA D region has been found to have a specific association with the sleep disorder NARCOLEPSY. (See also HLA-DR2.)

HLA-DR2 This stands for the human leukocyte antigen DR2, which is located on chromosome 6. This particular genetic marker has been reported to be nearly 100% associated with the disorder NARCOLEPSY. This high association has been found in Japanese patients, compared to only 85% of African-American patients with narcolepsy. In the United States, there is a 95% positivity of Caucasian patients with the HLA-DR2 antigen. The presence of this antigen indicates a genetic factor that is important in transmission of the narcolepsy disorder. It is possible that another factor, possibly infective or environmental, causes the expression of the disease in a susceptible individual. Persons who are DR2 negative are believed to be unable to develop narcolepsy.

HLA-DR2 testing may be helpful in the diagnosis of narcolepsy because DR2 positivity is supportive evidence to other clinical and electrophysiological features of the disorder. HLA-DR2 negativity should raise the possibility of a disorder other than narcolepsy to account for the patient's symptoms. HLA-DR2 testing may be useful in predicting whether a child of an affected parent has the likelihood of developing narcolepsy at a later date. However, the presence of HLA-DR2 positivity does not mean that the individual will develop narcolepsy, since approximately 25% of the general population is also HLA-DR2 positive.

Associated with HLA-DR2 positivity is the histocompatability antigen HLA DQ1. Every individual who is HLA-DR2 positive also has HLA DQ1. African-American patients with narcolepsy appear to have 100% positivity of HLA-DQ1, whereas HLA-DR2 positivity is present in only about 85%.

HLA-DR2 can be subdivided into two groups: DR15 and DR16. One-hundred percent of Japanese patients with narcolepsy have the DR15 subgroup. In addition, if the DR2 is subtyped according to a cytological and not a serological method, the subgroup Dw2 is also found in 100% of narcolepsy patients. (See also HISTOCOMPATABILITY ANTIGEN TESTING.)

Honda, Yutaka Dr. Honda (1929–) graduated in 1954 from the medical school of the University of Tokyo and received his Ph.D. degree in 1960 in clinical psychiatry from the graduate school, University of Tokyo. His doctoral dissertation was a clinical study of patients with both vegetative and mental symptoms (diencephalosis). That was the beginning of his clinical activities with narcoleptic and hypersomniac patients. His three major accomplishments in sleep research have been: the 1961 discovery, along with Dr. Yasuro Takahashi, of the effectiveness of imipramine and tricyclic antidepressants on cataplexy and hypnagogic hallucinations of narcolepsy; the 1968 discovery, along with Dr. Kiyohisa Takahashi, of sleep-induced secretion of growth hormone in normal subjects; and the 1984 discovery, in collaboration with Dr. Takeo Juji, of 100% positivity of HLA-DR2/Dw2 in narcolepsy.

Dr. Honda has been on the faculty of the University of Tokyo since 1959, except for several research fellowships in the United States from 1961 to 1963. Since 1969, he has been an associate professor of the Department of Neuropsychiatry at the University of Tokyo. Since 1985, he has been a director of the Neuropsychiatric Research Institute and a superintendent of its affiliated Seiwa Hospital.

Akimoto, H., Honda, Y. and Takahashi, Y., "Pharmacotherapy in Narcolepsy," *Disorders of the Nervous System* 21 (1960): 1–3.

Honda, Y., Takahashi, K., Takahashi, S. et al., "Growth Hormone Secretion During Nocturnal Sleep in Normal Subjects," *Journal of Clinical Endocrinology and Metabolism* 29 (1969): 20–29.

Horne, James Anthony Dr. Horne (1946–) obtained his Ph.D. degree in 1972 from the University of Aston in Birmingham in the field of psychophysiology of sleep loss. A psychologist and a biologist, Dr. Horne has been in the Human Sciences Department of Loughborough University in Leicestershire since 1973, first as a lecturer and, since 1989, as a professor in psychophysiology.

His principal fields of research have been in the physiology and psychology of human sleep, including its function, sleep loss and individual differences in circadian rhythms. Dr. Horne founded, and directs, the Sleep Research Laboratory at Loughborough University and is editor of the *Journal of Sleep Research*.

Horne, James, *Why We Sleep: The Functions of Sleep in Humans and Other Mammals*. London: Oxford University Press, 1988.

hygiene See SLEEP HYGIENE.

hyoid myotomy A surgical procedure that involves a repositioning of the hyoid bone to relieve upper airway obstruction associated with the OBSTRUCTIVE SLEEP APNEA SYNDROME. The tongue muscles often obstruct the airway because they are positioned posteriorly. The tongue is attached to the hyoid bone, which is tethered to the skull by several muscles. The hyoid myotomy operation involves release of these muscles.

The muscles attached to the hyoid bone, such as the sternohyoid, thyrohyoid and omohyoid, are several, and the hyoid bone is suspended to the mandible by strips of fascia, the muscle lining that has been taken from the thigh or temple muscles. Usually the hyoid myotomy is performed in conjunction with an osteotomy of the tip of the jaw. The tip of the jaw is moved anteriorly to advance the anterior attachment of the muscles of the tongue.

Many of the patients treated by this surgical procedure have also undergone the UVULOPALATOPHARYNGOPLASTY operation, with or without a TONSILLECTOMY AND ADENOIDECTOMY.

Hyoid myotomy is rarely performed now as it is not as effective as other surgical procedures.

hypercapnia Term describing an elevated blood-gas CARBON DIOXIDE level in the blood. (The carbon dioxide level during sleep may increase in patients who have SLEEP-RELATED BREATHING DISORDERS.) The level of carbon dioxide in the blood can be continuously measured during sleep by means of END-TIDAL CARBON DIOXIDE measurements, using an infrared carbon dioxide analyzer.

hypernycthemeral sleep-wake syndrome Term synonymous with NON-24-HOUR SLEEP-WAKE SYNDROME. The term *hypernycthemeral* is derived from the Greek word for *hyper,* meaning "above," and *nycthemeron,* meaning "pertaining to both night and day." This term was first proposed by Kokkoris, Weitzman and colleagues in 1978.

Kokkoris, C.P., Weitzman, E.D., Pollak, C.P., Spielman, A.J., Czeisler, C.A. and Bradlow, H., "Long-Term Ambulatory Temperature Monitoring in a Subject with a Hypernycthemeral Sleep-Wake Cycle Disturbance," *Sleep* 1 (1978): 177–190.

hypernycthemeral syndrome See NON-24-HOUR SLEEP-WAKE SYNDROME.

hypersomnia See EXCESSIVE SLEEPINESS.

hypertension An elevation of blood pressure typically seen in patients who have a diastolic blood pressure greater than 90 millimeters of mercury or a systolic blood pressure greater than 160 millimeters of mercury.

Hypertension has been reported in approximately 30% of patients with the OBSTRUCTIVE SLEEP APNEA SYNDROME. Studies of groups of hypertensive patients have demonstrated that between 25% and 30% have episodes of oxygen desaturation during sleep or an abnormal number of apneic episodes during sleep.

Treatment of the obstructive sleep apnea syndrome is typically associated with a lowering of blood pressure or improved blood pressure control.

Hypertension typically is asymptomatic and can be detected only by means of physical examination. Because of its association with the development of cardiac and vascular disease, elevated blood pressure requires treatment.

The majority of patients with hypertension have no known cause for the blood pressure elevation; however, some patients develop hypertension as a result of kidney disease, endocrine disorders or atherosclerosis.

Some medications used to treat hypertension can affect the sleep wake cycle. Beta blockers, such as propranol, can produce sleep disturbance that is characterized by INSOMNIA; and there is evidence that beta blockers may even worsen the obstructive sleep apnea syndrome. Other antihypertensive medications, such as clonidine, can produce excessive sleepiness.

Because of the high association between hypertension and the obstructive sleep apnea syndrome, patients with hypertension should be questioned as to the presence of snoring, obesity, disturbed sleep and the occurrence of apneic episodes during sleep to see if they have that disorder.

hyperthyroidism A disorder associated with excessive production of thyroid hormone from the thyroid gland in the neck. This is usually caused by enlargement or overactivity of the thyroid gland and produces characteristic symptoms of insomnia, weight loss, irritability, diarrhea, weakness, palpitations and tremulousness. Some patients with hyperthyroidism have a diffuse enlargement of the thyroid gland associated with antibodies that stimulate the thyroid gland. This disorder, which is termed Graves' disease, characteristically produces eye protrusion due to accumulation of excessive tissue behind the eyes.

The sleep disturbance associated with hyperthyroidism is typically one of difficulty in initiating and maintaining sleep. Sleep may be more restless and frequent arousals may be seen during polysomnographic testing. However, some patients have an increase in SLOW WAVE SLEEP.

Hyperthyroidism is treated by medications that suppress the activity of the thyroid gland, such as carbimazol, or by radioactive iodine, which destroys a portion of the thyroid gland. Surgical treatment may also be indicated. With treatment of the hyperthyroidism, the sleep disturbance usually resolves.

Following treatment for hyperthyroidism, sometimes the thyroid gland is rendered incapable of producing an adequate amount of thyroid hormone, thereby producing a deficiency in thyroid hormone. As a result, HYPOTHYROIDISM may occur many years after chemical treatment of hyperthyroidism. Hypothyroidism is associated with the development of excessive lethargy and sleepiness. Muscle changes associated with the lack of thyroid hormone can produce impaired respiration during sleep, with the development of CENTRAL SLEEP APNEA SYNDROME or hypoventilation during sleep.

hypnagogic Term applied to events occurring immediately prior to, or during, sleep onset; usually applied to dream activity during sleep onset, which is termed HYPNAGOGIC HALLUCINATIONS. Events that occur at the end of the sleep episode, in the transition from sleep to wakefulness, are called HYPNOPOMPIC.

hypnagogic hallucinations Visual images that occur at sleep onset; most typically associated with REM SLEEP. Hypnagogic hallucinations are a characteristic feature of the sleep onset REM period that occurs in patients with NARCOLEPSY. Occasionally the imagery may be extremely frightening, and such situations have been termed TERRIFYING HYPNAGOGIC HALLUCINATIONS. Images that occur upon awakening or at wake times are called HYPNOPOMPIC hallucinations.

hypnagogic hypersynchrony This term applies to rhythmical electroencephalographic activity of 5–6 Hz that occurs in the transition from wakefulness to sleep, which is present in infants after the first six months of life. Hypnagogic hypersynchrony usually disappears around six years, at which time it is replaced by increasing theta and delta activity, with a gradual loss of ALPHA ACTIVITY. The adult form of drowsiness, with alpha "drop out" and mixed frequency, low voltage activity, does not usually develop until early adolescence. (See also BETA RHYTHM, DROWSINESS, INFANT SLEEP, THETA ACTIVITY.)

hypnagogic jerk See SLEEP STARTS.

hypnagogic reverie Term applied to mentation that occurs at sleep onset; may comprise features of dream activity. It is most vivid at the onset of REM SLEEP but may occur at the onset of non-REM sleep. When frightening hypnagogic reverie occurs, the term TERRIFYING HYPNAGOGIC HALLUCINATIONS may be applied.

hypnagogic startle See SLEEP STARTS.

hypnalgia Term used for the occurrence of painful sensations induced by sleep. Many pains are increased in intensity during sleep; however, hypnalgias are pains that occur only during sleep. (See also CARPAL TUNNEL SYNDROME, SLEEP PALSY.)

hypnic jerks See SLEEP STARTS.

hypnic myoclonia See SLEEP STARTS.

hypnogenic paroxysmal dystonia The original term used for the disorder now called NOCTURNAL PAROXYSMAL DYSTONIA.

hypnogram This term is synonymous with POLYSOMNOGRAM but is less commonly used.

hypnograph This term is synonymous with the preferred term, "polysomnograph." (See also POLYSOMNOGRAM.)

hypnolepsy A term used for EXCESSIVE SLEEPINESS that resembles NARCOLEPSY. Hypnolepsy occurs as a result of a central nervous system lesion. The term is rarely used in current medical literature.

hypnology Term not widely used that refers to the science of the phenomena of sleep. It is derived from the Greek words *hypno,* meaning "sleep," and *ology,* meaning "study of."

hypnopedia This term refers to LEARNING DURING SLEEP.

hypnopompic Characteristic of events that occur in the transition phase from sleep to wakefulness, most commonly at the end of the main sleep episode. Occasionally, vivid hallucinations will be perceived at this time, particularly in patients with NARCOLEPSY. The term *hynopompic* is also commonly used to apply to seizures that occur at the time of awakening, or immediately thereafter. (See also HYPNAGOGIC HALLUCINATIONS.)

hypnos The ancient Greek god of sleep. Many words, such as *hypnosis, hypnology* and *hypnopedia,* have been derived form this Greek word.

hypnosis A mental state induced in individuals, who have increased suggestibility, by means of focusing attention and eliminating distracting environmental stimuli. An individual in the state of hypnosis does not usually go into sleep, although the relaxation can allow normal physiological sleep to occur. Typically, hypnosis produces a slowing of the encephalographic pattern; however, typical stage two features, such as SLEEP SPINDLES or the characteristic delta waves of SLOW WAVE SLEEP, do not occur.

Some of the features of hypnosis are very similar to sleep-related phenomena, such as the AUTOMATIC BEHAVIOR in SLEEPWALKING that typically would be seen in deep slow-wave sleep. These features are associated with the awake electroencephalographic pattern in hypnosis.

Hypnosis has been reported to be effective in treating some sleep disorders, such as sleepwalking or SLEEP TERRORS; however, other investigators have failed to find it a useful treatment.

hypnotic-dependent sleep disorder A sleep disturbance characterized by the intolerance for, or withdrawal of, HYPNOTICS. The sleep disturbance may be due to the chronic ingestion of hypnotic medications or their acute withdrawal. During chronic ingestion, the hypnotic effect tends to wear off and the underlying INSOMNIA may persist despite use of the medication. In some patients, there may be an increase in the metabolism of the hypnotic agent so that after an initial hypnotic effect in the first part of the night, there may be an increase in sleep disruption. After chronic ingestion of hypnotics, complete cessation of their ingestion leads to one or more nights of increased sleep fragmentation, which often results in the reinstitution of hypnotic therapy.

The medications most commonly associated with hypnotic-dependent sleep disorder are the BENZODIAZEPINES and BARBITURATES. However, other hypnotic agents may also produce this disorder.

Typically, the hypnotic agent is administered for an underlying insomnia disorder. So long as the cause of the insomnia is removed, an acute course of only a few days usually does not result in a hypnotic-dependent sleep disorder. However, if the drugs continue to be taken and the underlying insomnia disorder has not resolved, attempts to stop the medication are often associated with an increase in the insomnia, leading to an increased dosage of medication, or its continuation. Increased dosage often leads to accumulation of the active drug or its metabolites, particularly in the elderly population, resulting in daytime side effects. Excessive sleepiness, fatigue, tiredness, impaired cognitive and physical performance are typical features of medication accumulation.

Withdrawal of the hypnotic agent can lead to drug withdrawal effects during the daytime, such as nausea, restlessness, nervousness, anxiety, and an increase in sleep disruption following withdrawal, precipitating the patient into a depression, even with suicidal ideation. This psychiatric reaction is more liable to occur if the patient's original insomnia was related to an underlying DEPRESSION.

As a result of hypnotic-dependent insomnia, patients are often maintained on hypnotic medications for many years. This situation can arise from transient insomnia that may have occurred due to underlying stress, such as a bereavement or hospitalization. Hypnotic agents are often prescribed in a course that exceeds the typical duration of an ADJUSTMENT SLEEP DISORDER, so that instead of patients receiving a three to five day supply of medication, they may receive a month's supply. Unless normal sleep occurs, there is little inducement to the patient to stop the medication after the first few days following an acute emotional stress.

Although hypnotic-dependent sleep disorder can occur at any age, it is often seen in the geriatric population as their sleep tends to be more fragmented than that of younger patients. Therefore sleep disruption upon withdrawal of hypnotic medication is more common.

Patients receiving chronic hypnotic medications typically show alterations in the structure of sleep during polysomnographic monitoring. There may be a decrease in the slow wave and REM sleep stages and an increase in the lighter stage one and two sleep. There may be frequent sleep stage transitions, reduced K complexes, an increase in spindle activity, and the presence of an increased amount of alpha and beta activity. Hypnotic-dependent sleep disorder needs to be differentiated from insomnia due to other causes, such as the OBSTRUCTIVE SLEEP APNEA SYNDROME or PERIODIC LIMB MOVEMENT DISORDER. MALINGERERS seeking central nervous system depressant medications for drug abuse purposes must be distinguished from patients who have the hypnotic-dependent sleep disorder.

Treatment of hypnotic-dependent sleep disorder rests upon gradual reduction and withdrawal of the hypnotic agent, sometimes with the substitution of a medication with hypnotic properties but less dependency effects. For example, a tricyclic ANTIDEPRESSANT medication might be substituted. Encouragement of good SLEEP HYGIENE is essential during the withdrawal process. Patients need to be reassured and counseled about a temporary reoccurrence of insomnia during the withdrawal of the medication. (See also REBOUND INSOMNIA.)

Kales, Anthony, Bixler, E., Tan, T., Scharf, M. and Kales, J., "Chronic Hypnotic Drug Use: Ineffectiveness, Drug Withdrawal Insomnia and Dependence," *Journal of American Medical Association* 227 (1974): 511–517.

hypnotics Also known as sleeping pills, sedative medications and sedative-hypnotic medications, hypnotics are medications that induce drowsiness and facilitate the onset and maintenance of sleep. Typically, hypnotics will induce sleep similar to natural sleep in that normal REM/NREM sleep cycling occurs, and the person is able to be easily aroused from sleep.

Various potions have been used to induce sleep since antiquity; ALCOHOL was one of the most commonly used substances. Bromides were used as hypnotics in the middle of the 19th century, but chloral hydrate is the only hypnotic agent still in regular use that was introduced before the turn of the century.

During the first half of the 20th century, the most commonly used hypnotic medications were the approximately 50 derivatives of the BARBITURATES. The barbiturates were widely used for their central nervous system depressant effects and employed as antiepileptic agents, antianxiety medications, muscle relaxants and hypnotics. They were also effective in inducing anesthesia and are currently still used for their anesthetic effect.

Because of the unwanted sedative and sleep-inducing effects of the barbiturates, other non-sedative anticonvulsants were discovered in the 1930s and 1940s. Subsequently, the BENZODIAZEPINE hypnotics were introduced into clinical medicine in the 1960s. More than 3,000 benzodiazepine derivatives have been synthesized and about 25 are in current clinical use. The benzodiazepines have the advantage of being effective sedatives and hypnotics with little potential for serious side effects; in particular, they have low potential for producing serious central nervous system depression. The most common benzodiazepine hypnotics in the United States include flurazepam (Dalmane), temazepam (Restoril), triazolam (Halcion) and zolpidem (Ambien).

Although the barbiturates now comprise less than 10% of all prescription hypnotics, they are still very effective hypnotics. Because of their abuse potential, possible interaction with alcohol, the possibility of lethal overdose and their effect of inducing liver enzymes that can increase the metabolism of many medications, the barbiturates are of limited usefulness as everyday hypnotics. The barbiturates that have most commonly been used as hypnotics are secobarbital (Seconal), amobarbital (Amytal) and pentobarbital (Nembutal).

Other nonbarbiturate, nonbenzodiazepine hypnotic agents are also available and come from a variety of pharmacological groups. One of the most commonly prescribed agents is chloral hydrate (Noctec), which is a relatively mild hypnotic but is useful in the elderly because of its low potential for adverse reactions.

Chloral Hydrate

One of the oldest hypnotics, used for the treatment of insomnia. It is derived from chloral, a trichloroacetaldehyde, an unstable and unpleasant tasting oil that is produced in the hydrate form for more pleasant ingestion. As well as being a hypnotic agent, chloral hydrate has anticonvulsant properties.

This hypnotic has been shown to reduce SLEEP LATENCY and reduce the number of awakenings, with a variable change in the total sleep time. There is usually a slight decrease in SLOW WAVE SLEEP and variable suppression of REM SLEEP. The hypnotic effects of chloral hydrate disappear within two weeks of continuous use.

The main side effect is irritation of the mucous membranes and gastrointestinal tract. It can produce an unpleasant taste, nausea, vomiting and flatulence. There can be undesirable central nervous system effects, such as lightheadedness, malaise, ataxia and NIGHTMARES. Occasionally, allergic reactions can occur and there may be idiosyncratic reactions, such as paranoid behavior and SLEEPWALKING. Chloral hydrate is sometimes administered rectally because of the unpleasant taste and gastric irritation. The combination of chloral hydrate and alcohol led to the so-called Mickey Finn, a potion popularized in movies and crime fiction.

Habitual use of chloral hydrate can result in tolerance, dependence and addiction. Withdrawal after chronic addiction can lead to SEIZURES that can even result in death. Chloral hydrate is administered in doses of 0.5 gram to a maximum of 2 grams. The medication is best taken with milk or food in order to prevent gastrointestinal upset.

Ethchlorvynol

An oral hypnotic, brand name Placidyl, indicated for the management of insomnia as short-term hypnotic therapy for periods up to one week. Placidyl is available as dark red capsules containing either 200 milligrams or 500 milligrams of ethchlorvynol, or green capsules containing 750 milligrams of ethchlorvynol. It can cause gastrointestinal upset and hypersensitivity reactions.

Triclofos

Triclofos sodium is the sodium salt of chloral, which is a hypnotic agent limited in use because of its mild effects upon sleep and its gastrointestinal irritation. Chloral is more commonly used in the hydrate form called chloral hydrate.

L-tryptophan

A naturally occurring amino acid that is a precursor of the neurotransmitter serotonin (5-hydroxytryptamine). L-tryptophan (or tryptophan) can induce drowsiness and therefore has been used as a hypnotic agent. It typically is available in 500 milligram tablets, and up to five grams have been necessary to improve sleep. The effect of L-tryptophan upon sleep is controversial as some studies have shown little benefit in insomniac patients, whereas other studies have shown a reduced sleep latency and an increased depth of sleep. L-tryptophan also tends to have an irritant effect on the gastrointestinal tract and can produce nausea and vomiting.

In general, L-tryptophan has little usefulness in the management of chronic insomnia. The U.S. Centers for Disease Control (CDC) requested physicians to temporarily stop prescribing L-tryptophan in 1989 due to reports of 30 cases of eosinophilia-myalgia (some fatal). Three-quarters of those who developed this rare blood disorder were discovered to have been taking supplements of L-tryptophan.

Zaleplon

A novel pyrazolopyrimidine compound, brand name Sonata, that acts as a hypnotic by selectively binding to the BENZODIAZEPINE type-1 receptor situated on the alpha subunit of the GABA receptor complex. Zaleplon possesses attributes that many insomniacs would consider ideal: fast sleep onset, short duration, a low incidence of adverse effects and no residual effects four hours after dosing. Zaleplon has equal efficacy with TRIAZOLAM and zolpidem in decreasing time to sleep onset. It is safe and effective in the elderly at doses of 10 milligrams or less. There is no tolerance to the hypnotic effect, so the dosage does not need to be increased over time. There is no anterograde amnesia or residual sedative effects at doses of less than 20 milligrams four hours after administration. It has a very low potential for REBOUND INSOMNIA.

Zolpidem

A nonbenzodiazepine hypnotic agent that is the most widely used hypnotic in the United States. It has few side effects, does not cause rebound insomnia, and is safe if taken in overdose.

Zopiclone

A hypnotic medication derived from cyclopyrrolone that is not available in the United States but is available in Europe. This medication has properties that are similar to the more commonly-used benzodiazepine hypnotics, and it appears to bind to the same central nervous system receptor. Zopiclone produces an improvement in sleep efficiency, with an increased total sleep time and a decreased number of awakenings. It has few side effects but can cause a bitter taste in the mouth and difficulty with concentration during the daytime.

Other sedative medications that have hypnotic properties include glutethimide (Doriden), meprobamate (Miltown) and methyprylon (Noludar). Other agents that are now rarely prescribed as hypnotics because of their serious side effects include paraldehyde (Paral) and methaqualone.

A variety of nonprescription hypnotic medications are available as OVER-THE-COUNTER MEDICATIONS. Many of these medications are ANTIHISTAMINES that have sedative side effects, such as doxylamine, phenyltoloxamine and pyrilamine. These agents are not very effective in the treatment of INSOMNIA, can lead to the development of TOLERANCE and prominent residual daytime central nervous system depression, and are not recommended for general hypnotic use.

In recent years, there has been the realization that insomnia is not a primary diagnosis but rather a symptom of many underlying causes. Many of the causes of insomnia can be treated without the use of a hypnotic agent. The use of hypnotics for LONG-TERM INSOMNIA is to be avoided because of the potential problems of tolerance and the potential for drug abuse. Chronic insomnia can be managed by behavioral means, psychotherapy or non-hypnotic medications. The most appropriate use of hypnotic medications appears to be in the treatment of transient or SHORT-TERM INSOMNIA, such as JET LAG, where their use is for a few days only. The selection of a hypnotic is ideally made according to its duration of action so that people with daytime tiredness and fatigue are best treated by means of a short-acting hypnotic. Patients with mild features of anxiety are best treated by an intermediate-acting hypnotic, whereas patients with more severe anxiety are best treated by a long-acting hypnotic.

Darcourt, G., et al., "The Safety and Tolerability of Zolpidem: An Update," *Journal of Psychopharmacology* 13, no. 1 (1999): 81–93.

hypnotoxin Term applied to a substance presumed to be contained in the cerebrospinal fluid, which was able to produce sleep. In 1911, Henri Pieron demonstrated that the cerebrospinal fluid of sleep-deprived animals could induce sleep when injected into non-sleep-deprived animals and that a substance was transmitted capable of producing this sleep effect. The term SLEEP PROMOTING SUBSTANCE (SPS) is more commonly used than hypnotoxin. (See also SLEEP-INDUCING FACTORS.)

hypocretin (orexin) A peptide first identified in 1998. Produced by prehypocretin mRNA, hypocretin exists as two related peptides: hypocretin-1 (orexin A) and hypocretin-2 (orexin B). These neuropeptides are produced in neurons of the hypothalamus and affect two receptors: hypocretin receptor-1 and hypocretin receptor-2. The hypocretins are localized in the synaptic vesicles and possess neuroexcitatory effects.

An abnormal hypocretin receptor gene has been shown to be responsible for canine narcolepsy. Abnormalities of either the hypocretin receptor gene or of the production of hypocretins may be responsible for human NARCOLEPSY. Hypocretin cells are reduced or absent in patients with narcolepsy.

hypopnea An episode of shallow breathing during sleep that lasts 10 seconds or longer; associated with a reduction in airflow of 50% or more and a fall in the oxygen saturation level. The presence of some airflow distinguishes this event from apneic episodes. Hypopneas are usually seen in persons who have SLEEP-RELATED BREATHING DISORDERS, such as CENTRAL SLEEP APNEA SYNDROME or OBSTRUCTIVE SLEEP APNEA SYNDROME. (See also APNEA, APNEA-HYPOPNEA INDEX.)

hypothalamus A region at the base of the brain believed to have an important role in the maintenance of sleep and wakefulness. Original investigations by Constantin von Economo on patients suffering from ENCEPHALITIS LETHARGICA in the second decade of this century showed that the anterior hypothalamus was commonly responsible for INSOMNIA, whereas lesions of the posterior hypothalamus were associated with excessive sleepiness. The hypothalamus is also involved in many other autonomic processes including thermoregulation and control of food and fluid intake.

The hypothalamus has connections with the retino-hypothalamic tract, which leads from the retina to the optic chiasm, and synapses in the SUPRACHIASMATIC NUCLEI for the control of CIRCADIAN RHYTHMS. Isolation of the suprachiasmatic nuclei of the hypothalamus will disrupt circadian rhythmicity although the temperature rhythm will continue. Transplantation of fetal suprachiasmatic nuclei cells into other animals who have had the suprachiasmatic nucleus destroyed will return circadian rhythmicity.

Other experiments of either stimulating or lesioning cells of the hypothalamic region have demonstrated effects on sleep or sleepiness; however, the exact role of the hypothalamic centers in the control of sleep and wakefulness is unknown.

hypothyroidism A disorder characterized by a loss of production of thyroid hormone from the thyroid gland; caused by an intrinsic abnormality of the thyroid gland, or by reduced stimulation of the thyroid gland due to the loss of the brain thyroid-stimulating hormone. Thyroid deficiency can produce respiratory muscle failure with resulting OBSTRUCTIVE SLEEP APNEA SYNDROME or ALVEOLAR HYPOVENTILATION, which when severe may require the institution of mechanical ventilation. Hypothyroidism impairs the ventilation responses to HYPOXIA or HYPERCAPNIA and, in addition, leads to increased weight gain and deposition of mucopolysaccharides in the tissues of the upper airway.

Severe hypothyroidism can also produce tiredness, fatigue and sleepiness because of the reduced body metabolism. The diagnosis is made by the demonstration of a low free-thyroxine level in the blood, typically in association with an elevated, thyroid-stimulating hormone level. A thyroid scan is usually necessary to provide information on the function and anatomy of the thyroid gland. If the thyroid-stimulating hormone level is abnormally low, a brain CT scan, or MRI scan, is necessary to assess pituitary function.

The presence of sleep-related disorders, such as obstructive sleep apnea syndrome, can be confirmed by polysomnographic monitoring and the degree of daytime sleepiness by MULTIPLE SLEEP LATENCY TESTING.

The symptoms of hypothyroidism can be quite subtle, and it is therefore an important diagnosis to consider in any patient who has the obstructive sleep apnea syndrome. Thyroid levels should be checked in all patients, especially before surgical management of the syndrome.

Treatment of hypothyroidism involves replacement of thyroid hormone, typically with between 50 and 200 micrograms of thyroxine per day. The symptoms of daytime sleepiness and the features of SLEEP-RELATED BREATHING DISORDERS rapidly improve with replacement therapy. As hypothyroidism leads to a general increase in body weight, treatment often leads to weight reduction.

Severe hypothyroidism results in MYXEDEMA, which is characterized by generalized mucopolysaccharide accumulation throughout the body, resulting in thickening of the facial features and doughy induration of the skin. Respiratory depression is common in myxedema as are sleep-related breathing disorders, and the patient can lapse into myxedema coma, which is a hypothermic, stuporous state. Myxedema coma is frequently fatal. (See also POLYSOMNOGRAPHY, UPPER AIRWAY OBSTRUCTION.)

hypoventilation See ALVEOLAR HYPOVENTILATION.

hypoxemia A low level of oxygen in the blood. Hypoxemia during sleep typically occurs in patients with SLEEP-RELATED BREATHING DISORDERS such as the OBSTRUCTIVE SLEEP APNEA SYNDROME. The hypoxemia is usually detected by an oximeter, which measures the oxygen saturation of the hemoglobin. Hypoxemia can have important effects upon the body, particularly the cardiovascular system, as chronic hypoxemia can produce pulmonary hypertension that in turn can produce right-sided heart failure. Hypoxemia can also cause cardiac irritation, leading to cardiac irregularity or cardiac ischemia.

Assisted ventilation during sleep may be required for patients who have hypoxemia, by means of either CONTINUOUS POSITIVE AIRWAY PRESSURE (CPAP) or artificial ventilation devices. Oxygen therapy, respiratory stimulant medications or relief of UPPER AIRWAY OBSTRUCTION by surgery are other means employed to relieve hypoxemia in some patients.

hypoxia A reduction of oxygen supply to tissues below the level necessary to maintain normal cellular metabolism. Hypoxia can be produced either by a reduction in the oxygen level of the inspired air, such as that seen at high altitudes or due to UPPER AIRWAY OBSTRUCTION, or by means of an abnormality of the lung whereby oxygen is unable to adequately diffuse into the blood. Lung disease is a common cause of tissue hypoxia due to the deficient oxygenation of the blood (hypoxemia).

Hypoxia due to low inspired levels of oxygen can produce periodic breathing, which causes an alternating pattern of hyperventilation and hypoventilation that is a characteristic feature of ALTITUDE INSOMNIA (acute mountain sickness). Upper airway obstruction, which occurs in the OBSTRUCTIVE SLEEP APNEA SYNDROME, can be associated with a reduction in lung oxygen levels, thereby producing hypoxemia with resultant arousal and ventilatory stimulation.

Chronic lung disease, such as that seen in CHRONIC OBSTRUCTIVE PULMONARY DISEASE, particularly emphysema, is associated with impaired blood gas transfer and hypoxemia. Patients with chronic obstructive pulmonary disease can develop worsening hypoxemia during sleep, especially during REM sleep.

As a result of hypoxia, sleep becomes fragmented, with an increased number of arousals and awakenings related to the hypoxemia. The direct effects of hypoxemia can be detrimental on the cardiovascular as well as other body systems. (See also CHEYNE-STOKES BREATHING.)

Hz See HERTZ.

I

idiopathic hypersomnia Disorder associated with EXCESSIVE SLEEPINESS; believed to be of central nervous system cause. This disorder has similarities to narcolepsy but lacks the associated REM phenomena. Features such as CATAPLEXY, SLEEP PARALYSIS and HYPNAGOGIC HALLUCINATIONS do not occur in patients with idiopathic hypersomnia.

Idiopathic hypersomnia has its onset during adolescence and early adulthood and is characterized by gradually increasing daytime sleepiness. Typically, patients with idiopathic hypersomnia will take frequent NAPS, usually of one to two hours in duration. The major sleep episode may be of normal or longer than normal duration.

Polysomnographic studies (see POLYSOMNOGRAPHY) demonstrate a normal or prolonged total sleep time without evidence of sleep disruption. Daytime MULTIPLE SLEEP LATENCY TESTING demonstrates a mean sleep latency that is consistent with pathological sleepiness but is characterized by the absence of naps with REM sleep. Typically, patients with idiopathic hypersomnia will develop deep sleep stages, such as stage three or four sleep during nap opportunities.

Central nervous system tests, including brain imaging and encephalography, are usually normal.

Treatment is similar to that for improving alertness in patients with narcolepsy. It involves the use of STIMULANT MEDICATIONS, such as pemoline (Cylert), methylphenidate (Ritalin) or dextroamphetamine (Dexedrine). Treatment is initiated with pemoline and may be changed to methylphenidate or dextroamphetamine if pemoline does not give an adequate response. Usually treatment is lifelong; there is no evidence for remission of the underlying sleepiness.

Guilleminault, Christian, "Disorders of Excessive Daytime Sleepiness," *Annals of Clinical Research* 17 (1985): 209–219.

Roth, Bedrich, *Narcolepsy and Hypersomnia.* Basel: Karger, 1980.

idiopathic insomnia A lifelong form of insomnia that is believed to have a neurochemical basis; originally termed *childhood onset insomnia.* This insomnia is believed to be due to an inability to achieve a sustained high quality of sleep. Idiopathic insomnia is typically characterized by a prolonged SLEEP LATENCY, frequent awakenings at night and sometimes an EARLY MORNING AROUSAL. It is possible that people with idiopathic insomnia are those who comprise the lower 5% of the normal distribution of ability to have a normal quality sleep period. Elements of ANXIETY and hyperarousal may be present in such individuals, but there is no gross psychopathology warranting a diagnosis of ANXIETY DISORDER nor any evidence to suggest a diagnosis of DEPRESSION.

Idiopathic insomnia needs to be differentiated from PSYCHOPHYSIOLOGICAL INSOMNIA, which involves learned negative associations with sleep. Idiopathic insomnia is more likely to be stable over time, with poor quality sleep occurring in all sleep environments; the insomnia does not have the intermittent exacerbations that are seen with psychophysiological insomnia. Psychophysiological insomnia also rarely occurs from childhood. Individuals who are SHORT SLEEPERS typically awake refreshed in the morning and lack a complaint of poor quality sleep or of frequent awakenings as do those with idiopathic insomnia.

INADEQUATE SLEEP HYGIENE may be confused with idiopathic insomnia, although the intermittent nature of inadequate sleep hygiene contrasts with the more fixed complaint of idiopathic insomnia.

Polysomnographic studies of individuals with idiopathic insomnia have demonstrated severe sleep disruption, which is characterized by a long sleep latency and frequent arousals with early morning awakening. Sleep efficiencies are usually greatly reduced and there may be specific sleep stage abnormalities, such as reduction of spindle activity in stage two sleep or reduced rapid eye movements during REM SLEEP. As with psychophysiological insomnia, a reversed first night effect may be seen in which individuals sleep much better in the sleep laboratory on the first night because of the change in their habitual environment.

Idiopathic insomnia is typically lifelong and appears to be genetically transmitted. There is some suggestion that babies born during a difficult labor may be predisposed to developing this disorder. Its prevalence is unknown. There is some evidence to suggest an alteration in serotonin metabolism with inadequate production of serotonin.

Treatment of idiopathic insomnia is generally unsatisfactory. Attention to SLEEP HYGIENE and BEHAVIORAL TREATMENT OF INSOMNIA, such as STIMULUS CONTROL THERAPY and SLEEP RESTRICTION THERAPY, are useful.

imipramine See ANTIDEPRESSANTS.

impaired sleep-related penile erections The inability to achieve a penile erection during sleep. (This term is preferred to *sleep-related penile tumescence*.) All males, from infancy to old age, have penile erections that occur during REM SLEEP. The inability to achieve an adequate erection during sleep at night may help differentiate an organic from a psychogenic cause of impotence. MEDICATIONS and sleep disorders that disrupt REM sleep may also cause impaired sleep-related penile erections. The measurement of penile circumference and rigidity during sleep is an important test for differentiating organic impotence.

Diseases that affect the neurological or vascular supply of the penis can produce impaired erectile ability during sleep. In addition, neurotransmitter and endocrine disorders can also be contributing factors. Disorders such as diabetes mellitus and HYPERTENSION are common causes of organic impotence but other disorders, including renal failure, spinal cord injury, alcoholism, back injury and multiple sclerosis can also be common causes of impaired erections. Rarely, severe psychiatric disease, such as DEPRESSION, may be associated with impaired sleep-related penile erections. However, patients with PSYCHIATRIC DISORDERS are typically able to achieve several erections during REM sleep, although erections during wakefulness may be difficult to attain. Sleep-related impaired erections may occur following urogenital disorders such as prostatic hypertrophy or Peyrone's disease and following prostatic removal. Medications, particularly antihypertensives, ANTIDEPRESSANTS, narcotics or antipsychotic medications (see NEUROLEPTICS), may be associated with impaired erectile ability.

Impaired sleep-related erections may occur at any age; however, most commonly patients appear at a sleep disorders center with the problem after the age of 45 years.

The majority of patients with a complaint of impotence have impaired sleep-related penile erections demonstrated during polysomnographic evaluation. It is estimated that approximately 10% of adult males suffer from IMPOTENCE, the majority of whom have organic impotence.

Polysomnographic monitoring of erectile ability is obtained by the use of strain gauges placed around the penis and by the demonstration of adequate REM SLEEP. The absence of adequate penile erections either in rigidity or duration of erection is evidence for organic impotence. Typically erections during REM sleep will last longer than five minutes and erections of shorter duration are inadequate. The rigidity of the penis can be determined by a buckling pressure once the patient is awakened during sleep. If a pressure of less than 500 grams causes a buckling of the penis then this is evidence of an insufficient degree of penile rigidity. In most healthy males, the buckling of the penis will not occur unless the pressure exceeds 1,000 grams. Typically at least two nights of polysomnographic recording, with measurement of penile tumescence, is necessary in order to determine a diagnosis of organic impotence. However, many sleep laboratories require three nights of recording for confirmation.

If impaired sleep-related penile erections are present, other investigations, including penile blood pressure, penile neurodiagnostic tests and hormonal tests may be indicated in order to determine the cause of the impaired erectile ability. Occasionally, sleep disorders, such as OBSTRUCTIVE SLEEP APNEA SYNDROME, are associated with impaired sleep-related penile erections, which are improved by treatment of the sleep apnea syndrome. The medication Viagra is effective at improving erectile ability if taken one hour before sleep, in those who have erectile difficulties.

In many patients with organic impotence, the only means of treatment is by the surgical implantation of an artificial penile prosthesis. Patients with normal erectile ability during sleep, but with a complaint of impotence, may best be treated by means of sex, marital or psychiatric therapy. (See also ALCOHOLISM, SLEEP-RELATED PAINFUL ERECTIONS.)

Fisher, C., Schiavi, R.C., Edwards, S.A., Davis, D.M., Reitman, M. and Fine, J., "Evaluation of Nocturnal Penile Tumescence in the Differential Diagnosis of Sexual Impotence: A Quantitative Study," *Archives of General Psychiatry* 36 (1979): 431–437.

Ware, J.C., "Evaluation of Impotence—Monitoring Periodic Penile Erections During Sleep," *Psychiatric Clinics of North America* 10 (1987): 675–686.

impotence The inability to attain an adequate penile erection for sexual intercourse. Impotence may be due to psychological or psychiatric disorders, such as DEPRESSION or ANXIETY DISORDERS. Physical causes of impaired erectile ability commonly include vascular disorders, such as peripheral vascular disease of HYPERTENSION, or neurological disorders, such as peripheral neuropathies or spinal cord lesions (such as those due to a spinal cord injury). It is also a common manifestation of diabetes, probably because of a combination of vascular and neurological abnormalities associated with that disorder. Impotence also can occur in the OBSTRUCTIVE SLEEP APNEA SYNDROME, where it appears to have a higher prevalence than in the general population. Treatment of the obstructive sleep apnea syndrome leads to improve erectile ability.

The assessment of impotence involves an understanding of the patient's psychological and medical condition. Marital problems are a primary cause of sexual difficulty and treatment by a marriage guidance counselor may be indicated in such cases. If PSYCHIATRIC DISORDERS such as MOOD DISORDERS are present, then psychiatric treatment is usually necessary.

Patients with physical disorders, such as vascular disorders or diabetes, may require the implantation of an artificial penile prosthesis if Viagra is not effective. Penile prostheses are manufactured in two forms: an erect form, which is continuously erect, and an inflatable prosthesis that is made erect at the time of sexual activity. (See also IMPAIRED SLEEP-RELATED PENILE ERECTIONS, NOCTURNAL PENILE TUMESCENCE TEST, SLEEP-RELATED PENILE ERECTION.)

inadequate sleep hygiene Disturbance that results from practices that can have a negative effect on the sleep pattern. Improved SLEEP HYGIENE involves enhancing factors that will allow sleep to become more organized. Substances such as CAFFEINE, NICOTINE from cigarette SMOKING and other stimulants are likely to cause sleep onset difficulties or the inability to sustain quality sleep. ALCOHOL can also cause AROUSAL, but more commonly produces sedation followed by an arousal during the withdrawal phase.

Vigorous exercise before bedtime, intense mental stimulation late at night or late night social activities clearly increase arousal and reduce sleep quality. Spending an excessive amount of time in bed, irregular sleep onset and wake times or daily NAPS can all disturb the normal circadian pattern of sleep and wakefulness, leading to a breakdown in the sleep organization.

Inadequate sleep hygiene can lead to a persistent sleep disturbance, which develops into a PSYCHOPHYSIOLOGICAL INSOMNIA because of the learned negative associations due to the sleep disruption. Inadequate sleep hygiene can also accompany sleep disorders of other types. For example, INSOMNIA due to DEPRESSION may be complicated by spending an excessive time in bed and varying sleep onset and wake times. The start of the sleep disturbance typically occurs between young adulthood and old age; however, it can occur in adolescence.

Sleep studies document prolonged sleep latency, frequent nocturnal awakenings, early morning arousal and reduced sleep efficiency.

Treatment of inadequate sleep hygiene is to eliminate the negative behaviors, which usually leads to rapid resolution of the sleep disturbance.

Hauri, Peter, *The Sleep Disorders.* 2nd ed. Kalamazoo, Michigan: Academic Press, 1982.

Spielman, Arthur J., Saskin, Paul and Thorpy, Michael J., "Treatment of Chronic Insomnia by Restriction of Time in Bed," *Sleep* 10 (1987): 45–56.

incubus Latin term that applies to a form of nightmare that occurs in adults. The word comes from *in* and *cubare,* which signifies "to lie on." Incubus is an old term of SLEEP TERROR in adults. The term *incubus* refers to a demon lying on a sleeper and therefore causing the sleeper discomfort and pain. This is most clearly demonstrated in the painting entitled "The Nightmare," by Johann Heinrich Fuseli (1741–1825), located in the Detroit Institute of Art.

Closely related to the term *incubus* is the term *inuus,* which is the oldest of all Latin terms for "NIGHTMARE." This term was first used in Virgil's *Aeneid* (VI, 775) and may have led to the development of the word *incubus.*

indeterminant sleep Term applied to INFANT SLEEP that cannot be clearly differentiated into ACTIVE SLEEP or QUIET SLEEP. Typically, indeterminant sleep consists of a short episode of sleep, usually occurring between sleep changes or during the transition from wakefulness to sleep. Sometimes the term *intermediate sleep* has been used as synonymous with indeterminant sleep. (See also NON-REM-STAGE SLEEP, REM SLEEP, WAKEFULNESS.)

inductive plethysmography Noninvasive technique that has been used for the evaluation of ventilation during sleep. This device consists of a transducer of insulated wire placed around the chest to determine expansion of the lungs. A second loop of wire is placed around the abdomen; by utilizing the changes in electrical current generated by the movements of the bands of wire, tidal volume and evidence of UPPER AIRWAY OBSTRUCTION can be determined. During apneic phases, the excursions of the rib cage component in the abdomen are equal and in opposite directions, thereby causing a change in the measure that is typically called the sum. In a central apneic pause, all activity at the rib cage and abdomen is absent, and hence the sum tracing is without change.

Inductive plethysmography is most commonly used as a research procedure for the assessment of VENTILATION during sleep; however, it can also be used clinically in the evaluation of patients with SLEEP-RELATED BREATHING DISORDERS, not only of OBSTRUCTIVE SLEEP APNEA SYNDROME but also CENTRAL SLEEP APNEA SYNDROME and CENTRAL ALVEOLAR HYPOVENTILATION SYNDROME.

infant sleep Infant sleep is first recognized at a conceptual age of about 32 weeks. At this time, the infant state can be differentiated into WAKEFULNESS, QUIET SLEEP and ACTIVE SLEEP.

At the time of birth, the infant demonstrates a sleep pattern totaling 16 to 18 hours of sleep during the 24 hours. Sleep is achieved in short episodes of three to four hours, with brief awakenings. Sleep is evenly distributed over the day, and gradually the amount of sleep at night compared to during the daytime increases, so that a clear night-day differentiation is evident by three months of age.

The sleep episodes of the infant are characterized by approximately 50% of REM and 50% of non-REM sleep. Infants will go from wakefulness directly into REM sleep, a feature that is not seen in older children or adults unless some pathology is present. The NREM-REM SLEEP CYCLE is slower than that seen in adults, occurring approximately every 60 minutes.

The EEG pattern begins to resemble the sleep of adults by three months of age. SLEEP SPINDLE activity begins at this time and within the next few months K-COMPLEXES can be seen. The total amount of sleep gradually falls so that by six months the infant is sleeping approximately 15 hours per day. As the sleep-wake pattern becomes more consolidated at night, the latency into REM sleep becomes biphasic so that the shortest REM latencies are usually seen between 4 and 8 A.M. whereas the longer latencies are typically seen between midday and 4 P.M. Longer REM latencies become more apparent following longer periods of wakefulness, and the prevalence of REM sleep during the daytime gradually reduces over the first year of life.

Because REM and non-REM sleep cannot be thoroughly distinguished at this stage, the terms *active sleep* and *quiet sleep* are used. Active sleep is characterized by body movement activity with occasional vocalizations, whereas quiet sleep consists of cessation of body movements as well as the EEG features consistent with non-REM sleep. The characteristic EEG pattern of active sleep is a low voltage, irregular pattern with 5 to 8 Hz theta and 1 to 5 Hz delta activity.

Quiet sleep is characterized by high voltage, slow wave activity in the delta range. There is also the trace alternant pattern of high voltage slow waves mixed with rapid low voltage activity that occurs in bursts alternating with periods of low voltage "flat" periods. The eye movement activity is increased during active sleep and absent during slow wave sleep. The muscle tone activity is elevated during quiet sleep and relatively low during active sleep.

Some sleep is not able to be differentiated into active and quiet and is often called INDETERMINANT SLEEP. This type of sleep decreases as the infant develops. (See also ONTOGENY OF SLEEP, TRACE ALTERNANT.)

Hoppenbrouwers, T., Hodgman, J.E., Harper, R.N. and Sterman, M.B., "Temporal Distribution of Sleep States, Somatic Activity, and Autonomic Activity During the First Half Year Of Life," *Sleep* 5 (1982): 131–144.

infant sleep apnea A variety of respiratory disturbances that can occur in infants, predominantly during sleep. Infants who stop breathing during sleep often raise a fear of the SUDDEN INFANT DEATH SYNDROME (SIDS), in which otherwise healthy infants die suddenly during sleep. However, brief apneic pauses are common in infants; even for infants who have longer respiratory pauses, there is little evidence to substantiate that this is predictive of SIDS. Children who have very prolonged apneic pauses, greater than 20 seconds in duration, particularly premature infants, will have approximately a 5% greater risk of SIDS than otherwise healthy children. However, the observation of an infant who stops breathing and has some change in color, either by cyanosis or pallor, and who is often very limp at the time, is a frightening occurrence for a mother or father. Although the majority of such witnessed episodes are not associated with any significant cardiorespiratory events during infancy, there are a number of disorders in which respiration may be greatly compromised during sleep.

Infants who suffer other medical illnesses at the time of birth, either infection, trauma or hemorrhages, are more likely to develop respiratory irregularity that will be most prominent during sleep; in such circumstances some children may require aggressive intervention in order to maintain adequate VENTILATION. A number of sleep-related respiratory disturbances can occur in infants, such as the OBSTRUCTIVE SLEEP APNEA SYNDROME, CENTRAL SLEEP APNEA SYNDROME, CENTRAL ALVEOLAR HYPOVENTILATION SYNDROME and APNEA OF PREMATURITY. The obstructive sleep apnea syndrome is characterized by UPPER AIRWAY OBSTRUCTION that occurs predominantly during sleep, particularly during REM sleep, and is associated with a reduction in oxygen levels in the blood as well as increases in carbon dioxide values. Apneic episodes of similar duration can occur in the central sleep apnea syndrome, but in this disorder upper airway obstruction is not the primary event, although there is a decrease in central nervous system respiratory drive. This form of apnea is more common in infants who have central nervous system lesions. Some infants do not have apneic pauses but will have prolonged episodes of reduced ventilation during sleep, with associated oxygen desaturation and increases in carbon dioxide levels. This form of respiratory disturbance, termed *central alveolar hypoventilation syndrome–congenital type*, may require assisted ventilation until the infant is able to sustain ventilation spontaneously after maturation of the respiratory system.

infant sleep disorders INFANT SLEEP is very different from the sleep of young children or adults. It has a high percentage of REM sleep that fills 50% of the total sleep time, and sleep occurs in brief episodes throughout the 24-hour day. Approximately two-thirds of the day is spent in sleep.

During the first three months of life, the child's sleep appears to occur with a cyclical pattern that is slightly greater than 24 hours; therefore, the major sleep episode occurs slightly later on each successive day. This pattern, which is known as FREE RUNNING, is due to the underlying tendency of our biological circadian rhythms to have a PERIOD LENGTH slightly longer than 24 hours. This tendency in the infant is usually not a concern so long as the typical ENVIRONMENTAL TIME CUES are instituted to maintain the major sleep episode over the nighttime hours. If these environmental time cues, such as quieter nights and daytime stimulation, are not instituted, a delayed sleep pattern will develop. As a result, the major sleep episode occurs at a slightly later time and so the sleep episode will rotate around the clock. This is called the NON-24-HOUR SLEEP-WAKE SYNDROME and occurs in infants only if appropriate environmental cues are not instituted.

Colic is perhaps the most widely recognized cause of awakenings and crying at night in infants within the first four months of age. Usually colic occurs within the first three weeks of age and reduces in frequency so that about 50% of infants with colic will not have attacks after two months of age, and most infants will have outgrown colic by four months of age. The cause of colic is unknown and, although it is suspected of being due to stomach cramps, there is no scientific evidence to indicate that colic is of gastrointestinal cause. Current belief is that it is due to an immature central nervous system. There are some irregularities of behavior with increased arousal and sensitivity to environmental stimuli that cause the awakenings. Colic can lead to the development of more chronic sleep disturbances in the older infant if it is not appropriately managed in the first few months of life. The institution of good SLEEP HYGIENE and providing the appropriate sleep times is essential to ensure that more persistent sleep disturbances do not occur.

A benign form of abnormal movements can occur in newborn infants and is called BENIGN NEONATAL SLEEP MYOCLONUS. This disorder is associated with jerking movements of limbs, and even of the face or trunk, but is not associated with underlying epilepsy, and usually resolves within the first few weeks of life.

Usually the time between the second and sixth months of life is associated with a consolidated nighttime sleep episode and several daytime NAPS and is a relatively peaceful time for the mother. It is during this time that the major changes in the structure of the infant's sleep are occurring and so it is a critical time for the infant. Patterns of cortisol and growth hormone production are developing and become established by six months of age.

During the first six months of life, the respiratory system undergoes development. It is one of the most fragile body systems and is susceptible to variations that can be noted by the mother. Most healthy infants will have episodes of cessation of breathing that occur and last up to 20 seconds in duration. These episodes may concern a mother but may be a part of normal development and decrease in frequency as the child develops. Premature infants are more likely to have these apneas. A syndrome called APNEA OF PREMATURITY can exist where prolonged episodes may be associated with changes in oxygenation of the blood, and therefore a child may briefly turn blue or pale in color. Within the first few months of life, these episodes spontaneously decrease as a more healthy infant pattern of ventilation develops. Healthy premature infants with persistence of prolonged episodes of apnea may be predisposed to the SUDDEN INFANT DEATH SYNDROME, a disorder that is of concern to most mothers because it is sudden, unexpected and occurs in otherwise healthy infants.

At six months of age, the infant's sleep pattern becomes lighter and the number of awakenings can increase. It is at this time that the infant is becoming more aware of the world, and the frequent awakenings and difficulty in initiating sleep may cause the parents concern and anxiety. It is important during this time that positive sleep hygiene practices are put into place, particularly the institution of limits on the time that the child is put down for sleep and the time that the child is allowed to sleep undisturbed. An appropriate amount of daytime stimulation is necessary so that the development of a full period of wakefulness can gradually occur. Physical illnesses, such as ear or other infections, can cause the sleep pattern to be interrupted, but as long as the appropriate cues and positive associations with sleep are instituted, the disturbance is usually only temporary.

One form of insomnia, related to an allergy to cow's milk, is called FOOD ALLERGY INSOMNIA and can produce irritability in the infant, resulting in frequent arousals and crying. Very often there are other manifestations of the allergy, such as skin difficulties and gastrointestinal upset. The close association of the onset of the insomnia with the change from breast-feeding to cow's milk is the first indication that this form of sleep disturbance might be present. Elimination of cow's milk in the diet brings about a resolution of the insomnia.

The main forms of pathological sleep disturbance in the infant include ventilatory abnormalities, such as the obstructive sleep apnea syndrome, or neurological disorders, such as epilepsy. The SLEEP-RELATED BREATHING DISORDERS are evidenced by difficulty in breathing during sleep or prolonged episodes of cessation of breathing. Apneic episodes of greater than 20 seconds in duration are an indication of pathology, and may be due either to upper airway obstruction or a central cause. Typical obstructive sleep apnea syndrome is less likely to occur in the infant than in the older child who has enlarged tonsils. When upper airway obstruction occurs, it usually occurs in both wakefulness and sleep. Excessive sleepiness is not evident in the infant, and the main features of upper airway obstruction are difficulty in breathing and the change in coloration or heart rate. Upper airway obstruction is more common in infants with craniofacial abnormalities, such as those due to a small jaw or an enlarged tongue. Central apnea may be due to neurological disorders that may be have occurred during the time of a difficult delivery, such as an intracerebral hemorrhage. Central nervous system lesions can affect the control of breathing and lead to frequent episodes of breathing cessation during sleep, commonly called the CENTRAL SLEEP APNEA SYNDROME.

Many illnesses of an infective, biochemical or anatomical nature can predispose the infant to central apnea. For most infants, treatment of the underlying medical disorder will lead to resolution of the apneic episodes. However, some infants with primary respiratory difficulty may need to have artificial ventilation until the respiratory symptom has improved so that spontaneous control is possible. There has not been demonstrated a clear association between infants with apneic episodes of less than 20 seconds in duration and the subsequent development of sudden infant death syndrome.

Central nervous system disorders, such as epilepsy, can cause abnormal movements in infants during sleep. These episodes are often the result of central nervous system lesions, such as an intracerebral tumor. Metabolic abnormalities due to a change in the blood electrolytes are a common cause of seizures in the newborn infant, and with correction of the biochemical changes the seizure manifestations resolve. Sometimes epilepsy can be the cause of apneic episodes.

Ferber, Richard, *Solve Your Child's Sleep Problems.* New York: Simon and Schuster, 1985.

Guilleminault, C., ed., *Sleep and Its Disorders in Children.* New York: Raven Press, 1987.

initiating and maintaining sleep See DISORDERS OF INITIATING AND MAINTAINING SLEEP (DIMS).

insomnia Term derived from the Latin words *in,* meaning "no," and *somnus,* meaning "sleep." Insomnia strictly means the inability to sleep.

Insomnia is applied to people who have a complaint of unrefreshing sleep, or difficulty in initiating or maintaining sleep. Although the term has been used to refer to a disorder in which sleep disturbance can be objectively documented, it is more generally used for any disorder associated with a complaint of disturbed or unrefreshing sleep.

Most, but not all, patients with insomnia have daytime effects of the disturbed nighttime sleep, such as fatigue, tiredness, irritability or inability to concentrate, that can impair the ability to work or socialize. Insomnia has been used as a diagnosis in the past, but in recent years, with the recognition of the many different causes of insomnia, the term is now largely applied to the symptom complaint of the patient and should not be viewed as a specific disorder. With the development of SLEEP DISORDERS MEDICINE, many new disorders have been recognized that can produce a complaint of insomnia. The physician should determine the exact cause of the symptom in order to initiate appropriate treatment.

It is difficult to determine the prevalence of insomnia; however, it is clearly a widespread complaint. Everyone, at some point, has experienced insomnia, if only temporarily. National surveys have reported that up to one-third of the population has some degree of insomnia, and 50% of that third regard the insomnia as serious. Ten percent of people reporting severe insomnia have been prescribed HYPNOTICS and 5% have used OVER-THE-COUNTER MEDICATIONS.

In general, insomnia has not been well treated in the past because clinicians lacked a good understanding either of its causes or of the different treatment options available. Although it was clear that PSYCHIATRIC DISORDERS were associated with insomnia, particularly the MOOD DISORDERS, such as DEPRESSION or the ANXIETY DISORDERS, there was little understanding of the importance of physical causes of insomnia.

Research studies have demonstrated that the total amount of sleep does not necessarily correlate with the complaint of insomnia. Many patients who complain of insomnia have an amount of sleep that would be regarded as normal, and some patients very clearly have normal sleep without any interruptions or disruptions. Insomnia may also be related to impaired perception of sleep quality; for example, an infant may be brought to medical attention by a mother who complains that the child has frequent awakenings at night, which may be entirely normal in number and duration.

Therefore, the assessment of insomnia is most important, as treatment depends upon the cause of the insomnia and may vary from simple reassurance to behavioral, pharmacological or mechanical means. The age of the patient will influence the likelihood of certain sleep disorders being responsible for the complaint of insomnia. A clear understanding of the nature of the complaint and, when indicated, further investigations, such as polysomnographic monitoring, may be required to determine the exact cause of insomnia in order to develop a successful treatment plan.

Although many different classifications of insomnia have been developed, the differential diagnosis developed in the *International Classification of Sleep Disorders* has been clinically very useful. However, insomnia can be divided into slightly different groups associated with the following causes: behavioral or psychophysiological causes; psychiatric causes; environmental causes; drug-dependent factors; those associated with respiratory or movement disorders; those associated with alterations in the timing of the sleep-wake pattern or associated with the parasomnias or neurological disorders; those without any objective sleep disturbance; idiopathic insomnia; and a miscellaneous group of other causes of insomnia.

Insomnia Associated with Behavioral or Psychophysiological Causes

Insomnia associated with behavioral or psychophysiological causes includes ADJUSTMENT SLEEP DISORDER, PSYCHOPHYSIOLOGICAL INSOMNIA, INADEQUATE SLEEP HYGIENE, LIMIT-SETTING SLEEP DISORDER, SLEEP-ONSET ASSOCIATION DISORDER, NOCTURNAL EATING (DRINKING) SYNDROME.

These disorders often respond to the institution of SLEEP HYGIENE or BEHAVIORAL TREATMENT OF INSOMNIA.

Insomnia Associated with Psychiatric Disorders

Includes the mood disorders, such as depression or manic-depressive disease, PSYCHOSES, anxiety disorders, including PANIC DISORDERS, and ALCOHOLISM. Specific treatment of the psychiatric state is required; good sleep hygiene and behavioral treatments of insomnia can assist the resolution of the sleep complaint.

Environmental Factors

Particularly noise, temperature, or abnormal light exposure; may be important in the production of some forms of insomnia. The ingestion of some foods can produce a FOOD ALLERGY INSOMNIA, and toxins can produce a TOXIN-INDUCED SLEEP DISORDER.

Medications and Insomnia

Medications can be associated with the development of insomnia, with the chronic use of hypnotics leading to HYPNOTIC-DEPENDENT SLEEP DISORDER, which may exacerbate upon withdrawal of the hypnotic agent. The chronic use of stimulants, such as CAFFEINE, or weight-reduction medications, such as amphetamines, can produce a

STIMULANT-DEPENDENT SLEEP DISORDER. The chronic use of alcohol for sleep purposes can lead to an ALCOHOL-DEPENDENT SLEEP DISORDER. Gradual withdrawal of the offending agent under clinical supervision, with maintenance of good sleep hygiene, is usually all that is required for the treatment of these forms of insomnia.

Sleep-related Breathing Disorders

Can be associated with the complaint of insomnia, particularly in the elderly. OBSTRUCTIVE SLEEP APNEA SYNDROME, CENTRAL SLEEP APNEA SYNDROME and CENTRAL ALVEOLAR HYPOVENTILATION SYNDROME can all produce awakenings at night, with little evidence of daytime impairment of respiratory function. Polysomnographic investigation is usually necessary to understand the severity and extent of these disorders to determine appropriate treatment.

Other respiratory disorders, such as CHRONIC OBSTRUCTIVE PULMONARY DISEASE and SLEEP-RELATED ASTHMA, can have direct sleep effects. Insomnia may also be exacerbated by the RESPIRATORY STIMULANTS, such as the xanthines, that are used to treat these disorders.

Altitude Insomnia

Occurring at high altitudes and caused by the low level of inspired oxygen tension, which produces a periodic pattern of breathing often associated with insomnia. It usually resolves upon return to a lower altitude.

Insomnia and Abnormal Movement Disorders

Insomnia may be associated with abnormal movement disorders during sleep. Typical SLEEP STARTS, or hypnic jerks, can cause a sleep-onset insomnia, as can the RESTLESS LEGS SYNDROME, which is associated with disagreeable sensations in the legs. Rarely, nocturnal CRAMPS may cause sudden awakenings during sleep, leading to the complaint of insomnia.

The PERIODIC LIMB MOVEMENT DISORDER is a movement disorder that occurs solely during sleep. The patient may not be aware of it, but it is typically seen by a bed partner. It is associated with periodic movements of the limbs and disturbed quality of sleep, often leading to the complaint of insomnia or unrestful sleep.

The REM SLEEP BEHAVIOR DISORDER is associated with excessive movement and abnormal behavior during sleep. Insomnia also occurs in NOCTURNAL PAROXYSMAL DYSTONIA and RHYTHMIC MOVEMENT DISORDER, when it persists into adolescence or adulthood.

Insomnia Related to the Timing of Sleep

With the development of the science of CHRONOBIOLOGY, there has been the recognition that disorders of the timing of sleep are also associated with disturbed sleep quality. This is most evident to the general population through its awareness of TIME ZONE CHANGE (JET LAG) SYNDROME and SHIFT-WORK SLEEP DISORDER. A delay in the onset of sleep can produce a sleep onset insomnia in adolescence termed DELAYED SLEEP PHASE SYNDROME. In this disorder, the sleep pattern is delayed with regard to typical sleep times. Similarly, the opposite sleep pattern, the ADVANCED SLEEP PHASE SYNDROME, can cause an EARLY MORNING AROUSAL and a complaint of insomnia. Sleep occurs at an earlier time than desired. This particular sleep pattern is more common in the elderly, who find it difficult to stay awake late at night and yet awaken early in the morning, while it is still dark.

Behavioral or neurological disorders can produce an irregular sleep pattern characterized by frequently interrupted sleep episodes throughout the 24-hour day—the IRREGULAR SLEEP-WAKE PATTERN. Rarely, the NON-24-HOUR SLEEP-WAKE SYNDROME can occur; here, the sleep pattern continues to rotate around the clock, with a PERIOD LENGTH of 25, and not 24, hours.

Neurological Disorders and Insomnia

Neurological disorders are common causes of the inability to maintain sleep, and those most commonly seen, particularly in the elderly, include PARKINSONISM and DEMENTIA. Degenerative disorders and epilepsy are two other neurological disorders that commonly present with the complaint of disturbed sleep. Appropriate treatment of these neurological disorders includes attention to good sleep hygiene, with or without the use of hypnotic agents. FATAL FAMILIAL INSOMNIA, a rare form of insomnia, has a progressive deteriorating course that eventually leads to death. There is no known treatment.

Insomnia Associated with Parasomnias

Insomnia can be caused by PARASOMNIAS that do not typically produce complaints of insomnia or EXCESSIVE SLEEPINESS. CONFUSIONAL AROUSALS, SLEEP TERRORS, NIGHTMARES and SLEEP HYPERHIDROSIS (sweating) may cause awakenings that lead to insomnia.

Insomnia with No Objective Sleep Disturbance

A form of insomnia due to a misperception or misinterpretation of sleep. SLEEP STATE MISPERCEPTION, previously known as pseudoinsomnia, occurs when patients find sleep totally unrefreshing, when they deny having been asleep, despite having had a full night of good quality sleep. This unusual disorder is poorly understood and is often resistant to attempts at treatment.

Awakening at night with a sensation of an inability to breathe, termed the SLEEP CHOKING SYNDROME, can occur, yet polysomnographically documented sleep is entirely normal. This disorder might be an unusual manifestation of an anxiety or panic disorder.

Some people have a physiological requirement for less sleep than most and can be classed as SHORT SLEEPERS. However, the desire for longer sleep may lead to the complaint of insomnia. Reassurance that the short sleep is physiologically appropriate may be all that is required.

Idiopathic Insomnia

Some patients appear to have a lifelong inability to sustain good quality sleep, and the term IDIOPATHIC INSOMNIA (or childhood-onset insomnia) has been applied. This sleep disorder is believed to be due to a genetic or acquired abnormality in the sleep maintenance systems of the brain so that normal good quality sleep is never obtained. These patients are particularly susceptible to minor stressful or environmental stimuli, which cause an exacerbation of the insomnia. Lifelong attention to good sleep hygiene is necessary for such patients.

Other Causes of Insomnia

There are many other causes of insomnia, the majority of which are related to underlying medical disorders. Other causes of sleep disturbance that can lead to a complaint of insomnia include SLEEP-RELATED GASTROESOPHAGEAL REFLUX, FIBROSITIS SYNDROME, MENSTRUAL-ASSOCIATED SLEEP DISORDER, PREGNANCY-RELATED SLEEP DISORDER, TERRIFYING HYPNAGOGIC HALLUCINATIONS, SLEEP-RELATED ABNORMAL SWALLOWING SYNDROME and SLEEP-RELATED LARYNGOSPASM.

All of the above-mentioned sleep disorders need to be considered in the differential diagnosis of the patient presenting with insomnia. A detailed clinical and psychological history will often point to the cause of the insomnia without the need for objective polysomnographic evaluation (see POLYSOMNOGRAPHY); however, many of the above disorders need polysomnographic documentation. When there is no evident cause for the insomnia, polysomnographic monitoring may be indicated. Typically, the patient will be evaluated for the quality of sleep, as well as for abnormal physiological events during sleep. One or two nights of recording in a SLEEP DISORDER CENTER is usually necessary. This information, along with the historical information taken at the initial evaluation, usually leads to a precise diagnosis so an accurate treatment plan can be outlined.

Treatment

Most patients with insomnia deal with it without the need for professional help. The TRANSIENT INSOMNIA that occurs following stress usually lasts only a few days and then spontaneously resolves. However, the patient who suffers from continuing insomnia may be reluctant to seek medical help for fear of being prescribed medications with potential adverse side effects. Many people suffer from chronic insomnia in the hope that it will eventually spontaneously resolve itself.

If the insomnia does not resolve, the patient has several avenues to pursue for help. Popular books and articles on insomnia are a source of information that is commonly used; for many patients, they provide successful treatment strategies. Over-the-counter medications for the treatment of insomnia are plentiful and are widely publicized in the media. Some patients will find these over-the-counter medications helpful, although it is unclear whether the insomnia would have resolved spontaneously despite their use. However, many patients initially seek help from their physician, or turn to their physician after trying over-the-counter medications. In the past, physicians tended to take a brief history and considered prescribing hypnotic medications. But today, a more detailed history is usually taken to try to understand the source of the insomnia. If necessary, the patient will be referred to a specialist in sleep disorders medicine for further investigation or treatment.

If the insomnia is clearly related to a situational stress, such as bereavement, hospitalization or travel that included a time zone change, specific treatment is usually unnecessary since patients know that the insomnia will be temporary, but good sleep hygiene is still essential. However, if the condition is severe, treatment may be necessary, particularly with a short course of hypnotic medication. When insomnia lasts less than three weeks, but more than a few days, the term SHORT-TERM INSOMNIA is occasionally used, although it is clear that there may be many different causes of the onset of insomnia.

If the insomnia lasts longer than three weeks, then LONG-TERM INSOMNIA (or chronic insomnia) may develop, with specialist help and further investigation often warranted. At this time, consideration of the full differential diagnosis is necessary, and polysomnographic investigation may be needed. Treatment is usually directed to one or more of the above specific causes of insomnia and very often also requires instituting good sleep hygiene practices. Behavioral techniques that have been found to be useful for patients with behavioral or psychophysiological insomnia include STIMULUS CONTROL THERAPY, SLEEP RESTRICTION THERAPY, COGNITIVE FOCUSING, SYSTEMIC DESENSITIZATION, BIOFEEDBACK, AUTOGENIC TRAINING, PARADOXICAL TECHNIQUES and PROGRESSIVE RELAXATION. The judicious use of hypnotic medications can be helpful and consideration should be given to the use of appropriate psycho-pharmacological agents—such as the BENZODIAZEPINES, zolpidem or other antianxiety agents, or the tricyclic ANTIDEPRESSANTS—in patients with anxiety and depression. Antianxiety agents, or sedative antidepressants, can be useful when given at night to improve the quality of sleep and lead to resolution of the underlying psychiatric disorder. Occult sleep disorders, such as periodic limb movement disorder or obstructive sleep apnea syndrome, may require specific treatment by means of pharmacological or mechanical means, such as the use of CONTINUOUS POSITIVE AIRWAY PRESSURE (CPAP) devices.

Case History

A 50-year-old social worker had insomnia that had been present most of her life. Over the years, she had been treated by medications, mainly hypnotics, and had undergone behavioral therapy and psychotherapy. There had been little improvement in her sleep disturbance and in recent months she had been treated with a benzodiazepine antianxiety agent, alprazolam (Xanax). However, although this produced some slight improvement, she still could sleep only one-and-one-half to two hours at night and was extremely fatigued and tired during the daytime. She was aware of loud snoring, which had been commented upon by her husband, and she wondered whether the breathing difficulty contributed to her sleep disturbance. She had occasional feelings of restless leg syndrome; although she had been effectively treated with quinine for this symptom in the past, she did not require treatment at the current time.

She typically would go to bed around 12:30 at night and awaken at 6:30 in the morning. She had numerous awakenings during the night, and an assessment of her SLEEP LOG demonstrated that she had much variability in both the time of going to bed and the time of awakening in the morning. She also had bronchitis, for which she occasionally took bronchodilators; as these medications have a stimulant effect, they tended to exacerbate her sleep disturbance.

She had a number of other somatic complaints, which included mild generalized arthritis and gastrointestinal discomfort. She regarded herself as being a slightly tense and anxious person who was rather particular about things and a little compulsive.

Her examination revealed that she had normal blood pressure, and her breath sounds were rather harsh without any evidence of significant obstructive airways disease. Examination of the oropharynx revealed a long soft palate and the posterior pharyngeal wall was slightly difficult to visualize.

The initial impression was one of difficulty in initiating and maintaining sleep with mild daytime sleepiness. This disturbance appeared to be related to a number of factors, including her psychological state with the tendency for anxiety, and her physical illnesses, such as arthritis and bronchitis. And there was evidence to suggest she might have a mild degree of obstructive sleep apnea syndrome, and periodic limb movements in sleep with the presence of restless legs syndrome.

It was recommended that she should undergo polysomnography, which demonstrated 34 brief awakenings during the night, one of which was longer than five minutes in duration. However, her SLEEP EFFICIENCY was quite good at 86%. She had a few shallow episodes of breathing and one central apnea with a slight fall in oxygen but not below 91%. She had 41 periodic leg movements giving her an index of 6 episodes per hour of sleep. She had some restlessness of her legs, indicative of the restless legs syndrome, which was present during the recording.

A MULTIPLE SLEEP LATENCY TEST demonstrated a mean sleep latency of 7.3 minutes with one sleep onset REM period at 2 P.M., indicating a mild degree of daytime sleepiness. A second night of polysomnography confirmed the initial findings but demonstrated 177 periodic leg movements at a rate of 25 episodes per hour, confirming the presence of significant periodic leg movement disorder.

Treatment consisted of avoiding the use of bronchodilator medications for her bronchitis close to the time of sleep onset. The Xanax was continued at 0.5 milligrams, taken one hour before sleep in order to assist with treating the periodic leg movements. She was placed on a strict sleep restriction therapy schedule of going to bed at 1:30 A.M. and arising at 6:30 A.M.

After two weeks, her sleep pattern considerably improved. There was less variability in the time of going to bed and getting up, and the majority of her sleep was occurring between the hours of 1 and 6 A.M. Her sleep latencies, which consistently were more than 30 minutes in duration, and sometimes as long as four hours, gradually reduced so that after a period of two months of adhering to this regimen of sleep restriction her sleep latencies fell to less than 15 minutes. She consistently was getting about five hours of sleep and her sleep time was extended from 1:30 A.M. to 7 A.M. After several weeks on the sleep program, she progressed to getting between five and five-and-a-half hours of sleep, a great increase over the one and a half or two hours she was getting previously. The Xanax was continued throughout her treatment and she was delighted with her improvement and regarded her new sleep pattern as the best she could remember.

American Sleep Disorders Association, *International Classification of Sleep Disorders,* prepared by the Diagnostic Classification Steering Committee, Michael J. Thorpy, Chairman. Rochester, Minnesota: American Sleep Disorders Association, 1990.

Kales, Anthony and Kales, J.D., *Evaluation and Treatment of Insomnia.* New York: Oxford University Press, 1984.

Eddy, M. and Walbroehl, G.S., "Insomnia," *American Family Physician* 59, no. 1 (1999): 1911–1916, 1918.

Meyer, T.J., "Evaluation and Management of Insomnia," *Hospital Practice* 33, no. 12 (1999), 75–78, 83–86.

insufficient sleep syndrome Disorder characterized by EXCESSIVE SLEEPINESS during the day due to an inadequate amount of sleep at night; typically follows episodes of sleep deprivation that have reoccurred over weeks or months. Often the inadequate nocturnal sleep is unappreciated by the patient, who presents the complaint of excessive sleepiness of unknown cause. Examination of a SLEEP LOG may demonstrate the characteristic features: shorter than normal major sleep episode with a short latency to sleep onset; and an early morning awakening, usually by an alarm or other disturbance. Polysomnographic monitoring may be necessary if the cause of daytime sleepiness is unclear or if other disorders of excessive sleepiness are considered.

Typically, insufficient sleep syndrome is a disorder seen in adolescents or young adulthood; however, it can occur at any age. Usually it is associated with nocturnal or daily commitments that require an individual to go to bed or arise early.

This disorder needs to be differentiated from IDIOPATHIC HYPERSOMNIA, which is characterized by a normal or prolonged sleep episode at night, and from NARCOLEPSY, which is typically associated with

REM sleep phenomena such as CATAPLEXY, SLEEP PARALYSIS and HYPNAGOGIC HALLUCINATIONS.

Treatment rests upon a regular extension of TOTAL SLEEP TIME to ensure that the individual's sleep duration meets his or her physiological needs. The amount of sleep time required varies among individuals; for some it may need to be as long as nine hours on a regular basis. (See also DISORDERS OF EXCESSIVE SOMNOLENCE.)

Roehrs, Timothy, Zorick, F., Sickelsteel, R., Wittig, R. and Roth, T., "Excessive Daytime Sleepiness Associated with Insufficient Sleep," *Sleep* 6 (1983): 319–325.

interleukin-I (IL-I) A substance produced by the body in response to injury, inflammation and fever. It appears to be a single polypeptide or a group of factors that are produced in response to the stress. The most prominent effect of interleukin-I is to induce fever, but amongst its other effects is the induction of SLOW WAVE SLEEP. During the acute phase response of injury, there is an increased tendency for rest and sleep, possibly to allow affected cells to rest so repair is enhanced. Interleukin-I, when infused into rabbits, will induce slow wave sleep, along with fever. When interleukin-I is administered, along with an antipyretic medication, the body TEMPERATURE does not rise, but slow wave sleep increases, indicating that the temperature effect is not the primary cause of the sleep-inducing effect.

Blood levels of interleukin-I have been shown to increase shortly after sleep onset at a time that appears to coincide with the onset of natural slow wave sleep. When FACTOR S is injected into animals, it produces fever and slow wave sleep, a reaction that appears to be mediated by the production of interleukin-I. (See also SLEEP-INDUCING FACTORS.)

"intermediary" sleep stage See NON-REM-STAGE SLEEP.

intermediate sleep See INDETERMINANT SLEEP.

intermittent DOES (periodic) syndrome Term referring to a group of disorders characterized by RECURRENT HYPERSOMNIA. One form of this disorder, called the KLEINE-LEVIN SYNDROME, is distinguished by recurrent hypersomnia, gluttony and hypersexuality. A form of the disorder exists in which recurrent episodes only of hypersomnia occur at intervals of weeks or months. Each episode of hypersomnia lasts one to two weeks.

A form of recurrent hypersomnia occurs in association with the MENSTRUAL CYCLE and is called the MENSTRUAL-ASSOCIATED SLEEP DISORDER. This disorder can also be characterized by recurrent episodes of insomnia in association with the menses.

internal arousal Term occasionally used for the effect of excessive mental activity inducing insomnia. This process is a typical feature of PSYCHOPHYSIOLOGICAL INSOMNIA and is often produced by apprehension over the inability to sleep and conscious efforts to induce sleep.

internal arousal insomnia Term used for a state of heightened arousal that impairs the ability to fall asleep or to stay asleep. This form of heightened arousal is typically seen in insomnia disorders such as PSYCHOPHYSIOLOGICAL INSOMNIA, ANXIETY DISORDERS or agitated DEPRESSION. At the desired sleep time, patients become more alert with an increase in mental activity, because a flood of thoughts prevents them from "turning off" their minds. (See also INSOMNIA, MOOD DISORDERS.)

internal desynchronization During normal entrainment to a 24-hour day, or during the initial part of a FREE RUNNING experiment in TEMPORAL ISOLATION, all of an individual's biological rhythms are internally synchronized. During this time the rhythms have the same PERIOD LENGTH of approximately 24 hours; however, during prolonged studies of an individual in time-isolation, the biological rhythms may lose their synchrony and two or more rhythms will run at different period lengths. For example, the body temperature rhythm may continue with a period length of about 24 hours, whereas the sleep-wake cycle may have a period length of 33 hours. In humans, the two main rhythms are determined by the so-called x and y oscillators, which are believed to be two independent sets of processors that determine the rhythm of most physiological circadian rhythms. (See also BIOLOGICAL CLOCKS, CHRONOBIOLOGY, SUPRACHIASMATIC NUCLEUS.)

International Classification of Sleep Disorders In 1985, the ASSOCIATION OF SLEEP DISORDER CENTERS initiated the process of revising the original DIAGNOSTIC CLASSIFICATION OF SLEEP AND AROUSAL DISORDERS. The original classification was published in 1979 in the journal *SLEEP*. This classification has been very widely used throughout the world; however, with the recent advances in SLEEP DISORDERS MEDICINE it was believed that a revision was required.

A committee was headed by Michael Thorpy, M.D., and consisted of 18 clinical sleep disorder specialists who set about the process of revising the classification.

The classification scheme differs from that of 1979 in that it breaks the sleep disorders into four groups: the dyssomnias; the parasomnias; medical and psychiatric sleep disorders; and the proposed sleep disorders. This classification system differed from the original system in order to bring the classification more in line with the international classification of diseases. The original classification was considered most useful as a differential diagnostic listing for physicians but was not useful as an international classificational schema because many disorders were represented more than once. In the new classification system, each disorder has only one entry. In addition, the classification system differentiates those disorders that are primarily sleep disorders from those that are sleep disturbances associated with other medical disorders. (See Appendix III for outline of the international classification of sleep disorders.)

The development of the international classification of sleep disorders involved the cooperation of individuals in sleep societies from around the world and led to the recommendation that the name "International Classification of Sleep Disorders" be applied to the new system. The new classification was published in 1990 by the American Sleep Disorders Association, a member society of the ASSOCIATION OF PROFESSIONAL SLEEP SOCIETIES. A minor revision of the classification was carried out in 1998. (See also AMERICAN ACADEMY OF SLEEP MEDICINE, CIRCADIAN RHYTHM SLEEP DISORDERS, DYSSOMNIA, PARASOMNIAS, PROPOSED SLEEP DISORDERS, REM PARASOMNIAS, SLEEP-WAKE TRANSITION DISORDERS.)

international sleep societies A number of sleep societies have been developed around the world for the purposes of fostering sleep research or for promoting the development of clinical sleep disorders medicine. In the United States, the ASSOCIATION FOR THE PSYCHOPHYSIOLOGICAL STUDY OF SLEEP was founded in 1961, and it subsequently led to the ASSOCIATION OF PROFESSIONAL SLEEP SOCIETIES. The first society to be founded outside of the United States was the EUROPEAN SLEEP RESEARCH SOCIETY, in 1971, followed by the JAPANESE SLEEP RESEARCH SOCIETY in 1978, the BELGIAN ASSOCIATION FOR THE STUDY OF SLEEP in 1982, the SCANDINAVIAN SLEEP RESEARCH SOCIETY in 1985, the LATIN AMERICAN SLEEP RESEARCH SOCIETY in 1986 and the SLEEP SOCIETY OF CANADA in 1986. The bimonthly journal *SLEEP*, originally published by Raven Press, was sponsored jointly by the Association of Professional Sleep Societies, European Sleep Research Society, Latin American Sleep Research Society and the Japanese Sleep Research Society. The journal *Sleep* is now published by the AMERICAN ACADEMY OF SLEEP MEDICINE (AASM) and the SLEEP RESEARCH SOCIETY (SRS).

interpretation of dreams The most significant advance in the interpretation of DREAMS occurred with SIGMUND FREUD's psychodynamic writings on dreams in his initial publication *The Interpretation of Dreams*, published in 1900. Freud wrote: "*The Interpretation of Dreams* is the royal road to a knowledge of the part the unconscious plays in the mental life."

Dreams were regarded by Freud as protecting mental health by allowing sleep to continue while mental conflict was being expressed and managed without producing sleep disruption.

Freud also regarded dreams as being symbols of internal conflicts and a representation of deep-seated, unfulfilled desires, particularly of a sexual nature.

Although Freud's interpretation of dreams is still widely held, modern science has added neurophysiological information that refutes some of Freud's hypotheses. (See also REM SLEEP.)

Freud, Sigmund, *The Interpretation of Dreams*. New York: Basic Books, 1953; first published, 1900.

intrinsic sleep disorders Medical or psychological sleep disorders that originate or develop from within the body, or arise from causes within the body. Examples of intrinsic sleep disorders include PSYCHOPHYSIOLOGICAL INSOMNIA, NARCOLEPSY and OBSTRUCTIVE SLEEP APNEA SYNDROME. EXTRINSIC SLEEP DISORDERS, originating from causes outside of the body, the CIRCADIAN RHYTHM SLEEP DISORDERS and intrinsic sleep disorders are three groups within the category of the DYSSOMNIAS, disorders that produce difficulty in initiating or maintaining sleep, excessive sleepiness or both. (See also INTERNATIONAL CLASSIFICATION OF SLEEP DISORDERS, PSYCHIATRIC DISORDERS.)

inuus The oldest of all Latin terms for the NIGHTMARE, first used in Virgil's *Aeneid* (VI, 775). This term may have led to the development of the word *incubus*, a Latin term once used for nightmares occurring in adults. SLEEP TERRORS is now preferred over INCUBUS.

irregular sleep-wake pattern A sleep pattern without the usual circadian cycle of sleep and wakefulness. Episodes of sleep and wakefulness of variable duration occur throughout the 24-hour day, with sleep occurring unpredictably at any time of the day. However, in any 24-hour period, total sleep duration is normal.

This sleep pattern is commonly seen in individuals who are institutionalized, where there is a loss of the normal ENVIRONMENTAL TIME CUES to help maintain a regular sleep-wake cycle. In addition, such patients usually have neurological disorders that predispose them to an inability to maintain a normal sleep-wake cycle. But this pattern can also occur in non-institutionalized individuals who do not have strong environmental stimuli to ensure a regular sleep-wake cycle, such as persons who work or sleep on irregular schedules.

This chronobiological sleep disturbance differs from the ADVANCED SLEEP PHASE SYNDROME, DELAYED SLEEP PHASE SYNDROME and NON-24-HOUR SLEEP-WAKE SYNDROME in that these other disorders have regular sleep-wake cycles, although they may be temporarily displaced in relationship to a 24-hour clock time. Furthermore, patients with disorders producing EXCESSIVE SLEEPINESS during the day may show a similar pattern of frequent sleep episodes, but most disorders of excessive daytime sleepiness occur in the presence of a relatively intact nocturnal sleep period. However, NARCOLEPSY, which typically produces frequent daytime sleep episodes, can be associated with a disrupted nocturnal sleep pattern, particularly when the disorder is severe. Irregular sleep-wake pattern also has to be differentiated from irregular cycles due to either shift work (see SHIFT-WORK SLEEP DISORDER) or time zone changes (see TIME ZONE CHANGE [JET LAG] SYNDROME).

In irregular sleep-wake pattern, daytime sleepiness and complaints of INSOMNIA are common. Full alertness is usually decreased, and memory and other cognitive functions are often impaired. Because of the unpredictability of sleep episodes occurring throughout the 24-hour day, many individuals with this pattern tend to remain in an environment where they can be close to a bed. Elderly patients may become more housebound and less likely to expose themselves to environmental stimuli that, ironically, could help them to maintain a more regular sleep-wake pattern.

This sleep pattern may be induced by the use of medications that provoke daytime sedation, such as tranquilizers, or stimulants that can increase arousal at night.

This particular sleep disorder is relatively rare, although the prevalence in individuals with central nervous system dysfunction is thought to be greater than in other groups (although the exact prevalence is unknown). The pattern may occur at any age, although it is much more prevalent in the elderly. It does not appear to have any particular gender predominance.

Polysomnographic studies have demonstrated short (two-to-three-hour) episodes of sleep or wakefulness that occur at random throughout the 24-hour day. Sleep cycle monitoring is usually required for 48 hours or longer to substantiate this diagnosis. An alternative means of documenting this sleep-wake pattern is by using ACTIVITY MONITORS, which are movement detectors sensitive to the presence of sleep or wake episodes. Prolonged monitoring over days or weeks can be an effective way of documenting this sleep disorder. Because of the disruption of the sleep-wake cycle, the NREM-REM SLEEP CYCLE is often disrupted, and the ELECTROENCEPHALOGRAM may show a reduction in SLEEP SPINDLES and K-COMPLEX activity, as well as reduced SLOW WAVE SLEEP. REM SLEEP may also be disrupted.

Treatment of irregular sleep-wake pattern involves trying to maintain a regular major sleep episode at night and a full period of wakefulness during the day. In the institutionalized elderly, treatment includes providing stimulating activities during the day and preventing daytime sleep episodes. Appropriate environmental measures need to be in place to ensure a suitable nocturnal sleeping environment. Assistance in maintaining a good sleep episode at night might be brought about by the use of HYPNOTICS or, conversely, in order to assist alertness during the day, stimulant medications may be used. However, these medications are often of little assistance, and attention to the sleep-wake scheduling is usually most effective. Patients who have a central nervous system disease may lack the ability to maintain both a regular sleep episode at night and full awakeness during the daytime; therefore, attempts at correcting the irregular sleep-wake pattern may be unsuccessful.

J

Jacobsonian relaxation Term for relaxation methods proposed by Edmund Jacobson for promoting restful sleep. The relaxation methods involve sequential relaxation of muscle groups of the limbs and trunk in order to reduce heightened arousal and muscle tension. This form of relaxation is commonly recommended for patients who have INSOMNIA, either of psychophysiological cause or insomnia due to ANXIETY DISORDERS. (See also SLEEP EXERCISES.)

Jacobson, Edmund, *You Can Sleep Well.* London: Whittlesey House, 1938.

jactatio capitis nocturna This term is synonymous with HEADBANGING or RHYTHMIC MOVEMENT DISORDER. The term was first proposed in 1905 by Julius Zappert who provided the first clinical description of headbanging when he described six children with the disorder.

Japanese Sleep Research Society Founded in 1978, one of a number of sleep societies developed around the world to assist sleep research and promote the growth of clinical SLEEP DISORDERS MEDICINE. In the United States, the ASSOCIATION FOR THE PSYCHOPHYSIOLOGICAL STUDY OF SLEEP was founded in 1961, and it subsequently led to the ASSOCIATION OF PROFESSIONAL SLEEP SOCIETIES. The first society to be founded outside the United States was the EUROPEAN SLEEP RESEARCH SOCIETY, in 1978. (See also INTERNATIONAL SLEEP SOCIETIES.)

jet lag Term applied to symptoms experienced following rapid travel across multiple time zones. The term derives from jet air travel, which enables travelers to cross time zones much more quickly than by other, slower forms of transportation, such as by boat, where adaptation to the change in time occurs. The symptoms of jet lag include sleep disruption, gastrointestinal disturbances, reduced vigilance and attention span, and a general feeling of malaise. The severity of the symptoms depends upon the number of time zones crossed and usually occurs with a change of more than one or two hours. The symptoms gradually abate as adaptation to the new time zone occurs over the ensuing days. There is evidence to suggest that individuals may differ in their ability to adapt to the time zone changes. The ability to adapt is also dependent on the direction of travel, either eastward or westward: Studies of circadian rhythmicity suggest that adaptation occurs at a rate of 88 minutes per day after westbound travel, and only 66 minutes per day after eastbound travel. (See also ARGONNE ANTI-JET-LAG DIET, CIRCADIAN RHYTHM SLEEP DISORDERS, PHASE RESPONSE CURVE, TIME ZONE CHANGE [JET LAG] SYNDROME.)

Stone, B.M., et al., "Promoting Sleep in Shiftworkers and Intercontinental Travelers," *Chronobiology International* 14, no. 2 (1977): 133–143.

Jouvet, Michel Dr. Jouvet (1925–) attended medical school in Lyons, France. Since 1956, he has conducted research in neurophysiology, and since 1958 he has carried out research into the neurobiology of sleep. Professor and chairman of the Department of Experimental Medicine of Claude-Bernard University in Lyons, Dr. Jouvet was elected in 1977 to the French Academy of Sciences.

Through his research on cats, Dr. Jouvet's contributions to sleep have included the study of paradoxical sleep, the role of SEROTONIN and serotonergic neurons in the brain stem. (See also WILLIAM DEMENT, REM SLEEP.)

Jouvet, Michel, "Neurophysiology of the States of Sleep," *Physiological Review* 47 (1967): 117–177.

K

Kales, Anthony Dr. Anthony Kales (1934–) is coauthor, with Alan Rechtschaffen, Ph.D., of *A Manual of Standardized Terminology, Techniques, and Scoring Systems for Sleep Stages of Human Subjects,* published in 1968 by the Brain Information Service (Los Angeles, California).

Along with Joyce Kales, M.D., Dr. Kales founded the Sleep Disorders Clinic and Sleep Research and Treatment Center, initially located in 1962 at the University of Los Angeles and now at the Pennsylvania State University College of Medicine in Hershey, Pennsylvania. Dr. Anthony Kales is also professor and chairman of the Department of Psychiatry at Pennsylvania State University College of Medicine, and Dr. Joyce Kales is director of the Sleep Disorders Clinic and associate professor in the Department of Psychiatry.

Dr. Kales has been concerned with the diagnosis and treatment of sleep disorders, including insomnia, the parasomnias, enuresis, narcolepsy, and sleep apnea. Along with Dr. Ian Oswald, Dr. Kales pioneered the use of the sleep laboratory in assessing the effects of central nervous system-active drugs, such as the hypnotics and antidepressants.

Kales, Anthony and Kales, Joyce, *Evaluation and Treatment of Insomnia.* New York: Oxford University Press, 1984.

K-alpha A type of microarousal consisting of a K-COMPLEX followed by several seconds of ALPHA RHYTHM.

K-complex A high-voltage ELECTROENCEPHALOGRAM wave that consists of a sharp negative component followed by a slower positive component. K-complexes typically have a duration exceeding .5 second, occur during non-REM sleep, and are required for the definition of stage two sleep (see SLEEP STAGES). They can be detected by electrodes placed over a wide area of the scalp, but they are most clearly detected in the fronto-central regions. Frequently, K-complexes are associated with SLEEP SPINDLES.

K-complexes need to be distinguished from vertex sharp waves, which are usually short in duration (less than 0.3 second), low in amplitude and usually restricted to the vertex area of the skull. K-complexes are thought to be manifestations of central nervous system-evoked stimuli, and can be elicited during sleep by external stimuli, such as a loud noise.

Kleine-Levin syndrome Syndrome characterized by RECURRENT HYPERSOMNIA, gluttony and hypersexuality. This disorder was first described in part by Willi Kleine in 1925, and subsequently by Max Levin in 1929. Michael Critchley, in 1942, coined the term *Kleine-Levin Syndrome.* (See also DIET AND SLEEP).

Kleitman, Nathaniel Dr. Kleitman (1895–1999) is called "the father of modern sleep research"; in 1952, at the University of Chicago, along with Eugene Aserinsky and, later, WILLIAM DEMENT, Kleitman discovered the REM phase of sleep. Dr. Kleitman, who retired in 1960, stated for this encyclopedia: "After rediscovering the REM phase of sleep, with E. Aserinsky and W. Dement, my most significant contribution was to demonstrate the operation of a BASIC REST-ACTIVITY CYCLE during wakefulness as well as in sleep, where it is represented by REM-non-REM repetition—thus demystifying the function of REM sleep (reported in *Sleep,* 5[1982], 311–317)."

Dr. Kleitman received his Ph.D. from the University of Chicago and was a National Research Council Fellow in Utrecht, Paris and Chicago. Kleitman's 1939 work on sleep, in which he quoted more than 1,400 references (more than 4,300 in the revised edition), was the first comprehensive book on the subject. Until 1960, he was a professor of physiology at the University of Chicago.

Dr. Kleitman received the APSS Pioneer Award for his work in sleep research, as well as the 1966 Distinguished Service Award of the Thomas W. Salmon Committee on Psychiatry and Mental Hygiene of the New York Academy of Medicine. The AMERICAN ACADEMY OF SLEEP MEDICINE's annual award for outstanding contributions to sleep medicine was named after Kleitman and is called the Kleitman Award. Dr. Kleitman died in 1999 at the age of 104. (See also NATHANIEL KLEITMAN DISTINGUISHED SERVICE AWARD, REM SLEEP, SLEEP DEPRIVATION.)

Kleitman, Nathaniel, *Sleep and Wakefulness.* Chicago: University of Chicago Press, 1939; revised and enlarged, 1963.

Kleitman, Nathaniel and Kleitman, H., "The Sleep-wakefulness Pattern in the Arctic," *Scientific Monthly* 76 (1953): 349–356.

Kleitman, Nathaniel, Distinguished Service Award See NATHANIEL KLEITMAN DISTINGUISHED SERVICE AWARD.

Klonopin See BENZODIAZEPINES.

Kripke, David F. Dr. Kripke (1941–) received his medical degree from Columbia Medical School. He was a resident in psychiatry at Albert Einstein College of Medicine in New York (1968–1971). In 1972, he founded the Sleep Disorders Clinic at the San Diego Veterans Administration Medical Center in California. From 1979 to 1981 he was editor of *Sleep Research,* and he was the program chair of the Society for Light Treatment and Biological Rhythms. He has been professor of psychiatry at the University of California, San Diego, since 1982.

Dr. Kripke's sleep research areas, reflected in his more than 500 publications, have included chronobiology, light treatment, and sleep apnea.

Kripke, D.F., Simons, R.N., Garfinkel, L. and Hammond, E.C., "Short and Long Sleep and Sleeping Pills: Is Increased Mortality Associated?" *Archives of General Psychiatry* 36 (1979): 103–116.

Kryger, Meir H. Dr. Kryger (1947–) received his M.D. from McGill University in Canada. He is currently director of the Sleep Research Laboratory at the University of Manitoba and professor of medicine in the Department of Medicine at the same university, where he has been teaching since 1977. Dr. Kryger has been chairman of the Continuing Medical Education committee of the Association of Sleep Disorders Centers (1986–) as well as vice president of the Canadian Sleep Society (1986–). Dr. Kryger was the recipient in 1996 of the William C. Dement Award of the AMERICAN ACADEMY OF SLEEP MEDICINE (AASM).

Dr. Kryger's sleep research areas, represented in his more than 100 publications, are: sleep-related breathing disorders—such as hypoventilation, chronic airflow obstruction, the PICKWICKIAN SYNDROME and obstructive sleep apnea—as well as chronic mountain sickness.

Kryger, M., Roth, T. and Dement, W.C., eds., *The Principles and Practices of Sleep Disorders Medicine.* Philadelphia: Saunders, 1989.

Kryger, M.H., "Sleep Apnea: From the Needles of Dionysius to Continuous Positive Airway Pressure," *Archives of Internal Medicine* 143 (1983): 2301.

Kupfer, David J. Dr. Kupfer (1941–) received his M.D. from Yale University. He was a clinical fellow in psychiatry at Yale University School of Medicine, Department of Psychiatry (1966–67) and has been a professor in the Department of Psychiatry at the University of Pittsburgh School of Medicine, Western Psychiatric Institute and Clinic, since 1975, and chairman of the Department of Psychiatry since 1983.

Dr. Kupfer's sleep research areas have been sleep disturbances in patients with psychiatric problems (manic-depression, schizophrenia) and sleep disturbances in the elderly.

Kupfer, D.J., Grochocinski, V.J. and McEachran, A.B., "Relationship of Awakening and Delta Sleep in Depression," *Psychiatry Research* 19 (1987): 297–304.

kyphoscoliosis Curvature of the spine in the thoracic region that causes a backward and lateral curvature of the spinal column. The space available for the lungs is reduced and patients therefore are unable to adequately inflate the lungs, producing a restrictive lung disorder. The breathing pattern during sleep in patients with kyphoscoliosis may resemble a CHEYNE-STOKES RESPIRATION pattern—with or without central apneic episodes, solely with central sleep apnea, or even with obstructive sleep apnea. The breathing disturbance is greatest in REM sleep and is usually associated with blood oxygen desaturation.

The impairment of VENTILATION may produce daytime ALVEOLAR HYPOVENTILATION with a reduction in blood oxygen saturation and an elevation in carbon dioxide. More commonly, the ventilatory impairment may be restricted to sleep so that oxygen desaturation occurs solely during REM sleep. Kyphoscoliosis produces an increased number of awakenings and can lead to a complaint of disturbed nocturnal sleep due to the sleep-related breathing abnormalities. If the HYPOXEMIA is severe and the number of awakenings frequent enough, symptoms of daytime sleepiness may develop.

Treatment in the initial stages may include nocturnal oxygen therapy, although caution should be exhibited as this may exacerbate apneic episodes and lead to a dangerous rise in carbon dioxide. Assisted ventilation may be required for some patients, either by a negative pressure ventilation, such as a cuirass, or by means of a positive pressure ventilator applied to either a nasal mask or through a TRACHEOSTOMY. If patients with kyphoscoliosis have an obstructive sleep apnea component to their SLEEP-RELATED BREATHING DISORDER, then treatment by means of a CONTINUOUS POSITIVE AIRWAY PRESSURE (CPAP) device applied through a nasal mask can be effective in improving nocturnal oxygen saturation. Tracheostomy is usually not helpful unless there is a severe degree of obstructive sleep apnea syndrome present. RESPIRATORY STIMULANTS, such as medroxyprogesterone or acetazolamide, by themselves are not effective in improving ventilation in patients with kyphoscoliosis; however, there is some evidence to suggest that a combination of both might be useful in some patients.

Kryger, M.H., "Restrictive Lung Disease," in Kryger, M.H., Roth, T. and Dement, W.C., eds., *The Principles and Practices of Sleep Disorders Medicine.* Philadelphia: Saunders, 1989. pp. 611–616.

L

laboratory for sleep-related breathing disorders A medical facility providing diagnostic and treatment services for patients with SLEEP-RELATED BREATHING DISORDERS. The laboratory is under the directorship of a physician specializing in sleep-related breathing disorders, such as a pulmonary physician, and provides overnight polysomnographic services. Some laboratories also perform daytime MULTIPLE SLEEP LATENCY TESTS for EXCESSIVE SLEEPINESS.

Laboratories for sleep-related breathing disorders can be accredited by the AMERICAN ACADEMY OF SLEEP MEDICINE if they fulfill the standards and guidelines set by the association. However, these facilities are not required to have an accredited clinical polysomnographer on staff or the facilities for the diagnosis of other sleep disorders, such as INSOMNIA and excessive sleepiness. (SLEEP DISORDER CENTERS, comprehensive centers for patients with all forms of sleep disorders, provide appropriate services for such patients.)

lamboid waves See POSTS.

lark An early-to-bed-and-early-to-rise person. This term is used as the opposite of the EVENING PERSON or night owl, who is typically a person who goes to bed late at night and arises late in the day. The tendency for being a lark appears to increase with age as it is common for the elderly to fall asleep relatively early in the evening and awaken early in the morning. Some larks may erroneously think they have INSOMNIA due to the early hour of awakening. However, the duration of the sleep time is usually normal. (See also ADVANCED SLEEP PHASE SYNDROME, OWL AND LARK QUESTIONNAIRE.)

laryngospasm Term applied to acute and transient obstruction at the laryngeal level of the respiratory tract, most commonly due to vocal cord spasm. Laryngospasm is synonymous with the term *glottic spasm*. Laryngospasm can occur during wakefulness or sleep and may be induced by irritation of the vocal cords, anesthesia or psychogenic mechanisms.

Gastroesophageal reflux (see SLEEP-RELATED GASTROESOPHAGEAL REFLUX) can cause laryngospasm due to irritation of the vocal cords by gastric acid. Episodes of laryngospasm can be precipitated by gastroesophageal reflux in the OBSTRUCTIVE SLEEP APNEA SYNDROME. However, episodes of laryngospasm can occur during sleep independent of gastroesophageal reflux or the obstructive sleep apnea syndrome. In such patients, a psychogenic cause is suspected. Some patients can produce laryngospasm voluntarily, sometimes even to the point of producing loss of consciousness.

SLEEP-RELATED LARYNGOSPASM has some features in common with other forms of sleep-related ANXIETY DISORDERS, such as PANIC DISORDER. It is associated with panic and fear, which occurs out of sleep, and lasts only a few seconds before subsiding. However, in sleep-related laryngospasm, the stridor (high-pitched sound during inspiration of air) is a characteristic feature.

Laryngospasm due to gastroesophageal reflux is treated by the standard means of controlling gastroesophageal reflux, such as sleeping in a semi-upright position or taking medications such as Prilosec. Surgery on the lower esophageal sphincter may be required to prevent reflux. If obstructive sleep apnea is the cause of laryngospasm, then treatment is directed toward relief of the obstructive sleep apnea. Patients with the sleep-related laryngospasm of the idiopathic form, presumably psychogenic, have episodes so infrequently that specific therapeutic interventions have not been explored.

laser uvulopalatoplasty A surgical procedure that involves the removal of the uvula and a change in the shape of the soft palate. The procedure is performed for the relief of SNORING. It may also slightly reduce mild OBSTRUCTIVE SLEEP APNEA SYNDROME. The procedure is performed under local anesthesia in the physician's office and lasts about 20 minutes. It may need to be repeated several times until a satisfactory reduction in snoring is achieved. The main complication of the procedure is pain, which can be likened to a very bad sore throat that lasts for up to 10 days after the procedure.

latency to sleep See SLEEP LATENCY.

Latin American Sleep Research Society Founded in 1986, the Latin American Sleep Research Society is one of several sleep societies around the world founded to foster sleep research and the growth of clinical sleep disorders medicine. In the United States, the ASSOCIATION FOR THE PSYCHOPHYSIOLOGICAL STUDY OF SLEEP was founded in 1961, and it subsequently led to the ASSOCIATION OF PROFESSIONAL SLEEP SOCIETIES. The Latin American Sleep Research Society is one of the four international societies that originally sponsored the bimonthly journal *SLEEP*. (See also INTERNATIONAL SLEEP SOCIETIES.)

Lavie, Peretz Lavie (1949–) obtained his Ph.D. in 1974 in physiological psychology from the University of Florida at Gainesville. He became a lecturer in the unit of behavioral biology at the Faculty of Medicine, Technion, at the Israel Institute of Technology, and he has been a full professor there since 1989. From 1993 to 1999, he was the dean of the faculty of medicine at the Technion. Dr. Lavie was a member of the executive committee of the Sleep Research Society (1982–85; 1988–99) and vice president of the European Sleep Research Society (1988–90) as well as chairman of the scientific committee of the European Sleep Society (1998–2000). His areas of sleep research have included sleep disorders, chronobiology and dreaming. His book, *The Enchanted World of Sleep*, was originally published in Hebrew in 1993 and has since then been translated into 11 languages by Yale University Press.

Lavie P., "Ultrashort Sleep-waking Schedule. III. 'Gates' and 'Forbidden Zones' for Sleep," *Electroencephalography and Clinical Neurophysiology* 63 (1986): 414–425.

Lavie, P., Herer, P. and Hoffstein, V., "Obstructive Sleep Apnoea Syndrome as a Risk Factor for Hypertension: Population Study," *British Medical Journal* 320 (2000): 479–482.

L-dopa An antiparkinsonian medication that has been demonstrated to be effective in reducing the severity of episodes of RESTLESS LEGS SYNDROME and PERIODIC LEG MOVEMENTS during sleep. (See also BENZODIAZEPINES, PERIODIC LIMB MOVEMENT DISORDER, RESTLESSNESS.)

learning during sleep Some years ago, it was a vogue to try to develop ways of learning while asleep. But playing tape recordings through earphones that were plugged into sleeping subjects met with poor success. It is currently believed that exposure to auditory stimuli during sleep does not assist in learning. However, there is some evidence that learning during wakefulness immediately before sleep is often associated with better memory retention of information after several hours of sleep compared with learning following a similar number of hours of wakefulness. But, the difference is relatively small and is not thought to be of great benefit.

Material exposed to an awakened sleeper will be remembered more following awakenings from REM SLEEP than from awakenings out of SLOW WAVE SLEEP. However, there is no evidence to suggest that learning following an awakening from REM sleep poses any benefits over learning during usual wakefulness. Also, the element of sleep deprivation conveyed by awakening out of REM sleep may be detrimental to learning. EXCESSIVE SLEEPINESS can produce memory difficulties that may be due to the inability to retain information as a result of frequent microsleep episodes. (See also COGNITIVE EFFECTS OF SLEEP STATES, MICROSLEEP.)

Lemmi, Helio Dr. Lemmi (1929–) received his medical degree from the Faculdade de Medicina da Universidade de São Paulo in Brazil in 1955. Since 1976, he has been clinical professor of neurology at the University of Tennessee College of Medicine in Memphis, as well as director of the Sleep Disorders Center of Baptist Memorial Hospital (1977–). Dr. Lemmi was the recipient of the 1988 Nathaniel Kleitman Prize for Distinguished Service awarded by the Association of Sleep Disorder Centers.

Dr. Lemmi's main research contributions have been in the application of neurophysiological techniques in a variety of neurological and sleep disorders. He is a former chairman of the Accreditation Committee of the American Sleep Disorders Association. He retired from sleep medicine in 1999.

Lemmi, Helio, "Clinical, Neuroendocrine, and Sleep EEG Diagnosis of 'Unusual' Affective Presentations: A Practical Review," *Psychiatric Clinics of North America* 6 (1983): 69–83.

light sleep See STAGE ONE SLEEP.

light therapy Light has been shown to be effective in treating a number of psychiatric and sleep disorders. The effect of light is most evident in the treatment of SEASONAL AFFECTIVE DISORDER (SAD), which most commonly occurs in the mid- to late fall as the nights grow longer. The increased tendency for DEPRESSION is believed to be in part related to the reduced light exposure at that particular time of year. Those with SAD have other features of depression, such as increased weight gain, fatigue, loss of concentration and greater time spent in bed. Exposure to light of more than 2,000 lux for two or more hours in the morning, from, say, 6 to 8 A.M., can improve mood and decrease the seasonal affective disorder.

The individual with SAD may notice an improved daytime mood; however, there may be a mid-afternoon reduction in mood associated with the circadian variation in daytime alertness. Another exposure of light at that time, shorter than the first treatment, may improve the symptoms and reduce the need for a mid-afternoon nap.

Patients with DELAYED SLEEP PHASE SYNDROME can benefit from exposure to bright light toward the end of the habitual major sleep episode. The light exposure assists in producing a phase advance of the sleep period.

Bright light exposure may also be useful for treating sleep disorders due to shift work (see SHIFT-WORK SLEEP DISORDER) or jet lag (see TIME ZONE CHANGE [JET LAG] SYNDROME) as well as other causes of EXCESSIVE SLEEPINESS or INSOMNIA.

Although bright light systems are commercially available, natural bright light can also be utilized. In the course of good SLEEP HYGIENE, those prone to sleep disturbances should be exposed to natural light soon after awakening in the morning. Conversely, reduction of light exposure in the hours prior to bedtime can be useful in improving sleep onset.

The effect of light is believed to be mediated through the retino-hypothalamic pathway to the hypothalamus. In addition, light is known to affect the secretion of melatonin by the pineal gland, which may be important in the regulation of circadian rhythmicity. (See also CIRCADIAN RHYTHMS, MELATONIN, MOOD DISORDERS, PINEAL GLAND.)

Terman, Michael, "Light Therapy," in Kryger, M.H., Roth, Thomas and Dement, William C., *The Principles and Practices of Sleep Disorders Medicine.* Philadelphia: W.B. Saunders, 1989. pp. 771–772.

limit-setting sleep disorder A childhood sleep disorder characterized by inadequate limits on bedtime. A child who consistently refuses or stalls going to bed will delay bedtime—leading to resultant, insufficient TOTAL SLEEP TIME. When parents or caregivers institute limits, sleep normally occurs at the appropriate time. By adolescence, children are able to institute their own limits and this disorder does not occur. This disorder may be present in individuals who, for neurological or physiological reasons, are unable to institute their own bedtime.

In childhood, limit-setting sleep disorder generally begins once a child is at an age of being able to climb out of the crib, or is placed in a bed. The stallings are frequently associated with the need to either get something to eat or something to drink, to watch television or to play a game or to have a story read. These behaviors may progress to reporting unfounded fears regarding sleep, such as monsters in the bedroom.

The bedtime problem may be exacerbated by oversolicitous parents and is more likely to occur when both parents are working. They readily give in to the child's desire to spend extra time with the parents. Children with physical or mental handicaps may induce feelings of parental guilt, promoting inadequate limit-setting.

Parents may inadvertently contribute to limit-setting sleep disorder by allowing their school-age children to take a nap at any time during the day, which makes it more difficult to go to sleep at an appropriate hour at night. Furthermore, if parents have inconsistent evening schedules, or a child would miss seeing a working parent if he does go to bed at the designated hour, the parents may be unwittingly contributing to limit-setting sleep disorder. Allowing a drastically different bedtime on the weekends, versus weekday school nights, may also contribute to limit-setting sleep disorder.

The course of this sleep disorder varies upon whether caregivers institute and adhere to appropriate limits, or the child develops a sense of maturity related to school and other activities, which reinforces the need to set one's own limits. This type of sleep disorder may be more common in children who have a natural tendency to be "owls," either because of a genetic tendency or through learned behaviors due to parents tending to delay their own bedtime.

Limit-setting sleep disorder leads to inadequate sleep at night, with resulting irritability, fatigue, decreased attention, reduced school performances and tensions in interfamily social relationships.

Children with limit-setting sleep disorder generally show few abnormalities on polysomnography because appropriate limits are usually instituted in the course of performing sleep studies.

Treatment of limit-setting sleep disorder involves instituting, adhering to and enforcing appropriate bedtimes and wake times. A regular routine before sleep, as well as a consistent bedtime and wake time, will help to eliminate limit-setting sleep disorder.

This disorder needs to be differentiated from SLEEP ONSET ASSOCIATION DISORDER in which a bedtime object becomes necessary for good quality sleep and its withdrawal throws off the sleep pattern. Children who have the DELAYED SLEEP PHASE SYNDROME may have sleep onset difficulties. Limit-setting sleep disorder may develop into the disorder of INADEQUATE SLEEP HYGIENE if a child fails to assume responsibility for his own sleep hygiene and sleep pattern when it is appropriate to do so.

Ferber, Richard, *Solve Your Child's Sleep Problems.* New York: Simon & Schuster, 1985.

lithium Lightest of the alkali metals; in a form such as lithium carbonate, it is used for the treatment of mania in patients who have manic-depressive disease. Lithium has been shown to have beneficial effects upon the sleep-wake pattern, particularly in individuals who have sleep disturbances related to cyclical MOOD DISORDERS. Lithium increases the latency to REM sleep and enhances the amount of SLOW WAVE SLEEP. Wakefulness and lighter stage one sleep is usually reduced.

Lithium has been used in the treatment of the RECURRENT HYPERSOMNIA due to the KLEINE-LEVIN SYNDROME.

locus ceruleus A region of darkly stained cells that extends in two columns from the PONS to the midbrain. The cells of the locus ceruleus contain melanin, which causes its dark pigmentation. The locus ceruleus was originally thought to be primarily responsible for the generation of REM SLEEP, but recent evidence has indicated that the area ventral to the locus ceruleus, the nucleus reticularis pontis oralis (RPO), is the area primarily responsible for its generation. However, the caudal third of the locus ceruleus is important in the maintenance of REM sleep atonia.

The cells of the locus ceruleus contain the neurotransmitter noradrenalin and their stimulation induces wakefulness. The region around the locus ceruleus and the pons is important in the maintenance of the atonia of REM sleep, and destruction of this area leads to an increase in muscle tone. Experimental lesions in cats produce a state in which cats move around during REM sleep. A similar state has been described in some humans who have brain stem lesions. The pontine region around the locus ceruleus stimulates the medullary area of Magoun and Rhines, causing inhibition of the spinal motor neurons, resulting in muscle atonia. (See also PGO SPIKES, RAPHE NUCLEI, SLEEP ATONIA.)

long sleeper Term for someone who has a habitual sleep episode longer than the average for someone of the same age group. The quality of the sleep episode and the timing of sleep is normal. A long sleeper has a usual sleep duration of 10 hours or greater. Someone with a physiological need for a long sleep episode may regularly reduce the total sleep time by one or more hours, thereby leading to a state of chronic SLEEP DEPRIVATION, which may be compensated for on the weekends with longer sleep episodes.

Long sleepers have EXCESSIVE SLEEPINESS during the day if they get less sleep than they require. Full daytime alertness with a long sleep episode is necessary to confirm the diagnosis.

The sleep pattern of the long sleeper has usually been present since childhood and persists throughout life. Polysomnographic studies have demonstrated normal amounts of the deeper stages three and four sleep, but increased amounts of REM sleep and stage two sleep. The MULTIPLE SLEEP LATENCY TEST demonstrates normal daytime alertness without pathological sleepiness.

Long sleepers need to be differentiated from patients with other causes of excessive nocturnal sleep that typically can be due to impaired sleep quality. Disorders such as OBSTRUCTIVE SLEEP APNEA SYNDROME or PERIODIC LEG MOVEMENTS during sleep may produce a long sleep episode. In addition, a tendency to sleep later in the day may be due to DELAYED SLEEP PHASE SYNDROME, but those with delayed sleep phase syndrome fall asleep at a later hour than those who are long sleepers. Patients with NARCOLEPSY generally lack a long sleep episode and have other features indicating the diagnosis, such as CATAPLEXY and sleep attacks.

A diagnosis of a long sleeper is determined by the documentation of daily prolonged sleep episodes over a two- to four-week period.

Treatment is usually not required and individuals need to be reassured that their long sleep episode reflects one end of a continuum or pattern of normal sleep durations. Long sleepers may need to be counseled to maintain a regular full sleep episode at night to avoid sleep deprivation with resulting daytime sleepiness. Stimulant medications should not be given.

long-term insomnia Term proposed by the consensus development conference convened by the National Institute of Mental Health and the Office of Medical Applications of Research of the National Institutes of Health in November of 1983. The summary statement of the conference broke down insomnia into TRANSIENT, SHORT-TERM and LONG-TERM. Long-term insomnia was defined as insomnia that lasted more than three weeks. The conference suggested that nondrug strategies, such as SLEEP HYGIENE or BEHAVIORAL TREATMENT OF INSOMNIA, be the initial approach to treating this type of insomnia. In addition, a short trial of a sleep-promoting medication (see HYPNOTICS) could also be indicated. "Long-term insomnia" is not a specific diagnostic entity but rather refers solely to duration. A large number of sleep disorders, such as PSYCHOPHYSIOLOGICAL INSOMNIA or insomnia due to psychiatric disorders, can produce insomnia, and can produce long-term insomnia. (See also ADJUSTMENT SLEEP DISORDER, DISORDERS OF INITIATING AND MAINTAINING SLEEP, PSYCHIATRIC DISORDERS.)

L-tryptophan See HYPNOTICS.

L-tyrosine See STIMULANT MEDICATIONS.

lucid dreams DREAMS in which the dreamer is actually aware of dreaming, as though the dreamer is almost conscious—although he or she is in a state of REM SLEEP. Lucid dreams are more likely to happen in the later REM sleep episodes of the night, and they happen only infrequently. Some individuals seem to be particularly susceptible to having lucid dreams. Attempts to increase lucid dreams have been partially successful by means of certain training procedures, including posthypnotic suggestion and somatosensory stimulation. However, auditory information, when presented to the dreamer, does not appear to induce lucid dreaming.

There is no evidence that there are differences in personality features of lucid dreamers compared with those who do not have lucid dreams; there are differences in alpha activity of lucid dreamers.

Lugaresi, Elio Professor Lugaresi (1926–) obtained his degree in medicine and surgery in 1925. From 1977 to 1988 he headed the Department of Neurology of the Faculty of Medicine of Bologna University. His numerous professional appointments include president of the Italian Society of EEG and Neurophysiology (1969–1972), president of the Italian League against Epilepsy (1972–1975), and president of the Italian Society of Neurology (1984–1987). In 1983, he received a special award for his work on sleep medicine from the Association of Sleep Disorder Centers. In 1996 he received the Pisa sleep award of the European Sleep Research Society. In 1997 he was awarded the Potamkin Prize of the American Academy of Neurology and the Giuseppe Moruzzi award of the World Federation of Clinical Neurophysiology. Dr. Lugaresi's major fields of investigation have been clinical EEG, epilepsy and sleep disorders, and he was one of the first to polysomnographically study patients with the obstructive sleep apnea syndrome. Dr. Lugaresi has authored or edited 18 books.

Lugaresi, E., Cirignotta, F. and Montagna, P., "Nocturnal Paroxysmal Dystonia, " *Journal of Neurology, Neurosurgery, and Psychiatry* 49 (1986): 375–380.

Lugaresi, E., Pazzaglia, P. and Tassinari, C.A., *Evolution and Prognosis of Epilepsies*. Bologna: Aulo Gaggi, 1973.

Lugaresi, E., Medori, R., Montagna, P. et al., "Fatal Familial Insomnia and Dysautonomia with Selective Degeneration of Thalmic Nuclei, " *New England Journal of Medicine* 31 (1986): 997–1003.

Lugaresi, E., Tobler, I., Gambetti, P. and Montagna, P., "The Pathophysiology of Fatal Familial Insomnia," *Brain Pathology* 8 (1998): 521–526.

Provini, F., Plazzi, G., Tinuper, P., Vandi, S., Lugaresi, E. and Montagna, P., "Nocturnal Frontal Lobe Epilepsy: A Clinical and Polygraphic Overview of 100 Consecutive Cases," *Brain* 122 (1999): 1017–1031.

lung disease Many medical disorders are associated with impaired lung function. Disorders can be due to impaired respiration as a result of central nervous system, spinal cord, nerve or muscle diseases. Typically, these disorders are associated with hypoventilation during sleep (see ALVEOLAR HYPOVENTILATION) which may take the form of CENTRAL SLEEP APNEA SYNDROME OBSTRUCTIVE SLEEP APNEA SYNDROME, or nonapneic hypoventilation. KYPHOSCOLIOSIS due to thoracic spine curvature as a result of bone or neurological disease also results in sleep-related hypoventilation with HYPOXEMIA and HYPERCAPNIA. Restrictive lung disease can be produced by kyphoscoliosis as well as by other disorders that impair the ventilation of the lungs, such as severe OBESITY. Obstruction to airflow may be due to UPPER AIRWAY OBSTRUCTION as a result of lesions that produce the obstructive sleep apnea syndrome. Small airways disease, such as that seen in patients with asthma or CHRONIC OBSTRUCTIVE PULMONARY DISEASE, or destruction of lung tissue, such as seen in patients who have emphysema, can also produce hypoventilation during sleep. Interstitial lung disease is associated with the abnormal accumulation of cells, tissues or fluid in the lung, thereby impairing gas transfer. Many disorders, including idiopathic pulmonary fibrosis, sarcoidosis, malignancy, adverse effects of medications or other toxic effects on the lung, can produce interstitial lung disease.

Treatment depends upon the cause of the respiratory disturbance and may involve the use of MEDICATIONS or oxygen therapy, or artificial ventilation devices, such as CONTINUOUS POSITIVE AIRWAY PRESSURE devices or negative pressure ventilators. Surgery that may relieve upper airway obstruction by means of TRACHEOSTOMY or UVULOPALATOPHARYNGOPLASTY, thoracic spine straightening, diaphraghmatic pacemaker stimulation or reduction of obesity by gastric surgery are other alternatives. (See also SLEEP-RELATED BREATHING DISORDERS.)

Fletcher, E.C., ed., *Abnormalities in Respiration During Sleep: Diagnosis, Pathophysiology, and Treatment*. Orlando, Florida: Grune and Stratton, 1986.

M

maintenance of wakefulness test (MWT) A test of the ability to maintain alertness during the daytime. The maintenance of wakefulness test is carried out in a manner similar to the MULTIPLE SLEEP LATENCY TEST (MSLT) in that there are five nap opportunities, two hours apart, each 20 minutes in duration. However, the difference between these two tests is that in the MWT, the patient is encouraged to try to stay awake, whereas in the MSLT, the patient is encouraged to relax and fall asleep.

In the maintenance of wakefulness test, the patient is seated in a semi-reclining position in a darkened room. The latency from lights out to sleep onset is recorded (see SLEEP LATENCY). Electrodes are placed on the head in order to electrophysiologically determine sleep onset.

For an individual who usually sleeps from 11 P.M. to 7 A.M., the five nap opportunities are carried out at 10 A.M., 12 noon, 2 P.M., 4 P.M. and 6 P.M. The average sleep latency over the five naps is recorded. Average latencies of 10 minutes or longer indicate normal daytime alertness, and latencies of less than 10 minutes indicate pathological sleepiness.

The maintenance of wakefulness test is most useful in determining treatment response to STIMULANT MEDICATIONS, such as Cylert or Ritalin, to determine whether treatment of EXCESSIVE SLEEPINESS has been effective.

Although the maintenance of wakefulness test has less diagnostic usefulness than the multiple sleep latency test, it is sometimes performed along with the MSLT in order to determine whether a patient with a disorder of excessive sleepiness has the ability to remain awake. This assessment can be useful for determining an individual's ability to drive a vehicle or operate dangerous machinery.

malingerers Persons pretending to have sleep disturbances for such self-serving reasons as wanting medications that may be abused. A malingerer may complain of INSOMNIA to obtain prescriptions for HYPNOTICS, which will really be used for recreational purposes. Alternatively, some individuals report EXCESSIVE SLEEPINESS and falsify the symptoms of NARCOLEPSY in an attempt to obtain STIMULANT MEDICATIONS. A patient may even go so far as to attempt to falsify the results of polysymnographic testing in order to convince a physician of the presence of a sleep disorder. However, if someone is suspected of being a malingerer, careful analysis of POLYSOMNOGRAPHY, which cannot be falsified, will confirm or refute such suspicions.

Thorpy, Michael, Wagner, D.R., Spielman, Arthur J. and Weitzman, E., "Objective Assessment of Narcolepsy," *Archives of Neurology* 40 (1983): 126–127.

mandibular advancement surgery Surgery occasionally performed for individuals with OBSTRUCTIVE SLEEP APNEA SYNDROME produced by a retroplaced lower jaw. This procedure consists of a sliding osteotomy that is a splitting of the mandible so that the anterior half can be moved forward. It is primarily performed on patients who have retrognathia (a jaw that is placed posteriorally), which produces either facial abnormalities or severe obstructive sleep apnea.

This procedure usually requires long orthodontic preparation, which may include temporarily advancing the jaw by means of rubber bands attached to teeth clips. Repeated polysomnographic evaluation is usually necessary, with the jaw temporarily advanced to determine the likelihood of surgical success. Postoperatively, patients have the teeth wired together until the healing is complete.

Mandibular advancement surgery has few acute or long-term complications, and its main disadvantage is the prolonged preoperative assessment and postoperative recovery periods.

mastoids Protuberances of the skull that are situated behind the ear canals. The mastoids form the standard placement for reference electrodes, particularly in the monitoring of the ELECTRO-OCULOGRAM.

maxillo-facial (maxillofacial) surgery In SLEEP DISORDERS MEDICINE, maxillo-facial surgery is performed to prevent UPPER AIRWAY OBSTRUCTION during sleep in patients with the OBSTRUCTIVE SLEEP APNEA SYNDROME. Surgery may involve moving the jaw forward by means of a surgical procedure called MANDIBULAR ADVANCEMENT SURGERY. This surgery involves splitting of the mandible to produce a sliding osteotomy so that the anterior portion of the jaw can be advanced. Alternatively, a small portion of the tip of the jaw, which contains the attachments of the tongue muscle, can be advanced to bring the tongue muscle forward. Sometimes the maxilla needs to be advanced to obtain appropriate dental relationships in conjunction with the mandibular advancement surgery. HYOID MYOTOMY is sometimes performed in conjunction with the anterior advancement of the tip of the jaw. This procedure allows the muscles of the tongue to be advanced anteriorly to prevent obstruction at the base of the tongue during sleep. (See also SURGERY AND SLEEP DISORDERS.)

Coleman, J., "Oral and Maxillofacial Surgery for the Management of Obstructive Sleep Apnea Syndrome," *Otolaryngologic Clinics of North America* 32, no. 2 (1999): 235–241.

mazindol See STIMULANT MEDICATIONS.

McCarley, Robert William Dr. McCarley (1937–) received his M.D. from Harvard Medical School. Since 1984, he has been professor of psychiatry at Harvard Medical School, as well as director of the Laboratory of Neuroscience at Harvard Medical School Department of Psychiatry, among other academic and hospital appointments. Dr. McCarley was president of the Sleep Research Society in 1991 and in 1995 he received its Distinguished Scientist Award.

Dr. McCarley's sleep research contributions, reflected by his more than 160 journal articles, his books, and contributions to books, include cholinergic and monaminergic brain stem mechanisms of REM sleep and adenosine as a non-REM sleep factor. He has also written on dreams and depression as related to sleep, and neuroimaging in schizophrenia.

McCarley, R.W., "Neurophysiology of Sleep: Basic Mechanisms Underlying Control of Wakefulness and Sleep," In Chokroverty, S., ed., *Sleep Disorders Medicine.* 2nd ed. Boston: Butterworth-Heinemann, 1999. pp. 21–50.

McCarley, R.W., Ito, K. and Rodrigo-Angulo, M.L., "Physiological Studies of Brainstem Reticular Connectivity: II. Responses of mPRF Neurons to Stimulation of Mesencephalic and Contralateral Pontine Reticular Formation," *Brain Research* 409 (1987): 111–127.

Steriade, M. and McCarley, R.W., *Brainstem Control of Wakefulness and Sleep.* New York: Plenum Press, 1990.

medications Most medications can have an effect on sleep either by disturbing the quality of nighttime sleep or by producing impaired alertness or drowsiness during the daytime. The HYPNOTICS, including the BARBITURATES and BENZODIAZEPINES, have a profound effect on inducing sleepiness and therefore are given at night to improve the quality of nighttime sleep. If given during the daytime, these medications are less effective in inducing sleep, although they will allow underlying sleepiness to occur.

In general, the effect of hypnotic medications on nighttime sleep is short-lasting, and they are not recommended for chronic INSOMNIA. There may also be daytime side effects, such as impaired alertness, a particular concern in the elderly, especially with long-acting hypnotic medications. Some medications, such as the short-acting benzodiazepines, have been reported to increase the level of alertness during the daytime but can also induce feelings of ANXIETY and tension.

The other group of medications that have profound effects upon the sleep-wake cycle are the

STIMULANT MEDICATIONS, including the amphetamines and their derivatives used for the treatment of disorders of EXCESSIVE SLEEPINESS. RESPIRATORY STIMULANTS, such as the xanthines, are used for the treatment of CHRONIC OBSTRUCTIVE PULMONARY DISEASE. When administered at night, they can impair the ability to fall asleep.

The stimulant medications, when given during the daytime, increase the level of arousal, causing patients with disorders such as narcolepsy to be less likely to have undesired sleeping episodes. However, these medications have only a small effect on preventing sleepiness, so that someone with a disorder of excessive sleepiness will find it relatively easy to fall asleep if put in a situation conducive to sleep. When the stimulant medications are taken too close to nighttime sleep, they will impair the ability to stay awake at night and lead to frequent interruptions and awakenings of nighttime sleep. A new medication, MODAFINIL, is called a "wake-promoting agent" as it improves alertness by decreasing sleepiness. It is not a stimulant and therefore has little in the way of side effects.

Medications used for other medical disorders, such as the treatment of PSYCHIATRIC DISORDERS, also impair the ability to stay awake. The NEUROLEPTICS, which include medications such as the phenothiazines, and the minor tranquilizers, such as the benzodiazepines, will enhance sleep onset in some people and may lead to impaired alertness during the daytime. Some of these medications are used for their hypnotic properties in the treatment of patients with abnormal behavior during sleep, for example, haloperidol and chlorpromazine. As with other medications with hypnotic properties, TOLERANCE to their beneficial effects may develop in time.

Medications used for weight reduction purposes are often amphetamine derivatives, and therefore these medications can have an ability to impair the quality of nighttime sleep or reduce the tendency for daytime sleepiness. Medications such as mazindol and diethylpropion have been used for the treatment of excessive sleepiness due to disorders such as narcolepsy, even though their primary use is for the treatment of obesity.

Most other groups of medications have effects on the sleep-wake cycle that are predominantly side effects or adverse reactions. ANTIHISTAMINES are typically associated with the production of DROWSINESS or sleepiness, and sometimes this side effect has been used for sleep-inducing purposes. One of the most commonly used hypnotic medications in childhood is chlorpheniramine. Promethazine, a phenothiazine derivative used for its antihistamine effects in the treatment of upper respiratory tract infections, also has sedative effects.

The use of antihistamines as hypnotics is not considered appropriate because more specific hypnotics are available, if necessary (though rarely required in childhood).

Anticonvulsant and analgesic agents can have sedative properties that impair daytime alertness, such as the benzodiazepines or barbiturates, which can cause increased sedation at night or in the daytime. Similar effects can occur with the analgesics, which can impair VENTILATION during sleep. The opioid analgesics, such as MORPHINE, and the sedative anticonvulsives are therefore contraindicated in patients with breathing disorders, such as the obstructive sleep apnea syndrome.

Cardiac medications, particularly the beta-blockers (drugs commonly used to treat hypertension or cardiac irregularities), can have detrimental effects upon the quality of nighttime sleep by increasing the number of arousals and awakenings. Medications such as propranolol and metoprolol are particularly associated with disturbed sleep at night. Sometimes the beta-blocker medications will increase dreaming at night and lead to more frequent nightmares. Excessive sleepiness during the daytime may occur either because of the impaired quality of sleep at night or as a direct effect of the medication during the daytime. The hypertensive medication clonidine, which has the effect of stimulating adrenoreceptors, can produce sleepiness.

Another group of medications that can have a profound effect on sleep and wakefulness are the ANTIDEPRESSANTS, particularly the tricyclic antidepressant medications, such as amitriptyline. These medications are commonly used for their sedating effects in improving the nighttime sleep of patients with depression. When administered during the daytime, they can produce unwanted sedation. When given at night, the tricyclic antidepressants suppress REM sleep; their abrupt withdrawal can lead to a REM sleep rebound with associated NIGHTMARES.

Because many medications can disturb nighttime sleep and daytime alertness, the role of medication should be considered in any patient presenting with symptoms related to sleep and alertness. SLEEP HYGIENE practices, along with alteration in the timing or dosage of medications, may have a very beneficial effect on the sleep complaints.

Nicholson, A.N., Bradley, C.M. and Pascoe, P.A., "Medications: Effect on Sleep and Wakefulness," in Kryger, M.L., Roth, T. and Dement, W.C., *The Principles and Practices of Sleep Disorders Medicine.* Philadelphia: Saunders, 1989. pp. 228–236.

medroxyprogesterone See RESPIRATORY STIMULANTS.

melatonin A neurohormone that is found primarily in the PINEAL GLAND at the back of the brain. The pineal gland releases melatonin at night, in darkness, and its level in the blood reaches a peak between 1 A.M. and 5 A.M. The secretion of melatonin is inhibited by light through pathways that extend from the retina through the SUPRACHIASMATIC NUCLEUS to the pineal gland. The secretion of melatonin changes over life and appears to be maximal around the time of puberty, at which time it appears to be important in the development of sexual maturation.

The neurotransmitter serotonin is converted into melatonin in the pineal gland; therefore, medications that effect the synthesis of serotonin will also effect melatonin synthesis. Beta-blocker medications used in the treatment of cardiac disorders will suppress melatonin levels, whereas agents that stimulate serotonin production, such as 5-hydroxytryptophan (5-HT), will increase secretion.

Melatonin appears to be important in giving seasonal time cues. In animals, its administration can be used to affect the breeding season by inducing breeding behavior at an earlier time. Melatonin may also be able to alter circadian rhythmicity, as it appears to be able to synchronize the rest-activity cycle of animals. Attempts at manipulating the sleep-wake cycle by the administration of melatonin in humans have produced variable results.

Zisapel, N., "The Use of Melatonin for the Treatment of Insomnia," *Biological Signals and Receptors* 8, nos. 1–2 (1999): 84–89.

MEMA See MIDDLE EAR MUSCLE ACTIVITY.

Mendelson, Wallace B. Dr. Mendelson (1945–) received his M.D. from Washington University School of Medicine in St. Louis in 1969. From 1982 to 1987, Dr. Mendelson was chief of the Section on Sleep Studies at the Clinical Psychobiology Branch of the National Institute of Mental Health in Bethesda, Maryland. Dr. Mendelson, a past president of the Sleep Research Society, is currently a professor of psychiatry, medicine and clinical pharmacology at the University of Chicago as well as director of the Sleep Research Laboratory.

Dr. Mendelson's sleep research areas of interest, reflected in his numerous books and publications, are the neuropharmacology of sleep and wakefulness and clinical sleep disorders.

Mendelson, W.B., Owen, C., Skolnick, P., Paul, S.M., Martin, J.V., Ko, G. and Wagner, R., "Nifedipine Blocks Sleep Induction by Flurazepam in the Rat," *Sleep* 7 (1984): 64–68.

menopause Gradual reduction in ovarian function occurs in late to middle age in women associated with symptoms of emotional variability, depression and autonomic disturbances, such as hot flashes and night sweats. There is atrophy of estrogen-dependent tissues, such as breast tissue and the vaginal lining. Sleep becomes more fragmented, with awakenings often related to hot flashes or night sweats. These symptoms are partially relieved by estrogen replacement treatment. (See also MENSTRUAL-ASSOCIATED SLEEP DISORDER, MENSTRUAL CYCLE.)

menstrual-associated sleep disorder A disorder of unknown cause characterized by INSOMNIA or EXCESSIVE SLEEPINESS related to the menses or menopause. This disorder exists in three main forms: insomnia or hypersomnia, related to the MENSTRUAL CYCLE; and insomnia related to the MENOPAUSE. Insomnia, when it occurs in relation to the menses, usually occurs during the week prior to the onset of the menses. The insomnia is characterized by an inability to fall asleep, frequent awakenings at night and the inability to maintain sleep. Hypersomnia can also occur intermittently, but not necessarily during the week prior to the onset of the menses. There is no evidence of sleepiness at any other time of the menstrual cycle.

Insomnia related to the menopause is characterized by other features of the menopause, such as hot flashes and night sweats. The insomnia is primarily a maintenance insomnia with frequent awakenings rather than a sleep onset insomnia.

Polysomnographic monitoring has demonstrated fragmented sleep with prolonged awakenings and reduced SLEEP EFFICIENCY in the premenstrual insomnia form. Polysomnography during premenstrual hypersomnia demonstrates a normal major sleep episode. MULTIPLE SLEEP LATENCY TESTING can demonstrate increased sleepiness during the symptomatic time. Spontaneous awakenings with features of night sweats or temperature variation are seen in menopausal insomnia.

Menstrual-associated sleep disorder needs to be differentiated from PSYCHIATRIC DISORDERS producing insomnia or hypersomnia. In particular, the premenstrual syndrome, which is associated with marked emotional liability, may produce an insomnia in addition to other symptoms, such as excessive fluid gain, emotional symptoms of irritability, ANXIETY or DEPRESSION.

The menstrual-associated sleep disorder may be improved by the use of replacement hormone medications, such as progesterone or estrogen. Estrogen replacement also improves insomnia in some menopausal women. Attention to good SLEEP HYGIENE is helpful, and occasionally a short course of a hypnotic medication given premenstrually may be useful. (See also DISORDERS OF EXCESSIVE SOMNOLENCE, DISORDERS OF INITIATING AND MAINTAINING SLEEP, HYPNOTICS.)

Billiard, M., Guilleminault, C. and Dement, W.C., "Menstruation-Linked Periodic Hypersomnia," *Neurology* 25 (1975): 436–443.

Ho, A., "Sex Hormones in the Sleep of Women," in Chase, M.H., Stern, W.C. and Walter, P.L., eds., *Sleep and Research,* vol. 1. Los Angeles: Brain Information Service/Brain Research Institute, UCLA, 1972. p. 184.

menstrual cycle Studies of sleep during the menstrual cycle have shown that during the premenstrual time, when progesterone and estrogen levels are high, there is a decrease in SLOW WAVE SLEEP. The amount of wake time during the major sleep episode is also increased during the premenstrual week. However, the change in healthy females is relatively small. There are slight differences in the amount of REM sleep throughout the menstrual cycle. (See also MENOPAUSE, MENSTRUAL-ASSOCIATED SLEEP DISORDER.)

methylphenidate hydrochloride See STIMULANT MEDICATIONS.

methylxanthines See RESPIRATORY STIMULANTS.

micrognathia A term used to describe a small lower jaw. People with micrognathia are more liable to have UPPER AIRWAY OBSTRUCTION due to posterior positioning of the tongue when the mouth is closed. The upper airway obstruction may induce the OBSTRUCTIVE SLEEP APNEA SYNDROME, and treatment by means of surgery, such as MANDIBULAR ADVANCEMENT SURGERY, may be necessary to bring the anterior attachment of the tongue forward.

Micrognathia should be differentiated from retrognathia, which refers to a normal-sized lower jaw that is situated posteriorly in relation to the maxilla or the base of the skull.

microsleep An episode of sleep lasting only a few seconds that occurs during wakefulness. Microsleep episodes are associated with disorders of EXCESSIVE SLEEPINESS during the day and may impair the ability to form new memory, and hence are a cause of AUTOMATIC BEHAVIOR. They most typically occur in patients with NARCOLEPSY; however, they can also be seen in patients with other disorders of excessive sleepiness.

middle ear muscle activity (MEMA) Middle ear muscle activity (MEMA) has been reported during sleep and has been correlated with RAPID EYE MOVEMENTS during REM SLEEP. This MEMA is thought to reflect the phasic muscle activity that is characteristic of REM sleep. However, middle ear muscle activity occurs simultaneously with rapid eye movements only 34% of the time. The muscle activity can therefore also occur during the tonic phase of REM sleep. Skeletal muscle activity that can occur during REM sleep includes the rapid eye movements, diaphragmatic activity and middle ear muscle activity.

migraine Vascular headaches that are usually unilateral but can also be bilateral. These headaches can occur during sleep and, if so, are often associated with REM SLEEP. Migraine headaches are often characterized by a throbbing sensation that can awaken an individual from sleep—with the usual migrainous prodrome of visual aura with flashes of light followed by the development of the headache, most commonly in the fronto-temporal region of the head. Anorexia (loss of appetite), nausea, vomiting and photophobia (eyes sensitive to bright light) may develop in association with the migraine headaches. There may also be other neurological features, such as paresthesiae or muscular weakness. (See also SLEEP-RELATED HEADACHES.)

Mirapex See PRAMIPEXOLE.

Mitler, Merrill M. Born in Racine, Wisconsin, Mitler (1945–) received a Ph.D. in psychology from Michigan State University. While a postdoctoral fellow from 1973 to 1976 at the Sleep Research Center at Stanford University School of Medicine, Dr. Mitler helped to found the first Sleep Disorders Center, under Dr. WILLIAM C. DEMENT, and served as administrative director from 1977 to 1978. In 1978, Dr. Mitler relocated his research activities to the State University of New York at Stony Brook, where he founded the SUNY-Stony Brook Sleep Disorders Center. In 1983, Dr. Mitler moved to Scripps Clinic and Research Foundation in La Jolla, California. For 12 years, Dr. Mitler served as executive secretary-treasurer of the Association of Sleep Disorder Centers, later known as the American Sleep Disorders Association and now the AMERICAN ACADEMY OF SLEEP MEDICINE. Dr. Mitler is currently a professor in the Department of Neuropharmacology at the Scripps Research Institute as well as a clinical professor of psychiatry in the Department of Psychiatry, University of California, San Diego.

Dr. Mitler's sleep research contributions include new methods of daytime testing for excessive somnolence, efficacy studies of drug treatments for a variety of sleep disorders, and, along with Dr. William Dement, the discovery of narcolepsy in dogs.

Dr. Mitler has been actively involved with public policy and sleep, and he authored the often-cited committee report on the relationship between sleep and health risk.

Mitler, Merrill M., Boysen, B.G., Campbell, L. and Dement, William C., "Narcolepsy-cataplexy in a Female Dog," *Experimental Neurology* 45 (1974): 332–340.

Mitler, Merrill M., Carskadon, M.A., Czeisler, C.A., Dement, W.C., Dinges, D.F. and Graeber, R.C., "Catastrophes, Sleep and Public Policy: Consensus Report," *Sleep* 11 (1988): 100–109.

modafinil (Provigil) A unique compound for the treatment of NARCOLEPSY. It has become the first-line treatment for narcolepsy in the United States since being made available early in 1999.

Animal studies suggest that modafinil may act in part through gamma-aminobutyric acidergic (GABA) systems and does not interact with central alpha 1-adrenergic, beta-adrenergic, serotonergic, opioid or cholinergic systems. Recent research has indicated that modafinil inhibits the tuberomammillary nucleus (TMN). The TMN is an important nucleus that causes arousal by means of histamine.

Modafinil's pharmacologic profile is distinctly different from amphetamine and methylphenidate (see STIMULANT MEDICATIONS). The compound has low abuse potential in humans. It is less effective at relieving sleepiness than amphetamine but has a better safety profile. It is well tolerated. The most frequent adverse event reported is headache, which is usually mild and transient. Other effects include dry mouth and nausea.

Mogodon See BENZODIAZEPINES.

Monday morning blues The feelings experienced at or soon after awakening on a Monday morning;

characterized by difficulty in awakening, tiredness, fatigue and grogginess. The symptoms are due to an insufficient amount of sleep that occurs because the sleep pattern has been shifted to a later phase over the prior Friday and Saturday nights. (Many people prefer to go to bed later on a Friday and Saturday night compared to their usual time of going to bed during the workdays or school days of the week.) The sleep pattern shift on the weekend causes difficulty in initiating sleep at an earlier time on Sunday night, resulting in a later-than-desired sleep-onset time. This is compounded by the fact that the time of arising on Monday is typically earlier than that which occurred on the prior Saturday and Sunday mornings. As a result, the total sleep duration prior to awakening on Monday morning is less than is required for full alertness.

Ensuring regular sleep hours seven days a week will prevent the Monday morning blues. Otherwise, a brief Monday afternoon nap will lessen some of the sleepiness.

The natural tendency to delay the timing of the sleep pattern, and the difficulty in making an adequate advancement, is due to the chronobiological PHASE DELAY of the sleep pattern. There is less physiological capability to make phase advances of the sleep episode. (See also DELAYED SLEEP PHASE SYNDROME, FREE RUNNING, PHASE RESPONSE CURVE, SUNDAY NIGHT INSOMNIA.)

monoamine oxidase inhibitors A group of drugs that have the ability to block the breakdown of the metabolism of naturally occurring monoamines. These medications are primarily used when the tricyclic ANTIDEPRESSANTS are ineffective in treating depression. However, the monoamine oxidase inhibitors are limited in their usefulness because there are often severe and unpredictable interactions between the monoamine oxidase inhibitors and many drugs and foods. In particular, foods containing tyramine, such as cheese, are liable to produce a hypertension crisis. The monoamine oxidase inhibitors can also produce excessive central nervous system stimulation, with the production of INSOMNIA or excessive sweating. Severe hypotension can occur. Other side effects, such as dizziness, headache, difficulty in urination, weakness, dry mouth, constipation and skin rashes, are common.

The monoamine oxidase inhibitors have been shown to be very powerful REM SLEEP suppressant medications. Nocturnal use of monoamine oxidase inhibitors can induce total suppression of REM sleep at night. The REM sleep suppressant effect of the monoamine oxidase inhibitors is thought to be related to their effectiveness as antidepressants. The withdrawal of monoamine oxidase inhibitors can be associated with exacerbation of REM sleep phenomena, such as NIGHTMARES, SLEEP PARALYSIS and HYPNAGOGIC HALLUCINATIONS. In NARCOLEPSY there can be an exacerbation of CATAPLEXY.

The monoamine oxidase inhibitors exist in two forms, types A and B, that affect the two isoenzymes. The type A inhibitors, such as phenelzine (Nardil), have been shown to be more effective in the treatment of narcolepsy than the type B inhibitors, such as selegiline (Deprenyl). However, because of their potential for side effect, the monoamine oxidase inhibitors have a very limited role in the treatment of narcolepsy.

montage The manner in which a variety of physiological variables are displayed on the polysomnograph paper. The montage defines not only the number of physiological variables measured but also the sequence in which they are displayed. For example, in epilepsy recordings the electrodes may be connected to each other in varied sequences.

mood disorders PSYCHIATRIC DISORDERS characterized by a partial or a full manic or hypomanic episode, or by one or more episodes of DEPRESSION. A common feature of mood disorders is sleep disturbance characterized primarily by INSOMNIA but also by EXCESSIVE SLEEPINESS. Mood disorders comprise a variety of disorders, including bipolar disorder, cyclothymia, major depressive disorders or dysthymia.

Patients with bipolar disorder have episodes of mania or hypomania. The patient has a degree of inflated self-esteem, is more talkative than usual, has a flight of ideas, is more distractible, has an increase in goal-directed activity, and has a heightened involvement in pleasure activity. In addition to episodes of mania, there are often episodes of depression. However, during the manic episode the sleep disturbance is characterized by a reduced sleep duration, often requiring only three or four hours of sleep, and at times going without sleep for several days in a row. In contrast, at times of depression, excessive time may be spent in bed, with feelings of fatigue, tiredness and sleepiness that occur throughout the daytime.

Patients with cyclothymia have numerous episodes of mania that are less intense (hypomania) and alternate with numerous episodes of depressive symptoms. The sleep pattern of those with cyclothymia may fluctuate between a night with one short sleep duration and one with much longer sleep durations.

Those with major depression have one or more episodes of depressed mood, with loss of interest in pleasurable activities, that lasts at least two weeks. During this time, sleep is commonly disturbed, with insomnia as the typical complaint. There is difficulty in initiating and maintaining sleep, with a characteristic EARLY MORNING AROUSAL. Sometimes patients with major depression also complain of excessive sleepiness or tiredness during the daytime and may spend prolonged periods in bed. Excessively long sleep durations are more commonly seen in adolescents with major depression. This severe depression is seen in individuals who have dysthymia in whom the depressed mood is constantly present, with features of poor appetite, low energy, low self-esteem, feelings of hopelessness and poor concentration. Sleep disturbance in such dysthymic patients is similar to that seen in individuals with major depressive disorders and is characterized by insomnia but occasionally by the complaint of excessive daytime sleepiness.

Polysomnographic features of patients with major depressive disorder particularly show changes in REM SLEEP. Typically, sleep latency is increased and there may be frequent awakenings and an early morning awakening; however, there is often reduced slow wave sleep and an increased amount of REM sleep. The first REM period of the major sleep episode often occurs earlier than normal, with a short first non-REM sleep period. The density of rapid eye movements, particularly in the first REM period, is increased. Patients with depression may show a sleep onset REM period, and there may be more sleep disruption with low REM sleep percentages, particularly in older patients.

Patients with bipolar depression may have an improved sleep efficiency, with a longer total sleep time than that seen in patients with a more typical major depression. However, bipolar patients typically will complain of feeling unrefreshed upon awakening. There may also be complaints of excessive daytime sleepiness, especially during the depression phases. During the manic phases, REM sleep, as well as stage three/four sleep, may be greatly reduced, as may the total sleep time.

Polysomnographic features, particularly those of REM sleep, may be useful in confirming a diagnosis of depressive disorder and may be helpful in differentiating a diagnosis of depression from DEMENTIA in elderly patients.

The treatment of the mood disorder is primarily by the use of psychoactive medications, particularly the ANTIDEPRESSANTS, including the tricyclic antidepressants, the serotonin reuptake inhibitors and the MONOAMINE OXIDASE INHIBITORS. In addition, electroconvulsive therapy and psychotherapy may be helpful in some patients. Patients with bipolar disorder may be helped with the use of mood stabilizing medications such as lithium carbonate. In addition to medication directed to the underlying mood disorder, the sleep disturbance can be helped by means of attention to SLEEP HYGIENE and behavioral treatments, such as STIMULUS CONTROL THERAPY and SLEEP RESTRICTION THERAPY. Because DELAYED SLEEP PHASE SYNDROME may be associated with atypical depression, treatment by means of CHRONOTHERAPY may be useful in patients who have a sleep phase delay.

Other sleep disorders that produce a complaint of insomnia or excessive sleepiness must be considered in any patient with a mood disorder who complains of sleep disturbance. SLEEP-RELATED BREATHING DISORDERS and PERIODIC LIMB MOVEMENT DISORDER may produce tiredness and fatigue, which may be confused with depression. The effects of medications and drugs such as ALCOHOL should also be considered to be a complicating factor in the sleep disturbance. Patients who have NARCOLEPSY not uncommonly will have depression secondary to the excessive sleepiness. If not recognized as due to the narcolepsy, excessive sleepiness may erroneously be ascribed solely to depression. Patients with other disorders of excessive sleepiness, such as IDIOPATHIC HYPERSOMNIA, can easily be misdiagnosed as having depression as the cause of their daytime sleepiness. Other sleep disorders are common causes of sleep symptoms similar to that seen in depression and, when appropriate, polysomnographic monitoring may be indicated to help arrive at an accurate diagnosis.

Gillin, J.C., Duncan, W., Pettigrew, K.D., Frankel, B.L. and Snyder, F., "Successful Separation of Depressed, Normal, and Insomniac Subjects by EEG Sleep Data," *Archives of General Psychiatry* 36 (1979): 85–90.

Reynolds, C.F. and Kupfer, D.J., "Sleep Research and Affective Illness: State of the Art Circa 1987," *Sleep* 10 (1987): 199–215.

morning person Term applied to persons who go to bed early and awaken earlier than what is typical for the general population. Morning persons awaken early because their sleep pattern is advanced—the pattern of body temperature and other circadian rhythms are ahead of most other people's. A morning person conforms to the "early to bed, early to rise" maxim.

Morpheus The Greek god of dreams. The word MORPHINE was derived from Morpheus. (See also HYPNOS, SOMNUS.)

morphine A derivative of the opium poppy, *papaver somniferum,* which in 1806 was one of the first substances to be isolated from opium. It was named after MORPHEUS, the Greek god of dreams. Morphine has been used in medicine primarily as an analgesic to relieve PAIN but also as a treatment for acute congestive heart failure. It has sedative and respiratory depressant effects that limit its use in medicine. Morphine is also a drug that is abused for its euphoric properties, often being administered by intravenous injection in drug addicts.

Morphine has sedative effects that are associated with increasing SLOW WAVE SLEEP, often at the expense of REM SLEEP. Following morphine's administration, mental impairment commonly occurs and is characterized by learning and memory difficulties, as well as impaired psychomotor function and mood changes.

Morphine may be dangerous to patients with impaired ventilation. The combination of morphine with other sedative medications is particularly dangerous and can lead to respiratory arrest. (See also SLEEP-RELATED BREATHING DISORDERS.)

morphology The shape of a particular wave form or tracing recorded during POLYSOMNOGRAPHY. The morphology of ALPHA ACTIVITY is a sinusoidal wave form, whereas that of a K-COMPLEX is a biphasic slow wave. The morphology of abnormal EEG waves can help in determining the type of seizure and its location.

mountain sickness See ALTITUDE INSOMNIA.

movement arousal A lightening of sleep associated with a body movement; typically defined as an increase in EMG (ELECTROMYOGRAM) activity in association with a change in pattern seen in another recorded channel of either the EEG (ELECTROENCEPHALOGRAM) or ELECTRO-OCULOGRAM.

movement time When a subject moves during a polysomnographic recording, the tracing pen will move widely, obscuring the recording of sleep stages. Movement time must last at least 15 seconds to be scored as movement time. Movement time is usually not counted with either sleep or wake time but is scored as a separate state, unless sleep can be scored for more than half of the epoch. In that case, the record is scored according to the prevailing sleep stage. If wake time precedes or follows the movement activity, then movement time is scored as wake time.

multiple sleep latency testing (MSLT) First developed in 1978 by MARY CARSKADON as a means of determining levels of daytime sleepiness. This test measures an individual's ability to fall asleep when given five nap opportunities throughout an average day. Naps would typically occur at 10 A.M., 12 noon, 2 P.M., 4 P.M. and 6 P.M. for an individual on an average 11 P.M. to 7 A.M. sleep schedule. Electrodes are attached to the head for the measurement of the ELECTROENCEPHALOGRAM, ELECTRO-OCULOGRAM and ELECTROMYOGRAM in order to determine the onset and type of sleep. The patient is asked to lie down in a darkened room and the time from lights out to the start of stage one sleep is the sleep latency on a particular nap. The patient is usually given a 20-minute opportunity to fall asleep. If sleep does not occur during this time, the test is terminated until the next nap opportunity. If sleep occurs, the individual is given a 10-minute opportunity to continue sleeping in order to determine the type of sleep that occurs. If sleep does not occur, then the latency is scored as lasting 20 minutes, and at the end of the five nap opportunities, the mean SLEEP LATENCY is determined. A mean sleep latency of greater than 10 minutes over the five naps is regarded as being normal. Values of less than 10 minutes indicate pathological sleepiness, and those less than five minutes indicate severe daytime sleepiness. The presence of two or more sleep-onset REM periods on a multiple sleep latency test following a night of documented normal sleep is indicative of NARCOLEPSY.

muramyl dipeptide (MDP) A compound found primarily in bacterial cell walls. This substance came to attention when FACTOR S was found to be similar to muramyl dipeptide. Muramyl dipeptide, when infused into the brains of rats, has been shown to increase non-REM sleep and, in addition, appears to increase body temperature. Muramyl dipeptide appears to increase serotonin turnover in the brain, and may therefore have its effect on sleep primarily by means of a serotonergic mechanism. (See also DELTA SLEEP-INDUCING PEPTIDE, SLEEP-INDUCING FACTORS.)

muscle tone Term applies to resting muscle activity that is measured by means of the ELECTROMYOGRAM. Muscle tone is usually present during wakefulness but decreases during non-REM sleep stages. During REM sleep, muscle tone activity is almost absent.

myocardial infarction Commonly known as a heart attack; occurs when the blood supply to a portion of the heart muscle is impaired, leading to necrosis of the heart muscle. Acute myocardial infarction is associated with a 35% mortality. There is a circadian pattern of myocardial infarction with an increase in episodes occurring between 6 A.M. and 12 noon. The cause of this circadian variability is unknown but may be related to factors set in process by sleep mechanisms or may be related to the sudden increase in activity upon awakening following a relatively quiet state during sleep. Infarction may also be related to circadian changes in biochemical, platelet and fibrinolytic factors.

Following myocardial infarction, patients typically have poor quality sleep, which is characterized by an increased number of awakenings, reduced REM sleep and reduced sleep efficiency. Daytime sleep episodes are also more common in such patients. SLEEP-RELATED BREATHING DISORDERS have been implicated as a cause of myocardial infarction during sleep due to the associated HYPOXEMIA. Cardiac ARRHYTHMIAS are known to be more common in patients with sleep-related breathing disorders. (See also VENTRICULAR ARRHYTHMIAS, DEATHS DURING SLEEP, OBSTRUCTIVE SLEEP APNEA SYNDROME.)

myoclonus Term that refers to brief muscle contractions detectable by electromyographic recording. The term is used to denote muscle activity that lasts less than one second in duration. However, in sleep-related NOCTURNAL MYOCLONUS or PERIODIC LIMB MOVEMENT DISORDER, the muscle activity exceeds one second in duration and has a recurring pattern of characteristic frequency (20 to 40 seconds). (See also PERIODIC LEG MOVEMENTS.)

myxedema A severe form of HYPOTHYROIDISM that is characterized by generalized accumulation of mucopolysaccharide. A patient with myxedema will have a bland, expressionless face, doughy induration of the skin and hypothermia. Myxedema coma may result in a hypothermic, stuporous state that is often fatal. SLEEP-RELATED BREATHING DISORDERS and EXCESSIVE SLEEPINESS are typical features of patients with myxedema.

N

nadir The lowest point of a biological rhythm. The nadir may be applied to a CIRCADIAN RHYTHM, such as body TEMPERATURE, which has its nadir during the major sleep episode, typically two to three hours before awakening. (See also ACROPHASE, CHRONOBIOLOGY.)

naps Brief sleep episodes taken outside of the major sleep episode. Naps vary in duration, from five minutes to four or more hours. The time that naps are most likely to occur is in the mid-afternoon, when there is a reduced degree of alertness because of the biphasic circadian pattern of alertness. Some cultures will take a SIESTA in the mid-afternoon; consequently, nighttime sleep is reduced in duration.

Frequent daytime naps are seen in sleep disorders, particularly those associated with EXCESSIVE SLEEPINESS. The naps that occur in NARCOLEPSY are typically short in duration—often five minutes of sleep will be refreshing—and are characterized by the presence of REM SLEEP. Naps taken by persons with disorders that cause fragmentation and disruption of nighttime sleep, such as the OBSTRUCTIVE SLEEP APNEA SYNDROME, are commonly of longer duration, lasting 30 minutes or more, and are largely composed of non-REM sleep. The refreshing quality of naps varies from individual to individual, but typically naps in narcoleptics are found to be very refreshing, whereas the naps in patients with obstructive sleep apnea syndrome are often perceived as inducing even greater sleepiness and sometimes are associated with headaches upon awakening.

Persons who go into deep, SLOW WAVE SLEEP in naps are often difficult to awaken until their time of spontaneous awakening. If aroused prior to that time, they often feel very lethargic, confused and unrefreshed.

Naps are to be discouraged in individuals who have a primary complaint of INSOMNIA, particularly PSYCHOPHYSIOLOGICAL INSOMNIA or insomnia related to psychiatric disorders. Any daytime sleep will take away sleep from the nighttime sleep episode, thereby leading to greater nighttime sleep disturbance.

Naps commonly occur in children from infancy and gradually reduce in number and in duration as the child develops. Young children who have disturbed nighttime sleep often benefit from a daytime nap, and the elimination of the nap may contribute to sleep difficulties at night. However, in some children excessive sleeping during the daytime contributes to nighttime sleep disturbances. Napping in children has been shown largely to be culturally determined, particularly in older children. For example, in a study of children in Zurich, 21% at age five had daytime naps compared with 5% of five-year-olds surveyed in Stockholm.

As multiple daily naps are indicative of a sleep disturbance, one should consider disorders of excessive sleepiness as being the cause. Naps that are taken at times when maximal alertness is to be expected, for example about two hours after awakening and about four hours before the time of usual sleep onset at night, are particularly important in considering whether napping behavior is reflective of an underlying sleep disorder. Mid-afternoon naps are of less significance.

narcolepsy A disorder of excessive sleep that is associated with CATAPLEXY and other REM sleep phenomena, such as SLEEP PARALYSIS and HYPNAGOGIC HALLUCINATIONS. This disorder was first described by JEAN GELINEAU in 1880. Since that time it has been recognized as a common cause of excessive sleepiness. The sleepiness is characterized by brief episodes of lapses into sleep that occur throughout the day, usually lasting less than an hour. Sometimes only five or 10 minutes of sleep is sufficient to refresh the patient with narcolepsy.

The daytime episodes of sleep are often accompanied by DREAMS and a sensation of inability to move the body (sleep paralysis) upon awakening, which are typically associated with RAPID EYE MOVEMENT (REM) SLEEP. The sleepiness in narcolepsy usually becomes manifest when the individual is in a quiet situation, such as relaxing, reading or watching television, as well as in situations with minimal participation, such as while attending meetings, movies, theater or concerts. Sleep is also liable to be induced when the patient with narcolepsy travels in a moving vehicle, such as an automobile, train, bus or airplane. Due to the induction of sleepiness while driving, motor vehicle accidents are more common in individuals who have narcolepsy.

Sometimes the episodes of sleep that occur during the daytime occur quite suddenly and the individual is unable to prevent them, in which case they are often termed "sleep attacks." When the sleepiness is severe, it can occur while the individual is talking, eating, walking or actively conversing.

In addition to the excessive sleepiness, the characteristic and unique feature of narcolepsy is the presence of cataplexy, the onset of muscular weakness that occurs with emotional stimuli. A sudden, intense emotional response, such as laughter, anger, surprise, elation or pride, can induce a loss of muscle tone manifested by a weakness in the legs, with an occasional fall to the ground. If the precipitating stimulus continues, the sufferer may have a continuing state of paralysis that affects all skeletal muscles, and the individual will be completely paralyzed, in a state sometimes called "status cataplecticus." During episodes of cataplexy, consciousness, memory and the ability to breathe and move the eyes are retained. In milder forms of cataplexy, the weakness may occur in one or more groups of muscles, so that the jaw may droop or the head may sag or the wrist may go limp. Sometimes the weakness is not evident to observers, but is perceived as an unusual sensation by the sufferer. The symptoms of cataplexy can be dramatically eliminated by the use of tricyclic ANTIDEPRESSANTS, including protriptyline, clomipramine and imipramine. Other medications that have been shown to be helpful in the treatment of cataplexy are gamma-hydroxybutyrate and L-tyrosine. (See STIMULANT MEDICATIONS.) Episodes of cataplexy may be rare or infrequent, or may occur on a daily basis, causing severe incapacity.

In addition to excessive sleepiness and cataplexy, patients with narcolepsy often have other features indicative of an abnormality of REM sleep, such as sleep paralysis and hypnagogic hallucinations. Sleep paralysis is an inability to move upon awakening from sleep and is often perceived as a frightening sensation of being unable to breathe. Episodes usually last only a few seconds following which the individual comes to full wakefulness and is able to move. These episodes are thought to be partial manifestations of REM sleep that occur in the transition from REM sleep to wakefulness.

In addition, when REM sleep occurs at the onset of sleep, vivid, dreamlike images are often perceived. Termed hypnagogic hallucinations, these images may be frightening. The sufferer may imagine that someone is in the bedroom or the house is on fire, yet have difficulty in being able to respond to these images. These images occur in the transition from wakefulness to sleep, usually during nocturnal sleep, but they also occur during sleep episodes in the daytime. Less frequently the episodes will occur upon awakening from a sleep episode, at which time the episodes are termed hypnopompic hallucinations.

An additional feature of narcolepsy is AUTOMATIC BEHAVIOR, which is characterized by a seemingly normal behavior that occurs when an individual is tired or sleepy. These episodes of behavior are not recalled afterward. An example: When driving a car and arriving at a destination the individual may not recall the trip. Sometimes rather unusual behavior can occur during such states, so that a narcoleptic patient may erroneously put clothing in a refrigerator or stove and afterward not recall having done so. These episodes of inappropriate behavior are less common than normal behavior for which the individual is amnesiac.

Patients with narcolepsy will note disruption of nocturnal sleep that is characterized by frequent awakenings and the inability to continuously sustain normal sleep. The treatment of the nocturnal sleep disruption can lead to some improvement in the daytime sleepiness but does not eliminate daytime sleepiness, even if nocturnal sleep is returned to an entirely normal pattern. Some patients with narcolepsy may require treatment of severe nocturnal sleep disruption.

Narcolepsy generally occurs around the time of puberty (usually just after puberty, but occasionally before). Initially, excessive sleepiness is the presenting complaint and cataplexy occurs either concurrently or a period of months or years afterward. Due to the gradual onset of symptoms and the difficulty of diagnosis in the early years, most patients present in early adulthood, at which time the diagnosis is made. The disorder is lifelong and reaches a peak in middle age; however, there is considerable individual variability, and occasionally patients have maximal symptoms around the time of onset, with a gradual decrease over a lifetime.

The complete disappearance of daytime sleepiness is not, however, thought to occur. Much of the improvement in symptoms is the individual's learning to cope with the disability and the development of either denial for symptoms or subconscious unawareness of symptoms that may be seen by others.

Narcolepsy is thought to occur in approximately 40 per 100,000 of the general population, a prevalence rate similar to multiple sclerosis. Some ethnic groups appear to have a lower incidence of narcolepsy, such as Israeli Jews. The disorder affects both males and females equally, and there does seem to be a familial tendency, with a narcoleptic patient's child having an eight-times-greater risk of developing the disorder than the child of a non-narcoleptic.

Narcolepsy is of unknown origin but is believed to be due to a central nervous system abnormality. Some alterations in neurotransmitter levels, such as for dopamine, have been found to be in the fluid that bathes the brain (cerebrospinal fluid); however, an exact site of neuroanatomical abnormalities has not been determined.

Narcolepsy greatly affects an individual in almost every situation. Children with narcolepsy may have great difficulty in concentration, with memory difficulties that lead to impaired education. Adults will have frequent job changes and are prone to accidents due to sleepiness while driving a car or operating dangerous equipment.

The diagnosis of narcolepsy is made by a clinical history of excessive sleepiness or the presence of cataplexy. In the absence of a clear history of cataplexy, objective confirmation of the diagnosis by polysomnographic testing (see POLYSOMNOGRAPHY) is essential. Polysomnographic testing typically will show a reduced SLEEP LATENCY at night, often with the appearance of a sleep-onset REM period. Nocturnal sleep is also characterized by an increased amount of the lighter stage one sleep but normal amounts of deep sleep and REM sleep. There may be a disruption of the sleep-wake cycle, with frequent intermittent awakenings. Daytime sleepiness is demonstrated by the MULTIPLE SLEEP LATENCY TEST (MSLT), which usually shows a mean sleep latency of less than 10 minutes (typically below five minutes), indicating severe sleepiness. Also, the presence of two or more sleep-onset REM periods during a five-nap multiple sleep latency test is diagnostic and characteristic. Polysomnographic testing must be performed while the patient is on the usual sleep-wake pattern and free of medications that influence sleep and wakefulness.

Disorders such as PERIODIC LIMB MOVEMENT DISORDER and CENTRAL SLEEP APNEA SYNDROME are more liable to occur in patients with narcolepsy but are not the primary cause of the daytime sleepiness.

Recent evidence has demonstrated the presence of a specific genetic marker in patients with narcolepsy. Histocompatibility typing (see HLA-DR2) has demonstrated the presence of the DR2 and DQ1 groupings in nearly every patient with narcolepsy. But since these histocompatibility characteristics are also present in 25% to 30% of the general population, some additional factor must also be present to cause narcolepsy. It is believed that the presence of this genetic marker suggests that certain individuals are predisposed to developing narcolepsy; and the addition of another factor, possibly another viral or genetic factor, may be responsible for the expression of the disease. The presence of DR2 positivity varies with ethnic groups, being approximately 100% associated in the Japanese population, approximately 96% in the Caucasian population and about 85% associated with the African-American population. The HLA testing may be useful in aiding the diagnosis of individuals where there is some uncertainty as to the nature of the disorder producing excessive daytime sleepiness, or can be useful in determining if children of narcoleptic patients are predisposed to developing the disorder. A DR2 negative child is unlikely to ever develop narcolepsy. The allele HLA DQB1-0602 is the genetic factor most highly associated with narcolepsy.

In 2000 it was discovered that most narcoleptic patients are deficient in HYPOCRETIN, and pathological studies have demonstrated the loss of hypocretin cells in the hypothalamus.

The presence of cataplexy is a major factor in differentiating this disorder from other disorders of excessive sleepiness. In the absence of cataplexy, other disorders, such as idiopathic hypersomnia, subwakefulness syndrome, obstructive sleep apnea syndrome, periodic limb movement disorder, insufficient sleep syndrome, psychiatric disorders, recurrent hypersomnia and menstrual-associated sleep disorder must be considered as possible causes.

Treatment of narcolepsy is mainly symptomatic and consists of the use of STIMULANT MEDICATIONS for daytime sleepiness. The amphetamines, methylphenidate hydrochloride (Ritalin) and pemoline (Cylert), are often used. Dextroamphetamine is used less commonly now than in the past. These medications appear to have the ability to improve arousal during the daytime so the individual can prevent himself from falling into sleep episodes; however, these medications appear to have less effect in preventing sleep episodes when the individual is relaxed and in a situation conducive to sleep. In other words, these medications improve the ability to remain awake but do not impair the ability to fall asleep. The medication MODAFINIL (PROVIGIL), a wake-promoting agent, is effective at reducing sleepiness in patients with narcolepsy. The medication is replacing the use of Cylert and methylphenidrate for many patients.

Even with adequate dosages of medications, individuals with narcolepsy are still often handicapped by the tendency to fall asleep easily. However, the medications can greatly improve functional performance and allow an individual to maintain regular employment and social contacts. As well as the treatment of excessive sleepiness, other medications are required for the treatment of cataplexy. Tricyclic ANTIDEPRESSANTS are the most effective, with protriptyline, clomipramine and imipramine being the most commonly used medications. Recently the amino acid L-tyrosine has been reported to be effective in relieving cataplexy and improving daytime alertness in some patients with narcolepsy. Other effective medications include GAMMA-HYDROXYBUTYRATE, which can also improve cataplexy. Viloxazine has been shown to be effective in the treatment of cataplexy in patients with narcolepsy. Viloxazine hydrochloride is a derivative of propranolol, the beta-adrenergic-blocking cardiovascular drug used for the treatment of hypertension. The medication is available in Europe but not in the United States.

In addition to the treatment by medications, attention has to be given to SLEEP HYGIENE, with the maintenance of regular sleep onset and wake times, as well as an appropriate nocturnal sleep duration. Naps during the daytime should be kept to less than 20 minutes and should not be prolonged or they may cause a breakdown of the nighttime sleep pattern.

Case History

A 35-year-old fireman presented with a history of excessive sleepiness that had been present since his teenage years. This sleepiness had become more severe during the three years prior to presentation at the SLEEP DISORDER CENTER. The pattern of sleepiness was somewhat complicated by the irregular shift work that was necessary as a fireman. However, it was clear to himself and others around him that he would fall asleep more readily than other firemen who were on similar shift work. On several occasions, he had been erroneously accused of taking drugs or having alcohol, as he appeared to be extremely drowsy and lethargic. His work was in jeopardy; his sleepiness was clearly excessive and he was not allowed to drive the fire truck.

However, when he was aroused he was fully alert and could actively and accurately perform his duties.

The sleepiness affected his social life in that he would fall asleep very easily when sitting and talking, watching television or reading. When he went to the movies, he would always fall asleep within the first 20 minutes of the picture. When he went out for a drive with friends, he would let them drive because he was too sleepy to do so.

He also noticed the onset of a weakness that would come on when he became emotional, particularly with anger and to a lesser extent with laughter. He felt a very strange sensation that was unpleasant and he would try to fight it internally by suppressing his emotions; however, he would eventually have to sit or lie down. Although he was close to falling on many occasions, he never did so. These episodes were extremely embarrassing.

He had very excessive dreams and regarded himself as being the world's greatest dreamer. Usually the dreams were of pleasant events; however, many were characterized by a perception of flying through the air while viewing himself lying in bed. (This perception has been called an "out-of-body" experience.) At times he also would see hallucinations of people or events just before falling asleep at night.

The patient underwent polysomnographic testing that showed a rapid onset of REM sleep on the nighttime test, with a high amount of stage one sleep—features that were consistent with the diagnosis of narcolepsy. His sleep otherwise was normal; however, during a daytime multiple sleep latency test he fell asleep in less than two minutes on average of the five naps, and during four of the naps he went into REM sleep. These features on both the polysomnographic tests were diagnostic for narcolepsy.

He was initially treated with Cylert, which in his particular case was only partially effective, and at times he needed the extra help of a short-acting stimulant. Ritalin was occasionally used in conjunction with a background, stable dosage of Cylert. His cataplexy episodes were completely controlled by the use of Vivactil.

He gave up his job as a fireman and trained as a mechanical engineer serving home electric equipment, a position more appropriate for someone with narcolepsy as it kept him active during the day and also enabled him to have a more regular sleep-wake pattern. (See also AMERICAN NARCOLEPSY ASSOCIATION, HISTOCOMPATIBILITY ANTIGEN TESTING, NARCOLEPSY NETWORK, NARCOLEPSY PROJECT, SLEEP ONSET REM PERIOD.)

Altrich, M.S., "Diagnostic Aspects of Narcolepsy," *Neurology* 50, no. 2, Suppl. 1 (1998): S2–S7.

Guilleminault, C., Passouant, P. and Dement, William C., *Narcolepsy.* New York: Spectrum, 1976.

Mitler, Merrill, Nelson, S. and Hajdukovic, R., "Narcolepsy: Diagnostic, Treatment, and Management," *Psychiatric Clinics of North America* 10 (1987): 593–606.

Roth, B., *Narcolepsy and Hypersomnia.* Basel: Karger, 1988.

Wise, M.S., "Childhood Narcolepsy," *Neurology* 50, no. 2, Suppl. 1 (1998): S37–S42.

Narcolepsy and Cataplexy Foundation of America Nonprofit organization, based in New York City; founded in 1975 by Professor Helen Demitoff, R.N., Ph.D. Its purpose is the dissemination of information on NARCOLEPSY to the public and to physicians. (See also AMERICAN NARCOLEPSY ASSOCIATION, NARCOLEPSY NETWORK, NARCOLEPSY INSTITUTE.)

narcolepsy-cataplexy syndrome See NARCOLEPSY.

Narcolepsy Institute A state-funded program developed in 1985 by Michael Thorpy, M.D., at the Sleep-Wake Disorders Center of Montefiore Medical Center in New York City; it provides support services to individuals who have NARCOLEPSY as well as to their families. Originally called the Narcolepsy Project, it was renamed the Narcolepsy Institute in 1997.

The project serves all five boroughs of New York City, with counseling and crisis intervention programs for individuals or groups who are diagnosed as having, or suspected of having, narcolepsy. It provides basic information and helps individuals and their families to develop skills necessary to cope with the social and physical impact that this condition has on their lives.

The project is directed and run by professionals in counseling; it also offers training in counseling as well as research opportunities in the area of the psychosocial factors of narcolepsy. The program produces educational materials for patients that include videotapes, patient handbooks and a regular newsletter called *Perspectives.*

For information, contact the Narcolepsy Institute, Montefiore Medical Center, 111 E. 210th Street, Bronx, New York 10467.

Narcolepsy Network Incorporated as a not-for-profit organization in 1986 and organized on a local, state and national basis. Its motto, "CARE" (Communication, Advocacy, Research and Education), embodies its goals of sharing information about NARCOLEPSY, advocating for needs at all levels, supporting and encouraging narcolepsy research and helping to make the general public aware of narcolepsy and its consequences.

Persons having narcolepsy, their families, friends and those interested in narcolepsy and related daytime sleepiness disorders are welcome to attend meetings and to become active members. The organization publishes a newsletter, *The Network,* as well as numerous other printed and taped educational materials. Contact Narcolepsy Network, 227 Fairfield Road, Suite 310B, Fairfield, New Jersey 07004. (See also AMERICAN NARCOLEPSY ASSOCIATION, NARCOLEPSY INSTITUTE, NARCOLEPSY AND CATAPLEXY FOUNDATION OF AMERICA.)

Narcolepsy Project See NARCOLEPSY INSTITUTE.

narcotics The word "narcotic" is derived from the Greek word *narkosis,* meaning a benumbing. Narcosis is a nonspecific and reversible form of depression of the central nervous system, marked by stupor that is produced by drugs. The term "narcotics" primarily refers to the opioid derivatives of opium. The opioids include MORPHINE, pentazocine, oxycodone, heroin and CODEINE. The narcotic derivatives have been used in sleep medicine for the treatment of RESTLESS LEGS SYNDROME, particularly the medication oxycodone. Codeine has been shown to be helpful in improving sleepiness in some patients with NARCOLEPSY; however, because of its potential for addiction it is rarely used.

The narcotic derivatives mainly affect the central nervous system and can induce analgesia, sleepiness, mood changes, respiratory depression, constipation, nausea and vomiting. These medications affect specific receptors in the central nervous system that can be blocked by agents such as naloxone. (See also MORPHEUS.)

nasal congestion Normally breathing occurs through the nose during sleep, unless there is upper airway obstruction—when mouth breathing is necessary. Nasal congestion produces impaired nasal breathing during sleep, whether the congestion is due to acute nasal stuffiness or allergic rhinitis. It can also exacerbate preexisting OBSTRUCTIVE SLEEP APNEA SYNDROME or can induce apneas in a person who otherwise does not have apnea during sleep. Nasal infection and congestion need to be treated in any patient with obstructive sleep apnea syndrome to avoid a worsening apnea.

Nasal congestion can be treated surgically by submucous resection, the removal of polyps or treatment with mucosal medications. Medications used to treat allergic rhinitis include ANTIHISTAMINES, topical steroids and related medications.

Patients with the obstructive sleep apnea syndrome who are treated by CPAP (CONTINUOUS POSITIVE AIRWAY PRESSURE) may have an exacerbation or a new onset of allergic rhinitis. Initial treatment by nasal decongestants often will settle the nasal congestion; however, medications such as the antihistamines, anticholinergics or steroids may be required to allow the patients to continue the CPAP. (See also NASAL SURGERY.)

nasal positive pressure ventilation (NPPV) A new treatment modality that can be useful for patients who have SLEEP-RELATED BREATHING DISORDERS that are not responsive to CONTINUOUS POSITIVE AIRWAY PRESSURE devices (CPAP). Nasal positive pressure ventilation (NPPV) consists of the application of intermittent positive pressure ventilation through a nasal mask. Because of the increased ventilatory pressure, compared with continuous positive airway pressure devices, the lungs can be inflated in patients who otherwise have difficulty inspiring. This method is particularly useful for the treatment of CENTRAL SLEEP APNEA SYNDROME, especially in those with NEUROMUSCULAR DISEASES that prevent adequate VENTILATION during sleep, as well as for patients with KYPHOSCOLIOSIS.

nasal surgery Occasionally performed to relieve SNORING or the OBSTRUCTIVE SLEEP APNEA SYNDROME. Surgery to reduce the bulk of the nasal mucosa, submucuous resection, produces initial improvement in the severity of obstructive sleep apnea. However, it is unusual for the syndrome to be completely relieved by this procedure. As a result, submucous resection has infrequently been performed for the obstructive sleep apnea syndrome. It can be useful in combination with other surgical treatments, such as the UVULOPALATOPHARYNGOPLASTY (UPP) operation.

Submucuous resection in combination with UPP is only useful for those patients with a major degree of NASAL CONGESTION. Some patients who are prescribed the nasal CPAP (CONTINUOUS POSITIVE AIRWAY PRESSURE) system find that the nasal congestion prevents the routine use of CPAP. Surgical management of mucous congestion can improve airflow, thereby allowing the patient to tolerate CPAP more easily.

Submucous resection is required for sleep apnea due to severe deviation of the nasal septum. A major improvement in nasal breathing can result from the surgery. Mild septal deviation does not require corrective surgery because little beneficial effect on the sleep apnea is likely to be seen.

Nasal obstruction may occur at the nares, particularly in patients who have previous submucous resection with a subsequent nose droop. Choanal obstruction at the posterior nasopharynx may also be treated and is more likely to occur in patients who have cranial facial abnormalities contributing to the obstructive sleep apnea syndrome. (See also AIRWAY OBSTRUCTION, PHARYNX, SURGERY AND SLEEP DISORDERS.)

Nathaniel Kleitman Distinguished Service Award ". . . created in 1981 to honor service to the field of sleep research and sleep disorders medicine, especially generous and altruistic efforts in the areas of administration, public relations, and legislation. Whereas research and academic contributions produce their own rewards in publications, tenure, and recognition, the achievements of those who toil in the above areas may go unnoticed."

The award, presented by the ASSOCIATION OF PROFESSIONAL SLEEP SOCIETIES, was named for NATHANIEL KLEITMAN, Ph.D., one of the founders of modern sleep research, who at the University of Chicago, along with Eugene Aserinsky and WILLIAM C. DEMENT, discovered the REM phase of sleep.

Recipients of the Nathaniel Kleitman award have included: David P. White, M.D. (2000); John Sassin, M.D. (1999); Mark Mahowald, M.D. (1998); Paul Fredrickson, M.D. (1997); Alan Pack, M.B., Ch.B., Ph.D. (1996); James Walsh, Ph.D. (1995); Richard Ferber, M.D. (1994); Michael Thorpy, M.D. (1993); Phillip Westbrook, M.D. (1992); Mary Carskadon, Ph.D. (1991); Thomas Roth, Ph.D. (1990); Peter Hauri, Ph.D. (1989); Helmut Schmidt, M.D. and Helio Lemmi, M.D. (1988); William C. Dement, M.D., Ph.D. (1987); Christian Guilleminault, M.D. (1986); Alan Rechtschaffen, Ph.D. (1985); Mitchel B. Balter, Ph.D. and Merrill M. Mitler, Ph.D. (1984); Elliot D. Weitzman, M.D. (1983); William C. Dement, M.D., Ph.D. (1982); Ismet Karacan, M.D. and Howard P. Roffwarg, M.D. (1981).

National Commission on Sleep Disorders Research Established on November 4, 1988, with a mandate to conduct a comprehensive study of the knowledge of the incidence, prevalence, morbidity and mortality resulting from sleep disorders and of the social and economic impact of such disorders. In addition, the commission was to evaluate the public and private facilities and resources (including trained personnel and research activities) available for the diagnosis, treatment and research into sleep disorders. It also was developed to identify programs, including biological, physiological, behavioral, environmental and social by which improvements in the management of sleep disorders could be accomplished.

The commission conducted an extensive survey to determine the total sleep-related health needs of the American public. Many areas of government were involved in this commission, including the Department of Health and Human Services, with all of its agencies and institutes. Many other federal departments, including those of Defense, Transportation, Commerce, Energy, Labor and Education were involved in providing information for the National Commission on Sleep Disorders Research.

The commission represented the entire field of sleep disorders medicine, and over three years documented the impact of sleep research and SLEEP DISORDERS MEDICINE to the United States population.

National Narcolepsy Registry A registry of patient information and DNA samples established by the NATIONAL SLEEP FOUNDATION to further genetic research of NARCOLEPSY. This confidential registry will enable researchers to construct family trees, coordinate family history data and establish cell lines for DNA analysis. The registry's ultimate goal is to improve treatment of narcolepsy by identifying the gene or genes associated with the disorder. The registry is housed at the Sleep-Wake Disorders Center at Montefiore Medical Center in New York. The director is Michael Thorpy, M.D. The blood samples are stored and the DNA extracted at the Human Genetics Program of the Department of Molecular Genetics at Albert Einstein College of Medicine under the chairmanship of Raju Kucherlapati, Ph.D.

The National Narcolepsy Registry establishes cell lines on all affected patients and all DNA produced. The laboratory of Dr. Emmanuel Mignot, M.D., at Stanford University in Palo Alto, California, analyzes DNA samples for HLA DQB1-0602. DNA samples are available to any approved research study for genetic analysis. Requests for information on how to apply for samples must be forwarded to the National Sleep Foundation.

As of February 1998 more than 800 patients had volunteered for the registry. Emphasis is primarily on obtaining at least 100 sibling pairs and multiplex with narcolepsy, but all affected individuals and their families are encouraged to participate.

The registry is overseen by an advisory group established by the National Sleep Foundation composed of experts in science, research, ethics, advocacy, treatment and patient support.

For additional information, contact the National Narcolepsy Registry, c/o The National Sleep Foundation, 1552 K St. NW, #500, Washington, D.C. 20005. E-mail: natsleep@erols.com; Web: www.sleepfoundation.org.

National Sleep Foundation (NSF) A nonprofit organization dedicated to improving the quality of life for the millions of Americans who suffer from sleep disorders and to the prevention of catastrophic accidents related to sleep deprivation or sleep disorders. The NSF was founded in 1990 with a grant from the American Sleep Disorders Association (now called the AMERICAN ACADEMY OF SLEEP MEDICINE). The first executive director was Carol Westbrook. The first president was Tom Roth, followed by John Hoag (1994), Alan Pack (1995) and Lorraine Wearley (1996). Originally established in Los Angeles, the NSF moved to Washington, D.C., in October 1994.

The foundation seeks public and private funding to support research, education, training and information programs. Programs have included: the "Drive Alert—Arrive Alive" campaign to reduce the high incidence of sleep-related auto crashes; publications designed to inform and educate primary care physicians on the diagnosis and treatment of sleep disorders; educational symposia for physicians; public education; research grants; and partnerships with business and government to extend educational reach.

In 1996 the NSF sponsored the development of a NATIONAL NARCOLEPSY REGISTRY at Montefiore Medical Center in New York, to help determine the genetic cause of narcolepsy. The NSF established the Pickwick Club for physicians and other health care workers to assist in providing funds for research and other foundation activities. The Pickwick Club hosts an annual dinner at the ASSOCIATION OF PROFESSIONAL SLEEP SOCIETIES annual meeting to solicit corporate and individual donations for research. For further information, contact the National Sleep Foundation, 1522 K Street NW, #500, Washington, D.C. 20005. E-mail: natsleep@erols.com; Web: www.sleepfoundation.org.

neuroleptics Medications that have beneficial effects upon mood and thought and are used primarily to treat severe PSYCHIATRIC DISORDERS. This group of drugs, also known as the antipsychotic medications, has side effects that are characterized by abnormal neurological function. The neuroleptic medications include the phenothiazines and medications such as haloperidol. These medications can have pronounced sedative effects and are often used for patients with psychiatric disorders to control the underlying psychiatric state and also to improve sedation at night. The haloperidol and thioridazine are also commonly used for patients with DEMENTIA in order to produce nocturnal sedation. (See also CEREBRAL DEGENERATIVE DISORDERS, MOOD DISORDERS, NOCTURNAL CONFUSION.)

neuromuscular diseases Term applied to those disorders that are due to an abnormality of the muscle or its nerve supply. Typically these disorders will lead to muscle weakness and feelings of fatigue. Many neuromuscular disorders affect the muscles of VENTILATION, and SLEEP-RELATED BREATHING DISORDERS occur.

Neuromuscular disorders that affect ventilation in sleep include: lesions that affect the peripheral nerves, such as those due to poliomyelitis; viral infections, such as Landry-Guillain-Barre syndrome; and spinal cord lesions, such as myelopathies, trauma and vascular diseases of the spinal cord.

Muscle disorders, such as the dystrophies, dystonia myotonica and acid maltase deficiency, can all be associated with sleep-related breathing disorders.

Typically the neuromuscular diseases will produce a decrease of ventilation during REM sleep, with the development of HYPOXEMIA and sometimes HYPERCAPNIA. Depending upon the course of the neuromuscular disorder, treatment can be by oxygen, RESPIRATORY STIMULANTS, assisted ventilation devices or diaphragmatic pacemakers. (See also ALVEOLAR HYPOVENTILATION, CENTRAL SLEEP APNEA SYNDROME, PULMONARY HYPERTENSION.)

nicotine Stimulant that can interfere with the quality of sleep. It may produce a SLEEP ONSET INSOMNIA if taken immediately prior to the sleep episode, or it may prevent sleep from recurring if a cigarette is smoked during the night. People who have disorders of EXCESSIVE SLEEPINESS, such as OBSTRUCTIVE SLEEP APNEA SYNDROME, are liable to fall asleep while smoking in bed. A fire may result and can be a major cause of accidental death during sleep.

Nicotine is contained in cigarette tobacco. The content of nicotine in tobacco varies between 1% and 2% and the average cigarette delivers approximately 1 milligram of nicotine (range 0.05 to 2.0 milligrams). Nicotine is also present in chewing tobacco and can be obtained in a gum form (Nicorette). Nicorette has 2 milligrams of nicotine contained in small pieces of gum and is often used by smokers in an attempt to prevent or decrease some of the withdrawal effects when trying to stop smoking.

Nicotine produces an alerting pattern in the ELECTROENCEPHALOGRAM. In addition, it can produce hand tremor, decreased skeletal muscle tone and reduction in deep tendon reflexes.

TOLERANCE develops to some of the effects of nicotine with chronic use. Withdrawal syndromes may occur in individuals who are chronic smokers and are characterized by daytime DROWSINESS, headaches, increased appetite and sleep disturbances.

Help for quitting the cigarette habit is available from a variety of programs or organizations, such as Smokenders, the American Lung Association, ASH (Action on Smoking and Health), based in Washington, D.C., the American Cancer Society's FreshStart Program, and local or state affiliates of GASP (Group Against Smoking Pollution). A popular book about the history of the cigarette in America and the development of the cigarette habit is Robert Sobel's *They Satisfy* (Garden City, New York: Anchor Books/Doubleday, 1978). (See also INSOMNIA, SMOKING.)

United States Surgeon General, *The Health Consequences of Smoking: The Changing Cigarette.* Washington, D.C.: U.S. Government Printing Office, 1981; Department of Health and Human Services Publication No. (pHs) 81-50156.

night blindness A disorder of persons who have difficulty seeing at night but whose vision is relatively normal during the daytime or when in bright light. Night blindness is an early symptom of deficiency of vitamin A, a vitamin that is important in maintaining the integrity of the retina. With vitamin A deficiency, the retina degenerates and vision decreases. In addition, there usually are changes of the conjunctiva, which becomes dry, and there may be accumulations of foam-like lesions on the surface of the conjunctiva. These lesions, called Bitot's spots, can deteriorate and cause ulceration, with breakdown of the cornea, resulting in complete blindness.

Vitamin A deficiency occurs in developing Third World countries, and blindness in children is not uncommon. Night blindness usually responds well to the daily administration of 30,000 IU of vitamin A for one week. (See also NYCTALOPIA.)

night fears Fears common in children, particularly around the time of nursery school. The fears usually represent insecurity about some aspect of growing up, whether it is beginning school or being left with a baby-sitter, which leads to the development of fears at bedtime. Anxiety may not be apparent during the daytime; however, when the child goes to bed and is alone in the dark, mental images may begin and turn into fantasies. Commonly, a child may say there is a monster under the bed or hiding behind the curtains. In such situations, the parent should reassure the child that there is nothing to be afraid of; however, exhaustive searches in the bedroom are unnecessary and will not aid in relaxing the child. The best way to manage these concerns is for the parents to demonstrate love and concern for the child, and look for the daytime anxieties that are the cause of the nighttime fears.

Fear of the dark is also common in older children and the fear can be exacerbated by some event during the daytime, such as watching a scary movie. The parents should not insist that the child sleep in the dark but should accommodate the child by leaving a door partly open or using a night-light in the bedroom or hall. The sounds of other family members moving around the house can reassure the child that he or she is protected by the parents, which will help to reduce some of the fears of the dark.

NIGHTMARES commonly occur in children, and bad DREAMS are associated with the REM state of sleep. Nightmares may be a reflection of daytime concerns. Because nightmares are so common, reassurance at the time is all that is required to settle the child. The child may come into the parent's bedroom and wish to remain for the night, particularly if the dream was especially frightening, but this is to be discouraged (see FAMILY BED).

Sometimes night fears are a technique used to stall going to bed at night, and parents should be aware if their children are using these fears to manipulate their bedtime hours. It is important for the parents to establish limits, and if parents suspect this is the cause of the night fears, then appropriate management may be necessary or a form of LIMIT-SETTING SLEEP DISORDER may develop.

A child with recurrent or frequent fears or nightmares may require intervention with psychological counseling, but this is unnecessary for the majority of healthy children. (See also CONFUSIONAL AROUSALS, REM SLEEP, SLEEP TERRORS, SLEEP ONSET ASSOCIATION DISORDER.)

Ferber, Richard, *Solve Your Child's Sleep Problems.* New York: Simon and Schuster, 1985.

nightmare A frightening dream that usually produces an awakening from the dreaming stage of sleep. It often consists of having been chased or of personal injury. The nightmare sufferer will sit upright in bed in an intensely scared state. Dream recall is immediate, and the person is fully awake, often with a petrified look, breathing rapidly and with a rapid heart rate. Sometimes the nightmares may not cause awakenings, and the frightening content of the dream will be recalled upon awakening the next morning.

Nightmares are very common in childhood, particularly between the ages of three and six years; however, it is not uncommon for nightmares to be reported from the age of two years. Nightmares appear to be a common phenomenon, occurring in 10% to 50% of children between the ages of three and five years; treatment is usually unnecessary. The child should be reassured and usually can return to sleep without great difficulty.

The tendency for nightmares appears to decrease with increasing age; however, episodes commonly occur after the age of 60 years. When episodes occur in adulthood they may be associated with underlying PSYCHIATRIC DISORDERS, particularly borderline personality disorders, schizophrenia or schizoid personality disorder. However, 50%

of adults with nightmares have no psychiatric diagnosis. Emotional stress is clearly associated with an increased frequency of nightmares, as well as traumatic event stress. The use of medications, especially L-DOPA and the beta adrenergic blockers, used for the treatment of hypertension or cardiac disease, are often precipitants of nightmares.

There does not appear to be any gender difference in the incidence of nightmares in childhood; however, in adulthood, nightmares appear to be frequent in women. There is little evidence of any familial predisposition.

Polysomnographic monitoring of nightmares demonstrates an abrupt arousal occurring out of REM sleep. Episodes will usually occur after a prolonged period of REM sleep, and there may be an increased number of rapid eye movements and a variation in the heart and respiratory rates. Nightmares can also occur from REM sleep that is present in daytime NAPS.

Nightmares should be differentiated from SLEEP TERRORS, which are abrupt awakenings from the deep stage three or four sleep, usually heralded by a loud, piercing cry. The features that differentiate nightmares include the full awakening that is present in nightmares, whereas arousal is difficult in someone suffering from sleep terrors. Frightening dream content is always present in nightmares, whereas no dream content is typical for sleep terrors. Very often an individual with a sleep terror will go back to sleep and not recall the episode the next morning, whereas this is extremely unusual following nightmares.

Episodes of REM SLEEP BEHAVIOR DISORDER may have features similar to a nightmare; however, in REM sleep behavior disorder there is more "acting out" of the dream content, with less fear and panic. Usually sufferers of REM sleep behavior disorder do not fully awaken during the behavior.

Treatment for nightmares is not necessary in childhood, whereas adults can benefit from attempts to reduce emotional stress or withdrawal of precipitating medications. In some instances, suppression of episodes can occur with medications such as the tricyclic ANTIDEPRESSANTS. However, their abrupt withdrawal may lead to an increase in the nightmare frequency. (See also REM SLEEP, STRESS.)

Fischer, C.J., Byrne, J., Edwards, T. and Kahn, E., "A Psychophysiological Study of Nightmares," *Journal of the American Psychoanalytic Association* 18 (1970): 747–782.

Hartmann, E., "Nightmare After Trauma as Paradigm for All Dreams: A New Approach to the Nature and Functions of Dreaming," *Psychiatry* 61, no. 3 (1998): 223–238.

night owl See EVENING PERSON.

night person See EVENING PERSON.

night shift Work during the nocturnal hours, typically from 11 P.M. through to 7 A.M. (Work from 3 P.M. till 11 P.M. is usually called an EVENING SHIFT.) Night shift workers typically have disturbed chronobiological rhythms because of the altered sleeping pattern. A night worker will usually attempt to sleep upon returning home from the night work but often has a short sleep period of four hours (from about 8 A.M. to 12 noon). A nap in the late afternoon or evening is usually required before going to work.

Typically, night shift workers will revert to a normal time of sleeping, from 11 P.M. to 7 A.M., on the days off work. However, because of the fluctuating time for sleep, the sleep pattern is usually disrupted on the days off, and brief sleep episodes can occur at other times of the day. Most shift workers find it very difficult to maintain full alertness during the night shift-work, particularly if the work is monotonous and boring. However, if the shift worker has a circadian drop of body temperature that occurs during the shift work hours, it may be extremely difficult to maintain full alertness, particularly between 4 A.M. and 7 A.M. Studies of night shift work have failed to show complete adaptation to the shift work, even after 10 years of shift-work experience. (See also CHRONOBIOLOGY, SHIFT-WORK SLEEP DISORDER.)

night sweats See SLEEP HYPERHIDROSIS.

night terrors See SLEEP TERRORS.

nitrazepam See BENZODIAZEPINES.

noctambulation Term derived from the Latin word *noctambulatio* and synonymous with SLEEPWALKING. Noctambulatio is from the Latin words *nox,* for "night," and *ambulare,* "to walk."

Noctec See HYPNOTICS.

noctiphobia Term synonymous with nyctophobia; refers to an irrational fear of night and darkness that may be a manifestation of ANXIETY DISORDERS. Some children may experience noctiphobia during their early childhood, but they outgrow it. (See also ANXIETY, NIGHTMARE.)

nocturia Term referring to frequent urination at night, compared with the daytime; synonymous with nycturia. Patients with nocturia will have a full bladder, causing them to arise several times from sleep to go to the bathroom. Urinary frequency may be due to a variety of urological problems, including infections, local tumors, such as bladder or prostate tumors, bladder prolapse or other disorders affecting sphincter control. Patients with sleep disturbance typically will have an increase in the number of episodes of nocturia at times of the sleep disturbance. Some patients with insomnia may arise five or six times at night to go to the bathroom, and each time will typically void only a small amount of urine.

There is a strong association between the development of OBSTRUCTIVE SLEEP APNEA SYNDROME and the need for nocturia. Relief of the obstructive sleep apnea syndrome relieves the nocturia, as does the treatment of insomnia in patients who have nocturia related to insomnia. If urinating occurs during sleep, then the term SLEEP ENURESIS is used.

Many other medical disorders can produce nocturia, such as diabetes and bladder disorders, as well as medications, particularly diuretics.

nocturnal Pertaining to night, night-related. It does not necessarily imply a sleep-related phenomenon. Although many nocturnal disorders are sleep-related, some occur during the night hours, when the person is either awake or asleep, such as nocturnal epilepsy. The term is used to differentiate night from day, and is the opposite of the word "diurnal."

nocturnal angina See NOCTURNAL CARDIAC ISCHEMIA.

nocturnal cardiac ischemia Ischemia (lack of oxygen that causes damage to the tissue) of the myocardium (heart muscle) that occurs during the major sleep episode. Cardiac ischemia may be symptomatic, in which case it is often termed nocturnal angina, or the ischemia may be asymptomatic. It may be detected by electrocardiographic monitoring during sleep, either by Holter monitoring (a 24-hour electrocardiograph) or during nocturnal polysomnographic monitoring. When symptomatic, cardiac ischemia produces a chest pain that is described as a tightness within the chest, often like a vise. The pain may be felt in the jaw, left arm or the back. The pain may be mild, in which case the person may not believe it is of cardiac origin, or it may be severe, requiring acute medical attention.

Patients who have nocturnal cardiac ischemia will also usually have daytime ischemic episodes. However, nocturnal cardiac ischemia may be independent of any prior or current daytime ischemic features, and it may be related solely to underlying pathological disorders that occur during sleep, such as the OBSTRUCTIVE SLEEP APNEA SYNDROME. Episodes of nocturnal cardiac ischemia are more common in the later half of the night, particularly during REM SLEEP. Severe cardiac ARRHYTHMIAS and even sudden DEATH DURING SLEEP may result.

Cardiac ischemia is usually a feature of coronary artery disease—either intrinsic disease, such as atherosclerosis or coronary artery spasms, or valvular disease, such as aortic stenosis.

Patients at most risk for coronary artery disease are overweight males. Other risk factors include HYPERTENSION, cigarette smoking, a family history of cardiac disease and an elevated cholesterol level.

Electrocardiographic monitoring during sleep may demonstrate cardiac ischemia, which is evidenced by ST wave changes of 1 millimeter or greater, either elevation or depression. Polysomnographic monitoring may demonstrate either the cardiac ischemia or predisposing disorders, such as SLEEP-RELATED BREATHING DISORDERS.

Patients demonstrating cardiac ischemia require further cardiac investigations, which may include cardiac exercise testing with echocardiography or coronary angiography.

Nocturnal cardiac ischemia needs to be differentiated from other causes of chest pain that occur during sleep, such as left ventricular failure producing PAROXYSMAL NOCTURNAL DYSPNEA, gastroesophageal reflux or peptic ulcer disease.

Treatment of nocturnal cardiac ischemia rests on treatment of the underlying cardiac disease. Antianginal agents, such as long acting nitroglycerine, may need to be given before bedtime. Other medications and surgical management of coronary artery disease need to be considered. If underlying sleep-related disorders induce cardiac ischemia, such as the CENTRAL SLEEP APNEA SYNDROME, OBSTRUCTIVE SLEEP APNEA SYNDROME or CENTRAL ALVEOLAR HYPOVENTILATION SYNDROME, then treatment of these disorders is necessary.

Nowlin, J.B., Troyer, W.G., Jr., Collins, W.S. et al., "The Association of Nocturnal Angina Pectoris with Dreaming," *Annals of Internal Medicine* 63 (1965): 1040–1046.

Burack, B., "Hypersomnia Sleep Apnea Syndrome: Its Recognition in Clinical Cardiology," *American Heart Journal* 107 (1984): 543–548.

nocturnal confusion A typical occurrence in patients who have DEMENTIA. Patients will arise from sleep at night in a confused state, not knowing where they are, and start to behave as if it is daytime rather than nighttime. The activity of such patients may pose some major problems for caretakers and often can lead to institutionalization of the patient. The nocturnal confusion can be worsened by some HYPNOTICS or acute underlying medical illnesses. Attention to good SLEEP HYGIENE and the judicious use of sedative medications may be helpful.

nocturnal dyspnea Respiratory difficulty that occurs during sleep at night. This commonly occurs in association with lung or cardiac disease. Nocturnal dyspnea (also known as paroxysmal nocturnal dyspnea) is typically seen in patients who have left-sided heart failure that causes fluid to accumulate in the lungs, thereby producing discomfort and difficulty in breathing and leading to an awakening with a sensation of respiratory distress. It may also be due to other disorders that produce difficulty in breathing at night, for example, CENTRAL ALVEOLAR HYPOVENTILATION SYNDROME, CHRONIC OBSTRUCTIVE PULMONARY DISEASE or OBSTRUCTIVE SLEEP APNEA SYNDROME.

Marked OBESITY can cause compression of the lower lung fields, thereby leading to impaired VENTILATION during sleep and a sensation of dyspnea. Most often, individuals with nocturnal dyspnea will use several pillows in order to sleep in a semireclining position, which assists in improving ventilation during sleep. Sometimes nocturnal dyspnea may be so severe that a person needs to sleep upright in a chair for the entire night.

Treatment of many sleep-related respiratory disorders will relieve nocturnal dyspnea and allow improved quality of nocturnal sleep.

nocturnal eating (drinking) syndrome Disorder characterized by one or more awakenings that occur during the night with a desire for food or drink. Sleep cannot be reinitiated until the intake has been completed, after which sleep occurs easily. This sleep disorder usually occurs in children, although it can occur in adults. Typically, an infant would require nursing at the breast, or bottle feeding, after which the baby will return to sleep. The older child may request something to eat or drink and is unable to sleep until the requested food or drink has been taken. This disorder is also seen in adults who occasionally will awaken with a strong desire to eat. Again, sleep cannot be initiated until the desired food or drink has been ingested.

An infant's ability to sleep through the night without the need for food or drink is usually attained by the age of six months. Frequent awakenings may lead to the production of a disturbed sleep-wake pattern, with the need for sustenance at frequent intervals.

The need for food or drink in infants generally persists until the child is weaned completely, typically by age three to four months. However, if bottle feeding or drinks are allowed to be given throughout the night until an older age, then the sleep disturbance may occur.

Caregiver factors are very important in the development of this sleep disorder. In infants and children, the caregiver needs to recognize appropriate hunger signals; repeated demands without true need should not be complied with.

The increased weight gain may be a source of concern, anxiety and depression.

Approximately 5% of the population from six months to three years of age may exhibit the nocturnal eating (drinking) syndrome and the prevalence in adults is unknown.

Adults who ingest more than 50% of their caloric intake during the sleeping hours are regarded as having the nocturnal eating (drinking) syndrome. This condition is frequently associated with increasing weight gain and concern over frequent nocturnal awakenings.

Treatment of this disorder involves weaning the young child from the breast or bottle, the recognition of any true need for sustenance during sleep, the elimination of compliance with the false demands of children, behavior modification with sleep consolidation, and eliminating the need in adults to awake and eat or drink. There have been reports that there may be benefits from reducing carbohydrate intake, and increasing protein intake, before sleep. In the adult, hypoglycemia can occur during sleep and, if indicated, a glucose tolerance test may be necessary to explore this possibility. (Hypoglycemia is a disorder that is associated with intermittent low blood sugar levels. Treatment may require an adult to eat small portions of food at frequent intervals to stabilize the blood sugar level.)

nocturnal emission Ejaculation of sperm that occurs during sleep in relationship to a dream that is sexually motivated. (A common term for this phenomenon is "wet dream.") According to the Kinsey study of American males, approximately 85% of the male population will experience one or more "wet dreams" during their lifetime. The highest incidence of nocturnal emissions occurs during the late teens and diminishes with age. Nocturnal emissions occur in association with the SLEEP-RELATED PENILE ERECTIONS that occur during REM SLEEP.

Kinsey, A.C., Pomeroy, W.B. and Martin, C.E., *Sexual Behavior in the Human Male*. Philadelphia: W.B. Saunders, 1948.

nocturnal enuresis See SLEEP ENURESIS.

nocturnal leg cramps A painful feeling associated with muscle tightness or tension in the calves of the legs, but occasionally in the feet. The tightening of the muscle lasts a few seconds and usually stops spontaneously, but the discomfort may persist for up to about 30 minutes. When the nocturnal cramps occur during sleep, they will cause an awakening. Episodes may also occur during the daytime; however, patients with daytime cramps rarely have episodes during sleep. Some patients have a predisposition for having only sleep-related cramps.

Nocturnal cramps have also been called by the term "charley horse," derived from the old term for a horse that was lame due to the stiffness of its muscles.

The cause of the muscle cramps is poorly understood, but metabolic disturbances, such as diabetes or calcium abnormalities, can contribute. The cramps also appear to be more common during pregnancy.

The peak age of onset of nocturnal cramps appears to be in adulthood, but they can occur in children. However, this type of cramping has never been reported in infants or very young children.

This discomfort can be relieved by stretching the involved muscle, by movement and massage of the muscle, or by local heat to the affected area. Quinine is an effective medication.

The disorder needs to be distinguished from other forms of muscle disorder that can occur during sleep, such as PERIODIC LIMB MOVEMENT DISORDER, sleep-related seizures, NOCTURNAL PAROXYSMAL DYSTONIA and sleep-related tonic spasms, which all have differing clinical features and history.

Saskin, Paul, Whelton, Charles, Moldofsky, Harvey and Akin, Frank, "Sleep and Nocturnal Leg Cramps" (Letter to the Editors), *Sleep* 11 (1988): 307–308.

Simons, D.G., et al., "Understanding and Measurement of Muscle Tone as Related to Clinical Muscle Pain," *Pain* 75, no. 11 (1998): 1–17.

nocturnal myoclonus Term applied by Charles Symonds in 1953 for repetitive leg jerks that occur during sleep. The movements are 0.5 to 5 seconds in duration and occur at an interval of 20 to 40 seconds. The movements can occur simultaneously or asynchronously in either leg or both, or simultaneously in the upper limbs. As the movements are of longer duration than typical myoclonic jerks, the term PERIODIC LEG MOVEMENTS is preferred. When the movements reach sufficient frequency to disrupt sleep, the resulting disorder is called the PERIODIC LIMB MOVEMENT DISORDER. (See also RESTLESS LEGS SYNDROME.)

nocturnal paroxysmal dystonia (NPD) A neurological disorder that produces abnormal movement activity during sleep, particularly non-REM sleep. This disorder produces dystonic or dyskinetic movements that are characterized by a twisting or writhing type of movement. Nocturnal paroxysmal dystonia appears to be of central nervous system origin (caused by mechanisms inside the brain) and seems to have a long course lasting many years without spontaneous resolution.

There are two forms of nocturnal paroxysmal dystonia that are differentiated by the duration of the abnormal movement activity. One form, with short-lasting episodes, generally has movements that last only one minute or less, and episodes can occur up to 15 times every night. They are usually preceded by evidence of an arousal or an awakening that occurs immediately prior to the onset of the abnormal movements. Typically the patient will open his eyes during the arousal and then the movements will occur. They usually consist of writhing or twisting movements of the arms or legs. Following an episode, the patient is able to go back to sleep without difficulty. These brief episodes are believed to be manifestations of frontal lobe epilepsy.

Another form of nocturnal paroxysmal dystonia has long episodes that are more than two minutes in duration. These long episodes tend to occur less frequently and there may be only two or three episodes in a night. They are also characterized by the writhing and twisting movements of the limbs. This type of dystonia has been known to occur before the onset of other degenerative neurological disorders, such as Huntington's chorea.

Episodes of nocturnal paroxysmal dystonia can lead to severe sleep disruption and therefore a complaint of INSOMNIA. The patient will feel tired and not rested upon awakening in the morning. Also, because of the movements, the sleep of the bed partner can be disturbed and injuries can occur, either to the patient or the bed partner.

Short-lasting episodes rarely occur during the daytime, and generalized tonic-clonic seizures have also been reported.

Episodes of nocturnal paroxysmal dystonia have occurred in infancy or can occur for the first time as late as the fifth decade. It appears to have an equal prevalence in men and women, and episodes do not subside spontaneously but have been known to occur for at least 20 years.

Polysomnographic investigation has demonstrated that the episodes occur during stage two sleep and rarely can occur in stages three and four sleep; they do not occur during REM sleep. Immediately prior to the onset of the abnormal motor movement activity the ELECTROENCEPHALOGRAM shows evidence of an arousal or a brief awakening. Other forms of investigation, including brain imaging, have failed to reveal any specific central nervous system pathology to account for the disorder. Patients with generalized tonic-clonic seizures may have abnormal epileptiform activity seen on routine daytime electroencephalograms.

The abnormal movement needs to be differentiated from other forms of sleep-related movement disorders, such as the REM SLEEP BEHAVIOR DISORDER, which occurs predominantly during REM sleep and can be easily discerned by polysomnography. Other forms of parasomnia activity, including SLEEP TERRORS and SLEEPWALKING, are easily differentiated by their characteristic features. There may be difficulty in differentiating from SLEEP-RELATED EPILEPSY, particularly that of frontal lobe origin. Electroencephalographic patterns consistent with epilepsy are rarely seen in paroxysmal dystonia and suggest that nocturnal paroxysmal dystonia is not an epileptic phenomenon. Polysomnographic documentation of episodes has failed to show any preceding or following epileptic features.

Nocturnal paroxysmal dystonia is responsive to the anticonvulsive medication CARBAMAZEPINE (Tegretol).

Bhatia, K.P., "The Paroxysmal Dyskinesias," *Journal of Neurology* 246, no. 3 (1999): 149–155.

Lugaresi, E. and Cirignotta, F., "Hypnogenic Paroxysmal Dystonia: Epileptic Seizures or a New Syndrome?" *Sleep* 4 (1981): 129–138.

nocturnal penile tumescence (NPT) This term is usually applied to the NOCTURNAL PENILE TUMESCENCE (NPT) TEST, a test of the ability to obtain an adequate erection during sleep.

nocturnal penile tumescence (NPT) test A test of the ability to attain an adequate erection during sleep. This test involves monitoring the erectile ability during an all-night polysomnogram (see POLYSOMNOGRAPHY). Usually two or three nights of recording are required to adequately determine whether normal erections occur during sleep. All healthy males from infancy to old age have erections during REM sleep. If there is an inadequate amount or reduced quality of REM sleep, normal erections will not occur. The NPT test is used to help differentiate organic causes of erectile dysfunction from psychological causes. Impaired sleep-related erections during normal REM sleep are indicative of an organic cause of impotence.

nocturnal sleep episode The typical nighttime or major sleep episode that is determined by the daily rhythm of sleep and wakefulness. The nocturnal sleep episode is the conventional or habitual time for sleeping. For the majority of individuals, the nocturnal sleep episode lasts eight hours and commonly occurs between the hours of 11 P.M. and 7 A.M. The nocturnal sleep period usually consists of alternating cycles of REM and non-REM sleep and typically is comprised of about 5% stage one sleep, 45% stage two sleep, 5% stage three sleep, 15% stage four sleep and 30% REM sleep. There are usually four to six cycles of non-REM/REM sleep (see SLEEP STAGES). The percentages of each sleep stage and the duration of the nocturnal sleep episode vary according to age; in addition, there are individual differences at any one age.

An infant's sleep duration can be a total of 16 hours; however, the sleep is spread throughout the 24-hour period and consists of a higher percentage (about 50%) of REM sleep. In young adolescents, the percentage of REM sleep falls to about 20% of the total sleep time and remains at that level throughout adulthood and into old age. The amount of stage three and four sleep increases in percentage, to 30% of total sleep time in the prepuberty age groups, diminishes through adulthood to old age and is typically not present after 60 years. The total sleep time decreases from 16 hours per day in infancy to between 6.5 and 8.5 hours in adolescence and through adulthood to old age. The number of awakenings and arousals during the sleep period is typically at a minimum around the time of puberty and increases in middle age to old age.

The nocturnal sleep episode may be reduced in duration in some ethnic groups or in some individuals who prefer to take prolonged daytime NAPS (SIESTA) that can last two to four hours. Then the nocturnal sleep episode is reduced by the amount of time of the siesta. In such individuals, the typical nocturnal sleep episode duration is only four to six hours. (See also ONTOGENY OF SLEEP, SLEEP DURATION.)

NoDoz See OVER-THE-COUNTER MEDICATIONS.

noise A common cause of sleep disturbance. Environmental noise, due to traffic, aircraft or neighbors, can cause a person to have difficulty in initiating or maintaining sleep and can contribute to an EARLY MORNING AROUSAL. It is one of many environmental effects that can produce an environmental sleep disorder. In addition to its more obvious effect of causing awakenings and insomnia, noise can also disturb the quality of sleep by inducing brief arousals, which do not lead to full awakenings. This disturbance may lead to EXCESSIVE SLEEPINESS that can be documented by a MULTIPLE SLEEP LATENCY TEST.

Environmental noise can be eliminated from the bedroom by ensuring tight seals around windows and doors and the use of heavy curtains. Earplugs or the use of a white noise machine can be helpful for some patients. (Overuse or improper use of ear plugs, however, can lead to a buildup of wax, which might necessitate removal by a physician.) Alternatively, HYPNOTICS, which prevent the arousals and the awakenings, can be useful, particularly in the short term.

The subjective assessment of noise can vary among individuals. Some good sleepers may be totally oblivious to loud sounds during the night and sleep is undisturbed. However, others find even the quietest sounds especially disturbing. It is well-recognized that the mother of the newborn infant is able to sleep yet responds to the softest whimper of her baby, which may not be heard by her sleeping spouse. Patients who, for other reasons, have impaired sleep quality at night characterized by a complaint of insomnia are usually especially sensitive to environmental sounds.

SNORING, which can reach very loud levels, as high as 80 or 90 decibels, is a common cause of disturbance to a sleeping spouse. Although many bed partners are able to sleep beside a snorer without being bothered, loud snoring is usually very disruptive. Often there will be complaints not only from the bed partner but also from other people sleeping in the house, either children or relatives. Snoring may be of concern even to strangers, particularly when the snorer sleeps in a hotel or motel room. Loud snoring is commonly associated with the OBSTRUCTIVE SLEEP APNEA SYNDROME. Snoring not associated with the syndrome is often termed PRIMARY SNORING.

Lukas, J.S., "Noise and Sleep: A Literature Review and a Proposed Criteria for Assessing Effects," *Journal of the Acoustical Society of America* 58 (1975): 1232–1242.

nonfocal activity See DIFFUSE ACTIVITY.

non-REM intrusion Imposition of non-REM sleep during the REM SLEEP stage. Typically, a component of non-REM sleep, such as the SLEEP SPINDLE, SLOW WAVE SLEEP or K-COMPLEX, may intrude during REM sleep. Non-REM intrusion is generally associated with sleep disruption and is due to non-REM sleep occurring at a time of the sleep-wake cycle when it would otherwise not normally occur.

non-REM-REM sleep cycle See NREM-REM SLEEP CYCLE.

non-REM-stage sleep Sleep is composed of two main sleep stages: non-REM and REM sleep. Non-REM is further divided into stages one, two, three and four sleep. (See also SLEEP STAGES.)

nonrestorative sleep Sleep regarded as nonrefreshing or insufficient to produce full daytime alertness. Many disorders that produce sleep interruption, such as the OBSTRUCTIVE SLEEP APNEA SYNDROME and PERIODIC LIMB MOVEMENT DISORDER, can produce unrestful sleep. But in SLEEP STATE MISPERCEPTION sleep may be normal and full, yet the patient may awaken with the complaint of not feeling fully refreshed.

non-24-hour sleep-wake syndrome Characterized by a regular pattern of one-to-two-hour delays in the sleep onset and wake times; also known as the hypernyctohemeral syndrome. (*Hyper,* over, above; *nychthemeron,* a full period of a night and a day.) This rare disorder is one of the CIRCADIAN RHYTHM SLEEP DISORDERS. The non-24-hour sleep-wake syndrome is a sleep pattern that is similar to that seen in human subjects who live in a time isolation facility, free of ENVIRONMENTAL TIME CUES. Such subjects have a sleep-wake 25-hour pattern induced by the time period of the ENDOGENOUS CIRCADIAN PACEMAKER. Such patients complain of difficulty in falling asleep at night, or difficulty in awakening in the morning. Typically, this pattern is most disruptive when the major sleep episode occurs during the daytime and is least disruptive when the sleep episode occurs during the nocturnal periods. Attempts to control the sleep pattern by the use of HYPNOTICS are usually unsuccessful.

Because the sleep pattern severely interferes with daytime activities, individuals with this pattern are either self-employed or have flexible work patterns.

Some individuals with this sleep pattern have psychopathology characterized by being schizoidal or having an avoidant personality disorder. The syndrome is also present in blind adults and has been described as occurring congenitally in blind infants.

Polysomnographic studies have rarely been reported but would be expected to show normal sleep duration and quality that occurs with a progressive daily delay in sleep onset time.

The differential diagnosis of non-24-hour sleep-wake pattern includes DELAYED SLEEP PHASE SYNDROME, which is characterized by a stable sleep onset and awake time. The IRREGULAR SLEEP-WAKE PATTERN has a variable sleep onset time, with occasional sleep episode advances.

There are few reports of treatment attempts in patients with the non-24-hour sleep-wake syndrome, but recent evidence about LIGHT THERAPY being able to advance or delay sleep-onset time holds promise of enabling maintenance of a stable sleep-wake pattern. (See also FREE RUNNING, TEMPORAL ISOLATION.)

Kokkoris, L.P., Weitzman, E.D., Pollack, L.P. et al., "Long-term Ambulatory Monitoring in Subject With a Hypernychthemeral Sleep-wake Cycle Disturbance," *Sleep* 1 (1978): 177–180.

noradrenaline See NOREPINEPHRINE.

norepinephrine A neurotransmitter, also known as noradrenaline, that is widely found within the central and peripheral nervous system. Although norepinephrine was originally believed to enhance sleep, it is now believed to be an important agent in the activation of wakefulness. It is probable that norepinephrine works in conjunction with ACETYLCHOLINE in order to produce wakefulness. Studies with agents that inhibit the synthesis of norepinephrine have shown an initial increase in REM sleep, but then REM sleep appears to be suppressed. It is possible that the norepinephrine in the LOCUS CERULEUS is important in the maintenance of wakefulness and the production of REM sleep. The receptors known as the alpha 2 adreno-receptors appear to be most important in the regulation of sleep and wakefulness.

Studies of pharmaceutical agents have demonstrated that the role of norepinephrine in the control of sleep and wakefulness is very complex and poorly understood; further research is needed to define its exact role.

Medications that have an effect on norepinephrine synthesis, such as the MONOAMINE OXIDASE INHIBITORS, can markedly suppress REM sleep. However, these inhibitors have effects other than their effects upon norepinephrine synthesis. Clonidine, an antihypertensive agent, stimulates the adreno-receptors, and yet REM sleep is inhibited by very small doses of clonidine. However, clonidine also has an effect on wakefulness in that wakefulness can be increased with relatively small doses of clonidine, but high doses seem to inhibit wakefulness.

Gaillard, J.M., "Biochemical Pharmacology of Paradoxical Sleep," *British Journal of Clinical Pharmacology* 16 (1983): 205–230.

nosology The science of the classification of disease. The term is derived from the Greek word *nosos*, meaning disease. Many classification systems have been developed over the years for the sleep disorders; however, the system most commonly used was developed in 1979 by the Association of Sleep Disorder Centers and was published in the journal *SLEEP*. The DIAGNOSTIC CLASSIFICATION OF SLEEP AND AROUSAL DISORDERS has been widely used as the main classification for sleep disorders, not only in the United States but also internationally. In 1985, the process of redefining the names and classification of sleep disorders was undertaken by the American Sleep Disorders Association (now called the AMERICAN ACADEMY OF SLEEP MEDICINE). In 1990, the INTERNATIONAL CLASSIFICATION OF SLEEP DISORDERS was published by the American Sleep Disorders Association. It contains an extensive listing of all sleep disorders.

NPD See NOCTURNAL PAROXYSMAL DYSTONIA.

NPPV See NASAL POSITIVE PRESSURE VENTILATION.

NPT See NOCTURNAL PENILE TUMESCENCE.

NREM-REM sleep cycle This term denotes a recurrent cycle of non-REM alternating with REM sleep that occurs throughout the major sleep episode. This term is synonymous with the terms sleep cycle and sleep-wake cycle. Any non-REM sleep stage may alternate with REM sleep to form the NREM portion of the NREM-REM sleep cycle. In a typical adult sleep period of 6.5 to 8.5 hours, there are five non-REM-REM sleep cycles. The duration of the cycle increases from about 60 minutes in infancy to 90 minutes in young adulthood. (See also NON-REM-STAGE SLEEP, REM SLEEP.)

NREM sleep See NON-REM-STAGE SLEEP and SLEEP STAGES.

NREM sleep period Usually applies to the NREM sleep portion of the NREM-REM SLEEP CYCLE. The non-REM period usually consists mainly of stages two, three and four sleep. (See also NON-REM-STAGE SLEEP.)

nutrition and sleep See DIET AND SLEEP.

nyctalgia This word refers to pain that occurs in sleep only. The word is developed from the Greek NYCTOS, meaning night, and *algia,* referring to pain. This term is synonymous with HYPNALGIA.

nyctalopia Synonymous with the term NIGHT BLINDNESS. It is developed from the Greek *nyctos,* meaning "night," and *alaos,* meaning "blind."

nyctohemeral A full cycle of night and day. Nyctohemeral is derived from the Greek *nyctos,* for "night," and *hemera,* meaning "a day." This term is occasionally used in regard to sleep reversal, meaning that the night and day sleep pattern is reversed. The word is also used for a specific disorder where an individual has a day that is slightly longer than 24 hours, the NON-24-HOUR SLEEP-WAKE SYNDROME, which is synonymous with hypernycthemeral syndrome.

nyctophilia Derived from the Greek *nyctos,* meaning night, and *philein,* meaning to love. This term refers to a preference for night over day and could be applied to individuals who prefer socializing or working at night rather than during the day.

nyctophobia See NOCTIPHOBIA.

nycturia See NOCTURIA.

Nytol See OVER-THE-COUNTER MEDICATIONS.

O

obesity Defined as a body weight that is greater than the ideal body weight. The Metropolitan Life Insurance Co. weight tables are a commonly used source of determining ideal weight; these tables determine weight according to the patient's age, weight, sex and height. Morbid obesity is regarded as 100 pounds of weight over the ideal body weight as expressed on the Life tables.

Obesity is a common feature of OBSTRUCTIVE SLEEP APNEA SYNDROME and is most graphically portrayed in the story of Joe the Fat Boy in *The Pickwick Papers* by Charles Dickens. The PICKWICKIAN SYNDROME, which applies to persons with obesity, sleepiness and evidence of right-sided heart failure, was reported in the medical literature in 1954; since that time the relationship between obesity and sleepiness has been increasingly recognized.

Up to 80% of patients with obstructive sleep apnea syndrome are overweight, and the syndrome itself is exacerbated by obesity. Reduction of body weight sometimes reduces the severity of obstructive sleep apnea syndrome, although this is not a universal finding. Many patients find that there is a critical weight at which symptoms of obstructive sleep apnea become evident, and there may be little improvement in the symptoms until that weight is reached. For some people, reduction of body weight by as little as five or 10 pounds causes a major degree of improvement in symptoms, whereas in other patients even 100 pounds of weight loss may not produce any useful improvement.

In general, because there is a possibility that the obstructive sleep apnea syndrome can be improved, all patients are recommended to obtain an ideal body weight. For some morbidly obese patients, weight reduction by surgical means has been shown to produce a profound weight loss with a major degree of clinical improvement in obstructive sleep apnea syndrome.

The theory that effective treatment of obstructive sleep apnea syndrome would increase activity, and thereby lead to improved weight reduction, has not been demonstrated in research studies. Even following a TRACHEOSTOMY, which is usually performed in the most severe cases of the syndrome (the majority of whom are obese), five and 10 years after the surgery a significant loss of weight is not seen. Some patients, despite optimum treatment of their sleep apnea syndrome, will put on more weight.

Obesity appears to affect obstructive sleep apnea in three ways: it may contribute to the narrowing of the upper airway by increasing the bulk of tissues in the pharyngeal and neck region; the increased bulk of tissues may cause the tongue to prolapse back, thereby contributing to the blockage (occlusion) of the upper airway during sleep. Second, the excessive weight on the chest wall may contribute to impaired VENTILATION during sleep; this appears to be a more significant factor in females with large, pendulous breasts. Third, the large abdominal size affects diaphragm function.

For most patients with obstructive sleep apnea syndrome, obesity impairs diaphragmatic function during sleep, thereby impairing the function of the lungs (perfusion of the basal lung fields). The resulting right-to-left shunt allows unoxygenated blood to pass through the heart, which in turn causes arterial oxygen desaturation. Many extremely obese patients find they are unable to breathe adequately when lying on their backs because of this effect and therefore sleep in a semireclining or even in a sitting position.

In addition to surgical management of the obesity, which is typically reserved for patients over

300 pounds in weight, dietary programs, such as liquid diets, can be very effective in producing a rapid weight reduction. However, the long-term effects of the liquid diet programs have not been demonstrated, and initial results tend to suggest an early recurrence of the lost weight. Some patients find the more well-known dietary programs to be very effective, such as Weight Watchers or Overeaters Anonymous. Dietary suppressant medications, such as the amphetamine derivatives, are not only ineffective but are also potentially dangerous, as their cardiac stimulant properties may lead to serious cardiac ARRHYTHMIAS.

Although weight reduction is important for all overweight patients with obstructive sleep apnea syndrome, it cannot be relied upon as a primary form of treatment except in the mildest cases. As a primary treatment strategy weight reduction is poorly achieved by patients, and during the weight reduction attempts the patient's life may be at risk because of the effects of obstructive sleep apnea syndrome. Therefore, any recommendations for weight reduction must be pursued concurrently with effective treatment of the obstructive sleep apnea syndrome, which is most commonly carried out by either a CONTINUOUS POSITIVE AIRWAY PRESSURE device or upper airway surgery. (See also DIET AND SLEEP, SURGERY AND SLEEP DISORDERS.)

Whittels, E.H., "Obesity and Hormonal Factors in Sleep and Sleep Apnea," *Medical Clinics of North America* 69 (1985): 1265–1280.

Chin, K. and Ohi, M., "Obesity and Obstructive Sleep Apnea Syndrome," *Internal Medicine* 38, no. 2 (1999): 200–202.

obesity hypoventilation syndrome Applied to the condition of obese individuals who suffer severe hypoventilation during sleep and wakefulness. The hypoventilation causes a lowering of the oxygen level and an elevation of carbon dioxide, usually above 60 millimeters of mercury. The term describes any number of disorders characterized by hypoventilation during sleep, including OBSTRUCTIVE SLEEP APNEA SYNDROME, CENTRAL SLEEP APNEA SYNDROME and CENTRAL ALVEOLAR HYPOVENTILATION SYNDROME.

obstructive sleep apnea syndrome A disorder characterized by repetitive episodes of UPPER AIRWAY OBSTRUCTION that occur during sleep and are usually associated with a reduction in the blood oxygen saturation. It is synonymous with upper airway sleep apnea. The clinical features of this disorder were clearly described by Charles Dickens in his novel *The Pickwick Papers*. It was only in the 1960s that its pathophysiological basis could be understood.

Several hundred apneic episodes can occur during a night of sleep, thereby leading to severe sleep disruption and fragmentation, with the development of EXCESSIVE SLEEPINESS during the daytime. The apneic episodes are most severe during the REM stage of sleep, in part due to the associated loss of muscle tone, but also because of the change in metabolic control of VENTILATION.

The disorder is associated with loud SNORING, which is indicative of intermittent upper airway obstruction that at times can be complete and cause a cessation of airflow and obstructive apnea. The loud snoring is disturbing to bed partners or others, which often leads to the presentation of the patient to a SLEEP DISORDERS CENTER.

A typical feature of obstructive sleep apnea syndrome is excessive sleepiness. Sleepiness occurs whenever the patient is in a relaxed situation, varies from mild to severe and can lead to automobile ACCIDENTS. Typically patients with the obstructive sleep apnea syndrome fall asleep while reading, watching TV or even while attending business or social meetings. The patient may purposefully take a daytime nap, but the NAPS are usually not sufficiently refreshing. Awakenings are associated with a dull, groggy feeling and sometimes a headache.

Obstructive sleep apnea syndrome is also associated with very restless sleep, particularly in children who have varied positions in bed, often sleeping on their hands and knees. Occasionally the restlessness can result in a fall out of bed, but more typically movements of the arms and legs greatly disturb the sleep of a bed partner.

Primary or secondary enuresis can occur during sleep, particularly in children. (See SLEEP ENURESIS.) Gastroesophageal reflux may also be produced by obstructive sleep apnea syndrome.

The apneic events occur during NREM or REM sleep, but they are usually more severe in REM sleep. Repetitive episodes of upper airway obstruction last from 20 to 40 seconds. Apneic episodes as long as several minutes in duration can occur and are associated with a severe drop in blood oxygen and an increase in carbon dioxide. The apneic episode is terminated by an arousal, which leads to an awakening with return of increased muscle tone and several large breaths. After several breaths, sleep returns and another apneic event will occur.

Obstructive sleep apnea syndrome can be investigated by means of all-night POLYSOMNOGRAPHY, with appropriate measurement of breathing, oxygen saturation and heart rate. All-night polysomnography confirms the diagnosis and also allows determination of its severity. Apneic episodes of more than 60 seconds in duration, oxygen desaturation that falls below 70% and an APNEA-HYPOPNEA INDEX of greater than 50 episodes per hour of sleep are features that indicate severe obstructive sleep apnea syndrome.

Electrocardiographic changes typically occur in association with apneas and oxygen desaturation. A slowing of the heart rate during the apneic pause followed by reflex tachycardia (ARRHYTHMIA characterized by speeding of the heart rate) during the few breaths of hyperventilation commonly occurs and is termed the brady-tachycardia (arrhythmia characterized by slowing and speeding of the heart rate) syndrome. This electrocardiographic pattern, when it occurs solely during sleep, is diagnostic of obstructive sleep apnea syndrome. Occasionally, sinus pauses lasting 10 or more seconds, episodes of atrial tachycardia or VENTRICULAR ARRHYTHMIAS can occur.

Other investigations include documentation of the degree of severity of daytime sleepiness by means of the MULTIPLE SLEEP LATENCY TEST (MSLT). Mean sleep latencies of less than five minutes are commonly seen in patients with severe sleep apnea syndrome. Studies of the upper airway, including FIBEROPTIC ENDOSCOPY, can determine both the site of upper airway obstruction and the potential for success of operative procedures such as UVULOPALATOPHARYNGOPLASTY or TONSILLECTOMY AND ADENOIDECTOMY.

In addition, CEPHALOMETRIC RADIOGRAPHS of the upper airway will help demonstrate skeletal abnormalities and also the soft tissue changes of the upper airway.

Consequences of the obstructive sleep apnea syndrome include social difficulties related to the snoring and excessive daytime sleepiness; increased risk of motor vehicle accidents because of the sleepiness; cardiovascular consequences, which can include a MYOCARDIAL INFARCTION during sleep or sudden death during sleep; severe oxygen desaturation during sleep, which can be associated with development of pulmonary hypertension and right-sided heart failure.

Treatments of obstructive sleep apnea syndrome include behavioral as well as medical or surgical measures. Weight reduction is an essential recommendation for any overweight patient (see OBESITY) with obstructive sleep apnea syndrome. SMOKING may cause irritation and swelling of the upper airway, thereby exacerbating the upper airway obstruction as well as impairing pulmonary function, leading to deterioration of blood-gas exchange.

ALCOHOL exacerbates obstructive sleep apnea syndrome by causing central nervous system depression resulting in the increasing severity of apneic events.

The most effective medical treatment for obstructive sleep apnea syndrome is by use of a nasal CONTINUOUS POSITIVE AIRWAY PRESSURE (CPAP) device. CPAP provides an air splint of the upper airway preventing collapse of the soft tissues and thereby eliminating the apneic events. Unfortunately, up to 40% of the patients are unable to use the CPAP device, either for psychological reasons or because of medical complications of the treatment. Chronic rhinitis is a common cause of inability to use nasal CPAP and may result from irritation of the nasal tissues by the airflow. A variation of CPAP allows the air pressure to be reduced during expiration. These devices offer bilevel control of positive pressure. One device is called a BiPAP.

Surgical management of obstructive sleep apnea syndrome includes adeno-tonsillectomy—uvulopalatopharyngoplasty surgery in which the soft tissue at the level of the soft palate is removed. Other surgical procedures involve enlarging the air space at the back of the tongue by jaw surgery; this may be indicated in some patients who have severe obstructive sleep apnea syndrome. TRACHEOSTOMY is also an effective treatment for severe obstructive sleep apnea syndrome, particularly for those who are unable to respond to nasal CPAP therapy.

RESPIRATORY STIMULANTS can be partially effective in treating the obstructive sleep apnea syndrome. Medroxy-progesterone and protriptyline are most commonly used but have the potential for complications and may not be entirely effective.

Excessive daytime sleepiness due to obstructive sleep apnea syndrome needs to be distinguished from other disorders of excessive sleepiness. NARCOLEPSY and PERIODIC LIMB MOVEMENT DISORDER can produce excessive sleepiness and can occur concurrently with the obstructive sleep apnea syndrome. Other breathing disorders, such as CENTRAL SLEEP APNEA SYNDROME or CENTRAL ALVEOLAR HYPOVENTILATION SYNDROME, can be differentiated from obstructive sleep apnea syndrome by polysomnography. Patients who present with the primary complaint of INSOMNIA need to be differentiated from patients with other insomnia disorders, such as PSYCHOPHYSIOLOGICAL INSOMNIA or insomnia associated with psychiatric disorders.

Effective treatment of obstructive sleep apnea syndrome can lead to a dramatic resolution of the clinical symptoms and features. Respiration during sleep will return to normal without apneic episodes or oxygen desaturation. Electrocardiographic changes can be improved.

Case History

A 45-year-old tour guide noticed the gradual onset of excessive sleepiness over a five-year period. He was also a very loud snorer and the snoring, as well as the excessive sleepiness, were major concerns. The snoring bothered his wife, who had to sleep in another room because the snoring would disturb her sleep. As he was a tour guide, and often slept in hotels, he was unable to share a room with others because of the loudness of his snoring. During a trip to eastern Europe, the hotel maid had awoken him in the middle of the night because of complaints about his snoring from people in other rooms. He recalled that 25 years earlier, during a ski trip, he had to be separated from the rest of the group because of his snoring.

His daytime sleepiness would occur whenever he was in a quiet situation. He would fall asleep when sitting and watching TV in the evening or while reading. He was a smoker and, as a result of dropping cigarettes beside his favorite chair, had burnt holes in the carpet. He had fallen asleep while driving on at least two occasions and frequently would find himself veering to the side of the road because of sleepiness while driving. His wife was particularly concerned about his driving and therefore did most of it herself when they were together in the car.

He was a very restless sleeper and this contributed to his wife seeking refuge in another bed in another room. He also had a dry mouth upon awakening and occasionally would have severe morning headaches that would last for one to two hours. He was 5 feet 10 inches tall and weighed 210 pounds, which was the heaviest that he had ever been. Five years previously he had weighed 185 pounds and had tried to lose weight but found it very difficult to do so.

A physical examination showed an elevated blood pressure with diastolic level of 95. He had a very compromised posterior oropharynx, which appeared to be the site of his upper airway obstruction. He had bilateral conjunctivitis that was probably due to the chronic and constant sleep disturbance.

He underwent polysomnographic evaluation and had 222 obstructive sleep apneas, the longest being 66 seconds, and he had 161 episodes of shallow breathing (HYPOPNEAS). The oxygen saturation value fell from a baseline level of 93% while awake, to a low of 77% during the most severe apneas. He underwent a daytime multiple sleep latency test, which confirmed severe sleepiness with a mean sleep latency of 5.3 minutes. However, he did not have any REM sleep during the naps.

He underwent a repeat night of polysomnographic monitoring while using a nasal continuous positive airway pressure (CPAP) device. During the recording he had only 10 obstructive sleep apneas during the adjustment phase. When the CPAP system was adjusted to a pressure of 10 centimeters of water, he was entirely free of apnea episodes. His oxygen level did not fall below 90% at that pressure. The study demonstrated a great improvement in the quality of sleep, with a REM sleep rebound as well as a great increase in the amount of slow wave sleep. Upon awakening in the morning he felt much more alert and was energetic for the rest of the day.

He was prescribed a CPAP system to use on a regular basis at night and with this treatment his sleepiness was eliminated. He was able to drive without getting sleepy and stay up and watch his favorite TV programs without falling asleep. In addition to the improvement in his breathing at night and his sleepiness, the CPAP system also eliminated his snoring and restlessness, and his wife was able to return to sleeping in the same bed.

Henderson, J.H., II, and Strollo, P.J., Jr., "Medical Management of Obstructive Sleep Apnea," *Progress in Cardiovascular Diseases* 41, no. 5 (1999): 377–386.

obtundation Term applied to a reduced level of mental acuity often associated with decreased psychomotor activity. The alertness and awareness of the environment are reduced, although the patient may act in an appropriate manner to various internal needs and stimuli. The quiet state is often characterized by drowsiness and a tendency for excessive sleepiness. This altered state of consciousness may be due to metabolic, pharmacologic or intracerebral lesions. (See also COMA, DELIRIUM, STUPOR.)

Ondine's Curse From Act III of *Ondine* by Jean Giraudoux; means the inability to breathe during sleep.

> Ondine: Hans, you too will forget.
>
> Hans: Live! It's easy to say. If at least I could work up a little interest in living, but I'm too tired to make the effort. Since you left me, Ondine, all the things my body once did by itself it does now only by special order . . . It's an exhausting piece of management I've undertaken. I have to supervise five senses, two hundred bones, a thousand muscles. A single moment of inattention and I forget to breathe. He died, they will say, because it was a nuisance to breathe . . .

It was first described by John Severinghouse and Robert Mitchell in 1962 in three patients who had long episodes of cessation of breathing that occurred particularly while asleep. They needed assisted ventilation during sleep, but the patients were able to breathe voluntarily during the day. The term CENTRAL SLEEP APNEA SYNDROME is now most commonly used to refer to similar forms of sleep-induced apnea.

A number of neurological disorders have been associated with Ondine's Curse, such as brain stem lesions affecting the respiratory centers or spinal cord lesions. Patients with Ondine's Curse require assisted VENTILATION at night, usually by means of a positive pressure ventilator.

Giraudoux, Jean, *Ondine*, adapted by Maurice Valency. New York: Random House, 1954.

Severinghouse, J.W. and Mitchell, R.A., "Ondine's Curse: Failure of Respiratory Center Automaticy While Awake," *Clinical Respiratory* 10 (1962): 122.

oneiric Derived from the Greek *oneirus*, which means a dream; an event or activity pertaining to dreaming. Oneirism refers to an abnormal dream-like state of consciousness and is occasionally used to describe the unusual behavior that occurs in REM SLEEP in disorders such as REM SLEEP BEHAVIOR DISORDER and FATAL FAMILIAL INSOMNIA.

ontogeny of sleep There are major changes in sleep from infancy to old age. It is uncertain when sleep first occurs in infants; however, differentiation of an infant's state into WAKEFULNESS, ACTIVE SLEEP or QUIET SLEEP cannot be made until around 32 to 35 weeks of age. Because sleep in the infant is immature, it cannot be clearly differentiated into REM and non-REM and therefore the terms *active* and *quiet sleep* reflect the state of EEG and body activity. These terms are believed to be synonymous with REM and non-REM sleep, respectively. (See INFANT SLEEP.)

The total amount of sleep gradually decreases over the first decade and the percentage of non-REM sleep reaches a peak around the middle of the first decade. Normal developmental behavioral phenomena that occur from SLOW WAVE SLEEP, such as SLEEPWALKING and SLEEP TERROR episodes, are commonly seen at this time.

The total duration of sleep by around the time of puberty is seven to nine hours, with the onset of the teenage years often associated with a tendency to go to bed later, which may lead to SLEEP DEPRIVATION. The amount of REM sleep reaches 20% and 25% around the time of puberty and stays at that level in adulthood.

Throughout adulthood, sleep remains relatively stable, with the exception of a gradual reduction in the total amount of stages three and four sleep and an increase in the number of arousals and awakenings during sleep. By age 60, less than 10% of nocturnal sleep is slow wave sleep, and there are greater amounts of wakefulness and an increasing tendency for daytime sleepiness after this age. Pathological disturbances in sleep become more common, such as obstructive or central apneas and periodic limb movements. (See also ELDERLY AND SLEEP.)

Roffwarg, Howard P., Muzio, J.N. and Dement, William C., "Ontogenetic Development of the Human Sleep-Dream Cycle," *Science* 152 (1966): 604–619.

oral appliances Appliances that are indicated for use in patients with primary snoring or mild OBSTRUCTIVE SLEEP APNEA SYNDROME (OSAS) who do not respond to or are not candidates for treatment with behavioral measures such as weight loss or sleep-position change. Patients with moderate to severe OSAS should have an initial trial of nasal CONTINUOUS POSITIVE AIRWAY PRESSURE (CPAP) because greater effectiveness has been shown with this intervention than with the use of oral appliances.

Oral appliances are indicated for patients with moderate to severe OSAS who are intolerant of or refuse treatment with nasal CPAP. Oral appliances are also indicated for patients who refuse treatment or are not candidates for TONSILLECTOMY AND ADENOIDECTOMY, craniofacial operations or TRACHEOSTOMY.

At least 37 different oral appliances have been developed to maintain airway patency during sleep. They can be categorized into two groups: devices that hold the mandible anteriorly in relation to the maxilla, and devices that hold the tongue in an anterior position. Commercially available oral appliances include the following: Herbst Appliance, Mandibular Repositioner, Nocturnal Airway Patency Appliance, Snore Guard, TONGUE RETAINING DEVICE, Klearway, PM Positioner and Therasnore.

Herbst Appliance

An oral appliance developed from an orthodontic appliance that has been used for many years. It holds the jaw forward in both the open and closed positions. It has the advantage of allowing jaw opening during sleep. The Herbst Appliance usually holds the jaw open 75% of the patient's maximal protrusion and can be adjusted to allow further protrusion if it initially is ineffective. Polysomnographic studies have shown improvement in obstructive sleep apnea indices in patients using this appliance.

Mandibular Repositioner

A device that primarily moves the mandible forward to prevent tongue occlusion of the posterior airway. A rigid mandibular positioner moves the jaw forward 3 to 12 millimeters and has been shown to be effective in improving obstructive sleep apnea syndrome in several studies.

Nocturnal Airway Patency Appliance (NAPA)

A device that advances the mandible 6 millimeters anteriorly and 9 millimeters inferiorly. It has an oral breathing beak to prevent the lips from closing, and it stabilizes the mandible in both the horizontal and vertical directions. The NAPA has been shown to be effective in obstructive sleep apnea syndrome in a small number of studies and was granted marketing clearance by the U.S. Food and Drug Administration (FDA) for snoring and OSAS.

Snore Guard

An appliance that positions the mandible 3 millimeters behind maximal protrusion and opens the jaw 7 millimeters. It is easy to fit, covers the anterior teeth only and is soft and comfortable. Studies have shown improvement in snoring and obstructive sleep apnea syndrome in most patients. It is FDA-approved for snoring only.

Therasnore

A mandibular repositioner. It is one of the few appliances that requires no laboratory construction and is easily fitted chairside from a boil-and-bite blank. This appliance retains the mandible in a protrusive position with pliable thermoplastic material and affords the wearer limited jaw movement. Protrusive adjustability is possible to a small degree. Data supporting the effectiveness of the Therasnore is not yet published. FDA marketing clearance for snoring has been granted.

PM Positioner

A mandibular repositioner that may be laboratory-constructed from thermoplastic material allowing for easy insertion and removal when warmed. It is tooth-retained via friction grip and may be constructed with unique acrylic projections located in the cervical areas of the posterior teeth to aid retention. Protrusive adjustability is made quick, easy and accurate by movement of two expansion screws located bilaterally in the buccal region. When indicated, patients may self-adjust the appliance at home. Its unique positioning of the expansion screws affords lateral and vertical movement to the mandible. Data demonstrating effectiveness of the PM Positioner has not yet been published. FDA marketing clearance is pending.

Tongue Retaining Device (TRD)

An appliance that holds the tongue forward in sleep by means of a suction effect on the tongue. The tongue fits into a bulge anteriorly. Lateral airway tubes can be added if necessary. The device has been extensively studied with and without additional behavioral measures such as position training and is effective in many patients both for snoring and obstructive sleep apnea syndrome. It has been granted FDA marketing clearance for snoring.

Klearway

An appliance with a unique mechanical protrusive mechanism that permits the lower jaw to be moved forward in small steps of 0.25 millimeter until symptoms abate. It permits 1 to 3 millimeters of vertical and lateral movement, which allows patients to yawn, swallow or drink water while the device is in place. Published studies have shown significant reduction in APNEA-HYPOPNEA INDEX (AHI), an improvement in sleep quality and fewer awakenings and arousals for obstructive sleep apnea syndrome. FDA approval has been obtained for snoring and OSAS.

Bennett, L.S., Davies, R.J. and Stradling, J.R., "Oral Appliances for the Management of Snoring and Obstructive Sleep Apnea," *Thorax* 53, Suppl. 2 (1998): S58–S64.

orexin See HYPOCRETIN.

orthopnea Term used for shortness of breath that occurs in the recumbent position, not necessarily associated with nocturnal sleep. (See also NOCTURNAL DYSPNEA, OBESITY.)

Oswald, Ian A recipient of degrees in medicine and experimental psychology from the University of Cambridge, Dr. Oswald (1929–) began sleep research in 1956, while he was in the Royal Air Force. From 1982 to 1989, Dr. Oswald was chairman of the Department of Psychiatry of Edinburgh University in Scotland.

Dr. Oswald's early sleep research included studies of drowsiness caused by monotony, the effects of sleep deprivation, and auditory discrimination during sleep. Other areas of special interest to him include the effects of hypnotic and antidepressant drugs on sleep and the restorative function of sleep.

Oswald, Ian, with Kirstine Adam, *Get a Better Night's Sleep*. London: Martin Dunitz, 1983.
Oswald, Ian, *Sleeping and Waking*. Amsterdam: Elsevier, 1962.

OTC See OVER-THE-COUNTER MEDICATIONS.

over-the-counter medications Medications that are available without a prescription. In sleep medicine, the medications commonly available include the sleep aids and the stimulants.

Sleep aids for those with INSOMNIA include Goody's PM Powder (Block), Sleepinal (Thompson Medical), Sominex (Beecham Products) and Unisom (Leeming).

Goody's PM Powder

Each dose contains 500 milligrams acetaminophen and 38 milligrams diphenhydramine citrate. This medicine is for temporary relief of occasional headaches and minor aches and pains with accompanying sleeplessness.

Nytol

Nytol is composed of the antihistamine diphenhydramine hydrochloride in a 25-milligram tablet. This medicine can induce drowsiness and may interact with other depressant drugs, including alcohol. It should not be given to children under 12 years of age. It has anticholinergic properties and is contraindicated if someone has asthma, glaucoma or prostatic enlargement. Other possible side effects include dry mouth, loss of appetite, nausea and hypotension.

Nytol Natural Tablets

Each tablet contains equal parts ignatia amara 3X (St. Ignatius bean) and aconitum radix 6X (aconite root). It is indicated for occasional treatment of sleeplessness.

Sleepinal

Contains 50 milligrams of diphenhydramine hydrochloride in a tablet form. This medication is a help for difficulty in falling asleep. The diphenhydramine is an antihistamine with anticholinergic effects and should not be given to children under the age of 12 years.

The anticholinergic effects can produce dry mouth, dilated pupils and constipation, and the medication is contraindicated in patients who have asthma, glaucoma or prostatic enlargement.

Sominex Original Formula Nighttime Sleep Aid

The pharmaceutical (Beecham Products) name for a 25-milligram tablet of diphenhydramine hydrochloride that has antihistamine and anticholinergic effects. Sominex is not recommended for children under 12, and there may be drug interactions with alcohol and other central nervous system medications.

Tylenol PM

Sold in caplet, geltab or gelcap form, each dose contains 500 milligrams acetaminophen plus 25 milligrams diphenhydramine. It is useful as a remedy for sleep onset difficulties, especially when pain is a problem.

Unisom

Unisom is a 25-milligram tablet of doxylamine succinate, which is an antihistamine with a sedative effect. Because of the possible anticholinergic side effects of this antihistamine it should not be used by persons with asthma, glaucoma or prostatic enlargement.

The stimulants most commonly used for those with EXCESSIVE SLEEPINESS include NoDoz (Bristol Myers) and Vivarin (Beecham Products).

NoDoz Maximum Strength Caplets

A tablet with 200 milligrams of CAFFEINE, used to counteract tiredness and sleepiness; often used by long-distance drivers. It can interact with such caffeine-containing beverages as coffee, tea or sodas and produce a greater level of stimulation. Caffeine may induce tachycardia, elevation of blood pressure and insomnia and may produce a drug dependency sleep disorder.

Vivarin Alertness Aid Tablets

A tablet with 200 milligrams of caffeine, used to improve daytime alertness and wakefulness. It may interact with such caffeine-containing beverages as coffee, tea or sodas and may produce a greater level of stimulation.

Caffeine may induce tachycardia, elevation of blood pressure, insomnia and drug dependency sleep disorders.

Tinsley, J.A. and Watkins, D.D., "Over-the-Counter Stimulants: Abuse and Addiction," *Mayo Clinic Proceedings* 73, no. 10 (1998): 977–982.

overlap syndrome Term used for patients who have a combination of OBSTRUCTIVE SLEEP APNEA SYNDROME and CHRONIC OBSTRUCTIVE PULMONARY DISEASE. This combination of disorders produces a more sustained degree of HYPOXEMIA during sleep and increases the risk of developing PULMONARY HYPERTENSION and right-sided cardiac failure. Most patients with this syndrome present with typical features of obstructive sleep apnea, including EXCESSIVE SLEEPINESS during the day and SNORING. Patients with the overlap syndrome may be more susceptible to developing elevations of carbon dioxide levels following the administration of OXY-

GEN during sleep. Following relief of the obstructive sleep apnea syndrome, REM sleep-related oxygen desaturation typical of chronic obstructive pulmonary disease can require treatment by the administration of oxygen.

Flenley, D.C., "Chronic Obstructive Pulmonary Disease" in Kryger, M.H., Roth, T. and Dement, W.C., eds., *The Principles and Practices of Sleep Disorders Medicine*. Philadelphia: Saunders, 1989. pp. 601–610.

owl and lark questionnaire Survey developed in 1977 by JAMES HORNE and Olov Ostberg to determine morning or evening activity preference. This questionnaire determines the time of day that individuals are most active, least active or sleeping. Individuals who are alert until late evening, and do not arise early in the morning, are termed owls, whereas those who are early to bed and awaken early in the morning are termed larks. There is a range of preference for morning or evening tendency, and the most extreme forms of evening tendency are seen in patients who have the DELAYED SLEEP PHASE SYNDROME. Conversely, the most extreme form of a tendency to being a morning person is seen in someone who has the ADVANCED SLEEP PHASE SYNDROME. (See also CIRCADIAN RHYTHM SLEEP DISORDERS, PHASE RESPONSE CURVE.)

oximetry The measurement of oxygen levels that reflects the oxygen presence in the blood. Two forms of oximetry are commonly used, the predominant form being an infrared oximeter that measures the oxygen saturation of the capillaries by infrared light waves. Typically, an infrared oximeter has a probe that attaches to a patient's ear and the infrared light shines through the tissues and gives an estimation of the oxygen saturation. Such oximeters are most accurate for oxygen saturation levels greater than 50%. They are routinely used during POLYSOMNOGRAPHY to determine oxygen saturation values in patients who have respiratory disturbance, such as patients with OBSTRUCTIVE SLEEP APNEA SYNDROME or CENTRAL SLEEP APNEA SYNDROME.

In infants, a transcutaneous partial pressure of oxygen oximeter is used that gives a more stable assessment of the blood oxygen level. These oximeters are less liable to damage the sensitive skin of infants compared with the probe of the infrared oximeters, which can get quite hot. The infrared oximeter can give a pulse to pulse determination of oxygen saturation according to each heartbeat, whereas the transcutaneous oximeter can give only a trend of oxygen change, which requires several minutes for equilibration.

oxycodone See NARCOTICS.

oxygen Oxygen is an effective treatment for some SLEEP-RELATED BREATHING DISORDERS associated with HYPOXEMIA. CHRONIC OBSTRUCTIVE PULMONARY DISEASE, OBSTRUCTIVE SLEEP APNEA SYNDROME, CENTRAL SLEEP APNEA SYNDROME and CENTRAL ALVEOLAR HYPOVENTILATION SYNDROME are disorders where the nocturnal use of oxygen may be indicated.

Studies of patients with chronic obstructive pulmonary disease have demonstrated that 15 hours of oxygen therapy at 3 liters per minute administered by nasal prongs is associated with improved survival. However, similar levels of oxygen given to patients with the obstructive sleep apnea syndrome have produced prolonged apneic episodes during sleep with elevations of carbon dioxide. Low-flow oxygen at approximately 0.5 or 1 liter per minute, however, can be useful for some patients with sleep apnea. But the reports are variable, and in some studies oxygen has not been beneficial; therefore it should initially be administered under polysomnographic control.

Some patients with obstructive sleep apnea treated by CONTINUOUS POSITIVE AIRWAY PRESSURE (CPAP) may still have sleep-related hypoventilation that is not caused by UPPER AIRWAY OBSTRUCTION. The administration of oxygen through the CPAP mask may be an effective way of dealing with this residual hypoxemia. (See also HYPOXIA.)

P

pacemaker In sleep medicine, this term is often used to denote a group of neurons responsible for maintaining a biological rhythm. Most often it is used for the circadian pacemaker, a term used to refer to the SUPRACHIASMATIC NUCLEUS, which determines the rhythms of sleep and wakefulness, or rest and activity in animals. Many pacemakers are present in the body for the timing of different rhythms, such as cardiac rhythm or the control of the MENSTRUAL CYCLE. Some pacemakers are believed to be a subtle network of cells, such as the system that may be responsible for the circadian rhythm of body TEMPERATURE.

The term *pacemaker* is used in cardiology for an artificial device that maintains cardiac rhythm. A cardiac pacemaker may be required for certain sleep disorders, such as REM SLEEP-RELATED SINUS ARREST, which may induce a fatal episode of sinus arrest. Sometimes patients with bradycardia occurring during sleep, due to the OBSTRUCTIVE SLEEP APNEA SYNDROME, have a pacemaker inserted as a temporary measure. Treatment of the obstructive sleep apnea syndrome will reverse the bradycardia and episodes of sinus arrest associated with the syndrome. However, when investigative facilities for obstructive apnea are unavailable or where treatment cannot be immediately initiated, a temporary pacemaker may be necessary. A permanent pacemaker usually is not required for cardiac ARRHYTHMIAS due to obstructive sleep apnea syndrome. (See also CIRCADIAN RHYTHMS, CIRCADIAN TIMING SYSTEM, NREM-REM SLEEP CYCLE.)

pain Pain is commonly thought to be a major cause of sleep disturbance; however, research studies have shown that most patients with chronic pain do not have complaints regarding sleep. Acute pain is associated with sleep disturbance, but psychological and environmental factors, such as hospitalization, probably add to the sleep disturbance for this group. In a study of patients with chronic pain compared with a group of patients with insomnia of psychiatric cause, the insomnia patients had more sleep disturbance than the patients with chronic pain.

Several disorders have sleep complaints that may have a basis in pain. Patients with rheumatoid arthritis have frequent awakenings and disturbed sleep; however, sleep is usually not greatly disturbed unless there is an acute exacerbation of the arthritis. Patients with FIBROSITIS SYNDROME complain of NONRESTORATIVE SLEEP, which is predominantly a complaint upon awakening. Polysomnographic studies show the presence of ALPHA ACTIVITY throughout the sleep recording of these patients.

Tricyclic ANTIDEPRESSANTS can be useful for treating pain and also for the sleep disruption and alpha sleep seen in patients with fibrositis syndrome. HYPNOTICS can be useful in improving the quality of sleep of the patient in acute pain, such as is seen postoperatively.

panic disorder A psychiatric condition characterized by discrete episodes of intense fear that occur unexpectedly and without any specific precipitation. Panic disorder can occur during sleep and is associated with a sudden awakening with intense fear. A number of somatic symptoms occur with panic disorder, including shortness of breath, dizziness, palpitations, trembling, sweating, choking, chest discomfort, numbness and a fear of dying. Panic attacks can be associated with the symptoms of agoraphobia, in which there is a fear of being in certain places or situations. For example, an individual may have the feeling of needing to escape when outside of the home alone, in wide open spaces, in a crowd or traveling in a vehicle. Most panic attacks occur during the daytime and only rarely do panic attacks occur during sleep.

A panic episode that occurs during sleep is characterized by a sudden awakening during NON-REM-STAGE SLEEP, particularly stage two sleep (see SLEEP STAGES), with a feeling of intense fear of dying. Other somatic symptoms may be present.

The panic disorders are most commonly seen in young adults. There may be a prior history of childhood separation anxiety, and the disorder tends to run in families; it is more common in females.

The cause of panic disorder is unknown; however, infusions of lactate can precipitate episodes in susceptible individuals.

Panic disorder needs to be differentiated from anxiety disorder, in which anxiety is generalized and less focused on a specific situation or place. Panic disorder also has to be distinguished from SLEEP TERRORS, which typically occur from stage three/four sleep and are heralded by a loud scream. Patients with sleep terror episodes are confused or disoriented compared with patients with panic disorders, who are more typically aware of their surroundings. Agoraphobia is also not a feature of patients who have sleep terror episodes. The SLEEP CHOKING SYNDROME has some features that are similar to panic disorder; however, the focus of the anxiety is on the symptom of choking that occurs during sleep, and agoraphobia is not present, nor are daytime panic attacks.

In addition to discrete episodes of panic occurring during sleep, patients with panic disorders may have other features of difficulty in initiating and maintaining sleep, and they demonstrate a prolonged sleep latency and frequent awakenings with reduced total sleep time on polysomnographic investigation. The sleep disturbance appears to parallel the course of the underlying panic disorder.

Treatment of panic disorder is mainly pharmacological. Alprazolam (see BENZODIAZEPINES) has been demonstrated to be effective in suppressing episodes. Tricyclic ANTIDEPRESSANTS and beta-blockers have also been reported as being effective.

Raj, A. and Sheehan, D.V., "Medical Evaluations of Panic Attacks," *Journal of Clinical Psychiatry* 48 (1987): 309–313.

Ballinger, J.C., "Pharmacotherapy of Panic Attacks," *Journal of Clinical Psychiatry* 47 (1986): 27–32.

paradoxical sleep See RAPID EYE MOVEMENT SLEEP.

paradoxical techniques Procedures commonly used for the treatment of INSOMNIA. These techniques involve instituting wakeful activity, such as reading, writing or watching television, whenever the patient is unable to sleep. The premise is that by trying to remain awake sleep will occur naturally. (Very often sleep disturbance may be due to the strong attempts made to fall asleep.) The patient undergoing a paradoxical technique of trying to remain awake, by diverting the attention away from sleep, allows sleep to occur more rapidly. (See also AUTOGENIC TRAINING, BEHAVIORAL TREATMENT OF INSOMNIA, BIOFEEDBACK, COGNITIVE FOCUSING, SLEEP RESTRICTION THERAPY, STIMULUS CONTROL THERAPY, SYSTEMIC DESENSITIZATION.)

parasomnia Term used for the disorders of arousal, partial arousal and sleep stage transition. A parasomnia represents an episodic disorder in sleep, such as SLEEPWALKING, rather than a disorder of sleep or wakefulness per se. The parasomnias may be induced or exacerbated by sleep but do not produce a primary complaint of INSOMNIA or EXCESSIVE SLEEPINESS. According to the INTERNATIONAL CLASSIFICATION OF SLEEP DISORDERS, the parasomnias are divided into four groups: the first, the disorders of arousal, comprises sleepwalking, SLEEP TERRORS and CONFUSIONAL AROUSALS; the second, the sleep-wake transition disorders, comprises SLEEP STARTS, SLEEP TALKING, NOCTURNAL LEG CRAMPS and RHYTHMIC MOVEMENT DISORDERS; the third, a group usually associated with REM sleep, consists of NIGHTMARES, SLEEP PARALYSIS, IMPAIRED SLEEP-RELATED PENILE ERECTIONS, SLEEP-RELATED PAINFUL ERECTIONS, REM SLEEP-RELATED SINUS ARREST and REM SLEEP BEHAVIOR DISORDER; and the fourth group of other parasomnias includes SLEEP BRUXISM, PRIMARY SNORING, SLEEP ENURESIS, SLEEP-RELATED ABNORMAL SWALLOWING SYNDROME, NOCTURNAL PAROXYSMAL DYSTONIA, SUDDEN UNEXPLAINED NOCTURNAL DEATH SYNDROME and BENIGN NEONATAL SLEEP MYOCLONUS.

The parasomnias comprise those disorders that are regarded as primary or major sleep disorders and do not comprise the occurrence of medical or psychiatric events during sleep that otherwise might not cause a complaint of insomnia or excessive sleepiness. Such disorders, for example, the tremor of Parkinson's disease, are not included in the section entitled "parasomnias."

Schenck, C.H. and Mahowald, M.W., "A Parasomnia Overlap Disorder Involving Sleepwalking, Sleep Terrors, and REM Sleep Behavior Disorder in 33 Polysomnographically Confirmed Cases," *Sleep* 20, no. 11 (1997): 972–981.

Wise, M.S., "Parasomnias in Children," *Pediatric Annals* 26, no. 7 (1997): 427–433.

Parkinsonism Group of neurological disorders characterized by muscular rigidity, slowness of movements and tremulousness. The term is derived from the most well-known neurological disorder that produces these symptoms, Parkinson's disease. Associated with the neurological disorders are sleep complaints, typically INSOMNIA. Patients often have difficulty in maintaining both a regular sleep pattern and a full period of wakefulness during the daytime. In addition, there may be specific complaints related to the lack of body movement that occurs during sleep, such as the inability to arise to go to the bathroom or the inability to turn over in bed. Muscular disorders, such as leg cramping or jerking of the limbs, can also occur during sleep. Vivid dreams and NIGHTMARES, and REM sleep behaviors, may occur in patients with Parkinsonism.

Parkinson's disease affects up to 20% of the population over 60 years of age. The disorder is associated with loss of the dopamine cells of the brain, particularly of the substantia nigra. Neurotransmitter abnormalities are present, particularly of dopamine, serotonin and norepinephrine, which may contribute to the sleep disturbance.

The disruption of nighttime sleep can often lead to increased sleepiness during the daytime. It is unclear whether the daytime sleepiness is primarily the result of impaired nighttime sleep or whether it is an affect of degenerative neurological systems responsible for maintaining a regular sleep-wake pattern.

Patients with Parkinsonism, particularly those with the Shy-Drager syndrome, can have respiratory disorders during sleep to the extent that the OBSTRUCTIVE SLEEP APNEA SYNDROME or CENTRAL SLEEP APNEA SYNDROME is present.

The medications used to treat Parkinson's disease can also play a part in disturbing sleep-wake patterns. Medications primarily involve the use of levodopa, which can decrease nighttime sleep and exacerbate abnormal movement activity during sleep. However, treatment of Parkinson's disease is essential to maintain mobility, full alertness and activity during the daytime and restfulness at night. SLEEP HYGIENE measures are essential to reinforce a good sleep-wake cycle.

Polysomnographic monitoring may demonstrate many features of disrupted sleep, including sleep fragmentation with increased numbers of awakenings and arousals, and prolonged wakefulness during the night with a reduced amount of REM sleep. Sometimes there is a reduced amount of stage three/four sleep (see SLEEP STAGES). Tremulousness occurs during wakefulness but usually disappears during sleep; however, it can reappear during brief arousals and episodes of awakening during the night. Sometimes patients can have abnormal movements such as myoclonic jerks or PERIODIC LEG MOVEMENTS that occur during sleep, and there can also be tonic contractions of the muscles. Disruption of REM sleep with frequent arousals, and features of REM sleep occurring during other sleep stages, is commonly seen. The presence of excessive dreaming and nightmares may lead to abnormal movement activities and behaviors during REM sleep. SLEEP SPINDLE activity is generally reduced in patients with Parkinsonism.

Episodes of hypoventilation with central or obstructive apneas are occasionally seen in patients with Parkinsonism but are more common in patients who have the Shy-Drager form.

Treatment of Parkinsonism is primarily through the use of levodopa or dopaminergic medications such as pramipexole or ropinerole. Other medications include anticholinergics, amantadine and bromocriptine. The treatment of the sleep disturbance involves good sleep hygiene and appropriate usage of the anti-Parkinsonism medications. Sometimes daytime STIMULANT MEDICATIONS, such as pemoline, methylphenidate or dextroamphetamine, can be useful; however, the benefits are often only temporary. The nighttime sleep may be helped by short-acting benzodiazepine hypnotics, and sometimes low doses of the sedative tricyclic antidepressant amitriptyline.

Nausieda, P.A., "Sleep Disorders." in Koller, W.C., *Handbook of Parkinson's Disease.* New York: Marcel Dekker, 1987.

Lowe, A.D., "Sleep in Parkinson's Disease," *Journal of Psychosomatic Research* 44, no. 6 (1998): 613–617.

paroxysmal nocturnal dyspnea Term referring to recurrent episodes of shortness of breath that occur when an individual lies in the recumbent position, typically during nocturnal sleep. This condition occurs in individuals with heart failure in whom the ventricular dysfunction causes an increase in the pulmonary venous pressure, thereby allowing fluid to pass from the blood vessels into the alveoli of the lung, impairing respiratory gas exchange. Upon assuming the sitting or standing position, the fluid is cleared from the lungs, and the shortness of breath diminishes. Individuals who suffer from paroxysmal nocturnal dyspnea require several pillows in order to be able to assume a semi-reclining position during sleep. In such a position, the accumulation of fluid in the lungs is reduced and sleep may occur with fewer disturbances. The term ORTHOPNEA is also used for shortness of breath that occurs in the recumbent position but is not necessarily associated with nocturnal sleep. (See also NOCTURNAL CARDIAC ISCHEMIA.)

paroxysmal nocturnal dystonia See NOCTURNAL PAROXYSMAL DYSTONIA.

paroxysmal nocturnal hemoglobinuria (PNH) An acquired chronic hemolytic anemia that is characterized by intravascular hemolysis, which is exacerbated during sleep and results in hemoglobinuria (blood in the urine).

The primary abnormality is an abnormal sensitivity of the red blood cells to complement (a medical term for a substance produced by a certain type of cell that is involved in the breakdown of other blood cells). The red cells undergo lysis (a medical term for the destruction of cells), thereby releasing hemoglobin into the blood and predisposing the individual to venous thrombosis (blood clot). The thrombosis is a common cause of death in patients who are severely affected by paroxysmal nocturnal hemoglobinuria.

The disorder is diagnosed by either the acid hemolysis test or the sucrose lysis test. The presence of low leucocyte alkaline phosphatase and low red blood cell counts are other features of diagnostic significance.

The association between hemolysis and sleep is somewhat tenuous. The increased hemolysis is often first noticed when awakening in the morning.

Sometimes referred to as sleep-related hemolysis, paroxysmal nocturnal hemoglobinuria is the preferred term.

Hansen, N.E., "Sleep Related Plasma Hemoglobin Levels in Paroxysmal Nocturnal Hemoglobinuria," *Acta Medical Scandinavia* 184 (1968): 547–549.

pavor nocturnus Term derived from the Latin *pavor,* for terror, and *nocturnus,* meaning at night; refers to night terrors. The term SLEEP TERRORS is now commonly used because it specifies that episodes occur out of sleep.

pemoline See STIMULANT MEDICATIONS.

penile erections during sleep See ERECTIONS DURING SLEEP.

peptic ulcer disease This disease can awaken individuals at night because of a pain or discomfort present in the abdomen. Spontaneous pain occurs during sleep that is typically a dull, steady ache, usually within one to four hours after sleep onset. The pain can produce arousals and awakenings during sleep that lead to a complaint of INSOMNIA.

Peptic ulcer disease can be associated with SLEEP-RELATED GASTROESOPHAGEAL REFLUX with acid indigestion, HEARTBURN, and a sour, acid taste in the mouth. The pain of peptic ulcer disease often radiates to the chest or back. There is typically a hunger-like sensation, often with nausea, and there may be a cramping discomfort. The pain becomes intense and constant if perforation of the ulcer occurs.

There are hereditary factors involved in the cause of peptic ulceration. Individuals whose relatives have peptic ulcers have an increased likelihood of developing peptic ulcers; cigarette smoking is associated with a greater risk of developing duodenal ulceration. Drug ingestion of anti-inflammatory agents is also associated with a greater chance of developing peptic ulceration.

Duodenal ulceration is most common at about 20 years of age whereas gastric ulcer peaks between 50 and 60 years of age. There is an increased male predominance of peptic ulceration, with a male to female ratio of 2.5 to 1.

Polysomnography demonstrates an awakening that occurs just prior to the sensation of abdominal discomfort. Confirmation of the peptic ulcer disease is usually made by the demonstration of an ulcer by radiological or endoscopic studies.

Treatment of peptic ulcer disease is by reduction of gastric acid secretion and by such medications as rantidine (Zantac) or cimetidine (Tagamet). (See also ESOPHAGEAL PH MONITORING.)

periodic breathing A breathing pattern that consists of shallow episodes alternating with an increased depth of breathing. This can be seen at any age and commonly is seen in infants with breathing disorders (see INFANT SLEEP DISORDERS). It is also a typical pattern of the SLEEP-RELATED BREATHING DISORDERS, such as the OBSTRUCTIVE SLEEP APNEA SYNDROME or CENTRAL SLEEP APNEA SYNDROME. The periodicity of the breathing may induce a slight reduction in central respiratory drive that allows the upper airway to collapse, thereby exacerbating or inducing an obstructive apneic event.

Periodic breathing is seen in normal, healthy individuals at high altitudes due to the low level of inspired oxygen. This pattern of breathing is usually relieved by the administration of oxygen or by treatment with medications such as acetazolamide.

A periodic pattern of breathing was first described by Cheyne and Stokes in patients with cardiac disease. It is a pattern of breathing that commonly occurs during non-REM sleep; it is believed to be produced by either an increased circulation time or intracerebral disease.

Periodic breathing is produced by alteration in the blood carbon dioxide and oxygen levels, which causes a cessation of breathing, thereby allowing a low carbon dioxide level to return to normal. HYPOXEMIA or HYPERCAPNIA produces respiratory stimulation with an increased depth and rate of breathing, which causes a lowering of the carbon dioxide level and an elevation of the blood oxygen level. These changes lead to a reduction of respiratory drive, thereby producing the oscillations of ventilation. (See also ALTITUDE INSOMNIA, CHEYNE-STOKES RESPIRATION, INFANT SLEEP APNEA.)

periodic hypersomnia See RECURRENT HYPERSOMNIA.

periodic leg movements This term is synonymous with periodic limb movements, nocturnal myoclonus and periodic movements of sleep. It refers to periodic leg movements that occur with a stereotyped pattern of 0.5 to 5 seconds duration in one or both legs. The movement is typically a rapid partial flexion of the foot at the ankle, extension of the big toe and partial flexion of the knee and hip.

periodic limb movement disorder A disorder of recurrent episodes of leg movements that occur during sleep that can be associated with a complaint of either INSOMNIA or EXCESSIVE SLEEPINESS. Episodes of leg movements may be infrequent during sleep or may occur up to several thousand times during a typical sleep episode.

The leg movements are of short duration, lasting 0.5 to 5 seconds, and recur repetitively at intervals of approximately 20 to 40 seconds. The movements can occur in either leg or both simultaneously or asynchronously. The episodes typically occur in non-REM sleep and are usually absent during REM sleep. Often they cluster throughout the night so that there may be a run of 50 movements followed by uninterrupted sleep before a second or even a third cluster of movements.

Patients with periodic limb movement disorder present with the complaint of being unrested upon awakening in the morning. There may be tiredness and fatigue during the day and there may be frequent awakenings during the major sleep episode. Typically this disorder has been present for many years, often having been present since childhood. If the frequency of the episodes is sufficient to cause severe disruption of the nocturnal sleep episode then daytime sleepiness may result. Usually this sleepiness is somewhat vague and nonspecific at the onset but may become more severe with the increasing duration of the disorder.

People with the RESTLESS LEGS SYNDROME will typically have periodic limb movement disorder during sleep. The episodes of limb movements can be exacerbated by metabolic disorders, such as chronic uremia or hepatic disease. Medications, such as the tricyclic ANTIDEPRESSANTS, can aggravate this disorder and the withdrawal of central nervous system depressants, such as the HYPNOTICS, BENZODIAZEPINES and BARBITURATES, can also exacerbate it.

Typically the patient is unaware of the leg movements, because they occur only during sleep; polysomnographic documentation may be required to establish the presence of the disorder. The leg movements are often associated with upper limb movements and hence the term periodic limb movement disorder is preferred over such terms as periodic leg movements in sleep.

Treatment may be by means of medications that suppress the arousals related to the movements or the use of the newer dopaminergic agents such as pramipexole.

Coleman, Richard, "Periodic Movements in Sleep (Nocturnal Myoclonus) and Restless Leg Syndrome," in Guilleminault, Christian, ed., *Sleeping and Waking Disorders: Indications and Techniques.* Menlo Park, California: Addison-Wesley, 1982. pp. 265–295.

periodic movements of sleep See PERIODIC LEG MOVEMENTS.

period length The interval between recurrences of a particular phase of a biological rhythm. It can be measured from peak to peak, or trough (low point) to trough, or at some other recurring point of the rhythm. The period length of the sleep-wake cycle is typically 24 hours. (See also CHRONOBIOLOGY, CIRCADIAN RHYTHMS, NREM-REM SLEEP CYCLE.)

persistent psychophysiological insomnia This term was first presented in the *Diagnostic Classification of Sleep Disorders* that was published in the journal *SLEEP* in 1979. The simpler term, PSYCHOPHYSIOLOGICAL INSOMNIA, is the preferred term for the persistent type of psychophysiological insomnia. (See also ADJUSTMENT SLEEP DISORDER.)

PGO spikes PGO is an acronym for pontogeniculooccipital spikes, which are generated from the pons immediately prior to the onset of REM sleep. They are rapidly conducted through the lateral geniculate body to the occipital cortex. PGO spikes appear to be produced by cells in the pons that have been called PGO "on" neurons. The spikes are associated with the development of phasic activity during REM sleep, such as rapid eye movements, and may be elicited by sensory stimulation, such as sound or touch.

Various explanations have been offered for the function of PGO spikes. It has been suggested that PGO spikes may be involved in alertness during REM sleep, general brain stimulation during REM sleep to enhance learning and memory, and may be important in the production of dream imagery during sleep. (See also DREAMS.)

pharynx Derived from the Greek for "the throat"; refers to the musculo-membranous passage among the mouth, posterior nares and the larynx and the esophagus. The pharynx is often divided into the portion above the level of the soft palate, which is called the nasopharynx, a lower portion between the soft palate and the epiglottis, called the oropharynx, and the hypopharynx, which lies below the tip of the epiglottis and opens into the larynx and esophagus. It has been suggested that the portion of the pharynx that lies behind the soft palate be called the velopharynx.

The pharynx is the prime site of obstruction in patients who have the OBSTRUCTIVE SLEEP APNEA SYNDROME. Evaluation of the pharynx may involve FIBEROPTIC ENDOSCOPY of the upper airway or CEPHALOMETRIC RADIOGRAPHS.

Most patients with obstructive sleep apnea syndrome have obstruction at the level of the soft palate caused by an elongated soft palate and narrowing of the air passage at that level. Patients with obstruction of the pharynx at the soft palate level may be suitable for the UVULOPALATOPHARYNGOPLASTY procedure for the relief of SNORING and the obstructive sleep apnea syndrome. Commonly the obstruction in the airway is at the oropharyngeal or hypopharyngeal level, in which case procedures to bring the tongue forward, such as HYOID MYOTOMY or mandibular advancement surgery, may be helpful. Mechanical devices, including the TONGUE RETAINING DEVICE, or other dental appliances, such as the EQUALIZER, can be useful in maintaining a patent posterior pharyngeal airway in some patients. A more effective means is by the use of a CONTINUOUS POSITIVE AIRWAY PRESSURE DEVICE, which applies a positive air pressure to the posterior pharynx, thereby preventing the collapse of the pharyngeal tissue.

phase advance A chronobiological term applied to an advancement of a rhythm in relationship to another variable, most commonly clock time. (See also PHASE DELAY, PHASE SHIFT.)

phase delay The delay of a rhythm in relation to another variable, usually clock time. (See also PHASE RESPONSE CURVE, PHASE SHIFT.)

phase response curve A plot of the change in the phase shift as a response to a stimulus given at different points of a biological cycle. The phase response curve demonstrates an animal's ability to advance or delay a particular rhythm, most commonly the rest activity or the sleep-wake cycle. (Although a phase response curve has not yet been documented in humans, there is evidence that a phase change of the sleep-wake cycle can be accomplished by altering the timing of exposure to bright light.)

The phase response curve demonstrates that phase delays occur when the light stimulus is presented early in the night, whereas phase advance shifts occur when the stimulus is presented late in the night; and little or no phase response shift occurs when the stimulus is presented during the day portion of the light-dark cycle. (See also PHASE SHIFT, LIGHT THERAPY.)

phase shift A displacement of a rhythm in relationship to some other variable, usually clock time.

phase transition This term is used to specify one of the two junctures between the major sleep episode and the major portion of wakefulness in the 24-hour sleep-wake cycle.

phasic event A brain muscle or autonomic event of an episodic or fluctuating nature that occurs during a sleep episode. Such a phasic event is seen during REM sleep and can comprise muscle twitches or the rapid eye movements. Usually, phasic events have a duration that is measured in terms of milliseconds, and they last one to two seconds at the most.

Phillipson, Eliot A. Born in Edmonton, Alberta, Canada, Dr. Phillipson received his doctor of medicine degree, with distinction, from the University of Alberta in 1963. Dr. Phillipson (1939–), who is now a professor in the Department of Medicine of the University of Toronto, contributed to sleep physiology by conducting the first systematic study of the regulation of respiration during non-REM and REM sleep, and by demonstrating fundamental differences in respiratory regulation between the two sleep stages. His 1977 paper on ventilatory and arousal responses to CO_2 in sleeping dogs demonstrated the powerful overriding effect of REM sleep on the metabolic respiratory control system. Phillipson's 1978 paper, with C.E. Sullivan et al., demonstrated the critical dependence of breathing on the metabolic respiratory control system during slow-wave sleep.

Phillipson, Eliot A. et al., "Ventilatory and Waking Responses to CO_2 in Sleeping Dogs," *American Review of Respiratory Disease* 115 (1977): 251–259.

Sullivan, C.E. et al., "Primary Role of Respiratory Afferents in Sustaining Breathing Rhythm," *Journal of Applied Physiology* 45 (1978): 11–17.

pH monitoring Technique used to evaluate the acidity of esophageal contents in order to determine if gastroesophageal reflux has occurred. A pH probe is usually placed through the nose approximately 5 centimeters above the esophageal sphincter. Esophageal pH is generally 7.0 and the reflux is associated with drop in the pH of the distal esophagus below the level of 4.0. Following a drop in the pH, clearance of the acid in the esophageal sphincter is associated with a rise to a pH of 5 or greater.

PH monitoring is usually performed over a 24-hour period or over the sleep episode to determine whether gastroesophageal reflux occurs in association with sleep or daytime activities. Esophageal reflux can be the cause of esophageal disorders, such as esophagitis, or sleep-related disorders, such as respiratory distress during sleep. (See also SLEEP-RELATED LARYNGOSPASM, SLEEP-RELATED GASTROESOPHAGEAL REFLUX, OBSTRUCTIVE SLEEP APNEA SYNDROME.)

photoperiod The duration of light in a light-dark cycle. Usually the photoperiod lasts approximately 12 hours; however, in environments where darkness does not occur until 10 P.M. and sunrise occurs at 4 A.M., the photoperiod will be 18 hours in duration. In the extreme polar regions, the photoperiod may last 24 hours when there is continuous light.

The photoperiod is often varied during experimental studies of the effects of light upon animals, and so the portion of light to dark is varied.

An abnormal photoperiod may be a factor in producing sleep disturbance, and some CIRCADIAN RHYTHM SLEEP DISORDERS, such as DELAYED SLEEP PHASE SYNDROME, may be induced by an abnormal photoperiod in the Arctic or Antarctic regions.

phylogeny The evolution or development of a plant or animal. The phylogeny of sleep is based on studies of the evolutionary physiology of vertebrate sleep, which have revealed three distinct phylogenetic stages. The first type of sleep, which is found in fish and amphibians, is termed "primary sleep" and comprises different sleep-like forms of rest. This type of sleep appears to be a non-differentiated form compared to the sleep patterns found in higher vertebrates. An "intermediate sleep" form is found in reptiles and is characterized by activated and nonactivated stages, which divide sleep into two distinct phases. Nonactivated sleep has a more pronounced, synchronized, electrical cerebral activity, with features that are indicative of SLOW WAVE SLEEP.

The third type of sleep, a "paradoxical phase of sleep" seen in birds, is characterized by desynchronization of the electroencephalogram and a reduction in muscle tone. Suggestive of REM SLEEP, this type of sleep is differentiated from the slow activity that is more pronounced in mammals.

On the evolutionary scale, slow wave sleep appears to have arisen about 200 million years ago, and paradoxical sleep approximately 50 million years later.

This evolution of sleep correlates with the degree of development of overall cerebral electrical activity and the level of development of the higher regions of the brain. The evolution of the thalamo-cortical system is of particular importance in the development of sleep. This system first began in amphibians, became more specialized in reptiles, and is most clearly developed in mammals. The development of mammalian sleep is clearly related to the development of the thalamo-cortical pathways. The development of REM sleep appears to arise from the early forms of activated sleep.

Pickwickian syndrome Term applied to individuals who are overweight, with ALVEOLAR HYPOVENTILATION, an elevated carbon dioxide level and abnormally low oxygen level in the blood, and, most commonly, to patients who have severe OBSTRUCTIVE SLEEP APNEA SYNDROME, who are sleepy during the daytime, are loud snorers, obese and have impairment of daytime blood gases. The term was derived from the description of Joe the fat boy in *The Posthumous Papers of the Pickwick Club,* published on March 31, 1836. Charles Dickens modeled his description of the sleepy boy upon someone who very clearly had all the typical features of obstructive sleep apnea syndrome.

Although the term *Pickwickian syndrome* had been used prior to the 1950s, it was brought to more general attention in a paper published in 1956 by Burwell et al. The term may apply to disorders of impaired respiration during sleep other than obstructive sleep apnea, and it frequently is used to describe people who have right-sided heart failure in association with the other typical features.

It is preferable to use more specific terms than Pickwickian syndrome to describe patients who have sleep disorders characterized by OBESITY, hypersomnolence, snoring and alveolar hypoventilation, such as the obstructive sleep apnea syndrome or CENTRAL ALVEOLAR HYPOVENTILATION SYNDROME.

Kryger, M.H., "Fat, Sleep, and Charles Dickens," *Clinics and Chest Medicine* 6 (1985): 555–562.
Dickens, Charles, *The Posthumous Papers of the Pickwick Club*. London: Chapman and Hall, published in serial form, 1836–1837.

pineal gland A small, pea-sized protuberance situated at the back of the brain above the brain stem. Rene Descartes in the 17th century regarded the pineal as the seat of the soul. The pineal gland is markedly influenced by light because its primary hormone, MELATONIN, is released at night and is suppressed during the day. The circadian pattern of melatonin levels peaks between 1 A.M. and 5 A.M. and is maximal around the time of puberty. Melatonin is an important hormone in the regulation of circadian rhythms. It also appears to be important in the control of reproduction and in normal sexual development.

The pineal gland is innervated (nerve fibers go to the gland) by sympathetic fibers that arise in the superior cervical ganglion of the neck. Light impulses from the retina pass through the SUPRACHIASMATIC NUCLEUS of the hypothalamus. Pathways extend from the suprachiasmatic nucleus to the spinal cord and innervate the superior cervical ganglion and from there pass to the pineal gland. (See also CIRCADIAN RHYTHMS.)

placebo A sham or false treatment that most commonly is in the form of a tablet with no effective ingredient, used for either the psychological effects or for control purposes in research studies. The term is derived from the Latin, meaning "I will please."

A placebo is also known as a "dummy medication." The placebo response depends upon the patient-physician relationship, with the sense of being helped by the physician an essential element to its effectiveness. The effects of a placebo are most commonly experienced as changes in mood or other subjective feelings. The response can be either positive or negative, depending upon the desired effect. Usually the response to a placebo cannot be taken to mean that the patient has either a "psychogenic" or "real" symptom. (See also MEDICATIONS.)

Placidyl (ethchlorvynol) See HYPNOTICS.

plethysmograph A biomedical instrument used for measuring changes in the volume of an organ or a part of the body. Plethysmography is used in SLEEP DISORDERS MEDICINE for determining changes in chest and abdominal volume and in the measurement of changes in TUMESCENCE (swelling) of the penis during sleep.

Plethysmography is most commonly performed for the determination of SLEEP-RELATED BREATHING DISORDERS by means of an inductive plethysmograph. Loops of insulated wire are placed around the rib cage and abdomen and connected to a transducer so that changes in impedance of the wire bands reflect changes in the volume of the chest or abdomen. Typically, an increasing lung volume is associated with a reduction in abdominal volume. However, if UPPER AIRWAY OBSTRUCTION occurs, there is a reduction of lung volume, with an increase in abdominal volume due to the diaphragm action. This paradoxical pattern of respiration is indicative of obstructive sleep apneic episodes, whereas a reduction of activity of both bands is representative of central apneic episodes.

Mercury-filled STRAIN GAUGES are placed around the penis in order to detect changes in the volume of the penis during sleep. Usually a strain gauge is placed around the base of the penis and another at the tip. During REM sleep all healthy males will have penile erections and the measurement of the size of the penile erection by plethysmography gives an indication as to whether the patient has the physiological capability of attaining normal erections in sleep (which helps to assess if impotence is of a physiological or psychiatric cause).

Respitrace is the trade name for an inductive plethysmograph that is capable of measuring changes in volume of the chest and abdomen to determine ventilation. (See also CENTRAL SLEEP APNEA SYNDROME, OBSTRUCTIVE SLEEP APNEA SYNDROME, SLEEP-RELATED PENILE ERECTIONS.)

poliomyelitis A viral infection that affects the nerves that innervate skeletal muscles. This disorder can affect the nerves within the brain stem or spinal cord, and as a result there can be wasting and atrophy of the muscles, leading to severe weakness or paralysis. Patients with severe poliomyelitis may have the inability to sustain respiratory movements on their own and therefore require assisted VENTILATION, particularly during sleep. The late effect of poliomyelitis may produce worsening of the muscle strength many years after the initial infective insult, and a picture of progressive ventilatory deterioration may be seen. Patients can present with increasing daytime sleepiness due to impairment of respiration during sleep, which leads to fragmented sleep with blood gas changes characterized by oxygen desaturation at night. In such cases, assisted ventilation during sleep may be necessary, and if daytime ventilation is impaired, assisted ventilation 24 hours a day may be indicated. (See also CENTRAL SLEEP APNEA SYNDROME, SLEEP-RELATED BREATHING DISORDERS.)

polycythemia An increase in the size of the red blood cell mass of the blood. Polycythemia is occasionally seen in patients with the OBSTRUCTIVE SLEEP APNEA SYNDROME, particularly when associated with chronic obstructive lung disease (the OVERLAP SYNDROME), which produces a more constant level of HYPOXEMIA. Approximately 7% of patients presenting with obstructive sleep apnea syndrome are found to have polycythemia. The chronic hypoxemia stimulates the red blood cell marrow to increase the number of red cells so that the oxygen-carrying capacity of the blood is increased. Treatment of the sleep-related hypoxemia leads to improvement of the polycythemia.

polysomnogram The continuous and simultaneous recording of physiological variables during sleep; includes the ELECTROENCEPHALOGRAM (EEG), the ELECTRO-OCULOGRAM (EOG) and the ELECTROMYOGRAM (EMG). In addition, the electrocardiogram (ECG) (a graph of the electrical activity of the heart) records respiratory airflow, respiratory movements, blood oxygen saturation and lower limb movement activity. Other commonly taken measures include intraesophageal pressure, intraesophageal pH changes, end-tidal carbon dioxide values and penile tumescence.

The polysomnogram is the recording upon which sleep disorder specialists rely in order to obtain objective documentation of a patient's physiological status during sleep. It typically consists of a paper tracing, approximately 1,000 pages long. However, it may be recorded on magnetic tape or on a computer disc.

The polysomnogram is scored in a standard manner according to epochs of 20 or 30 seconds in duration, and sleep is scored by the Alan Rechtschaffen and Anthony Kales method. (See also POLYSOMNOGRAPHY, SLEEP DISORDER CENTERS.)

Rechtschaffen, Alan and Kales, Anthony, *A Manual of Standardized Terminology, Techniques, and Scoring System for Sleep Stages of Human Subjects.* Los Angeles: Brain Information Service, 1968.

polysomnography Studies of sleep require the measurement of several physiological variables, including activity of the brain, the eyes and the muscles. Sleep is typically recorded on an electroencephalograph machine, which has the ability of measuring not only the ELECTROENCEPHALOGRAM (EEG) but also the electromyographic (EMG) (see ELECTROMYOGRAM) activity and electrooculography (EOG) (see ELECTRO-OCULOGRAM). The EEG records the brain activity, the EMG records the muscle activity and the EOG monitors eye movements.

The electroencephalogram electrodes are placed on the scalp in the routine manner; however, only a few electrodes are required. For reporting sleep, an electrode is centrally placed on the head (in the C3 or C4 position), and this electrode is referred to an electrically neutral lead usually placed on the mastoid bone behind the ear (at either A1 or A2 position). This produces a unipolar recording, which measures the difference in the electrical activity between the C3 position and the A1 electrode. The electrodes are usually attached to the head by means of collodion, a temporary glue, in order to prevent their dislodgment during a whole night's recording. (Electrodes may be attached to the face with surgical tape, but collodion is used to attach electrodes to the scalp.)

The electromyogram is usually recorded from chin-muscle activity. Two electrodes are placed just beneath the tip of the chin and the difference between recorded potentials is measured, giving a bipolar recording.

With the electro-oculogram, the electrodes are attached to the outer canthus of each eye to record eye movements. Usually two eye channels are measured, so when the eyes move conjugately, the tracings appear as mirror images of each other. The electro-oculogram electrodes are referred to a reference electrode. Because the retina is negatively charged with respect to the surface of the eye, movements of the eye induce a potential difference, which is recorded by the electrodes.

In addition to measuring sleep activity, polysomnography often involves the measurement of other physiological variables during sleep, such as respiratory movements, airflow, electrocardiogram, blood-oxygen saturation, carbon dioxide levels, urometry, skeletal muscle activity, pH monitoring and penile tumescence (erections of the penis) to help in analyzing the cause of impotence.

The electrical signals of a polygraph go in just one direction—from the patient to the polygraph—so there is little possibility of the patient receiving an electrical shock. The tracings for each sensor are recorded on a continuous roll of moving paper, which becomes the record of a night's sleep, and that record is known as a POLYSOMNOGRAM. Typically, a patient will be asked to come to the sleep laboratory an hour or two before the patient's usual bedtime. The electrodes are attached at the appropriate place to enable recording of each desired measure. An entire night of sleep will be recorded on the polygraph, creating almost a thousand pages of chart paper monitoring of EEG waves, eye movements, muscle activity and the other physiological variables.

For clinical or research studies, the different parameters can be measured according to different arrays called a MONTAGE, depending upon the clinician's preference and the particular variables under investigation. A standard recording for a patient with the disorder of OBSTRUCTIVE SLEEP APNEA SYNDROME might be as follows: two electroencephalogram measures, one at the C3 position and one at the O2 position, as well as electro-oculogram and chin electromyogram recordings. Leg movement activity can be recorded by means of electromyographic measures of the right and left anterior tibialis muscles in order to help confirm body movements associated with arousals that may occur because of apnea episodes. In order to determine airflow, THERMISTORS that determine temperature changes of inspired and expired air may be placed at both left and right nasal passages and another at the mouth. A small microphone may be utilized in order to determine sounds of SNORING. Respiratory movements are detected by means of bellows pneumographs placed around the abdomen and chest or, alternatively, mercury strain gauges can be placed on the chest and abdomen. An electrocardiogram is recorded by chest leads. An infrared, transcutaneous sensor may be used for recording oxygen saturation values, and end-tidal carbon dioxide levels may be recorded by means of a small tube placed in one of the nostrils attached to a capnograph.

Patients undergoing polysomnography for suspected seizure disorders may have additional electroencephalogram channels recorded, whereas a patient undergoing studies for SLEEP-RELATED PENILE ERECTIONS would have sleep measured along with measurements of penile tumescence during sleep.

Although patients typically undergo polysomnography over their habitual sleep period for a minimum of eight hours of recording, in many clinical situations it may be necessary for the patient to undergo more than one night of recording in order to obtain adequate information. (See also ACCREDITED CLINICAL POLYSOMNOGRAPHER, SLEEP DISORDER CENTERS.)

Chesson, A.L., Jr., et al., "The Indications for Polysomnography and Related Procedures," *Sleep* 20, no. 6 (1997): 423–487.

pons Region of the brain stem that lies between the medulla and the midbrain; important in the maintenance of sleep and wakefulness because it contains the LOCUS CERULEUS, RAPHE NUCLEI and reticular nuclei. Although the pons is clearly defined by the external anatomical landmarks, the nuclei extend across boundaries. Various and incompatible terms have been used to describe the reticular regions of nuclei.

The raphe nuclei, which are likely to be important in the regulation of phasic events of REM sleep, contain serotonin. Although the raphe nuclei of the pons were thought to be important in the maintenance of slow wave sleep, the region around the nuclei appears to be more important.

The pons is also the site of the pontogeniculooccipital (PGO) waves (see PGO SPIKES), which are large phasic potentials generated from the pons immediately prior to the onset of REM sleep. (See also SLEEP ATONIA.)

pontogeniculooccipital spikes (PGO) See PGO SPIKES.

Positive Occipital Sharp Transients of Sleep See POSTS.

POSTS POSTS is an acronym for Positive Occipital Sharp Transients of Sleep—a transient electroencephalographic potential that is commonly seen during stages two and three sleep in adolescents and young adults. There is no known cause or association of POSTS. (See also ELECTROENCEPHALOGRAM, NON-REM-STAGE SLEEP, SLEEP STAGES.)

post-traumatic hypersomnia A disorder of EXCESSIVE SLEEPINESS that occurs within 18 months of a traumatic event involving the central nervous system. This disorder may consist of a changed sleep pattern, such as a long sleep duration at night, as well as frequent sleep episodes during the day on a background of excessive sleepiness. The sleep disturbance typically occurs within months of the trauma and may resolve spontaneously within a period of weeks to months. However, sometimes the sleep disturbance may be long-lasting and may never resolve. This disorder is diagnosed in the presence of severe excessive daytime sleepiness if there are no other features of neurological deficit.

Certain parts of the central nervous system are more likely to induce this sleep disturbance if involved in the trauma, such as injury involving the hypothalamic or brain stem regions. Pathological studies have usually demonstrated widespread lesions throughout the central nervous system at autopsy so that the specific site causing post-traumatic hypersomnia is unknown.

Polysomnographic studies of this disorder have shown a slightly prolonged nocturnal sleep period or relatively normal nocturnal sleep with excessive sleepiness, evident on MULTIPLE SLEEP LATENCY TESTING. The daytime sleep episodes are generally of non-REM sleep. It is possible that some patients with this disorder have microsleep episodes that impair daytime functioning and may be detectable only by 24-hour polysomnographic monitoring.

Diagnosis of this disorder is made in part upon the temporal association with the head trauma. Other disorders of excessive sleepiness contribute to motor vehicle accidents, which may lead to head trauma. Patients suspected of having post-traumatic hypersomnia should have other disorders of sleepiness ruled out by appropriate polysomnographic investigation.

Treatment of post-traumatic hypersomnia is largely symptomatic and rests on the use of daytime STIMULANT MEDICATIONS, such as methylphenidate or pemoline, to alleviate the sleepiness.

Guilleminault, C., Faull, A.M., Miles, L. and Van den Hoed, J., "Post-traumatic Excessive Daytime Sleepiness: A Review of 20 Patients," *Neurology* 33 (1980): 1584–1589.

Hall, C.W. and Danoff, D., "Sleep Attacks: Apparent Relationship to Atlantoaxial Dislocation," *Archives of Neurology* 32 (1975): 57–58.

pramipexole A clinically effective nonergot dopamine agonist used in the treatment of RESTLESS LEGS SYNDROME (RLS). Pramipexole has preferential affinity to the D3 receptor subtype; the D3 receptor subtype seems to be the most important in suppressing the features of RLS. Pramipexole also interacts with D2 and D4 receptors. However, it has seven times greater affinity for the D3 receptor than it does for the D2 or D4 receptor. It has some affinity for norepinephrine receptors but little affinity for 5HT (SEROTONIN) receptors. Pramipexole may also provide neuroprotective effects through depression of dopamine metabolism, antioxidant effects and stimulation of trophic activity.

The limited studies available suggest that it is effective in treating restless legs syndrome and suppresses periodic limb movements. Its profile and side effect profile appear to be better than those of L-DOPA or pergolide: It causes less daytime augmentation of RLS than L-dopa and less nausea than does pergolide. The pharmacologic profile includes an elimination half-life of 12.9 hours. Pramipexole does not interact with cytochrome P450 enzymes and is not expected to alter responses to concomitant medications by interfering with their metabolism. It is an effective antiparkinsonian medication.

Doses are from 0.125 milligram to 4.5 milligrams. Side effects that have been encountered include nausea, constipation, and insomnia. Sleepiness and visual hallucinations occur more commonly than with placebo. The brand name for pramipexole is Mirapex. (See also L-DOPA, PERIODIC LEG MOVEMENTS.)

predormital myoclonus See SLEEP STARTS.

pregnancy-related sleep disorder Sleep disorder characterized by either EXCESSIVE SLEEPINESS or INSOMNIA occurring during the course of pregnancy. Typically the disorder is a biphasic one, with the onset of sleepiness during the first trimester and insomnia in the third trimester. In some women, parasomnia activity, such as NIGHTMARES and SLEEP TERRORS, can occur in association with the pregnancy.

Complaints of tiredness, fatigue and sleepiness are common during the first trimester, sometimes even before the pregnancy has been diagnosed. The TOTAL SLEEP TIME can be increased and a pregnant woman will frequently have the need to take a nap.

Normal pregnancy is associated with changes in the quality of nighttime sleep and an alteration in daytime alertness. Typically in the first trimester there is an increased sleepiness with a heightened desire to take a daytime nap. For some women who experience ANXIETY related to the pregnancy, insomnia may occur, related to the emotional components of the pregnancy and not due to any pregnancy-related physical condition. CAFFEINE or NICOTINE withdrawal may add to the sleep disruption.

During the second trimester, the tendency for daytime napping disappears; however, the quality of the nocturnal sleep episode starts to deteriorate. SLEEP LATENCY, the number of awakenings and the SLEEP EFFICIENCY tend to increase at this time.

Some of the sleep disturbances in the later months of the pregnancy may be related to the increase in the physical complaints at this time, such as an uncomfortable sleep position due to back discomfort, increased urinary frequency and fetal movements.

Because of increased abdominal pressure, it might be expected that sleep-related breathing abnormalities would increase. However, respiratory disturbance has not been described in pregnancy, and this may be due to the increased progesterone levels at this time that act as a respiratory stimulant. TIDAL VOLUME is increased by PROGESTERONE.

Polysomnographic studies have demonstrated a gradual reduction of deeper stages three/four sleep during the pregnancy (see SLEEP STAGES), with its absence in the later stage of pregnancy in some women. The sleepiness may be clinically evident and documented by MULTIPLE SLEEP LATENCY TESTING. The polysomnographic features of the nocturnal sleep disturbance are typically those of an increased sleep latency, frequent awakenings, increased stage one sleep and reduced sleep efficiency.

There is some evidence to suggest that postpartum psychoses may be related to the sleep state changes that occur in late pregnancy. Following delivery, REM sleep decreases markedly and normalizes over the subsequent two weeks, and there is a gradual recovery of stage four sleep after delivery.

Following delivery, the disturbed quality of sleep generally resolves itself unless other factors intervene, such as postpartum depression, in which case insomnia or hypersomnia due to MOOD DISORDERS may occur. There may now be sleep-related problems because of the frequent awakening of the newborn, but those problems are environmentally caused rather than a physical complaint associated with the post-pregnancy period. The new mother can minimize the effects of sleep deprivation that often occur because she interrupts her sleep to respond to the newborn, by taking turns with her spouse to respond to the newborn if the cries are not food-related, or, if she is bottle-feeding, by keeping the baby nearby so it is easier to go back to sleep after attending to the newborn, or by taking naps during the day at the same time that the newborn naps so that she does not try to get through the next night of interrupted sleep completely exhausted.

The onset of fatigue, tiredness and excessive sleepiness (of relatively short duration) in a woman of childbearing age should suggest the possibility of pregnancy-related sleep disorder. Other disorders contributing to sleep disruption, such as NARCOLEPSY or PERIODIC LIMB MOVEMENT DISORDER, should be considered in the differential diagnosis.

Treatment of pregnancy-related sleep disorder is purely supportive mainly by SLEEP HYGIENE measures. Pregnant women should not take hypnotic medications. However, if the sleep disturbance is associated with the development of severe anxiety or DEPRESSION, and the maternal or fetal well-being is at risk, sedative hypnotics may be indicated in the third trimester, but only under the guidance of an obstetrician. (See also INFANT SLEEP DISORDERS, INSUFFICIENT SLEEP SYNDROME, SLEEP-RELATED BREATHING DISORDERS.)

Karacan, I., Hine, W., Agnew, H., Williams, R.L., Webb, W.B. and Ross, J.J., "Characteristics of Sleep Patterns During Late Pregnancy and the Post Partum Periods," *American Journal of Obstetrics and Gynecology* 101 (1968): 579–586.

pregnancy and sleep See PREGNANCY-RELATED SLEEP DISORDER.

premature infant Infant born after the 27th week of pregnancy and before full term, who weighs between 1,000 grams (2.2 pounds) and 2,500 grams (5.5 pounds). Premature infants are more likely to have SLEEP-RELATED BREATHING DISORDERS characterized by APNEA. Apneic episodes occur predominantly during sleep but can also occur during wakefulness. This disorder, APNEA OF PREMATURITY, often spontaneously resolves as the infant ages. Premature infants have a greater risk of suffering from SUDDEN INFANT DEATH SYNDROME than full-term infants. (See also INFANT SLEEP, INFANT SLEEP APNEA, INFANT SLEEP DISORDERS.)

premature morning awakening See EARLY MORNING AROUSAL.

premature ventricular contraction See VENTRICULAR PREMATURE COMPLEXES.

primary insomnia See PSYCHOPHYSIOLOGICAL INSOMNIA or IDIOPATHIC INSOMNIA.

primary snoring A disorder characterized by loud sounds that come from the back of the mouth during breathing in sleep and in the absence of impaired breathing. This disorder is differentiated from the OBSTRUCTIVE SLEEP APNEA SYNDROME, in which loud snoring is associated with impaired VENTILATION during sleep, sleep disruption and abnormal cardiovascular features. Usually, primary snoring is noted by a disturbed bed partner. The snorer is typically unaware of the loud snoring; however, there may be a brief gasp or choking sensation at the termination of a loud snore.

The snoring is usually rhythmical, with a continuous sound made during inspiration and expiration that can be worsened by body position, such as sleeping on the back. (Sometimes this form of snoring is eliminated when the snorer lies on the side.)

Any disorder that produces narrowing of the upper airway, such as enlarged tonsils, acute rhinitis or upper respiratory tract infections, may exacerbate or bring out the tendency for primary snoring. Medications that impair arousal, such as HYPNOTICS or ALCOHOL, may also exacerbate the tendency for snoring. Often the development of snoring is associated with increasing weight gain and can be relieved in many patients by loss of body weight (see OBESITY).

Snoring is more common in males than in females and is most common for both groups in the elderly population over the age of 65 years. However, snoring may occur at any age and may be seen in infancy, but it is more commonly seen in children associated with tonsillar or ADENOID enlargement before or around the time of puberty.

Polysomnographic monitoring helps to distinguish primary snoring from the obstructive sleep apnea syndrome. UPPER AIRWAY OBSTRUCTION is not present during sleep, and the sleep episode is normal without arousals or awakenings, nor is there evidence of oxygen desaturation or associated cardiac ARRHYTHMIAS. Very often the snoring is more pronounced during REM SLEEP.

Snoring can produce social consequences, such as embarrassment and even marital discord. The sleep of a bed partner is liable to be disrupted, particularly if the bed partner is a light sleeper or has INSOMNIA. Primary snoring may be treated by means of behavioral measures, such as the avoidance of smoking, alcohol or large meals before sleep. Sleeping on the side rather than on the back often lessens the severity of snoring. It may be necessary for a bed partner to use earplugs or use a noise machine to muffle the sound of snoring. Sometimes a bed partner may try to fall asleep earlier in the night than the snorer so that the sounds of snoring do not interfere with sleep onset.

If the above behavioral means are ineffective in removing the snoring, consideration can be given to surgical relief of the upper airway obstructive lesions, such as removal of enlarged tonsils or redundant nasal mucosa. Treatment of upper respiratory tract infections, or the use of nasal decongestants or antihistamines, may be helpful. Specialized operative procedures, such as the UVULOPALATOPHARYNGOPLASTY operation, may be effective in reducing the snoring in many patients; however, careful selection is necessary as not all patients will respond to this procedure.

Lugaresi, E., Cirignotta, F., Coccagna, G. and Pinna, C., "Some Epidemiological Data on Snoring and Cardiocirculatory Disturbances," *Sleep* 3 (1980): 221–224.

progesterone A female sex hormone, used in sleep medicine in the form of medroxyprogesterone (see RESPIRATORY STIMULANTS), for stimulation of respiration to treat some SLEEP-RELATED BREATHING DISORDERS.

progressive relaxation The sequential relaxation of muscle groups to assist in sleep onset for those with INSOMNIA. This method of relaxation was first proposed by Edmund Jacobson and is occasionally referred to as JACOBSONIAN RELAXATION or SLEEP EXERCISES. (See also DISORDERS OF INITIATING AND MAINTAINING SLEEP, PSYCHOPHYSIOLOGICAL INSOMNIA.)

Project Sleep A program developed in 1979 by the United States Surgeon General's office to create materials and educate physicians and the general public about sleep and arousal disorders. This project was created in coordination with the ASSOCIATION OF SLEEP DISORDER CENTERS, the American Medical Association and members from the pharmaceutical industry, including the Upjohn Company.

In addition to disseminating printed information on sleep and arousal disorders, one of the program's major contributions was the production of a comprehensive series of slides with audio cassette tapes on sleep and sleep disorders. It was disseminated to medical schools and other interested parties throughout the United States.

prolactin A hormone released from the pituitary gland that accompanies GROWTH HORMONE release. This hormone is under the close control of the neurotransmitter DOPAMINE, which inhibits prolactin secretion. Prolactin is secreted during sleep and has a CIRCADIAN RHYTHM that is tied to the sleep-wake cycle but is not related to specific sleep stage activity.

Prolactin is secreted in higher amounts during pregnancy and lactation and also appears to be important in the maintenance of the reproductive system in both males and females.

Medications that affect dopamine levels will influence the secretion of prolactin. Phenothiazines (antipsychotic drugs) that inhibit dopamine action can produce elevated levels of prolactin whereas bromocriptine, a dopamine agonist (a drug that acts in the same manner as dopamine), will suppress the release of prolactin. (See also ADRENOCORTICOTROPHIN HORMONE, CORTISOL.)

Urade,Y. et al., "Prostaglandin D2 and Sleep Regulation," *Biochimica et Biophysica Acta* 1463, no. 3 (1999): 606–615.

proposed sleep disorders A category of the INTERNATIONAL CLASSIFICATION OF SLEEP DISORDERS that lists various disorders for which there is insufficient information available to substantiate the presence of a particular disorder. This category also contains newly described disorders not yet substantiated by replicated data in the medical literature—for example, the SLEEP CHOKING SYNDROME. In addition, disorders representing one end of the spectrum of normality are included here—for example, SHORT SLEEPER and LONG SLEEPER.

prostaglandins Chemicals (autocoid) derived from arachidonic acid (acid present in the body) that are widely distributed in almost every tissue and fluid in the body. The lipid-soluble acid was first identified in seminal fluid, which led to the name "prostaglandin." In addition to their widespread actions throughout the body, the prostaglandins are found in areas of the brain concerned with sleep mechanisms. The presence of prostaglandin D (PGD2) in the preoptic nuclei is associated with sleep induction and maintenance, whereas PGE2, which is found in the posterior thalamic nuclei, is believed to be responsible for wakefulness. These newly discovered neurotransmitters are major factors in the control of sleep and wakefulness. (See also SLEEP-INDUCING FACTORS.)

protriptyline See ANTIDEPRESSANTS.

Provera See RESPIRATORY STIMULANTS.

Provigil See MODAFINIL.

provisionally accredited sleep disorder center A category of accreditation phased out by the AMERICAN SLEEP DISORDERS ASSOCIATION in 1989; it was for sleep disorder centers that did not fully meet the standards and guidelines outlined by the association or centers that had not yet applied for accreditation. Centers now either meet all the standards and guidelines and become fully accredited or are not accredited at all. (See also ACCREDITATION STANDARDS FOR SLEEP DISORDER CENTERS, ASSOCIATION OF SLEEP DISORDER CENTERS.)

Prozac See ANTIDEPRESSANTS.

pseudoinsomnia See SLEEP STATE MISPERCEPTION.

psychiatric disorders A psychiatric diagnosis is the most frequent diagnosis given to patients with the complaint of INSOMNIA who are seeking help at SLEEP DISORDER CENTERS; almost all patients with DEPRESSION have some sleep complaint. (Insomnia due to acute situational stress is more common in the general population.)

The MOOD DISORDERS, typically disorders due to mania, hypermania or depression, are common causes of the complaint of insomnia, especially EARLY MORNING AROUSAL. Patients with bipolar disorder, such as manic-depressive disorder, will often show periods of short sleep duration during the manic episodes, alternating with episodes of EXCESSIVE SLEEPINESS during the depressive phase. Typically, patients with depression do not have true hypersomnia, that is, the total sleep time during a 24-hour period is not increased above normal levels. However, an excessive amount of time spent in bed is a common feature of depressed patients.

ANXIETY DISORDERS cause sleep disruption, characterized by prolonged sleep latency with frequent awakenings and poor sleep efficiency. These features are most commonly seen in patients who have general anxiety disorders; however, poor sleep quality is also seen in patients who have PANIC DISORDERS. More typically, panic disorder causes an acute event during sleep, with an awakening and feelings of fear and intense anxiety. These abrupt and infrequent episodes during sleep at night are usually accompanied by similar panic attacks during wakefulness. Patients with panic disorders may also suffer from agoraphobia, which is characterized by a fear of being in certain situations where escape may be difficult, such as in a crowded environment or a moving vehicle. The features of agoraphobia and daytime panic episodes are important in order to differentiate panic disorder from awakenings with panic due to other disorders, such as SLEEP TERRORS, which may have a similar presentation.

Patients with the PSYCHOSES, such as schizophrenia or schizoaffective disorder, may have very severe sleep disturbance. This disturbance is characterized by sleep onset difficulties, with small amounts of nocturnal sleep that can alternate with prolonged episodes of sleep. This pattern of sleep may lead to a complete sleep reversal, with no sleep at night and the major sleep episode during the day. Patients with a psychosis can have REM sleep disorders characterized by a reduced REM sleep latency and increased REM density, which is similar to that seen in patients with depression. However, these polysomnographic features are not invariably present, as they are in the depressive disorders.

ALCOHOLISM is associated with severe sleep disturbance due to the acute ingestion of alcohol; it is initially associated with an increase in SLOW WAVE SLEEP, but is followed by a withdrawal effect of sleep disruption, which is seen as the alcohol is metabolized. The chronic alcoholic who abstains from drinking alcohol will have severe sleep disruption. This may be characterized by disrupted REM sleep, hallucinations and NIGHTMARES, as well as disturbed sleep related to autonomic hyperactivity as a result of the alcohol withdrawal. Drinking alcohol during the day will cause impaired daytime functioning because of increased lethargy and sleepiness; that effect is often exacerbated if there was too little sleep the night before.

Other psychiatric disorders, such as substance abuse, adjustment disorder, dissociative and somatoform disorder, can also be associated with either difficulty in initiating and maintaining sleep or excessive sleepiness.

American Psychiatric Association, *Diagnostic and Statistical Manual of Mental Disorders,* 3rd ed., rev. Washington, D.C.: American Psychiatric Association, 1987.

Reite, M., "Sleep Disorders Presenting as Psychiatric Disorders," *Psychiatric Clinics of North America* 21, no. 3 (1998): 591–607.

psychophysiological insomnia A form of INSOMNIA that develops because of learned associations that negatively impact on sleep. Typically, individuals with psychophysiological insomnia tend to react to stress with an increased level of agitation and tension that is often evident by physiological arousal with increased muscle tension and vasoconstriction. With psychophysiological insomnia, there is an overconcern about the inability to fall asleep, which makes it harder to fall asleep. This apprehension may exist throughout the daytime when thinking about the likelihood of little sleep that night.

Sometimes individuals with psychophysiological insomnia can fall asleep at times when it is unexpected, such as relaxing in a chair in the early evening. This reflects their ability to fall asleep when unconcerned about sleep, but when in situations of wanting to fall asleep, the harder the person tries, the less likely it is that sleep will occur. Conditioning factors that contribute to this insomnia include lying in bed awake. The usual sleep environment becomes negatively associated with good sleep. Therefore many individuals with this type of insomnia find that when sleeping in bedrooms other than their own, sleep can occur relatively easily.

Psychophysiological insomnia may be precipitated by a stressful event and may develop subsequent to an ADJUSTMENT SLEEP DISORDER so that after the precipitating event has resolved, the negatively learned associations with sleep continue, and the insomnia becomes chronic. This type of insomnia often becomes fixed over a period of time as intermittent life stress may exacerbate or produce recurrence of psychophysiological insomnia.

Although elements of anxiety and depression are present, particularly in relation to the sleep period, there is little evidence of overt psychopathology. Patients with this form of insomnia do not meet standard psychiatric criteria for the diagnosis of a general anxiety disorder or depression.

Psychophysiological insomnia is uncommon in childhood or adolescence. It will usually present for the first time in the twenties or thirties. More typically, individuals will seek help in middle age. It appears to be more common in females, and there may be a familial tendency.

Polysomnographic monitoring of sleep usually demonstrates a prolonged sleep latency, multiple awakenings, early morning awakening and a reduced sleep efficiency. There may be an increase in the lighter stage one sleep and reduction in a deeper slow wave sleep. Increased muscle tension during sleep can be demonstrated by muscle activity monitoring. Not infrequently, individuals with psychophysiological insomnia will show a reversed "first night effect" in which they sleep much better in the lab on the first night because of the change in their habitual environment; however, the learned negative associations with sleep return by the second night, which demonstrates the reduced quality of sleep.

Psychophysiological insomnia needs to be differentiated from a number of other insomnia disorders. INADEQUATE SLEEP HYGIENE can produce a chronic form of insomnia due to alterations in the timing of sleep, excessive CAFFEINE intake, altered meal times or the ingestion of dietary factors that can adversely affect sleep (see DIET AND SLEEP). An environmental sleep disorder can develop because of such factors as light, noise, abnormal temperature or an uncomfortable or adverse sleeping environment. If anxiety or depression are major factors and warrant a psychiatric diagnosis of either anxiety or mood disorder, the appropriate psychiatric treatment is indicated. If the sleep disturbance is the result of an acute stressful situation, and lasts less than three weeks, then a diagnosis of adjustment sleep disorder is made.

Treatment of psychophysiological insomnia involves redeveloping positive associations with the sleeping environment. Attention to good sleep hygiene is essential, and behavioral management is the most appropriate form of treatment. Relaxation therapy, such as JACOBSONIAN RELAXATION, specific behavioral treatments that may involve STIMULUS CONTROL THERAPY or SLEEP RESTRICTION THERAPY can be helpful. A short or intermittent course of HYPNOTICS may be useful; however, chronic and long-term use of hypnotics is to be discouraged.

Haure, Peter and Fischer, J., "Persistent Psychophysiological (Learned) Insomnia," *Sleep* 9 (1986): 38–53.

Perlis, M.L. et al., "Psychophysiological Insomnia: the Behavioral Model and a Neurocognitive Perspective," *Journal of Sleep Research* 6, no. 3 (1997): 179–188.

psychoses PSYCHIATRIC DISORDERS characterized by the presence of delusions, hallucinations, inappropriate effect, incoherence and catatonic behavior, which lead to impaired social and work functioning. Sleep disturbance, either INSOMNIA or EXCESSIVE SLEEPINESS, is a common feature of these disorders.

Psychoses can be produced by organic neurological disorders, as well as by DEMENTIA, ALCOHOLISM, drug effects, schizophrenia, AFFECTIVE DISORDERS, paranoid states and autism.

The sleep disturbances associated with psychoses are typically sleep disruption, with a severe difficulty in initiating sleep. There may be an inadequate amount of sleep because of hyperactivity associated with the psychotic disorder, which leads to a partial or complete reversal of the sleep-wake cycle. Daytime sleepiness may result due to the disturbed sleep at night or the disrupted sleep-wake pattern.

Polysomnographic studies of patients with psychoses have shown varied sleep patterns; some patients will even show normal sleep. Typically there is an increased SLEEP LATENCY, decreased total sleep time, reduced SLEEP EFFICIENCY with frequent awakenings, and reduced SLOW WAVE SLEEP. There may be features of disturbed REM sleep, such as shortened REM latency, increased REM density and varied percentages of REM sleep.

Treatment of the psychoses is by pharmacological means and typically involves the use of phenothiazine medications. The drug therapy may produce sedation, insomnia or withdrawal syndromes. Institutionalization may be required for patients with psychoses who have a severe impairment of their ability to adequately function in society.

Kupfer, David J., Wyatt, R.J., Scott, J. and Snyder, F., "Sleep Disturbance in Acute Schizophrenic Patients," *MJ Psychiatry* 126 (1970): 1312–1323.

Zarcone, V.P., "Sleep and Schizophrenia," in Williams, R.L., Karacan, I. and Moore, C.A., eds., *Sleep Disorders: Diagnoses and Treatment.* New York: John Wiley, 1988. pp. 175–188.

pulmonary hypertension An increased pressure in the pulmonary arteries that leads to hypertrophy and dilation of the right side of the heart. The most potent stimulus for pulmonary constriction leading to pulmonary hypertension is alveolar HYPOXIA. Hypoxia may be produced by SLEEP-RELATED BREATHING DISORDERS that impair ventilation of the lungs. Pulmonary hypertension can be a consequence of severe OBSTRUCTIVE SLEEP APNEA SYNDROME or CENTRAL ALVEOLAR HYPOVENTILATION SYNDROME.

pupillometry The measurement of pupil diameter and activity. Large, stable pupils are associated with alertness, and small, unstable pupils are associated with decreased alertness and sleepiness. Variations and fluctuations in pupil size can be measured by a pupillometer. The pupillometry test is mainly used as a research procedure to determine sleepiness and has little diagnostic usefulness.

Q

quiet sleep Term used to describe NON-REM-STAGE SLEEP that is seen in infants and animals when the specific sleep phases from one through four are unable to be clearly determined. Quiet sleep usually refers to an encephalographic pattern of sleep in the absence of eye movement recordings or muscle tone recording. The term "non-REM" is preferred when specific SLEEP STAGES are able to be determined. Quiet sleep is distinguished from ACTIVE SLEEP, in which there is an increase in body movement and faster electroencephalographic patterns.

R

raphe nuclei Serotonin-containing neurons in two columns that extend from the medulla to the upper border of the PONS. This region was considered to be important in the maintenance of NON-REM-STAGE SLEEP and SLOW WAVE SLEEP because lesions in the area of the raphe nuclei produced INSOMNIA in cats. If the cells of the raphe nuclei are exposed to an anti-serotonergic agent that inhibits the production of SEROTONIN, such as parachorophenylalanine (PCPA), insomnia will result. However, more recent evidence has suggested that the serotonin-containing cells are not essential for the production of non-REM sleep. But the serotonin-containing neurons may facilitate the onset of slow wave sleep, possibly through a mechanism that stimulates synthesis of sleep factors. The serotonergic raphe neurons project to the hypothalamus, which is thought to be the primary site of the production of sleep factors.

Destruction of the raphe nuclei is associated with an increase in PGO waves, whereas stimulation of the raphe nuclei causes a reduction of PGO activity. It has been suggested that the role of the raphe nuclei is to inhibit the production of PGO waves during wakefulness and contain their activity to REM sleep. (See also LOCUS CERULEUS.)

rapid eye movements The presence of rapid eye movements during sleep was first discovered by Eugene Aserinsky and NATHANIEL KLEITMAN in 1953. This historic discovery of REM sleep led to the recognition that sleep was not a homogeneous state but consisted of two major divisions, REM sleep and non-REM sleep.

Rapid eye movements are seen during wakefulness but are also characteristic of the rapid eye movement stage of sleep (REM sleep). The EEG pattern and muscle tone distinguish the presence of REM sleep from wakefulness, although the pattern of the rapid eye movements usually differs and is characteristic in REM sleep. The movements often occur in discrete bursts in REM sleep. In addition, the presence of the sawtooth EEG pattern in association with the rapid eye movements assists in the determination of REM sleep. The eye movements are conjugate (move together) and can occur in a vertical, horizontal or diagonal direction. The rapid eye movements can be seen under the closed eyelids.

With the discovery of the association of dreaming and rapid eye movement sleep it was initially thought that the rapid eye movements reflected visual scanning of the content of dreams. Subsequent research suggested this was not the case; the rapid eye movements bore no relation to the dream content. (See also REM DENSITY, REM-OFF CELLS, REM-ON CELLS, REM PARASOMNIAS, REM SLEEP, REM SLEEP LATENCY, REM SLEEP ONSET, REM SLEEP PERCENT, REM SLEEP PERIOD.)

Aserinsky, Eugene and Kleitman, Nathaniel, "Regularly Occurring Periods of Eye Motility and Concomitant Phenomena During Sleep," *Science* 118 (1953): 273–274.

rapid eye movement sleep (REM sleep) One of the five stages of sleep that are scored according to the method of Alan Rechtschaffen and Anthony Kales. REM sleep is defined by the appearance of a relatively low voltage, mixed frequency EEG activity and episodic, rapid eye movements that occur simultaneously. The EEG pattern resembles stage one sleep (see SLEEP STAGES), with the exception that there are fewer vertex sharp transients and, sometimes, distinctive "saw tooth" waves. The muscle activity is usually at its lowest degree of tone as the skeletal muscles become paralyzed in this sleep stage (see REM ATONIA).

The loss of muscle tone is due to a hyperpolarizing inhibitory activation of the alpha motor neuron. The REM phasic activity is due to excitatory input on the motor-neurone, which is superimposed on a background of inhibitory input. All striated muscle is affected by the phasic jerks and twitches that occur during REM sleep. Rapid eye movements, contractions of the middle ear musculature and the irregular contractions of the respiratory muscles are all components of this phasic muscle activity.

REM sleep typically comprises about 20% to 25% of normal adult sleep. However, the percentage in childhood is greater, with up to 50% of sleep being REM sleep in infancy.

Usually there are five NREM-REM SLEEP CYCLES in a full night of sleep, with REM sleep occurring in episodes of increasing duration from 10 to 30 minutes.

REM sleep is also associated with other physiological changes, such as an increased oxygen consumption of the brain compared with that during non-REM sleep, variability of blood pressure and heart rhythm, variable respiratory rate and altered blood gas control. Body TEMPERATURE control also differs during REM sleep compared with non-REM sleep.

Certain pathological events are more likely to occur during REM sleep, such as obstructive sleep apneas (see OBSTRUCTIVE SLEEP APNEA SYNDROME) and blood oxygen desaturation. Some disorders occur solely during REM sleep, such as the REM SLEEP BEHAVIOR DISORDER, NIGHTMARES and SLEEP-RELATED PAINFUL ERECTIONS. The presence of penile erections during REM sleep is an important finding in the differentiation of IMPOTENCE due to organic versus psychogenic causes. Normal erections during REM sleep in a patient complaining of impotence generally reflect a psychogenic cause of the impotence.

Rechtschaffen, Alan and Kales, Anthony, eds., *A Manual of Standardized Terminology, Techniques, and Scoring System for Sleep Stages of Human Subjects.* Los Angeles: Brain Information Service, University of California, 1968.

Howland, R.H., "Sleep-Onset Rapid Eye Movement Periods in Neuropsychiatric Disorders: Implications for the Pathophysiology of Psychosis," *The Journal of Nervous and Mental Diseases* 185, no. 12 (1997): 730–738.

rebound insomnia INSOMNIA that occurs upon acute withdrawal of hypnotic medication. This form of insomnia more commonly occurs in persons who are on high dosages of HYPNOTICS, particularly short-acting hypnotics. It is less likely to occur in persons who take hypnotic agents for a brief period of time.

Rebound insomnia is characterized by increased sleep disruption with a greater number of awakenings and sleep stage changes that occur upon cessation of the medication. It can be reduced by a gradual decrease in dosage prior to withdrawal. All patients withdrawing from hypnotic medication should be reassured that some sleep disruption is likely for the first few days following cessation of drug treatment. But as long as good SLEEP HYGIENE is instituted, and other causes of insomnia are not present, sleep should return to normal within a few days. (See also BARBITURATES, BENZODIAZEPINES, HYPNOTIC-DEPENDENT SLEEP DISORDER.)

Rechtschaffen, Alan Dr. Rechtschaffen (1927–) received his Ph.D. in psychology from Northwestern University in 1956. In 1957, he became an instructor in psychology in the Department of Psychiatry at the University of Chicago. Beginning in 1968, he was a professor of psychology in the Departments of Psychiatry and Psychology at the University of Chicago. He is now retired.

Dr. Rechtschaffen's sleep research areas included the physiology of sleep and the effects of sleep deprivation, as well as work on dream psychophysiology and phylogeny of sleep. (See also WILLIAM DEMENT, DREAMS, NON-REM-STAGE SLEEP, REM SLEEP, SLEEP DEPRIVATION.)

Dr. Rechtschaffen received the Distinguished Service Award of the Sleep Research Society in 1989. He is also the recipient of the Lifetime Achievement Award from the WORLD FEDERATION OF SLEEP RESEARCH SOCIETIES.

Rechtschaffen, Alan, Gilliland, M.A., Bergmann, B.M. and Winter, J.B., "Physiological Correlates of Prolonged Sleep Deprivation in Rats," *Science* 221 (1983): 182–184.

Rechtschaffen, Alan and Kales, Anthony, eds., *A Manual of Standardized Terminology, Techniques, and Scoring System for Sleep Stages of Human Subjects.* Los Angeles: Brain Information Service, University of California, 1968.

reciprocal interaction model of sleep First proposed by J. Allan Hobson, Robert McCarley and Peter W. Wyzinski in 1975 to explain the cellular interactions in the regulation of REM sleep. They suggested that there are two sets of cells, the REM-OFF CELLS and REM-ON CELLS, that are located in the pontine region of the brain stem. The REM-on cells cause the initiation of REM sleep, and the REM-off cells cause the termination of REM sleep. The REM-on cells are situated near the REM-on cells in a similar region of the brain stem and include the serotonergic cells of the RAPHE NUCLEI. Since the original proposal, the model has been modified to include both explanations of non-REM sleep and waking. (See also GIGANTOCELLULAR TEGMENTAL FIELD, ASCENDING RETICULAR ACTIVATING SYSTEM, SEROTONIN.)

recurrent hypersomnia A group of disorders characterized by recurrent episodes of EXCESSIVE SLEEPINESS that occur weeks or months apart. These disorders may be associated with other symptoms, such as gluttony or hypersexuality. The combination of recurrent hypersomnia, gluttony and hypersexuality is also known as the KLEINE-LEVIN SYNDROME, which was first described by Willi Kleine in 1925 and Max Levin in 1929. However, a form of recurrent hypersomnia can exist without features of gluttony or hypersexuality; it is then called recurrent hypersomnia monosymptomatic type.

Recurrent hypersomnia more commonly occurs in adolescents or young adults. Typically an episode of excessive sleepiness will occur over a one-to-two-week period followed by weeks or months of normal daytime alertness. There often are personality disturbances, such as withdrawal, irritability and lethargy. Persons with this disorder may eat excessively and start to eat any food in sight. The hypersexuality is characterized by excessive discussion or display of sexual behavior along with public masturbation.

Episodes occur very infrequently and, on average, occur twice a year. Some patients may go many years without an episode or may have as many as one episode each month.

During the period of hypersomnolence, there can be great impairment of social and occupational functioning. The behavior changes can be so intense that the patient requires hospitalization.

Polysomnographic investigation has tended to show excessive sleepiness with high sleep efficiencies and reduced awake time during sleep. A loss of the deeper stage three and four sleep has been demonstrated; however, MULTIPLE SLEEP LATENCY TESTING during the daytime has shown the presence of sleep onset REM periods on one or more naps.

The disorder is believed to be in part due to a hypothalamic dysfunction. There have been some reports of abnormal hormone secretory patterns during sleep. GROWTH HORMONE and PROLACTIN secretion may be abnormal.

A recurrent form of hypersomnia, MENSTRUAL-ASSOCIATED SLEEP DISORDER, also occurs in relationship to the MENSTRUAL CYCLE and is characterized by insomnia and hypersomnia.

Recurrent hypersomnia needs to be differentiated from hypersomnias due to central nervous system tumors and other causes of excessive sleepiness, such as IDIOPATHIC HYPERSOMNIA, NARCOLEPSY and INSUFFICIENT SLEEP SYNDROME. Excessive sleepiness due to PSYCHIATRIC DISORDERS, such as major DEPRESSION or bipolar depression, may present similarly, with the exception of the gluttony and hypersexuality.

Treatment of recurrent hypersomnia is largely supportive. Lithium carbonate has been reported to stabilize the behavior in some patients but not in others. The effect of STIMULANT MEDICATIONS in improving alertness is usually only very temporary. (See also DISORDERS OF EXCESSIVE SOMNOLENCE, MOOD DISORDERS.)

Critchley, M. and Hoffman, H.L., "The Sojourn of Periodic Somnolence and Morbid Hunger (Kleine-Levin Syndrome)," *British Medical Journal* 1 (1942): 137–139.

Reynolds, C.F., Kupfer, D.J., Christianson, C.L. et al., "Multiple Sleep Latency Test Findings in Kleine-Levin Syndrome," *Journal of Nervous and Mental Disease* 172 (1984): 41–44.

relaxation exercises A variety of techniques to enhance muscle relaxation in order to reduce muscle tension and help sleep onset. Various forms of relaxation exercises are utilized; however, one of the most commonly used is the JACOBSONIAN RELAXATION method. BIOFEEDBACK exercises can also enhance relaxation. (See also SLEEP EXERCISES.)

REM atonia The atonia (loss of muscle tone) of REM sleep causes the skeletal muscles to become flaccid so that the arms and legs are paralyzed. REM sleep cannot be scored if the ELECTROMYOGRAM (EMG) muscle activity is increased. Only a few muscles have the ability to move during REM sleep, such as the eye muscles, the auditory muscles, and the diaphragm for respiration. Occasional phasic (short burst) muscle activity is seen during the atonia of REM sleep.

Some disorders, such as the REM SLEEP BEHAVIOR DISORDER, are associated with a variable degree of muscle activity that episodically occurs during REM sleep and leads to the behavior that is characteristic of the disorder. The polygraphic features of REM sleep behavior disorder indicate a disrupted and dissociated form of REM sleep. The REM behavior disorder is not too dissimilar to an experimental condition seen in cats with neurological lesions placed in the pontine region of the brain stem. Cats with such lesions have the absence of the REM atonia and are able to move around during REM sleep. It has been proposed that there are two systems in the nervous system that control muscle tone and movement during REM sleep: a locomotor system and a system that determines atonia. Usually the locomotor system is inhibited by REM sleep simultaneously with activation of the system producing the muscle atonia during REM sleep. (See also RAPID EYE MOVEMENT SLEEP.)

Morrison, A.R., "A Window on the Sleeping Brain," *Scientific American* (1983): 94–102.

REM-beta activity Beta rhythm that occurs during REM sleep. This particular electroencephalographic pattern can be seen in patients who have ingested medications, particularly the BENZODIAZEPINE hypnotics (see also HYPNOTICS), such as flurazepam. The presence of increased beta activity during REM sleep and other sleep stages may persist for as long as two weeks after the last ingestion of the hypnotic agent. (See also BETA RHYTHM, RAPID EYE MOVEMENT SLEEP.)

REM density The frequency of eye movements that occur during REM SLEEP; usually expressed as the number of eye movements per minute of REM sleep. REM density may be increased in patients with DEPRESSION; treatment with tricyclic ANTIDEPRESSANTS can reduce REM density. Although REM density can be an indicator of depression, it is less useful than the presence of a shortened REM SLEEP LATENCY in aiding the diagnosis of such patients.

REM-off cells Cells believed to inhibit the REM-ON CELLS and, by so doing, stop the occurrence of REM sleep. These cells are believed to be located in the pontine region of the brain stem and include the RAPHE NUCLEI. (See also GIGANTOCELLULAR TEGMENTAL FIELD, RECIPROCAL INTERACTION MODEL OF SLEEP.)

REM-on cells Cells believed to be responsible for the initiation of REM SLEEP; located in the GIGANTOCELLULAR TEGMENTAL FIELD of the pons. (See also RECIPROCAL INTERACTION MODEL OF SLEEP, REM-OFF CELLS.)

REM parasomnias Abnormalities that occur during sleep that are not associated with excessive sleepiness or insomnia but are usually associated with REM sleep; a subdivision of the parasomnias and the INTERNATIONAL CLASSIFICATION OF SLEEP DISORDERS. The parasomnias in this section include NIGHTMARES, SLEEP PARALYSIS, IMPAIRED SLEEP-RELATED PENILE ERECTIONS, SLEEP-RELATED PAINFUL ERECTIONS, REM SLEEP-RELATED SINUS ARREST, and REM SLEEP BEHAVIOR DISORDER.

REM rebound An increase in the amount, duration and density of REM sleep that occurs following the curtailment of a variety of techniques that have suppressed REM sleep. For example, REM rebound can occur following medication suppression of REM sleep by such drugs as the tricyclic ANTIDEPRESSANTS or MONOAMINE OXIDASE INHIBI-

TORS, commonly used for the treatment of DEPRESSION.

Another means of producing REM sleep deprivation is by mechanically arousing an individual whenever REM sleep is detected during a polysomnographic recording. This procedure not only reduces REM sleep but also causes frequent arousals during the major sleep episode. Following this method of REM sleep deprivation there is a rebound of REM sleep.

Some disorders, such as OBSTRUCTIVE SLEEP APNEA SYNDROME, can markedly interfere with the ability of the subject to maintain REM sleep; its relief by either TRACHEOSTOMY or CONTINUOUS POSITIVE AIRWAY PRESSURE devices can lead to an initial REM rebound. REM sleep episodes lasting several hours can sometimes be seen in these situations.

A REM rebound is often accompanied by an increase in awareness of having had long and complex DREAMS. Occasionally NIGHTMARE activity may be exacerbated by the REM rebound. ALCOHOL is also a REM suppressant drug and its withdrawal, particularly in the chronic alcoholic, can lead to a REM rebound, with an increase in nightmares.

REM sleep See RAPID EYE MOVEMENT SLEEP.

REM sleep behavior disorder Disorder characterized by the acting out of dream content during the dreaming stage (REM SLEEP) of sleep. Typically, affected persons will have a predominance of violent activity that occurs during sleep and involves punching, kicking, running or other movements of the limbs. These movements may injure a bed partner, which precipitates the disorder being brought to medical attention. The episodes usually occur about 90 minutes after the onset of sleep when the person goes into REM sleep; however, it can occur throughout the major sleep episode. Very often episodes may be precipitated by withdrawal from ALCOHOL or other HYPNOTICS. The disorder has also been described as occurring in association with NARCOLEPSY. There may be partial manifestations of the disorder, evidenced by episodes of SLEEP TALKING or limb movements that may antedate the development of the more physically active behavior.

The most common age of presentation is after age 60; however, episodes have been reported to occur in childhood and in individuals of any age with neurological disorders such as cerebral vascular disease, degeneration or tumors of the brain stem, and DEMENTIA. It has also been described in association with multiple sclerosis. Recent evidence indicates that REM sleep behavior disorder can be a precursor to the development of Parkinson's disease.

The majority of persons with REM sleep behavior disorder appear to be male, and there is some evidence to suggest a familial pattern.

An identical disorder has been described in animals who have suffered lesions in the brain stem. Cats with lesions affecting the locomotor inhibitory region of the brain stem often will have motor activity during REM sleep.

Polysomnographic monitoring of persons with this disorder has shown an intermittent absence of muscle tone. Concurrent rapid eye movements indicative of REM sleep alternate with high muscle activity lasting a few seconds prior to the immediate resumption of REM sleep. There may be an increase in the density of the rapid eye movements and also in the total amount of SLOW WAVE SLEEP.

REM sleep behavior disorder needs to be differentiated from SLEEP-RELATED EPILEPSY or other disorders of arousal, such as SLEEPWALKING or SLEEP TERRORS. Nightmares may be somewhat similar but are characterized by less motor activity and lack of the typical polysomnographic features of REM sleep behavior disorder.

Treatment of REM sleep behavior disorder involves securing the bedroom—such as removing sharp objects from nightstands—so the individual does not suffer injury. Clonazepam (see BENZODIAZEPINES) in a dose of 0.5 to 1 milligram, given before sleep at night, has been shown to be very effective in suppressing the behavior. Occasionally tricyclic antidepressants have been shown to be effective as well.

Case History

A 58-year-old real estate executive had episodes of excessive body activity in association with dreams at night. On occasion, he would hit the nightstand or his wife while moving about excessively during sleep. These episodes had occurred over the previous five years. He did have a history of sleepwalking as a child; however, this went away in adolescence and had never reoccurred. The current activity during sleep was characterized by a lot of violent activity, particularly boxing or fighting an individual, and was very different from his childhood sleepwalking episodes. At times, his wife, who was lying quietly beside him, would become the focus of his dream activity and occasionally would get in the way of some of his more violent movements. On one occasion, his activity caused him to fall out of bed and he cut his head on the nightstand. All of the activity was associated with dream content, and he appeared to be actually trying to act out dreams during sleep. He was on no medication at this time, and had sought help from several physicians. His baseline blood work and brain scan were normal. There was no evidence of any underlying neurological disorder. He underwent an all-night POLYSOMNOGRAM, which demonstrated much restlessness during REM sleep with an abnormal amount of muscle activity; REM sleep was very fragmented.

A diagnosis of REM sleep behavior disorder was made on the clinical history and the polysomnographic data. He was prescribed clonazepam (0.5 milligram) to take before sleep at night. With this medication, the activity abruptly subsided and he had a quiet night's sleep. The patient noticed considerable improvement over the subsequent two months; however, some activity reoccurred and the dosage was increased to 1 milligram, whereupon the episodes subsided and remained absent over the subsequent months.

Schenck, C.H., Bundlie, S.R., Patterson, A.L. and Mahowald, M.W., "Rapid Eye Movement Sleep Behavior Disorder: A Treatable Parasomnia Affecting Older Males," *Journal of American Medical Association* 257 (1987): 1786–1789.

REM sleep deprivation REM SLEEP deprivation can be produced by mechanically preventing REM sleep from occurring, or by the use of REM suppressant medications. A patient may be mechanically aroused whenever a polygraph shows that he is entering REM sleep; however, this tends to produce frequent arousals and therefore the effects of REM deprivation may be masked by the effects of the frequent arousals or awakenings. A variety of medications, including antidepressant medications such as tricyclic ANTIDEPRESSANTS or MONOAMINE OXIDASE INHIBITORS, as well as BENZODIAZEPINES, STIMULANTS and ALCOHOL, can usually inhibit REM sleep.

The initial effects of REM sleep deprivation are an increase in brain activity; aggressive and sexual behavior may be increased. Psychological difficulties have been reported as the result of REM deprivation; however, recent evidence tends to suggest that this is an unlikely effect.

Positive effects of REM deprivation can include improvement of DEPRESSION, and several studies have shown this to be clinically useful.

The most pronounced effect of REM sleep deprivation is REM REBOUND, with a dramatic increase in the amount and duration of REM sleep episodes. (See also DREAMS.)

REM sleep and dreaming In 1953, Eugene Aserinsky and NATHANIEL KLEITMAN at the University of Chicago made a major scientific development in the study of dreams when they recognized physiological changes during dreaming and rapid eye movements (REM). Over the next few years, joined by WILLIAM C. DEMENT, the researchers compared dream recall during REM versus NREM SLEEP PERIODS. By 1957, the results of these experiments were published: Subjects awakened 191 times during REM periods had dream recall 80% of the time, or in 152 of the awakenings. By contrast, subjects were awoken 160 times during NREM periods, with only 6.9% or 11 dream recalls. Dement writes in *Some Must Watch While Some Must Dream:* "When compared to the overall NREM results, the REM period was unquestionably established as the time when the probability of being able to recall a dream is maximal."

Dement further notes that persons who keep dream diaries at home will recall only one dream when interviewed the next morning about their dreams. By contrast, subjects in a laboratory, when awakened throughout the REM periods, will remember four out of the five dreams that occur during the REM period, forgetting only 20% of their dreams. (See also REM SLEEP.)

Dement, William C., *Some Must Watch While Some Must Dream*. New York: W.W. Norton, 1976.

REM sleep intrusion A brief episode of REM SLEEP that occurs during non-REM sleep. The term may also be applied to the occurrence of a single, disassociated component of REM sleep, such as eye movements or loss of muscle tone, that occurs in the absence of all typical features of REM sleep. It may also apply to a brief episode of REM sleep that occurs out of sequence with the normal NREM-REM SLEEP CYCLE. REM sleep intrusion may be seen in severe sleep disruption due to an INSOMNIA of many causes or in disturbances of REM sleep, such as fragmentation seen as a result of medication or other sleep disorders, such as NARCOLEPSY.

REM sleep latency The interval from sleep onset to the first appearance of REM sleep during a sleep episode. In normal, healthy adults, REM sleep usually occurs approximately 90 minutes after the onset of non-REM sleep. A short REM latency is seen in patients who have DEPRESSION and may be a biological marker of depression. Treatment of depression in such patients often leads to a normalization of the REM latency. REM latencies of less than 65 minutes are regarded as being shorter than normal. A short REM latency may also be seen in patients who acutely withdraw from a REM suppressant medication, such as tricyclic ANTIDEPRESSANTS, ALCOHOL or MONOAMINE OXIDASE INHIBITORS.

In NARCOLEPSY, the REM sleep latency is usually reduced. Patients may sometimes go directly into REM sleep. However, this is not always present. The presence of REM sleep during a daytime MULTIPLE SLEEP LATENCY TEST has more diagnostic usefulness. The occurrence of REM sleep within 10 minutes of initiating a daytime nap is regarded as supportive evidence of narcolepsy. Two or more sleep onset REM periods during a multiple sleep latency test that is performed following a night of normal sleep is diagnostic of narcolepsy.

Infants (see INFANT SLEEP) have a much greater percentage of REM sleep (in contrast to adults) and will frequently initiate their short sleep episodes by an immediate occurrence of REM sleep; therefore, a short REM sleep latency is commonly seen.

REM sleep-locked This term has been used for the close association between CHRONIC PAROXYSMAL HEMICRANIA (a type of headache) and REM SLEEP. Episodes of chronic paroxysmal hemicrania during sleep always occur in association with REM sleep. (See also SLEEP-RELATED HEADACHES.)

REM sleep onset The occurrence of REM sleep at sleep onset; occasionally used instead of the longer SLEEP ONSET REM PERIOD, which is the preferred term.

REM sleep percent The proportion of total sleep time that is filled by REM sleep. For adults, a typical night of sleep is comprised of 20% to 25% REM sleep; in an infant, REM sleep equals 50% of the total sleep time. The percentage of REM sleep falls slightly from young adulthood to old age. (See also RAPID EYE MOVEMENT SLEEP.)

REM sleep period Occasionally used for an episode of REM SLEEP that occurs during the major sleep episode. The term is discouraged from use because the word "period" implies a cyclical event; therefore, REM sleep period may be confused with the NREM-REM SLEEP CYCLE.

REM sleep-related sinus arrest A disorder of cardiac rhythm that produces episodes of sinus arrest during REM SLEEP in otherwise healthy individuals. This disorder has been described in young adults and appears to be associated with symptoms that include acute discomfort, sudden palpitations, light-headedness, feeling of faintness and blurred vision. Some individuals with this disorder have reported episodes of syncope (fainting) that have occurred during the nocturnal hours.

The diagnosis is based entirely upon the presence of episodes of sinus arrest of at least 2.5 seconds in duration, which suddenly occur during REM sleep. Episodes as long as 9 seconds have been reported. Additional investigations, including coronary angiography and electrical conduction studies, are normal.

The episodes of ARRHYTHMIA are not associated with sleep-related respiratory disturbance or oxygen desaturation. They occur in clusters and do not induce arousals or awakenings.

This disorder must be differentiated from the cardiac irregularity characterized by brady-tachycardia that is typically seen in the OBSTRUCTIVE SLEEP APNEA SYNDROME.

If the episodes are frequent in occurrence and long in duration, consideration should be given to implantation of a ventricular inhibited pacemaker in order to prevent episodes of cardiac arrest.

Guilleminault, Christian, Pool, P., Motta, J. and Gillis, A.M., "Sinus Arrest During REM Sleep in Young Adults," *New England Journal of Medicine* 311 (1984): 1006–1010.

RERA See RESPIRATORY EFFORT–RELATED AROUSAL.

respiratory disturbance index (RDI) Also known as APNEA-HYPOPNEA INDEX. RDI is a measure of the number of apneas, both central and obstructive, plus the number of hypopneas, expressed per hour of sleep. A respiratory disturbance index of greater than five is regarded as an abnormal frequency of respiratory events during sleep. This index is commonly used as a measure of the severity of the sleep apnea syndromes. Many authors regard the term RDI as preferable to the apnea-hypopnea index because it is more descriptive for those not familiar with the term HYPOPNEA. (See also APNEA, CENTRAL SLEEP APNEA SYNDROME, OBSTRUCTIVE SLEEP APNEA SYNDROME.)

respiratory effort Applies to respiratory muscle activity; typically measured during sleep to determine the degree of respiratory impairment. Patients who have cessation of respiratory movements during sleep, as is seen during an apneic episode, will have no respiratory effort, whereas patients with the OBSTRUCTIVE SLEEP APNEA SYNDROME may have an increased degree of respiratory effort, particularly immediately prior to the termination of the obstructive event. Respiratory effort does not imply that there is a transfer of air between the atmosphere and the lung because complete airway obstruction may occur despite the presence of respiratory effort.

Respiratory effort can be measured by means of a mercury-filled strain gauge, a bellows pneumograph or INDUCTIVE PLETHYSMOGRAPHY. (See also APNEA, CENTRAL SLEEP APNEA SYNDROME.)

respiratory effort–related arousal (RERA) An arousal associated with increasing negative esophageal pressure which is terminated by a sudden change in pressure to a less negative level with an arousal. The event lasts 10 seconds or longer.

Five or more RERAs per hour are regarded as abnormal and in association with other symptoms are sufficient to produce a diagnosis of OBSTRUCTIVE SLEEP APNEA SYNDROME. (See also CENTRAL SLEEP APNEA SYNDROME.)

respiratory stimulants Drugs used in SLEEP DISORDERS MEDICINE for the stimulation of VENTILATION in SLEEP-RELATED BREATHING DISORDERS such as CENTRAL SLEEP APNEA SYNDROME or OBSTRUCTIVE SLEEP APNEA SYNDROME.

Acetazolamide (Diamox)

A carbonic anhydrase inhibitor used as a respiratory stimulant for the treatment of breathing disorders such as central sleep apnea syndrome. This agent is primarily used for central sleep apnea syndrome due to central nervous system lesions or impaired circulation time. It is also an effective agent for the treatment of ALTITUDE INSOMNIA (acute mountain sickness) and may be partially beneficial in the treatment of the obstructive sleep apnea syndrome.

This drug affects carbonic anhydrase activity, leading to a rise in the carbon dioxide tension in the tissues that stimulates the chemoreceptors, resulting in increased respiratory stimulation.

Acetazolamide has diuretic properties and can cause an increase in NOCTURIA. Other side effects include paresthesia (abnormal sensory symptoms, such as numbness and tingling) and daytime DROWSINESS.

Medroxyprogesterone

Medroxyprogesterone acetate is a derivative of the naturally-produced hormone progesterone, which is used in sleep disorders medicine as a respiratory stimulant for the promotion of ventilation. Medroxyprogesterone has been demonstrated to be effective in some patients with the obstructive sleep apnea syndrome, although it may be more useful for patients who have central sleep apnea syndrome or CENTRAL ALVEOLAR HYPOVENTILATION SYNDROME. However, optimal therapy still does not completely eliminate the respiratory disturbance during sleep, and therefore other treatments for the sleep-related breathing disorders are preferable, such as assisted ventilation devices.

The effect of medroxyprogesterone appears to be by means of increasing respiratory center chemosensitivity to alterations in the blood gases.

Adverse side effects of medroxyprogesterone include reduced libido, fluid retention and an increased likelihood of thrombosis; therefore its usefulness is limited. Provera is the trade or pharmaceutical name for medroxyprogesterone.

Methylxanthines

A group of stimulant medications that includes CAFFEINE, theophylline and theobromine. These alkaloids occur in plants that are widely found in nature, and the leaves are often used to create beverages such as tea, cocoa and coffee.

The methylxanthines are used to stimulate the central nervous system in order to improve alertness but also to relax muscles, such as the muscle of the lung airways. Theophylline is particularly useful for the treatment of asthma and CHRONIC OBSTRUCTIVE PULMONARY DISEASE because of its effect of relaxing bronchial muscle. However, theophylline is an even stronger central nervous system stimulant than caffeine. It can stimulate the medullary respiratory center and can be useful for treating sleep-related breathing disorders of infants and also Cheyne-Stokes breathing. The methylxanthines also cause cardiac stimulation and theophylline can produce an increase in heart rate, even precipitating cardiac irregularity in some sensitive people. Theophylline, if taken for breathing disorders during sleep, can cause so much stimulation that INSOMNIA may result. (See also CHEYNE-STOKES RESPIRATION, INFANT SLEEP DISORDERS.)

restless legs syndrome A disorder associated with discomfort experienced in both legs as well as the uncontrollable urge to keep moving the legs. This discomfort is described as a crawling, tickling, itching sensation in the legs and is usually found in the calf, feet and sometimes in the thigh. It is rarely experienced as a pain. This syndrome was first described by K.A. Ekbom in 1945, and it is recognized as a cause of difficulty in falling asleep at night. The legs are moved around in bed to find a comfortable position, and often the patient has to get out of bed to walk around. Rubbing the calves and exercising the muscles often produces a temporary relief.

The discomfort is typically present at sleep onset, although it often can occur during wakeful episodes during the night. Sometimes the sensation is also experienced during the daytime when lying down or sitting.

The discomfort may be very intense and has been said to have driven sufferers, on rare occasion, to commit suicide.

Since restless legs syndrome is typically associated with PERIODIC LEG MOVEMENTS, treatment may be required for both conditions. Polysomnographic evaluation of restless legs syndrome demonstrates movement of the legs that occurs at sleep onset and a prolonged SLEEP LATENCY. There may be further episodes of leg movements occurring during wakeful episodes throughout the night. Intermittent periodic leg movements can be seen in sleep throughout the polysomnographic recording.

Restless legs syndrome needs to be differentiated from other disorders that produce abnormal movements during sleep. SLEEP STARTS are whole body jerks that occur only at sleep onset. The restless movements that occur during REM SLEEP BEHAVIOR DISORDER typically occur during REM sleep at night and are associated with more violent movements, reflecting the acting out of DREAMS. NOCTURNAL PAROXYSMAL DYSTONIA is a disorder associated with abnormal posturing of the limbs; it typically occurs during non-REM sleep and not at sleep onset.

Although the cause of this disorder is unknown, relief of the discomfort is available by using a variety of medications including the anticonvulsants as well as the HYPNOTICS. Carbamazepine (see ANTIDEPRESSANTS) may be helpful in some patients; however, many patients do not respond to this medication. The most effective BENZODIAZEPINE is clonazepam, which is also effective against the periodic leg movements that can occur in association with restless legs syndrome. However, other benzodiazepines, such as trizolam, and narcotic derivatives, such as oxycodone, have also been shown to be useful in some patients.

L-DOPA has been shown to be effective in reducing the number of episodes of both restless legs syndrome and periodic leg movement during sleep. Other dopaminergic agents such as PRAMIPEXOLE have also proved to be very effective and now have become the medications of choice.

Ekbom, K.A., "Restless Leg Syndrome," *Neurology* 10 (1960): 868–873.

Mahowald, M.W. et al., "Parasomnias Including the Restless Legs Syndrome," *Clinics of Sleep Medicine* 19, no. 1 (1998): 183–202.

Silber, M.H., "Restless Leg Syndrome," *Mayo Clinic Proceedings* 72, no. 3 (1997): 261–264.

restlessness Term applied to increased body movements occurring during sleep. Restlessness (a restless sleep) is often an indication of an underlying sleep disorder, and therefore investigation by appropriate polysomnographic studies may be indicated. Although occasional awakenings are not uncommon in normal, healthy sleepers, in general sleep should be relatively quiet for most individuals.

Restlessness predominantly occurs during disorders that produce INSOMNIA, such as PSYCHOPHYSIOLOGICAL INSOMNIA, or insomnia due to psychiatric disorders. However, it can also occur in other disorders that disrupt sleep, such as the OBSTRUCTIVE SLEEP APNEA SYNDROME, the REM SLEEP BEHAVIOR DISORDER and the RESTLESS LEGS SYNDROME.

Individuals who complain of insomnia will often describe how they stay motionless during sleep with the hope it will enhance sleep onset and reduce the amount of times they awaken during sleep. However, lying in bed awake often makes the individual aware of discomfort related to body position. Restlessness occurs because of the need to keep changing position. Some disorders may be directly associated with discomfort of body position, such as PREGNANCY-RELATED SLEEP DISORDER or the restless legs syndrome. However, in the majority of individuals who suffer from insomnia due to psychophysiological or psychiatric causes, the discomfort experienced is a result of being in a single position for a prolonged period of time while awake. Very often the discomfort is exacerbated by the increased muscular tension and ANXIETY that accompany insomnia. The generalized restlessness that accompanies insomnia often leads to the individual getting out of bed and going to another room or walking about for a period of time before returning to bed. Although the SLEEP SURFACE is sometimes responsible for the discomfort, in most cases it is not the primary cause unless there was a recent change in the sleep surface.

Patients with the obstructive sleep apnea syndrome can be particularly restless. The termination of the apneic events is associated with an increase in body movements, and not uncommonly there are reports of an arm being raised from the bed or the legs changing position. The movements may become excessive and lead the individual to fall out of bed. Not uncommonly, children will adopt a hands/knees position in order to improve their breathing at night.

In the elderly population, in addition to the increased number of causes of insomnia, the REM sleep behavior disorder is associated with increased motor activity during sleep. In this disorder, the individual will tend to act out DREAMS and so there may be quite violent arm and leg movements. Restlessness may be the primary complaint of a spouse.

The restless legs syndrome is characterized by a discomfort experienced in the legs in which the legs have to be moved to relieve the discomfort. Typically, patients will get out of bed in order to walk around thereby easing the pain. Once sleep onset has occurred, generally the legs are still; however, brief interruptions or awakenings of sleep will often be associated with an increase in the leg movements.

Although a number of parasomnias, such as SLEEPWALKING, can be associated with abnormal movement activity, restlessness is usually not a common feature, in part due to the episodic nature of the movements. SLEEP-RELATED EPILEPSY generally produces infrequent episodes during sleep, and therefore a complaint of restless sleep is uncommon.

Restoril See BENZODIAZEPINES.

reticular activating system See ASCENDING RETICULAR ACTIVATING SYSTEM.

reversal of sleep A 12-hour shift in the onset of the major sleep episode. Reversal of sleep has been performed experimentally to determine the effect on circadian rhythmicity. Sleep itself is less efficient when acutely moved, and there is usually a decrease in deep stages three/four sleep and REM sleep (see SLEEP STAGES). Total sleep time is shorter than before the shift, and the REM SLEEP LATENCY is reduced.

Following an acute reversal of the sleep pattern there are changes in underlying circadian rhythms in that some will shift with the change in the sleep pattern, but others will remain fixed at the previous phase. For example, the pattern of cortisol secretion and body temperature adjusts very slowly over a period of one to two weeks to the new time of sleep. Some body rhythms, such as urine volume and electrolyte excretions, shift to the new pattern of sleep within a few days, as does growth hormone secretion.

Reversal of sleep is also applied to individuals who are on a stable pattern of sleeping during the day and awakening at night. In such individuals, the pattern of circadian rhythmicity has adjusted to the new time of sleep and therefore there is no dissociation between circadian rhythms. This pattern is sometimes seen in individuals who have a severe form of the DELAYED SLEEP PHASE SYNDROME. An acute reversal of the sleep pattern also occurs in shift workers and individuals who cross many time zones. (See also CIRCADIAN RHYTHMS, SHIFT-WORK SLEEP DISORDER, TIME ZONE CHANGE (JET LAG) SYNDROME.)

Weitzman, Elliot, Kripke, B.F., Goldmacher, D., McGreagor, P. and Nogeire, C., "Acute Reversal of the Sleep-Waking Cycle in Man," *Archives of Neurology* 22 (1970): 483–489.

reversed first night effect Typically, sleep is of better quality on the first night of polysomnographic recording in the laboratory, and of much reduced quality during the second night. This pattern can be seen in patients with IDIOPATHIC INSOMNIA or PSYCHOPHYSIOLOGICAL INSOMNIA. (See also FIRST NIGHT EFFECT.)

rheumatic pain modulation disorder See FIBROSITIS SYNDROME.

rhythmic movement disorder A disorder characterized by repetitive abnormal movements during sleep such as HEADBANGING, BODYROCKING or leg rolling. These movements usually occur during the lighter stages of sleep or immediately prior to sleep onset; however, rarely they can occur during deep sleep stages or RAPID EYE MOVEMENT (REM) SLEEP. Usually treatment is limited to securing the environment so that banging into solid objects does not harm the individual. For example, a child in a crib may need to have padding affixed to crib bars to prevent injury. Medication treatment is usually not effective although the BENZODIAZEPINES have been helpful in some patients. See also HEAD ROLLING.

rhythms This term applies to a cyclical process and in sleep medicine mainly applies to the sleep-wake rhythm. Rhythms that occur within a 24-hour cycle are called CIRCADIAN RHYTHMS. Rhythms less than 24 hours are called ultradian (see ULTRADIAN RHYTHM), and those greater than 24 hours are called infradian.

The most frequently studied rhythms in human physiology are the circadian rhythms, of which the sleep-wake cycle, body TEMPERATURE and cortisol pattern are examples.

The term "biological rhythm" applies to the rhythmicity of biological variables; however, this is not to be confused with BIORHYTHM, a term that is not used in CHRONOBIOLOGY. Biorhythms are patterns of human behavior that are determined by astrological signs and have no scientific validity.

Rigiscan An ambulatory rigidity and tumescence monitor that is worn by the patient overnight to determine whether normal erections occur. This monitoring device is used to differentiate between IMPOTENCE of an organic or psychogenic cause. If full erections occur at night, then the problem is often considered to be due to psychogenic causes.

The Rigiscan consists of two loops: one is placed around the base of the penis, and the other around the tip of the penis. The loops are pulled at intermittent intervals to detect tumescence and rigidity. Some patients find the loops to be uncomfortable; however, most patients are able to sleep without difficulty while wearing the device. In some sleep laboratories, the Rigiscan has replaced the use of STRAIN GAUGES in the determination of NOCTURNAL PENILE TUMESCENCE. (See also IMPAIRED SLEEP-RELATED PENILE ERECTIONS, NOCTURNAL PENILE TUMESCENCE TEST, POLYSOMNOGRAPHY.)

Ritalin See STIMULANT MEDICATIONS.

Roffwarg, Howard Philip Dr. Roffwarg (1932–) obtained his undergraduate degree from Columbia University and his M.D. from the College of Physicians and Surgeons of Columbia University. Since 1977, he has been professor of psychiatry at the University of Texas Southwestern Medical Center at Dallas and director of the Sleep Research Laboratories at the University of Texas Southwestern Medical Center at Dallas, among other appointments.

In June 1988, Dr. Roffwarg became the president of the American Sleep Disorders Association (see AMERICAN ACADEMY OF SLEEP MEDICINE). Dr. Roffwarg is a past president of the SLEEP RESEARCH SOCIETY. He chaired the Diagnostic Classification Committee that produced the first major classification of the sleep disorders.

One of Dr. Roffwarg's earliest research studies was on the relationship of dream imagery to rapid eye movements of sleep. Dr. Roffwarg has also researched the relationship of depression to sleep and sleep markers, plasma testosterone and sleep, and the relationship of REM sleep to brain maturation in mammals, among other topics.

Giles, D.E., Roffwarg, H.P. and Rush, A.J., "REM Latency Concordance in Depressed Family Members," *Biological Psychiatry* 22 (1987): 910–914.

Roffwarg, H.P. (chairman, Association of Sleep Disorder Centers), "Diagnostic Classification of Sleep and Arousal Disorders," *Sleep* 2 (1979): 1–137.

Roth, Thomas Dr. Roth (1942–) received his Ph.D. in psychology in 1970 from the University of Cincinnati. Dr. Roth has worked extensively in sleep and sleep disorders medicine, publishing widely on sleep and breathing and the psychopharmacology of sleep. He is currently the chief of the Division of Sleep Medicine and director of research at Henry Ford Hospital in Detroit, Michigan, and clinical professor in the Department of Psychiatry at the University of Michigan School of Medicine in Ann Arbor, Michigan. Dr. Roth has served on the board of the SLEEP RESEARCH SOCIETY and is a past president of the American Sleep Disorders Association (now called the AMERICAN ACADEMY OF SLEEP MEDICINE.) He is past chairman of the Scientific Program Committee of the ASSOCIATION OF PROFESSIONAL SLEEP SOCIETIES. Since 1999 he has been editor in chief of the professional journal *SLEEP.*

Roth, Thomas, Roehrs, T., Koshorek, G. and Zorick, F., "Sedative Effects of Antihistamines," *Journal of Allergy Clinical Immunology* 80 (1987): 94–98.

Kryger, M., Roth, T. and Dement, W., eds., *The Principles and Practices of Sleep Disorders Medicine,* 2nd ed. Philadelphia: Saunders, 1994.

S

SAD See SEASONAL AFFECTIVE DISORDER.

sandman A personification of sleep or sleepiness that refers to someone who goes around sprinkling sand in the eyes as a way of inducing sleep. The term developed from the gritty sensation that often occurs in the eyes upon awakening in the morning. The term "dustman" was first reported in P. Egan's *Tom and Jerry* in 1821: "till the dustman made his appearance and gave the hint to Tom and Jerry that it was time to visit their beds." The term referred to getting sleepy and the sensation of dust being in the eyes. Over the years, "dustman" became associated with garbage and refuse, and therefore the term was changed from "dustman" to "sandman." The term "sandman" is still commonly used in children's fairy tales.

Sanorex See STIMULANT MEDICATIONS.

sawtooth waves A form of THETA ACTIVITY that occurs during REM SLEEP and is characterized by a notched appearance on the wave form. This notched appearance looks like the teeth of a saw, hence the term "sawtooth waves." These episodes of EEG activity occur in bursts that last up to 10 seconds and are a characteristic of REM sleep.

Scandinavian Sleep Research Society Founded in 1985, the Scandinavian Sleep Research Society is one of many sleep societies founded around the world to stimulate sleep research and the growth of clinical sleep disorders medicine. In the United States, the ASSOCIATION FOR THE PSYCHOPHYSIOLOGICAL STUDY OF SLEEP was founded in 1961 and subsequently led to the ASSOCIATION OF PROFESSIONAL SLEEP SOCIETIES. The first society to be founded outside the United States was the EUROPEAN SLEEP RESEARCH SOCIETY, in 1971.

schizophrenia Group of psychiatric disorders (see PSYCHOSES) characterized by disturbances of thought process, with delusions and hallucinations. Specifically there is a low level of intellectual and social functioning that typically occurs before middle age. Sleep disturbances are common in schizophrenic patients and are characterized by INSOMNIA or alterations in the sleep-wake cycle.

During acute schizophrenia, there may be a reduction in the TOTAL SLEEP TIME, and an alteration in the timing of REM SLEEP, with a short REM SLEEP LATENCY, similar to that seen in DEPRESSION. The amount of SLOW WAVE SLEEP may be reduced, but the amount of REM sleep is usually normal.

The sleep symptoms often parallel the course of the underlying schizophrenia, which usually requires psychiatric management.

SCN See SUPRACHIASMATIC NUCLEUS.

seasonal affective disorder (SAD) A disorder that most often occurs in the mid-to-late fall as the nights grow longer. The increased tendency for DEPRESSION is believed to be in part related to the reduced light exposure at that particular time of year. A clinical diagnosis of SAD is made if, for at least two consecutive winters, someone experiences being depressed, sleeping too much, overeating, craving carbohydrates, a diminished sex drive and working less productively. Such individuals are relatively depression-free during the rest of the year, when there is more light. Exposure to light of more than 2,000 lux (a unit of illumination) for two or more hours in the morning from 6 A.M. to 8

A.M. can improve mood and decrease the seasonal affective disorder. But there may be a mid-afternoon reduction in mood associated with the circadian variation in daytime alertness. A shorter exposure of light at that time may improve the symptoms and reduce the need for a mid-afternoon nap.

Although SAD is uncommon—an estimated half a million people are affected in the United States—a related seasonal condition has been found in 25% of the general population whereby clinically depression is absent but there are mood swings related to the winter and diminished light. In the northern United States, light deprivation and related mood swings seem to begin in October, achieve their most severe form in January and go into remission by the end of February. Bright light systems are commercially available. (See also CIRCADIAN RHYTHMS, LIGHT THERAPY, MOOD DISORDERS.)

sedative-hypnotic medications See HYPNOTICS.

sedative medications See HYPNOTICS.

seizures Term commonly used to denote a clinical manifestation of an epileptic discharge. (The term "epilepsy" applies to a disorder of abnormal brain electrical activity, whereas the term "seizure" applies to the clinical manifestation.) Patients may have epilepsy but may not have seizures if their disorder is under good control with anticonvulsant medications. Rarely some forms of epilepsy do not have seizure manifestations, such as ELECTRICAL STATUS EPILEPTICUS OF SLEEP.

Seizures may take many forms and may be associated with cognitive, motor or sensory symptoms. The most commonly recognized seizure manifestation is that of a tonic-clonic seizure disorder, which produces jerking movements of the arms and legs, often in association with loss of consciousness. However, focal forms of movement disorders are also seen in which only one limb or a portion of a limb may be involved in abnormal movement.

Sometimes the seizure manifestation is very subtle and may produce only blinking or a slight twitching of the mouth. This form of presentation of a seizure disorder is typically seen in patients with absence or petit mal disorder, which is associated with impaired cognition; its only outward manifestation may be blinking, lip smacking or repetitive hand movements. Other forms of disorders may be associated with more pronounced behavioral abnormalities, such as temporal lobe (psychomotor) seizures. Manifestations include walking movements that can occur out of sleep and appear similar to sleepwalking episodes. Frontal lobe seizures are typically associated with behavioral disorders or abnormal mentation. Autonomic seizures are characterized by changes in autonomic functions such as heart rate, respiratory rate, gastrointestinal function, sweating or pupil diameter. Some seizure disorders, such as tonic seizures, may produce a stiffening of the muscles that results in generalized increased muscle tone, and others, such as akinetic seizures, are often associated with loss of muscle tone producing falls to the ground.

Seizures often occur during sleep and are typically characterized by abnormal motor activity, sometimes producing SLEEPWALKING episodes or enuresis (bed-wetting, see SLEEP ENURESIS). Epilepsy is a major cause in children of secondary enuresis. Rarely SLEEP TERROR episodes may be due to epilepsy. Some abnormal movement disorders, such as NOCTURNAL PAROXYSMAL DYSTONIA, can occur during sleep and have features similar to those of seizures. These disorders can be differentiated from seizures by appropriate encephalographic monitoring during sleep.

Seizure disorders can affect an individual of any age; however, some seizures are more commonly seen in childhood. Infantile spasms associated with hypsarrhythmia (abnormal EEG pattern) or the tonic seizures of Lennox-Gastaut syndrome (atonic seizures) are seen in young children. Petit mal epilepsy and generalized tonic-clonic (grand mal) seizure disorder are common in prepubertal and postpubertal children.

In adults, including the elderly, partial complex seizures (temporal lobe or psychomotor) are more commonly seen. Generalized seizures can also occur as a result of central nervous system lesions, such as a stroke. A stroke typically produces a focal motor seizure that may become generalized, with whole body tonic-clonic movements similar to that seen in grand mal epilepsy.

Most seizure disorders can be adequately controlled by anticonvulsant medications such as phenytion, phenobarbital, or carbamazepine (see ANTIDEPRESSANTS). (See also BARBITURATES, BENIGN EPILEPSY WITH ROLANDIC SPIKES.)

Sterman, M.B., Shouse, M.N. and Passouant, P., *Sleep and Epilepsy.* New York: Academic Press, 1982.

selective serotonin reuptake inhibitors (SSRIs) See ANTIDEPRESSANTS.

serotonin A neurotransmitter that is found in cells of the central nervous system, particularly within the brain stem. Serotonin is a naturally-occurring agent in the blood that has the effect of producing vasoconstriction. It is believed to be involved in the regulation of sleep because inhibition of the synthesis of serotonin in animals has led to very profound INSOMNIA. MICHEL JOUVET in 1969 first proposed that serotonin is involved in the maintenance of sleep, particularly SLOW WAVE SLEEP. The RAPHE NUCLEI of the brain stem are the primary site of the serotonin-containing neurons that are involved in sleep regulation.

Precursors of serotonin, such as tryptophan, have been shown to induce drowsiness in animals; however, the effects in man are unclear. Research studies on L-tryptophan (see HYPNOTICS) have suggested a beneficial effect on reducing SLEEP LATENCY and improving the depth of sleep. L-tryptophan is a commonly used OVER-THE-COUNTER MEDICATION in patients who have sleep disturbance; however, it has a relatively weak hypnotic effect. L-tryptophan has recently been withdrawn from the market in the United States because of an association with potentially fatal eosinophilia-myalgia syndrome.

Several ANTIDEPRESSANTS that inhibit the reuptake of serotonin—the so-called serotonin blockers—tend to decrease REM SLEEP. Serotonin reuptake blockers, such as fluvoxamine, zimeldine, femoxitine and fluoxetine, have been reported to be effective in suppressing the CATAPLEXY of NARCOLEPSY. The tricyclic antidepressants that inhibit the uptake of serotonin have pronounced effects in decreasing REM sleep. It has been proposed that the antidepressant effect of these medications is due to this suppression effect on REM sleep.

Jouvet, M., "Biogenic Amines and the States of Sleep," *Science* 163 (1969): 32–41.

serotonin reuptake inhibitors See ANTIDEPRESSANTS.

SESE See ELECTRICAL STATUS EPILEPTICUS OF SLEEP.

settling Popular term that is often used to describe an infant who sleeps through the night and does not awaken for feedings during the night. Settling typically occurs within the first three months of life. (See also INFANT SLEEP, INFANT SLEEP DISORDERS.)

shift-work sleep disorder Disorder that affects workers who work the night shift and who typically have a disturbed sleep-wake pattern. Since most nighttime shift work is performed between 11 P.M. and 7 A.M., sleep is typically delayed until after the shift. SLEEP ONSET would begin anywhere between 6 A.M. and 12 noon. In addition, on days off the shift worker may attempt to return to a more normal sleep-wake pattern, with sleep occurring during the night hours when he would usually be working. As a consequence of the delayed sleep pattern when working the NIGHT SHIFT and the alteration and timing in sleep on days off, complaints of INSOMNIA or EXCESSIVE SLEEPINESS are common.

The duration of sleep after the night shift is reduced to between one and four hours, often at the expense of the lighter stages one and two sleep or rem sleep (see SLEEP STAGES). This sleep length is often found to be unrefreshing; a second sleep episode is often taken prior to commencing the next night of shift work. The second sleep episode may commence at approximately 8 P.M. and last for two hours. Despite these attempts to maintain a normal amount of sleep in a 24-hour period, a tendency to sleepiness exists throughout all periods of wakefulness, often impairing the mental ability of the night shift worker while working. Reduced ALERTNESS and errors are commonly reported as consequences of shift work.

In addition to disturbed sleep-wake patterns and reduced work capacity, there are medical and social consequences of shift work. Gastrointestinal disorders are reported as are drug and alcohol dependency induced by attempts to correct the disturbed sleep-wake pattern. The social consequences may include marital discord and impairment of other social relationships.

The disturbance of the sleep-wake pattern follows the shift work change. Rotating shifts will divide the day into three work periods: a night shift, day shift and EVENING SHIFT. A shift worker may rotate between one shift and another and typically will have less sleep-wake difficulties when on the day shift. After resuming the night shift, the first few days are associated with the most pronounced disturbance of the sleep-wake cycle, and after a few days there is a partial adaptation. This adaptation, however, is typically disturbed by the altered sleep-wake pattern that occurs on days off from work.

There is evidence to suggest that an individual who has been described as an "owl" or "night person" or EVENING PERSON is more able to adapt to shift work than an individual described as a "lark" or MORNING PERSON. With increasing age, shift workers find it more difficult to sustain an adequate sleep episode during the daytime after a night of shift work.

The prevalence of this sleep disorder is related to the number of shift workers in the community. Between 5% and 8% of the total population work the night shift.

Polysomnographic monitoring of the 24-hour day confirms the difficulty of maintaining an appropriate sleep duration during the morning after the shift work, and the tendency to sleepiness during the waking portion of the 24-hour cycle. Continuous monitoring of polysomnographic variables, or the use of an ACTIVITY MONITOR, can be helpful in documenting the tendency to sleepiness, and the pattern of sleep and wake episodes.

Other disorders of sleep and wakefulness must be considered as causes of sleep disturbance in shift workers. Patients with insomnia may adopt night work in order to help deal with their excessive wakefulness at night. Sometimes patients on shift work may present with a complaint of excessive sleepiness and be mistaken for having a disorder such as NARCOLEPSY. Very often, patients with narcolepsy may adopt shift work in an attempt to rationalize their excessive sleepiness. The temporal (time) association between the disturbance of sleep and wakefulness and the onset of shift work is an important variable in excluding other causes of insomnia or excessive daytime sleepiness. A secondary drug-dependent sleep disorder, or STIMULANT-DEPENDENT SLEEP DISORDER, may result from the disrupted sleep-wake patterns.

Treatment for shift-work sleep disorder requires attention to the sleep-wake pattern and also to the nature of the shift work. The daytime sleep episode should occur in an environment that is conducive to good sleep (see SLEEP HYGIENE). Elimination of daytime noise and light as well as attention to appropriate temperature control is important in order to assure a good sleep period during the daytime. In addition, if an adequate sleep period cannot be obtained following a night of shift work, it may be preferable to break the sleep period into two portions, with an initial four-hour sleep episode after the shift, in the morning, and another two-hour period, at night, prior to going to the shift. This particular sleeping pattern seems to be associated with improved alertness on the shift work. Also, the work performed on the night shift must be stimulating and not monotonous or boring in order to maintain full alertness. If the sleep pattern that is established can be maintained seven days a week, rather than five days a week, the shift worker is more likely to adapt to the altered sleep-wake pattern.

The direction of the rotation of shift work has been reported to influence a worker's adaptation to shift work. Rotations that occur in a clockwise direction are said to be preferable to those rotations that occur in an anticlockwise direction. (For example, a rotation from day to evening to night shift is clockwise.) In addition, there is a controversy over the duration of the shift rotation. Some specialists consider that a short and rapidly rotating shift period of only a few days on each night or day shift is preferable to one in which the night shift worker will work for several weeks on a particular shift. The tendency for sleepiness also increases with the length of the night shift so that 12-hour shifts are associated with a greater sleepiness in the final few hours of the shift than in shorter, six- or eight-hour shifts.

HYPNOTICS have been reported to be beneficial for the shift worker. A short course of a short-acting hypnotic can enhance a shift worker's daytime sleep episode and lead to improved alertness during the waking portion of the sleep-wake cycle. New treatments that are being explored include the use of MELATONIN to shift sleep and MODAFINIL to improve alertness. (See also CIRCADIAN RHYTHM SLEEP DISORDERS.)

Van Reeth, O., "Sleep and Circadian Disturbances in Shift Work: Strategies for Their Management," *Hormone Research* 49, nos. 3–4 (1998): 158–162.

short sleeper An individual who consistently sleeps less than someone of the same age. Typically, the total sleep time is less than 75% of the lowest normal sleep time for someone of that age. Although exact limits for the total sleep times of a particular individual are unknown, a sleep episode of less than five hours in any 24-hour day, before the age of 60 years, is regarded as an unusually short sleep episode. (After the age of 60, the nocturnal sleep period is usually reduced in duration, but daytime sleep episodes are more common, so the normal total sleep within any 24-hour period is still typically greater than five hours in duration.)

Sleep lengths in short sleepers may vary from two hours to five hours in duration; however, most short sleepers sleep for only three to five hours, without any tendency for daytime sleepiness. Monitoring of sleep-wake patterns by means of an activity monitor may be useful in documenting the sleep length of short sleepers over a period of weeks or months.

Short sleepers, because of a complaint of INSOMNIA at night, often have the expectation that they should sleep for eight hours. Excessive time spent in bed awake is considered an inability to fall asleep and, hence, induces a complaint of insomnia. Although the pattern of short sleep has its onset in early adolescence, when the more typical adult sleep pattern is being established, it is not usually regarded as a problem until adulthood, when a full eight-hour sleep period is desired. An adolescent short sleeper very often has fewer complaints about the sleep period and usually enjoys the luxury of being able to stay up late at night.

Studies have indicated that most short sleepers are males and the prevalence of this disorder is rare. There is some evidence to suggest it is more common in families.

A psychological profile of short sleepers by Ernest Hartmann, Frederick Baekeland and George Zwilling indicated that they generally are not psychiatrically disturbed but tend to be high achievers who are efficient and who have a tendency to hypomania, an increase in activity, with an elevated, expansive mood.

A survey by Daniel Kripke, R. Simons, L. Garfinkel and E. Hammond that involved over one million individuals indicated that people with a nocturnal sleep period of less than five hours had a shorter life expectancy than those with more usual sleep durations.

Objective documentation of the sleep patterns of short sleepers is relatively sparse. It is difficult to confirm the habitual tendency to short sleeping because of the difficulty in monitoring someone for 24 hours a day for many consecutive days. Studies that have been performed have tended to show normal amounts of stages three and four sleep, with reduced lighter sleep stages and REM sleep. There is no evidence for any sleep disorder causing disrupted nighttime sleep or for a tendency to daytime sleepiness.

Short sleepers need to be differentiated from individuals who have psychopathology that may cause a short-term reduction in total sleep time, such as is seen during the manic phase of manic-depressive disease.

Short sleepers also have to be differentiated from those who have short sleep but then make up for it by an excessively long sleep episode, such as on the weekends. Those individuals are classified as having insufficient sleep and may be chronically sleep deprived.

No treatment is indicated or necessary for a short sleeper other than the reassurance that the sleep length is normal for that individual and that an appropriate time spent in bed will allay concerns regarding insomnia. Many short sleepers, particularly in middle or old age, are concerned about being awake at night when others are sleeping; it should be suggested that they find activities to occupy them during their period of wakefulness.

(See also ACTIVITY MONITOR, INSUFFICIENT SLEEP SYNDROME, MOOD DISORDERS.)

Hartmann, E., Baekeland, F. and Zwilling, G.R., "Psychological Differences Between Long and Short Sleepers," *Archives of General Psychiatry* 26 (1972): 463–468.

Kripke, D.F., Simons, R.N., Garfinkel, L. and Hammond, E.C., "Short and Long Sleep and Sleeping Pills: Is Increased Mortality Associated?" *Archives of General Psychiatry* 37 (1979): 103–116.

short-term insomnia Term proposed by the consensus development conference that was held in November 1983 by the National Institute of Mental Health and the Office of Medical Applications of the National Institutes of Health. The conference summary suggested the terms "TRANSIENT INSOMNIA," "SHORT-TERM INSOMNIA" and "long-term insomnia." Short-term insomnia was defined as lasting up to three weeks, usually in association with a situational stress—such as an acute loss, work or marital stress—or due to a serious medical illness. SLEEP HYGIENE and nondrug procedures are primarily recommended for the treatment of this type of sleep disturbance. However, sleep-promoting medications, such as the BENZODIAZEPINES, could be considered. This form of insomnia is equivalent to ADJUSTMENT SLEEP DISORDER; however, other causes of insomnia, such as jet lag or shift work, when seen within three weeks of their onset, could also be regarded as short-term insomnia. (See also HYPNOTICS.)

SIDS See SUDDEN INFANT DEATH SYNDROME.

siesta A voluntary nap usually taken in the midafternoon by certain cultural and ethnic groups, such as the Latin Americans and the Spanish. Many societies adopt the midafternoon siesta to avoid the hottest part of the day, particularly in tropical environments. A siesta usually lasts two hours and is taken at a point in the biphasic circadian ALERTNESS cycle when there is an increased amount of sleepiness, typically between 2 P.M. and 4 P.M. Prolonged siestas are taken at the expense of nighttime sleep so that total sleep time within any 24-hour period is still one-third of the day, or about eight hours. Longer siestas of four hours may be accompanied by a short nocturnal sleep episode of a similar duration. Most persons in cultures where siestas are typical tend to stay up later at night because the NAP necessitates shorter nocturnal sleep.

There is some debate as to whether a pattern of daytime and nighttime sleep is preferable to a pattern of a single longer nocturnal sleep episode. The natural tendency for increased sleepiness twice during a 24-hour period tends to imply that a daytime siesta may be preferable. In addition, lunch has a soporific effect and although the tendency for sleepiness in the midafternoon is not entirely due to food intake at midday, it will exacerbate the tendency for tiredness. Many cultures that take a siesta will purposely have a large midday meal, which is an additional stimulus to taking a midafternoon nap. Consequently, the evening meal is often taken at a later hour, approximately 9 to 10 P.M.

It is believed by many that the sleep pattern seen in prepubertal children of eight or nine hours of nocturnal sleep along with a daytime of maximal alertness is preferable. Therefore in many societies the tendency for a daytime nap or siesta is discouraged. The avoidance of a midafternoon nap is especially important for persons who suffer from sleep disorders such as INSOMNIA, as it may lead to a further breakdown and disruption of nighttime sleep. (See also CIRCADIAN RHYTHMS, NAPS.)

Siffre, Michel A speleologist (cave expert) who began an experiment on July 16, 1962, of living in an underground cavern in the Alps between France and Italy. The underground cavern contained an ice glacier at a depth of 375 feet below the surface. Siffre stayed in a tent on the underground ice shelf for 59 days and recorded his sleep-wake pattern while isolated from ENVIRONMENTAL TIME CUES. The sleep-wake pattern showed a rhythm of 24 hours and 30 minutes over the course of the experiment. This study was one of the first demonstrations of man's FREE RUNNING pattern of sleep and wakefulness in an environment isolated from time cues. (See TEMPORAL ISOLATION.)

Siffre, Michel, *Beyond Time.* New York: McGraw-Hill, 1964.

sigma rhythm Previously-used term for SLEEP SPINDLES. Sigma rhythm is derived from the shape of the Greek "sigma" character.

situational insomnia See ADJUSTMENT SLEEP DISORDER.

sleep A behavioral state characterized by rest, immobility and reduced perception of environmental stimuli in which cognition and consciousness are suspended. Sleep occurs when the brain waves slow, and the erratic activity of many parts of the brain starts to coalesce into a coordinated synchronized background rhythm. The heart rate slows, the muscles relax, and the wakeful brain mentation calms to the point that a satisfying sense of contentment occurs as we mentally drift away from our environment into peaceful unconsciousness. See also BEDTIME, DREAM CONTENT, DREAMS, DREAMS AND CREATIVITY, SLEEP DEPRIVATION, SLEEP DURATION, SLEEP NEED, SLEEP ONSET, SLEEP STAGES.

Sleep A leading scholarly journal originally published bimonthly by Raven Press, Ltd., but now published by the AMERICAN ACADEMY OF SLEEP MEDICINE. The journal was initially sponsored jointly by the ASSOCIATION OF PROFESSIONAL SLEEP SOCIETIES, THE EUROPEAN SLEEP RESEARCH SOCIETY, the LATIN AMERICAN SLEEP RESEARCH SOCIETY and the JAPANESE SLEEP RESEARCH SOCIETY, but now it is the official journal of the American Academy of Sleep Medicine. A peer-reviewed journal, *Sleep* contains scholarly articles on all aspects of sleep (clinical, experimental, biochemical, etc.), reporting sleep research findings as well as announcements, book reviews and a bibliography of recent literature in sleep research. *Sleep* is listed in *Index Medicus, Current Contents* and *PASCAL/CNRS.*

sleep apnea Cessation of breathing that occurs during sleep. APNEA in association with complete cessation of respiratory movements is termed "central sleep apnea" whereas apnea that occurs in association with upper airway obstruction is called "obstructive sleep apnea." A mixed form of apnea may occur if there is an initial central apnea that is continuous with an obstructive apnea. Sleep apnea is differentiated from episodes of partial obstruction, which are termed HYPOPNEAS, in which there is an incomplete reduction of airflow (but a reduction of 50% or more) associated with a reduction in blood oxygen saturation.

Some people have frequent episodes of sleep apnea and may develop a sleep apnea syndrome. CENTRAL SLEEP APNEA SYNDROME or OBSTRUCTIVE SLEEP APNEA SYNDROME are the two apnea syndromes seen in infancy, childhood or adulthood. A physiological form of central sleep apnea may occur in premature infants and is called APNEA OF PREMATURITY. (See also INFANT SLEEP APNEA, SLEEP-RELATED BREATHING DISORDERS.)

sleep architecture The organization of the NREM-REM SLEEP CYCLE and wakefulness as it occurs during a sleep episode. The duration of SLEEP STAGES and the relationship to preceding and following wakefulness is recorded so that the structure of the sleep episode can be demonstrated, often as plotted in the form of a histogram.

The sleep architecture is often described as being disrupted if there are frequent sleep stage changes and a greater number than normal of arousals or awakenings. A sleep episode that is normal may be described as having a normal sleep architecture.

sleep atonia Term denoting the decrease of muscle activity during sleep. As sleep gets deeper, from the early stages of NON-REM STAGE SLEEP through to SLOW WAVE SLEEP, muscles reduce in activity and tone. The most pronounced reduction of muscle tone is during REM SLEEP, when the alpha motor neurons of the spinal cord are inhibited by the medullary region of Magoun and Rhines. The medullary inhibitory region is stimulated by the caudal region of the LOCUS CERULEUS.

Bilateral-lateral pontine lesions in cats can cause destruction of the region around the locus ceruleus, thereby preventing stimulation of the medullary inhibitory region, leading to a retention of muscle tone during REM sleep. Cats with such lesions will tend to "act out" DREAMS. A similar situation has recently been discovered in humans in whom muscle activity persists during REM sleep and the patient also "acts out" dreams. This disorder, which has been called the REM SLEEP BEHAVIOR DISORDER, is most commonly seen in persons over the age of 60 years, although it has been described in younger individuals, usually in association with neurological lesions of varied types. The majority of cases of REM sleep behavior disorder have no known neurological cause. (See also PONS.)

sleep bruxism Stereotyped movement disorder that involves clenching or grinding the teeth during sleep. Some individuals have bruxism when awake during the day; others have bruxism predominantly while asleep. When bruxism occurs during sleep, it commonly produces an unpleasant grinding sound that may be disturbing to a bed partner; it can also interfere with the sufferer's quality of sleep by causing brief arousals. When the grinding occurs over many years, the cusps of the teeth can be worn down, and this may be detected during a routine dental examination. The constant grinding during sleep often leads to discomfort in the muscles of the jaw and there may also be gum damage. Bruxism is a cause of an atypical headache and may also produce a temporomandibular joint discomfort.

Bruxism typically occurs in healthy adults or children, but it is more common in children who have a central nervous system disorder such as cerebral palsy. Exacerbation of the bruxism may occur with psychological stress.

Although the majority of the population will at some time grind their teeth, if only infrequently, up to 5% of the population have more persistent teeth grinding. The onset of teeth grinding among healthy infants occurs at a mean age of 10 months, affecting male and female children equally.

Studies of bruxism during sleep have shown that it can occur during all stages but is most common during stage two sleep (see SLEEP STAGES). Rarely will it occur predominantly in REM sleep.

Bruxism may be helped by the use of a dental appliance, the mouth guard, which is worn during sleep. Attention to underlying psychological stress by using appropriate psychological or psychiatric treatment may also be helpful. For many individuals, the disorder does not require a specific treatment. Particularly in children, it appears to be a transient phenomenon.

Funch, P. and Gile, E.N., "Factors Associated with Nocturnal Bruxism and Its Treatment," *Journal of Behavioral Medicine* 3 (1980): 385–397.

Ware, J.C. and Rugh, J., "Destructive Bruxism: Sleep Stage Relationship," *Sleep* 11 (1988): 172–181.

sleep choking syndrome Disorder characterized by choking episodes that occur during sleep and do not have an apparent organic or psychiatric cause. The patient awakens with a sudden and intense feeling of being unable to breathe associated with a choking sensation. The episodes occur typically in the early part of the night. Once awake, there is a sensation of fear, ANXIETY and the feeling of impending death. Within a few seconds, the anxiety abates as the awareness develops that breathing is unimpaired. This disorder commonly occurs either nightly or almost every night.

The sleep choking syndrome is not associated with any objective evidence of difficulty in breathing. There is no stridor, hoarseness or change in color noted in these patients. Bed partners are usually not aware of the episodes until reported to them the next morning.

The episodes most commonly occur in females in early to middle adulthood.

Polysomnographically, patients demonstrate no abnormalities and do not have choking episodes during the monitoring. Polysomnographic monitoring is usually necessary to exclude an organic cause and to have sufficient information to reassure the patient of the benign nature of the syndrome.

Episodes of awakening with a choking sensation need to be differentiated from several breathing disorders, including the OBSTRUCTIVE SLEEP APNEA SYNDROME, CENTRAL SLEEP APNEA SYNDROME and CENTRAL ALVEOLAR HYPOVENTILATION SYNDROME. Other disorders that can produce a sensation of difficulty in breathing and fear include PANIC DISORDERS, which are usually associated with agoraphobia and the presence of daytime panic episodes. SLEEP-RELATED LARYNGOSPASM can be differentiated by the absence of stridor, hoarseness, cyanosis or pallor in association with the episodes.

Treatment of the disorder is primarily by reassurance. However, antianxiety agents, or HYPNOTICS, may be required for some patients. The cause of the disorder is thought to be psychological.

sleep cure See SLEEP THERAPY.

sleep cycle See NREM-REM SLEEP CYCLE.

sleep deprivation One of the most intriguing questions in sleep research is, "Why do we need to sleep?" As this is a difficult question to answer, experimenters have studied the opposite phenomenon of what happens if you do not sleep. Sleep deprivation has been studied extensively to determine the effect of sleep loss, as well as the loss of specific components of sleep, such as REM SLEEP.

Although it is clear that most people who are deprived of sleep become sleepy, no one had ever tried staying awake for a prolonged period of time until 1959, when PETER TRIPP, a New York disc jockey, stayed awake for some 200 hours as a fund-raising publicity stunt. Toward the end of Tripp's 200-hour vigil, psychotic features became evident, with hallucinations. As a result of this unscientific experiment of sleep deprivation, it was erroneously believed that the loss of sleep would be accompanied by severe mental deterioration.

The first opportunity to scientifically study somebody who had been deprived of sleep occurred in 1964 when RANDY GARDNER, a San Diego resident, remained awake for 260 hours. During the later part of his stint of wakefulness, he was observed by the sleep researcher WILLIAM C. DEMENT, and subsequently studied by Dr. Laverne Johnson in the sleep laboratory at the San Diego Naval Hospital. Toward the end of the attempt at keeping awake, it was clear that Gardner was in a state of partial sleep and wakefulness that could not be separated. One of the intriguing questions that arose was whether he would have a prolonged sleep episode following the wakefulness. After the 11 days, Gardner slept for 14 hours and 40 minutes and appeared entirely refreshed upon awakening. He subsequently remained awake for 24 hours before having a second sleep episode of normal duration of approximately eight hours. Gardner did not have any psychiatric disturbance related to the sleep deprivation; subsequent sleep episodes demonstrated that the accumulated lost sleep was not made up by the body, as a short sleep episode appeared to be fully refreshing.

Subsequent research studies have given conflicting results, with some brief psychiatric disturbances following sleep deprivation of up to 10 days. However, prolonged and complete sleep deprivation is usually not possible because of the intrusion of brief sleep episodes, even though the subject is active and conversant.

There are major changes in mood and performance, with fatigue, irritability, impaired perception and orientation, and inattentiveness due to sleep deprivation. These features begin after about 36 hours of sleep deprivation and are most notable during the time that would usually be the time of the habitual sleep period. Even during the first night of sleep deprivation, subjects have great difficulty in maintaining full alertness at the time that correlates with the low point in body TEMPERATURE, typically between 4 A.M. and 6 A.M. This particular time is most crucial in studies of sleep deprivation because a few minutes of inattention will allow a nonactive subject to fall asleep.

Activity and mood following one night of sleep deprivation do not show a linear decrease from the time of the last sleep episode but rather there is a cyclical fluctuation in the relation to the circadian pattern of alertness and sleepiness. The mid-afternoon following a night of sleep deprivation is a time of increased sleepiness and decreased alertness, which is related to the physiological, biphasic pattern of alertness. However, there is increasing alertness in activity a few hours later although the level of activity may be much reduced.

There are some neurological features of sleep deprivation, such as weakness of the muscles and tremulousness of the limbs, as well as incoordination and unsteadiness.

Short episodes of sleep deprivation have been beneficial in some situations. It is often used as an activating procedure for the diagnostic monitoring of patients with suspected seizure disorders. Total sleep deprivation has also been demonstrated to improve mood in patients suffering from DEPRESSION.

Polysomnographic monitoring after a brief episode of sleep deprivation demonstrates a short SLEEP LATENCY with an increased amount of SLOW WAVE SLEEP that often occurs at the expense of REM sleep. On subsequent nights, there may be an increase in REM sleep until the pattern returns to normal sleep stage percentages (see SLEEP STAGES).

Studies of selective sleep deprivation are largely limited to suppression of slow wave sleep or REM sleep. It is almost impossible to suppress non-REM sleep due to its universal occurrence at sleep onset.

REM sleep deprivation is typically produced by an auditory or physical stimulus that mechanically awakens the subject whenever entering into the particular sleep stage as determined by polysomnographic monitoring. REM sleep deprivation is associated with an increased pressure for REM sleep that is evident during the subsequent sleep episode. The amount and percentage of REM sleep is increased, and there often is a short REM SLEEP LATENCY. These are features indicative of REM REBOUND.

REM sleep deprivation has been used as a treatment means for patients who have depression and has been found to be effective. The association between improved mood and reduction in REM sleep has led to the hypothesis that the tricyclic ANTIDEPRESSANTS work because they are effective REM sleep suppressants. MONOAMINE OXIDASE INHIBITORS, which are particularly powerful REM sleep medications, are also strong improvers of mood and depression and are usually associated with severe reduction and almost total elimination of REM sleep during their administration.

Animal studies with REM sleep deprivation in controlled experiments have recently suggested that deprivation of REM sleep may be associated with early death in animals, which may have relevance for humans as well.

Sleep deprivation as a clinical feature is common in disorders that affect the quality of nighttime sleep, leading to disruption of sleep stages. Disorders such as OBSTRUCTIVE SLEEP APNEA SYNDROME or PERIODIC LIMB MOVEMENT DISORDER produce EXCESSIVE SLEEPINESS due to the frequent disruption of sleep stages. However, patients with INSOMNIA typically do not have an increased amount of daytime sleepiness despite complaints of very little sleep. Research studies have demonstrated that the duration of sleep in patients with insomnia is only slightly shorter than that of the normal population, whereas the subjective assessment of sleep reduction is much greater.

Chronic sleep deprivation is a common feature of adolescents who go to bed late and have to rise early for school. Adolescents who get less sleep than is required develop sleepiness during the daytime, which may become manifest as daytime NAPS. People who live in tropical countries often take a mid-afternoon SIESTA, but subsequently have a shorter nighttime sleep episode with a later bedtime and an early time of arising. Such people have a total sleep time in a 24-hour period that is normal. Some people who do not allow themselves to take a daytime sleep episode can become chronically sleep-deprived by the limited amount of time they sleep at night. Sleep of five or less hours may produce severe chronic sleepiness in a person who usually requires seven hours of sleep. Chronic sleep deprivation needs to be differentiated from NARCOLEPSY or other disorders of excessive sleepiness. The INSUFFICIENT SLEEP SYNDROME is the term used for the disorder characterized by chronic sleep loss and excessive sleepiness.

Rechtschaffen, Alan, Bergmann, B.M., Everson, C.A., Kushida, C.A. and Guilland, M.A., "Sleep Deprivation in the Rat: X. Integration and Discussion of the Findings," *Sleep* 12 (1989): 68–87.

Horne, J.A., "Sleep Function: With Particular Reference to Sleep Deprivation," *Annals of Clinical Research* 17 (1985): 199–208.

sleep diary See SLEEP LOG.

sleep disorder centers Facilities designed for the diagnosis, evaluation and treatment of patients with sleep disorders. A comprehensive sleep disorder center has the expertise and facilities for diagnosing and evaluating disorders that occur during sleep as well as disorders of EXCESSIVE SLEEPINESS during the day. The disorders that are able to be evaluated cover all medical specialties and age groups from infancy to old age. The first sleep disorder center in the United States was developed in the early 1970s at the Stanford University Medical Center. By the end of 1988, 110 sleep disorder centers had been accredited in the United States. Similar centers are being developed in many other countries, including Japan, England and Germany.

A typical sleep disorder center comprises a specialist in SLEEP DISORDERS MEDICINE, usually a physician, and consultants from a variety of different medical specialties, including otolaryngology, pulmonary medicine, cardiology, neurology and psychiatry. Patients typically undergo a full clinical evaluation that may involve seeing a psychologist and, if necessary, patients will undergo polysomnographic testing.

A sleep disorder center will have at least one recording room for POLYSOMNOGRAPHY, and typically will have two or three rooms. These rooms consist of a hotel-like bedroom with specialized monitoring equipment housed in an adjacent control room. Patients will undergo all-night polysomnographic monitoring as needed, which may be followed by an assessment of excessive daytime sleepiness by MULTIPLE SLEEP LATENCY TESTING. Some patients require several nights of polysomnographic monitoring to determine an accurate diagnosis, or to provide for treatment under polysomnographic monitoring. Bathroom and kitchen facilities are usually available for the patient's comfort.

In addition to clinicians' offices and the polysomnographic recording areas, a sleep disorders center usually will have a conference room where multidisciplinary clinical case conferences are held.

The development of quality standards for sleep disorder centers throughout the United States is provided through the AMERICAN ACADEMY OF SLEEP MEDICINE. Sleep disorder centers are accredited if they meet the standards and guidelines of the American Academy of Sleep Medicine. (See also ACCREDITATION STANDARDS FOR SLEEP DISORDER CENTERS, FIRST NIGHT EFFECT, REVERSED FIRST NIGHT EFFECT.)

sleep disorder centers, accreditation standards for See ACCREDITATION STANDARDS FOR SLEEP DISORDER CENTERS.

sleep disorder clinics See SLEEP DISORDER CENTERS.

sleep-disordered breathing Term applied to a variety of breathing disorders that can occur during sleep, such as the OBSTRUCTIVE SLEEP APNEA SYNDROME, CENTRAL SLEEP APNEA SYNDROME or CENTRAL ALVEOLAR HYPOVENTILATION SYNDROME. Chronic respiratory diseases including nocturnal asthma can also produce sleep-related breathing abnormalities, characterized by reduction in blood oxygen saturation during sleep as well as disrupted sleep. Sleep-disordered breathing may consist of a pattern of hyperventilation or hypoventilation with or without apneic episodes. The term *sleep-disordered breathing* has also been applied to the APNEAS and HYPOPNEAS that occur during sleep and is often expressed as the RESPIRATORY DISTURBANCE INDEX. (See also CHRONIC OBSTRUCTIVE PULMONARY DISEASE, SLEEP-RELATED ASTHMA, SLEEP-RELATED BREATHING DISORDERS.)

sleep disorders medicine A clinical specialty concerned with the diagnosis and treatment of disorders of sleep and wakefulness. In the last 25 years, there has been a rapid development of this subspecialty area due to the recognition of the importance of sleep in health and disease. It is estimated that approximately 100 million people in all age groups in the United States have a disturbance of sleep and wakefulness, which can manifest itself in many different ways. SUDDEN INFANT DEATH SYNDROME affects some 7,000 normal infants every year. Approximately 250,000 people have a disorder of EXCESSIVE SLEEPINESS termed NARCOLEPSY, which causes them to have impaired ALERTNESS during the day—a lifelong and incurable disorder.

Approximately 18 million shift workers have disturbed sleep-wake patterns due to the altered relationship of sleep and their underlying circadian rhythms (see SHIFT-WORK SLEEP DISORDER). In recent years, it has become known that breathing disturbances during sleep can produce daytime sleepiness and are associated with sudden death during sleep; the OBSTRUCTIVE SLEEP APNEA SYNDROME is believed to occur in up to two million Americans. About 30 million people have INSOMNIA at some time of their lives that causes significant concern and stress. The recognition that these and other disorders are associated with the pathophysiology of sleep has led to the development of sleep disorders medicine.

Sleep disorders medicine in the United States has evolved from basic and clinical research of sleep disorders. Research programs were developed to understand the anatomy and physiology of normal sleep. In 1961, the first sleep research society, the ASSOCIATION FOR THE PSYCHOPHYSIOLOGICAL STUDY OF SLEEP, was developed; its name was subsequently changed to the SLEEP RESEARCH SOCIETY, out of which sleep disorders medicine arose. Sleep disorder centers were developed in the early 1970s and standards and guidelines for such facilities were established in 1975 by the ASSOCIATION OF SLEEP DISORDER CENTERS. This led to the development of the CLINICAL SLEEP SOCIETY, a society of clinicians from all medical specialties with a specific interest in sleep and sleep disorders medicine. The Association of Sleep Disorder Centers and the Clinical Sleep Society merged to form the AMERICAN ACADEMY OF SLEEP MEDICINE (formerly called the American Sleep Disorders Association), which currently oversees the standards and guidelines for the accreditation of sleep disorder centers and provides information and professional education in all aspects of patient care. The AMERICAN BOARD OF SLEEP MEDICINE has developed examinations for the certification of physicians in sleep medicine. In addition, the technologists trained in performing polysomnographic studies have formed the ASSOCIATION OF POLYSOMNOGRAPHIC TECHNOLOGISTS, which provides training courses and certification examinations for sleep technicians. In 1987, the three main sleep societies formed the ASSOCIATION OF PROFESSIONAL SLEEP SOCIETIES, which comprised the Sleep Research Society, the American Sleep Disorders Association and the Association of Polysomnographic Technologists. In 1995, the Association of Polysomnographic Technologists left the group to organize its own annual meeting.

Major events that impacted on the development of sleep disorders medicine included the discovery of REM SLEEP in the early 1950s, the recognition of the obstructive sleep apnea syndrome in the late 1960s, the development of the first diagnostic classification of sleep disorders in 1979 (see DIAGNOSTIC CLASSIFICATION OF SLEEP AND AROUSAL DISORDERS) and the development of physical facilities (see SLEEP DISORDER CENTERS) for the practice of sleep disorders medicine, with the capability of performing polysomnographic evaluations during sleep (see POLYSOMNOGRAPHY) and for assessing daytime sleepiness (see MULTIPLE SLEEP LATENCY TESTING). In 1989, the first comprehensive teaching text was developed, *The Principles and Practices of Sleep Disorders Medicine,* edited by Drs. MEIR KRYGER, THOMAS ROTH and WILLIAM C. DEMENT.

Sleep disorders medicine has clarified the many disturbances of sleep and wakefulness that not only threaten physical and emotional health and lives but also greatly impair the ability to adequately perform during the working part of the day.

sleep disorder specialist A physician (M.D.) who is trained and knowledgeable in the practice of SLEEP DISORDERS MEDICINE. In the United States, the majority of sleep disorder specialists have undergone appropriate certification by passing the examination in sleep medicine that is given by the AMERICAN ACADEMY OF SLEEP MEDICINE. Most sleep disorder specialists have polysomnographic monitoring equipment available to assist in the diagnosis and management of sleep disorders. Sleep disorder specialists usually practice in a SLEEP DISORDER CENTER, which is a comprehensive diagnostic and treatment facility capable of diagnosing and treating all types of sleep disorders.

sleep drunkenness Term applied to the condition of people who have difficulty awakening in the morning and who often awaken in a confused and disoriented state. Although originally proposed as a distinct disorder, sleep drunkenness is no longer thought to be a specific diagnostic entity. Instead, sleep drunkenness, or confusion and disorientation upon awakening, is a feature of many DISORDERS OF EXCESSIVE SOMNOLENCE, such as the OBSTRUCTIVE SLEEP APNEA SYNDROME, IDIOPATHIC HYPERSOMNIA, CONFUSIONAL AROUSALS or the SUBWAKEFULNESS SYNDROME.

sleep duration The time one spends sleeping varies according to age, and there are individual differences at any particular age. A number of factors can influence sleep duration, such as an individual's voluntary control of sleep duration (by going to bed earlier or later, or waking up earlier or later) and genetic determinants. Variation in sleep time may be determined by nighttime or daytime social or work commitments. When a short sleep episode persists on a regular basis it may impair daytime alertness and EXCESSIVE SLEEPINESS may occur. In such circumstances, the individual will have a tendency to fall asleep at inappropriate times and may take frequent daytime NAPS.

Sleep duration varies from approximately 16 hours in infancy (see INFANT SLEEP) to six hours in the elderly (see ELDERLY AND SLEEP). In general, there is a gradual decline in the sleep duration as one ages. Sleep in infancy is characterized by short episodes of REM and non-REM sleep that alternate with short episodes of wakefulness. Approximately seven episodes of sleep occur throughout the 24-hour day. The number of episodes decreases, and the duration of the nocturnal sleep episode increases, so that by one year of age a child may be sleeping nine hours at night with two short naps of about two hours each during the rest of the 24-hour day. By age four years, the major sleep episode comprises about 10 hours in duration and there may or may not be one nap. Most prepubertal children have a nocturnal sleep duration of approximately 10 hours without a tendency for daytime naps, and this length of nocturnal sleep gradually reduces to six hours after 60 years of age.

Most young adults sleep 7.5 hours each night, with a slight increase in sleep duration on weekends by approximately one hour. However, there is a normal distribution of sleep length across each age group, with some individuals having less than five hours of sleep a night and others having more than nine hours. Recent research has indicated that adults who receive less than five hours of sleep on a regular basis, or more than nine hours of sleep, have an increased mortality (see DEATHS DURING SLEEP).

In addition to a reduction of total sleep duration as one gets older, there is also a change in the ratio of REM to non-REM sleep. In infancy, about 50% of all sleep is REM SLEEP, and this percentage decreases as one gets older so that by age two years, about 25% of the sleep period is REM sleep and at age 60 years, about 20% is REM sleep. In addition, the frequency and number of awakenings during the major sleep episode increases from childhood through adulthood to old age.

In some societies, the nocturnal sleep episode is of shorter duration because a daytime SIESTA is taken. Siestas that last four hours may be accompanied by a nocturnal sleep episode that is only four to six hours long. The total amount of sleep within a 24-hour period is usually normal, and is equivalent to that seen in societies without a siesta.

Research has demonstrated that sleep duration may be reduced voluntarily if one gradually cuts back on the amount of sleep at night. This sleep reduction is done at the expense of the lighter stages of sleep and REM sleep, which become reduced. If sleep duration is reduced below the physiological need for an individual then excessive sleepiness will result. Many people who report a long sleep duration often spend an excessive amount of time in bed awake at night. Reduction in hours spent sleeping will eliminate this wake time and lead to more consolidated and efficient nocturnal sleep. Although individuals have been reported to sleep as little as two hours per night, this is very rare. (Individuals who have a genetic predisposition to less sleep are termed SHORT SLEEPERS.) In order to confirm a short sleep duration, an individual must be studied in an environment free of time cues (see ENVIRONMENTAL TIME CUES) for at least seven days so that both nocturnal and daytime sleep can be recorded. Some individuals report the complete absence of sleep for months and even years. Such people, when studied in the sleep laboratory, are seen to be sleeping, yet upon awakening do not perceive that they slept. This disorder is called SLEEP STATE MISPERCEPTION or pseudosomnia.

Some persons have a genetic tendency for a prolonged nocturnal sleep episode (greater than nine hours of sleep per day). For others, very often prolonged nocturnal sleep episodes occur at the expense of consolidated sleep so that frequent or lighter stages of sleep occur throughout the sleep episode. Long sleep episodes may alternate with short sleep episodes; this is particularly seen with people who have mental disease characterized by manic-depressive stages. Rarely, some people can extend their nocturnal sleep for one or two nights for periods as long as 15 hours in total duration. When an episode of prolonged sleep occurs, there is usually a return of stage three or four sleep toward the end of the sleep episode. Awakening from this sleep can lead to a complaint of fatigue, tiredness and DROWSINESS for the remainder of the day. Such prolonged sleep durations in healthy people rarely occur for more than two nights at a time. However, a genetic predisposition to long sleep rarely occurs and those individuals are termed LONG SLEEPERS.

Many sleep disorders can affect sleep duration. Patients with insomnia typically report a short sleep duration at night, although recent studies have shown that sleep duration in insomnia patients is very similar to people without a complaint of insomnia. Disorders that affect the quality of nocturnal sleep may lead to a change in sleep duration; for example, OBSTRUCTIVE SLEEP APNEA SYNDROME and PERIODIC LIMB MOVEMENT DISORDER are two disorders commonly associated with an increased nocturnal sleep duration. In addition, patients with the disorder IDIOPATHIC HYPERSOMNIA typically have a rather prolonged nocturnal sleep episode.

Roffwarg, Howard P., Muzio, J.M. and Dement, William C., "Ontogenic Development of the Human Sleep-Dream Cycle," *Science* 152 (1966): 604–619.

Hartmann, Ernest, Baekeland, F. and Zwilling, G.R., "Psychological Differences Between Long and Short Sleepers," *Archives of General Psychiatry* 26 (1972): 463–468.

sleep efficiency The amount of sleep that occurs during a sleep episode in relation to the amount of time available for sleep. During POLYSOMNOGRAPHY it is usually expressed as a percentage of TOTAL SLEEP TIME according to the TOTAL RECORDING TIME. The sleep efficiency is an indication of how much wakefulness occurred during the time available for sleep. Usually a sleep efficiency of greater than 80% is regarded as normal in the sleep laboratory. Efficiencies greater than 95% are indicative of an abnormally high sleep efficiency and are typically seen in patients with NARCOLEPSY or IDIOPATHIC HYPERSOMNIA. Sleep efficiencies of less than 80% are typical of disorders that produce a complaint of INSOMNIA.

sleep enuresis Also known as bed-wetting, this is a disorder that is characterized by urinating during sleep. This disorder can occur in both children and adults, although it is much more common in children. Usually sleep enuresis is not considered to be a diagnosis before the age of five; up to that time frequent bed-wetting may be a normal developmental behavior. Primary enuresis indicates that control of urination at night has never occurred and therefore bed-wetting has occurred since infancy. Secondary enuresis indicates that there has been a period of time when complete urinary control has occurred during sleep but then some factor caused the control of urination to become disturbed, and bed-wetting occurred. At least three to six months of dryness is considered necessary before the term secondary enuresis is used.

Polysomnographic studies of bed-wetting have indicated that it occurs in any stage of sleep, most commonly at the end of the first third of the night. As children between the ages of five and eight years of age have a larger percentage of stage three/four sleep at night than adults, it is more likely that an episode of enuresis will occur during stage three/four sleep (see SLEEP STAGES). Originally it was thought that there might be a specific sleep stage association with enuresis; however, this has not been proven. Bed-wetting episodes appear to occur in relation to the amount of time that has passed since the last episode of voiding urine and are not due to a particular sleep stage.

It is estimated that approximately 10% of all six-year-old children are enuretic and this percentage decreases with age to 3% of 12-year-olds. In early adulthood, approximately 1% to 3% continue to be enuretic. Primary enuresis comprises the majority of all enuretic patients—up to 90%—the remainder being secondary enuretics. The male to female ratio is three to two.

The cause of primary enuresis is unknown. Current theories suggest it is due to a central nervous system maturational defect, as it spontaneously resolves with age. Rarely enuresis may be due to bladder abnormalities, such as a small bladder or urinary sphincter abnormalities. In the adult, secondary enuresis may be caused by a variety of disorders, including urinary tract infections, and lesions that affect the urinary sphincter mechanism, such as local bladder or prostatic tumors. Sleep disorders may increase the frequency of NOCTURIA, although enuresis during sleep does not occur. However, OBSTRUCTIVE SLEEP APNEA SYN-

DROME is a common cause of secondary enuresis in both children and adults. Rarely enuresis may be related to emotional immaturity. It may be seen in the child who demonstrates regression or passive-aggressive behavior due to family or social stresses.

Treatment is not required before age five, and if there is evidence that the frequency of urination is decreasing, treatment may be unnecessary even after age five. Studies have demonstrated that patients who undergo treatment by a variety of different means can usually be helped. However, approximately 15% of all patients will have a spontaneous remission of the enuresis.

Bladder training exercises such as controlling urination by preventing frequent daytime urination may be helpful. It is reported that up to 30% of children are helped by such exercises. Sphincter training exercises—where the child is asked to interrupt the urinary stream repeatedly, approximately 10 times for each voiding of the bladder—have also been reported to be helpful. A variety of conditioning processes have been utilized, such as using an alarm system. These means are often successful but require motivation on the part of the enuretic. Reinforcement of positive urinary control during sleep by means of a star chart or other reward system is helpful.

Along with any management of enuresis it is very important that the individual is supported by other members of the family. A loss of the support will often lead to the relapse of urinary control. Other positive reinforcement processes, such as removing the child from diapers or transferring from a crib to a bed, can often be positive steps in encouraging emotional maturation.

Medication can be useful for patients who have not responded to behavioral techniques. The tricyclic ANTIDEPRESSANTS, such as imipramine, may be useful in some patients, as also an anticholinergic medication, such as oxybutynin chloride (Ditropan). Antidiuretic hormones have also been shown to be useful, such as the intranasal desmopressin (DDAUP). Although medications are not the complete answer to treatment of enuresis, they can be useful, particularly for a child who may be staying over at a friend's place or staying at overnight camp. Other causes of enuresis must be excluded. Urinary tract infections must be treated, and if obstructive sleep apnea is present, treatment of this disorder can lead to resolution of the enuresis.

Cendron, M., "Primary Nocturnal Enuresis: Current Concepts," *American Family Physician* 59, no. 5 (1999): 1205–1214, 1219–1220.

Ferber, Richard, "Sleep-Associated Enuresis in the Child," in Kryger, M., Roth T. and Dement, W., eds., *The Principles and Practices of Sleep Disorders Medicine.* Philadelphia: Saunders, 1989. pp. 643–664.

Forsythe, W.F. and Redmond, A., "Enuresis and Spontaneous Cure Rate: Study of 1129 Enuretics," *Archives of Disease in Childhood* 49 (1974): 259–263.

Mikkelsen, E.J. and Rappoport, J.L., "Enuresis: Psychopathology, Sleep Stage, and Drug Response," *Neurological Clinics of North America* 7 (1980): 361–377.

sleep exercises Exercises prior to sleep at night are often recommended for patients who have an increase in muscle tension and a difficulty in relaxing that impairs the ability to fall asleep. The exercises are composed of relaxation techniques that lower arousal so that natural sleep can occur. They can be performed during the daytime (wakefulness) to assist in recognizing when muscle tension is high, and prior to the sleep episode to relax the tension and facilitate sleep onset. BIOFEEDBACK techniques have also been developed to aid in recognizing when muscle tension is high.

Typical relaxation exercises involve tensing and tightening up one or more muscles and then perceiving the sensation that occurs when they relax. Relaxation exercises can be performed while lying on the back with the eyes closed and the legs uncrossed. They should last at least 30 minutes; however, up to 60 minutes may be necessary if a great deal of muscle tension is present. Exercises of the legs involve bending both feet downward at the ankles and clawing the toes at the same time. The knees are straight and should not bend. The feet and toes are then allowed to go limp suddenly. Several minutes of relaxation should then occur before repeating the tension and relaxation phase of the feet. Following relaxation of the legs, the rest of the body, including the arms, should be relaxed. Similar exercises can be used for other muscles in the legs, arms, trunk, head and neck.

The muscle exercises proposed by Edmund Jacobson in 1983 have been found useful by many patients with increased muscle tension (see JACOBSONIAN RELAXATION).

sleep hygiene A variety of different practices that are necessary in order to have normal, good quality nocturnal sleep and full daytime alertness. These practices ensure that a regular pattern of sleep and wakefulness will occur in association with a pattern of underlying circadian rhythms. ENVIRONMENTAL TIME CUES are an important component of ensuring that the sleep-wake cycle maintains a normal rhythm and timing; disturbances of these cues will lead to a weakening of the circadian rhythmicity with consequent disturbances of the sleep-wake pattern.

The strongest environmental time cues are those that occur around the time of awakening and involve the maintenance of a regular wake time with adequate exposure to light.

Practices that are associated with a normal sleep-wake pattern are: avoidance of napping during the daytime; regular wake and sleep onset times; ensuring that an appropriate length of time is spent in bed, which is neither too short nor too excessive; avoidance of stimulants such as CAFFEINE, NICOTINE and ALCOHOL in the period immediately preceding bedtime; avoidance of stimulating exercise before bedtime; an adequate relaxation period before bedtime; avoidance of emotionally-upsetting activities or conversations immediately before bedtime; avoidance of activities associated with wakefulness in bed, for example, watching television or listening to the radio; a pleasant sleep environment, which includes sleeping on a comfortable mattress with adequate bed covers, and ensuring that the bedroom environment is not too cold, too hot or too bright; avoidance of dwelling on mental problems in bed. (See also INADEQUATE SLEEP HYGIENE.)

sleep hyperhidrosis Term for profuse sweating that occurs during sleep; also known as night sweats. The patient may have an excessive amount of sweating during daytime hours as well. This disorder can produce discomfort due to the excessive wetness of the bed clothes, which may need to be changed several times throughout the night. In some patients, the disorder can be relatively brief in duration, but in others it is a lifelong tendency. Excessive sweating can be exacerbated by chronic febrile (feverish) illness and a variety of other disorders, including diabetes insipidus, hyperthyroidism, pheochromocytoma, hypothalamic lesions, epilepsy, cerebral and brain stem strokes, cerebral palsy, CHRONIC PAROXYSMAL HEMICRANIA, spinal cord infarction, head injury and spontaneous periodic hypothermia. Sleep hyperhidrosis can also be a feature of pregnancy and can be induced by the use of antipyretic medications.

There does not appear to be any gender difference in the presence of this disorder, and it can be seen at any age but most commonly is seen in early adulthood. Sleep hyperhidrosis can occur in older age groups in association with the development of the OBSTRUCTIVE SLEEP APNEA SYNDROME.

Treatment is dependent on the cause of the sweating. Some patients may respond to amitriptiline or clonidine given before sleep. However, for many patients no cause can be determined; for most patients, treatment is not required. (See also PREGNANCY-RELATED SLEEP DISORDER.)

Lea, M.J. and Haber, R.C., "Descriptive Epidemiology of Night Sweats Upon Admission to a University Hospital," *Southern Medical Journal* 78 (1985): 1065–1067.

sleep hypochrondriasis See SLEEP STATE MISPERCEPTION.

sleep-inducing factors Various natural factors that are produced by the body are thought to have the effect of inducing sleep. The presence of these factors was first suggested by Henri Pieron in 1913 when the cerebrospinal fluid of a sleep-deprived dog had induced sleep in another dog after being injected into the ventricles of the brain. Since that time, studies have confirmed the presence of sleep-inducing properties of natural fluids, and various substances have been isolated that appear to have a sleep-inducing property. In 1967, Pappenheimer took spinal fluid from sleep-deprived goats and injected it into the ventricles of other animals and found that sleep could be induced. The compound that was known as FACTOR S was eventually isolated from the urine of healthy males and this compound, when injected into rabbits, produced SLOW WAVE SLEEP. Since that time, a variety of other sleep-promoting peptides have been discovered, including delta-sleep-inducing peptide (DSIP) and SLEEP-PROMOTING SUBSTANCE (SPS). Factor S appears to be very similar to a substance, which is found in bacterial cell walls, called MURAMYL DIPEPTIDE (MDP). This compound, when infused into animals, has been shown to increase NON-REM-STAGE SLEEP. However, it also affects increasing body TEMPERATURE. Further work with MDP suggested a relationship between the immune system and sleep because the compound INTERLEUKIN-I, a polypeptide, is produced in the acute phase response to injury and has marked slow wave sleep–inducing properties.

Other natural compounds that may have a sleep-inducing effect include CHOLECYSTOKININ (CCK), which is a peptide that is found in both the gastrointestinal tract and the brain. Injection of CCK into animals has produced a reduction in the SLEEP LATENCY. However, it may be associated more with behavioral sedation rather than the induction of true sleepiness.

Somatostatin is another agent that has been localized to the cells in the brain stem that are associated with the induction and maintenance of sleep. It may well have a direct effect on the regulation of sleep.

Various neurotransmitter agents, including SEROTONIN, NOREPINEPHRINE and ACETYLCHOLINE, are known to be agents that have a pronounced effect on inducing alertness or sleep; agents such as prostaglandin-D2 and uridine also have been demonstrated to have some sleep-inducing properties.

Thus a variety of agents are believed to be involved in the regulation of sleep and wakefulness, and the exact role of each has yet to be elucidated. However, it is clear that the control of sleep and wakefulness is a complex system that involves numerous neurochemical agents.

sleepiness Difficulty in maintaining the alert state so that, if an individual is not kept active and aroused, he will readily fall into sleep. Sleepiness is not just a form of tiredness and fatigue, but a reflection of a true need for sleep. When sleepiness occurs in situations where sleep would be inappropriate, such as during the day, it is termed EXCESSIVE SLEEPINESS. A variety of disorders that affect the quantity or quality of nocturnal sleep can lead to excessive sleepiness; however, normal sleepiness occurs in relation to the major sleep episode at night. Although sleepiness may be predominant, the arousal system can allow the individual to maintain full alertness, despite there being a strong physiological need for sleep. For example, this occurs in individuals working the night shift or in individuals staying up late at night because of work commitments or social interactions.

sleeping pills See HYPNOTICS.

sleeping sickness Also known as trypanosomiasis (brucei), sleeping sickness is an acute infection caused by a protozoan that induces sleepiness associated with a chronic meningoencephalomyelitis. This protozoan is transmitted to humans by the tsetse fly. There are two main forms of the disease: the *Gambian,* or West African type; and the *Rhodesian,* or East African type. Trypanosomiasis differs in its sensitivity to medication, and the Rhodesian form is often more severe, and more often fatal, than the Gambian form.

The infection usually presents in the acute phase with high fever and lymphadenopathy, often accompanied by severe headaches. Gradually the major sleep episode becomes disrupted and EXCESSIVE SLEEPINESS develops. The central nervous system features may develop several years after the onset of the acute infection. Seizures, coma and eventually death can occur if the disorder is untreated.

Sleeping sickness can be diagnosed by demonstrating the presence of the trypanosome in the blood, lymph nodes or spinal fluid. Serum abnormalities include increases in the IgM, and there is an increase of cerebrospinal fluid protein with central nervous system involvement. The disease is easily recognized if there has been exposure in endemic areas.

Polysomnographic studies demonstrate that the non-REM sleep loses its characteristic features of spindle activity (see SLEEP SPINDLES) and K-complexes, and the SLEEP STAGES become unrecognizable. However, REM sleep maintains its polysomnographic features, but sleep onset REM periods may be present during daytime episodes of sleepiness.

Early in the disease, suramin is the most effective medication; however, melarsoprol is recommended once there is central nervous system involvement. An alternative medication is alpha-difluoromethylornithine (DFMO), which has recently been shown to be more effective and less toxic than melarsoprol.

Mhlanga, J.D. et al., "Neurobiology of Cerebral Malaria and African Sleeping Sickness," *Brain Research Bulletin* 44, no. 5 (1997): 579–589.

Schwartz, B.A. and Seskande, C., "Sleeping Sickness: Sleep Study of a Case," *Electroencephalography and Clinical Neurophysiology* 3 (1970): 83–87.

sleep interruption A break in the SLEEP ARCHITECTURE that results in an arousal or an episode of wakefulness. Sleep interruption occurs in persons who have disorders during sleep that lead to an arousal or an awakening, such as INSOMNIA, OBSTRUCTIVE SLEEP APNEA SYNDROME or PERIODIC LIMB MOVEMENT DISORDER.

sleep latency The amount of time from lights out, or bedtime, to the commencement of the first stage of sleep, either non-REM or REM sleep. The sleep latency is usually within 20 minutes in normal sleepers and is typically 30 minutes or longer in persons suffering from INSOMNIA. Short sleep latencies of less than 10 minutes are usually seen in disorders of EXCESSIVE SLEEPINESS, such as NARCOLEPSY or OBSTRUCTIVE SLEEP APNEA SYNDROME. This term is preferred over the term "latency to sleep."

sleep log A written record for 24 hours or longer of a person's sleep-wake pattern. Sleep logs typically comprise information on sleep for at least two weeks. The information recorded includes the BEDTIME, SLEEP ONSET time, SLEEP DURATION, awake times, final wake-up, ARISE TIME and the timing and length of daytime NAPS. Other information can also be recorded, such as the use of sleep-inducing or STIMULANT MEDICATIONS, and the nature of wakeful activities. Sleep log is synonymous with the term "sleep diary."

sleep maintenance (DIMS) This term applies to people who complain of INSOMNIA and have difficulty in maintaining sleep once it has been initiated. Sleep maintenance insomnia can comprise either awakenings during the sleep episode or an early final awakening. It is a common feature of most forms of insomnia with the exception of the DELAYED SLEEP PHASE SYNDROME, which is characterized by a prolonged SLEEP ONSET without any sleep maintenance difficulty. The 1979 edition of the DIAGNOSTIC CLASSIFICATION OF SLEEP AND AROUSAL DISORDERS listed nine major groups of disorders of initiating and maintaining sleep.

sleep medicine and clinical polysomnography examination This examination was held for the first time in 1990 for applicants with a degree in the health field. Applicants can be either a Ph.D., M.D. or D.O. This examination replaces the previous accredited CLINICAL POLYSOMNOGRAPHER EXAMINATION. Physicians can receive certification in both sleep medicine and clinical polysomnography, and Ph.D.s can receive certification in clinical polysomnography.

Physician applicants for the examination are required to hold an M.D. or D.O. and be licensed to practice medicine in a state, commonwealth or territory of the United States or Canada. They must have undergone a one-year training in SLEEP DISORDERS MEDICINE or POLYSOMNOGRAPHY under the supervision of a board-certified sleep specialist and at least two years of an accredited residency program.

Both part one and part two of the examination were reorganized to be more specific to the applicant's background training. Part one is entirely multiple-choice questions; however, the questions focus on medical, diagnostic and treatment decisions for the physician.

Applicants for the Ph.D. examination need a Ph.D. degree with doctoral specialization in the health field and two years of clinical experience. They must have one year of training in clinical polysomnography under the supervision of an accredited clinical polysomnographer. (See also

ACCREDITATION STANDARDS FOR SLEEP DISORDER CENTERS, AMERICAN ACADEMY OF SLEEP MEDICINE, CLINICAL POLYSOMNOGRAPHER.)

sleep mentation The imagery and thinking experienced during sleep. Sleep mentation usually consists of a combination of thoughts and images that can occur during REM SLEEP. The imagery is most vividly expressed in DREAMS, which are clear representations of waking activity. This form of imagery is usually expressed during REM sleep, but it may occur less vividly during NON-REM-STAGE SLEEP, particularly during stage two sleep (see SLEEP STAGES). Sometimes mentation and dream imagery can occur at SLEEP ONSET and may be termed HYPNAGOGIC REVERIE.

sleep need Like the need for air and water, sleep is a necessity for humans, not an optional activity or even a skill that has to be learned. About a third of our lives is spent sleeping. It is possible for a short while to get by on less sleep, or to put off sleeping, but the need to sleep will eventually force anyone to succumb (see SLEEP DEPRIVATION).

The question "Why do we need to sleep?" is one that has intrigued scientists over the centuries, ever since Aristotle, in the fourth century B.C., noted that afternoon sleepiness appeared to follow midday meals. Lucretius in 55 B.C. perceived a connection between sleep and wakefulness.

We know that all animals, and fish, sleep for part of the 24-hour day, yet there is little understanding about why sleep is necessary.

There are currently three main theories about why we need to sleep. The first, the Restorative Theory, hypothesizes that sleep restores some component of our physiology that is used up during wakefulness. This restoration may be of a physical, chemical or mental nature. However, no one has yet been able to determine exactly what might be lost during wakefulness that is restored during sleep.

Studies have centered around trying to determine if there is any direct association between daytime physical activity and nighttime sleep. But investigations into athletes who are well-trained have failed to show any association between increased daytime activity and improved quality or duration of nighttime sleep. Some studies, however, have tended to show that there is an increase in stage three/four sleep, particularly if the exercise is performed in the late afternoon. However, other studies have tended to show different results with delay and decrease in REM sleep. The means of analyzing electroencephalographic sleep may affect these results because more specialized forms of analysis (by means of spectral analysis, EEG frequency analysis) have given different information than studies that have been scored by more traditional methods. The spectral analysis studies have tended to give support to the restorative theory of exercise and SLOW WAVE SLEEP by demonstrating improved slow wave sleep.

A second theory, called the Cleansing Theory, was first proposed in 1958 by Hughlings Jackson, a neurologist. The Cleansing Theory suggests that sleep affects memory, it cleans away unwanted memories and allows consolidation of memories that are important and need to be retained. The theory has been extended by others, including Francis Crick in 1983, who has proposed that it is the REM sleep that is particularly valuable in cleaning out unwanted memories, perhaps by a mechanism that involves dreaming.

The third theory of sleep need is the Circadian Theory developed in the 1970s. This theory hypothesizes that sleep is necessary in order to maintain CIRCADIAN RHYTHMS. It has been proposed that the interaction of the circadian rhythms is the most effective and efficient means of maintaining physiology in a state so that it can adequately adapt to changes in environmental or internal factors. A normal sleep-wake cycle has been shown to promote the maximal and ideal rhythm amplitude and phase relationships. Body temperature has its nadir during sleep and rises to a maximum amplitude 12 hours later. The strength of the cyclical pattern is diminished by a disrupted sleep pattern. (See also AGE.)

sleep onset The transition from wakefulness to sleep that usually comprises stage one sleep. In certain situations, particularly in infancy (see INFANT SLEEP) and in NARCOLEPSY, sleep onset may occur with REM SLEEP. Sleep onset is usually characterized by: a slowing of the ELECTROENCEPHALOGRAM (EEG); the reduction and eventual disappearance of ALPHA ACTIVITY; the presence of EEG vertex sharp transients; and slow rolling eye movements. Although an EPOCH (one page of a POLYSOMNOGRAM) of stage one sleep is usually required as documentation for sleep onset, some researchers prefer to take the first epoch of any stage of sleep other than stage one as being the criterion for sleep onset. The reason is that stage two sleep is more associated with subjective recall of sleep onset. Sometimes the sleep onset will be regarded as the onset of continuous sleep, which may comprise the beginning of three or more continuous epochs of stage one or other stages of sleep.

Sleep onset usually occurs within 20 minutes of the bedtime; however, people who complain of INSOMNIA may have a sleep onset that occurs 30 minutes or longer from the attempt to initiate sleep. Sleep onset may occur rapidly in disorders characterized by EXCESSIVE SLEEPINESS during the day or by hypersomnia, such as OBSTRUCTIVE SLEEP APNEA SYNDROME or narcolepsy. (See also SLEEP LATENCY, SLEEP STAGES.)

sleep onset association disorder Primarily a disorder of childhood where a child typically needs to have a favorite object (teddy bear, stuffed toy, blanket or bottle) or behavior (rocking in a mother's arms, hearing lullabies) for SLEEP ONSET to occur. In adults, the associated behavior may be the use of a television or a radio. When the object or behavior is not present, sleep onset becomes more difficult, and awakenings may occur throughout the night.

The sleep onset association is often reinforced by a caregiver. A child may be put to bed with a pacifier or a bottle, and the pattern or association with sleep becomes fixed until the child reaches a level of independence when it can maintain its own sleep pattern without the use of the object. If the behavior is not spontaneously eliminated with increasing maturity, it may be necessary to actively limit the introduction of the object.

This form of sleep disorder can be present from the first few days of life, but most commonly it becomes set between six months and three years of age. The disorder can occur for the first time at any age, and it is frequently seen in adulthood to old age, when falling asleep to a television or radio is typical.

This sleep disturbance can also occur at any age in response to a household disturbance, such as a move to a new home, marital difficulties, sibling rivalries or other forms of emotional stress that necessitate getting a comforting object in order to initiate sleep.

Polysomnographic monitoring demonstrates essentially normal sleep patterns, particularly if the sleep onset association object is present. However, sleep onset difficulties and an increase in the frequency and duration of awakenings at night may occur if the object is unavailable.

This form of sleep disturbance needs to be differentiated from LIMIT-SETTING SLEEP DISORDER where inadequate limits on bedtimes and wake times are the primary cause of the sleep disturbance. It also needs to be distinguished from PSYCHOPHYSIOLOGICAL INSOMNIA in the adult, in which negative associations to sleep are developed rather than the positive associations seen in sleep onset association disorder.

Treatment involves a gradual withdrawal of the object so that positive associations are developed to sleep, in the sleeping environment, without the need for a specific object. During the time of withdrawal of the object, good SLEEP HYGIENE measures are essential in order to prevent a breakdown of the sleep pattern or the development of psychophysiological insomnia.

sleep onset insomnia A form of insomnia characterized by difficulty in initiating sleep; there is an increased SLEEP LATENCY, but once sleep is initiated, little, if any, sleep disruption occurs. Sleep onset insomnia is typically seen in patients with the DELAYED SLEEP PHASE SYNDROME, where the timing of sleep is altered in relationship to the 24-hour day. There may be a prolonged sleep latency but, once sleep is initiated, sleep is normal in quality. Rarely, a sleep onset insomnia may be produced as a result of a PSYCHOPHYSIOLOGICAL INSOMNIA or an ANXIETY DISORDER; a pure sleep onset insomnia is also a rare feature of DEPRESSION. Some disorders, such as the RESTLESS LEGS SYNDROME or excessive SLEEP STARTS, may also be associated with a sleep onset insomnia.

sleep onset nightmares See TERRIFYING HYPNAGOGIC HALLUCINATIONS.

sleep onset REM period (SOREMP) Typically the onset of REM SLEEP is 90 minutes after sleep onset. But a sleep onset REM period is characterized by the initiation of REM sleep within 20 minutes of sleep onset. Sleep onset REM periods are a characteristic feature of NARCOLEPSY during the major sleep episode as well as during daytime NAPS. Two or more sleep onset REM periods seen during a daytime MULTIPLE SLEEP LATENCY TEST, in an individual who otherwise has a normal preceding night of sleep, may be diagnostic of narcolepsy. However, sleep onset REM periods may also be seen in other disorders of disrupted REM sleep, such as in severe OBSTRUCTIVE SLEEP APNEA SYNDROME.

Most patients with narcolepsy will have three sleep onset REM periods during a five-nap multiple sleep latency test; however, not uncommonly five sleep onset REM periods will occur. A single sleep onset REM period, particularly on the first or second nap of the multiple sleep latency test, may be seen in normal individuals who otherwise do not have a sleep disorder. However, two or more sleep onset REM periods are regarded as being distinctly abnormal for people without a sleep disorder.

sleep palsy A muscle weakness, present upon awakening, that is associated with pressure over nerves supplying a particular muscle or group of muscles. Some nerves in the limbs, such as the ulnar, radial and peroneal, are superficially placed in the limbs and therefore are liable to compression interfering with their conductive properties. A sleep palsy is commonly experienced if the limb is not moved and pressure is sustained over the nerve for half an hour or longer.

Sleep palsies generally resolve within a few minutes after resuming a more comfortable position; however, if an individual sleeps deeply and does not awaken because of the discomfort, the muscle weakness that results may last hours, days or even weeks. A typical form of sleep palsy occurs in individuals who have their arousal threshold increased because of drinking ALCOHOL. The so-called Saturday night palsy is related to excessive alcohol consumption, causing sleep to occur with the person in an unusual position, often with the radial nerve of the arm being compressed, leading to paralysis of the muscles supplied by that nerve. Typically a wrist drop will result after sleep has occurred in a chair and the arm is draped over the hard chairback. (See also CARPAL TUNNEL SYNDROME.)

sleep paralysis A condition of whole body muscle paralysis that occasionally may be present at the onset of sleep, or upon awakening during the night or in the morning. It is a manifestation of the muscle atonia (loss of muscle activity) that occurs in association with the dreaming (REM) stage of sleep (see DREAMS). Dream activity can accompany the limb paralysis; however, the patient is usually awake and fully conscious during the phenomenon. Typically an individual will attempt to move a limb and, finding an inability to do so, will feel fear, panic and at times the sensation of impending death. Respiratory movements are usually unimpaired, but the sensation of an inability to breathe is common.

The episodes last from seconds to several minutes and usually terminate spontaneously. The individual may make some moaning sounds during the episode, which may attract the attention of the bed partner; being touched or some other stimulus will assist in terminating the episode.

The condition, when seen frequently in any individual, raises the possibility of the diagnosis of NARCOLEPSY and typically is associated with EXCESSIVE SLEEPINESS during the day and CATAPLEXY. Unless the condition is associated with narcolepsy, it usually does not warrant therapeutic intervention. Reassurance is often required, and the initial episodes are often those of most concern, since in time recognizing the benign nature of the episodes reduces the concern.

A familial form of the condition has been recognized that is unaccompanied by other abnormal neurological features.

Sleep paralysis can sometimes be seen where there has been insufficient or poor-quality nocturnal sleep, such as with patients who have been sleep deprived (see SLEEP DEPRIVATION) or who have OBSTRUCTIVE SLEEP APNEA SYNDROME.

If the treatment is indicated, a REM suppressant medication, such as one of the tricyclic ANTIDEPRESSANTS, may be useful.

Goode, G. B., "Sleep Paralysis," *Archives of Neurology* 6 (1962): 228–234.
Hishikawa, Y., "Sleep Paralysis." in Guilleminault, Christian, Dement, William C. and Passouant, P., eds., *Narcolepsy.* Vol. 2: *Advances in Sleep Research.* New York: Spectrum, 1976. pp. 97–124.
McKecknie, J., "Incidence and Diagnosis of Sleep Paralysis," *Nursing Times* 94, no. 22 (1998): 50–51.
Roth, B., Bruhova, S. and Berkova, L., "Familial Sleep Paralysis," *Archives Suisses Neurological Neurochir Psychiatry* 102 (1968): 321–330.

sleep pattern A person's routine of sleep and waking behavior that includes the clock hour of BEDTIME and ARISE TIME, as well as NAPS and time and duration of sleep interruptions. A typical 24-hour sleep pattern comprises eight hours of sleep at night, followed by 16 hours of wakefulness. A biphasic sleep pattern is seen in individuals who have a prolonged sleep episode in the late afternoon, such as a SIESTA, in association with a major sleep episode at night. (See also CIRCADIAN RHYTHMS, SLEEP DURATION, SLEEP INTERRUPTION.)

sleep-promoting substance (SPS) SPS has been isolated from the brains of rats that have been sleep deprived. This agent, when infused intracerebrally into rats, produces an increase in SLOW WAVE SLEEP and REM SLEEP. This substance has not yet been chemically identified and other researchers have failed to confirm its existence. (See also SLEEP-INDUCING FACTORS.)

sleep-regulating center Term proposed by Constantin Von Economo following his careful anatomic studies of patients with ENCEPHALITIS LETHARGICA. He believed that a sleep-regulating center was present in the upper brain stem in the posterior hypothalamus.

sleep-related abnormal swallowing syndrome Disorder that occurs during sleep in which there is aspiration of saliva that produces coughing and choking episodes, due to inadequately swallowed saliva that collects in the pharynx and erroneously passes into the larynx and trachea. This choking and coughing can cause INSOMNIA.

This disorder was first described by CHRISTIAN GUILLEMINAULT in 1976 as an unusual cause of insomnia. The patient described by Guilleminault had frequent episodes of coughing and gagging that were associated with "gurgling" sounds, probably due to the pooling of saliva in the lower part of the pharynx. Because of the frequent aspiration, patients with this disorder may be prone to respiratory tract infections that can be worsened by increased use of HYPNOTICS, which may be prescribed to help the insomnia.

Polysomnographic studies have demonstrated a very disturbed sleep pattern with frequent awakenings occurring throughout all the sleep stages; however, deep SLOW WAVE SLEEP does not occur. This disorder needs to be differentiated from other disorders that cause choking episodes during sleep, in particular, OBSTRUCTIVE SLEEP APNEA SYNDROME. Episodes of SLEEP-RELATED GASTROESOPHAGEAL REFLUX can also lead to coughing and choking during sleep, but daytime episodes of acid reflux associated with heartburn, chest pain and other features indicative of reflux are usually present in such patients. Patients with SLEEP-RELATED LARYNGOSPASM may appear to have a disorder similar to sleep-related abnormal swallowing syndrome; however, the episodes of laryngospasm are rare, and between episodes patients are typically asymptomatic.

The pathology of sleep-related abnormal swallowing syndrome is unknown; however, abnormalities in either the swallowing reflex, its motor component or the protective mechanism guarding the larynx are considered to be possible causes.

Treatment is largely symptomatic, and one can consider the use during sleep of anticholinergic agents, such as amitriptyline (see ANTIDEPRESSANTS), which reduce upper airway secretion.

Guilleminault, C., Eldridge, F.L., Philipps, J.R. and Dement, W.C., "Two Occult Causes of Insomnia and their Therapeutic Problems," *Archives of General Psychiatry* 33 (1976): 1241–1245.

sleep-related asthma Frequent asthmatic attacks that occur during sleep. Typically these episodes will lead to an arousal or an awakening from sleep.

The awakenings are characterized by difficulty in breathing, wheezing, coughing, gasping for air and chest discomfort. Often there may be excessive mucus produced during these episodes. Typically the patient will use a medication, such as a bronchodilator, that relieves the acute episodes.

Asthma attacks during sleep appear to be more common in children, and it is reported that up to 75% of asthmatic patients have some nighttime episodes. Generally the severity of the sleep-related asthma parallels the severity of daytime asthma.

The cause of sleep-related asthma is unknown; however, circadian factors are thought to play a part. There is a circadian variation in bronchial resistance, which tends to be increased in the early morning hours, and there may also be a circadian change in the intensity of airway inflammation at night. There are also nighttime reductions in the serum level of epinephrine (chemical produced by the adrenal gland) and CORTISOL (hormone produced by adrenal gland) that may predispose an individual to an asthmatic attack. In addition, the effect of medications during the daytime may wear off during the nocturnal sleep episode.

Polysomnographic evaluation of persons with sleep-related asthma tends to show that episodes are more likely to occur during the second half of the sleep episode. However, there does not appear to be a specific sleep stage relationship.

Episodes of acute difficulty in breathing at night need to be differentiated from a variety of other SLEEP-RELATED BREATHING DISORDERS, as well as SLEEP-RELATED GASTROESOPHAGEAL REFLUX, SLEEP-RELATED LARYNGOSPASM or the SLEEP CHOKING SYNDROME.

Treatment of sleep-related asthma involves appropriate management of daytime asthma. Appropriate treatment of the acute sleep-related attacks is also required. In addition, elimination of any potential bedroom allergens may reduce the frequency of sleep-related asthma.

Clark, T.J.H., "The Circadian Rhythm of Asthma," *British Journal of Chest Disease* 79 (1985): 115–124.

D'Ambrosio, C.M. et al., "Sleep in Asthma," *Clinics of Sleep Medicine* 19, no. 1 (1998): 127–137.

Martin, R.J., "Nocturnal Asthma and the Use of Theophylline," *Clinical & Experimental Allergy* 28, Suppl. 3 (1998): 64–70.

———, "Nocturnal Asthma," in Martin, Richard J., ed., *Cardiorespiratory Disorders During Sleep*. New York: Futura Publishing Company, 1984. pp. 119–146.

sleep-related breathing disorders This term applies to breathing disorders that are induced or exacerbated during sleep. Although many different respiratory disorders are affected by sleep, the three main syndromes associated with sleep are the OBSTRUCTIVE SLEEP APNEA SYNDROME, CENTRAL SLEEP APNEA SYNDROME and the CENTRAL ALVEOLAR HYPOVENTILATION SYNDROME.

The obstructive sleep apnea syndrome is characterized by UPPER AIRWAY OBSTRUCTION that occurs during sleep, leading to a change in the arterial blood gases. HYPOXEMIA produces cardiac effects and disrupts sleep, leading to the development of EXCESSIVE SLEEPINESS during the day.

Central sleep apnea syndrome is characterized by cessation of breathing that occurs without upper airway obstruction and leads to blood gas changes that also can produce disrupted sleep and daytime sleepiness.

Central alveolar hypoventilation syndrome is due to shallow breathing that occurs during sleep, with associated blood gas changes. Typically there is the development of daytime sleepiness but sometimes a complaint of INSOMNIA.

The sleep-related breathing disorders can occur at any age, from infancy through old age, and can have a spectrum of severity ranging from very mild to life threatening.

Treatment varies depending upon the primary cause of the respiratory disturbance but can range from behavioral techniques, such as weight loss, the use of RESPIRATORY STIMULANTS, the use of mechanical devices to prevent upper airway obstruction, or assisted ventilation, to surgical treatments (see SURGERY AND SLEEP DISORDERS) ranging from TONSILLECTOMY to TRACHEOSTOMY, in order to relieve the upper airway obstruction.

Fletcher, E.C., ed., *Abnormalities of Respiration During Sleep: Diagnosis, Pathophysiology, and Treatment.* Orlando: Grune and Stratton, 1986.

sleep-related cardiovascular symptoms Symptoms that arise from a variety of cardiac disorders, including those that affect cardiac rhythm and cardiac output. The symptoms are primarily discomfort or pain in the chest, or respiratory difficulty.

One of the most common symptoms related to cardiovascular disease is PAROXYSMAL NOCTURNAL DYSPNEA, which is shortness of breath related to recumbency (lying down), which is usually associated with sleep. This symptom is indicative of heart failure as a result of either myocardial or valvular disease and features difficulty in breathing and a sensation of suffocation that induces the patient to sit up or get out of bed. There may be a sensation of needing air, "air hunger," and persons may need to open a window in order to inspire cooler air. Due to the difficulty in breathing when lying down, a large proportion of the night may be spent sleeping in a semi-reclining or sitting position. The shortness of breath while lying flat is called ORTHOPNEA.

Chest pain may occur during sleep. The terms "nocturnal angina" or NOCTURNAL CARDIAC ISCHEMIA have been used to describe the chest pain that occurs in sleep at night. Precipitation of chest pain during sleep may be the result of REM sleep features, such as variability in blood pressure and heart rate. It is also possible that the lowering of blood pressure during SLOW WAVE SLEEP may precipitate coronary artery insufficiency, leading to angina.

Sleep disorders, such as the SLEEP-RELATED BREATHING DISORDERS, in particular the OBSTRUCTIVE SLEEP APNEA SYNDROME, are also believed to be a cause of nocturnal angina and cardiac ischemia during sleep. Cardiac ARRHYTHMIAS may also be precipitated by sleep-related breathing disorders and may induce symptoms of chest discomfort or shortness of breath.

Some cardiovascular disorders during sleep are essentially asymptomatic; for example, REM SLEEP-RELATED SINUS ARREST generally does not have any sleep-related symptoms. Individuals who die from SUDDEN UNEXPLAINED NOCTURNAL DEATH SYNDROME (SUND) are asymptomatic prior to the terminal event.

Patients with sleep-related cardiovascular symptoms need to undergo electrocardiography throughout sleep, in association with POLYSOMNOGRAPHY, to determine oxygen saturation levels and the presence of sleep-related breathing disorders. Correction of the sleep-related breathing disorders can reduce symptoms during sleep and reduce the likelihood of a catastrophic cardiovascular event. Patients with REM sleep-related sinus arrest may require the insertion of a permanent pacemaker as a preventative measure.

Chest discomfort during sleep may be due to a number of different sleep disorders. SLEEP-RELATED GASTROESOPHAGEAL REFLUX commonly produces chest discomfort that may be difficult to distinguish from that of a cardiac cause. Difficulty in breathing at night is commonly produced by the sleep-related breathing disorders, such as obstructive sleep apnea syndrome, CENTRAL SLEEP APNEA SYNDROME and CENTRAL ALVEOLAR HYPOVENTILATION SYNDROME. Occasional awakening with the sensation of the heart having stopped is not uncommon in patients who have ANXIETY DISORDERS, PANIC DISORDER or SLEEP TERRORS. Choking episodes during sleep can also be seen in patients with the SLEEP CHOKING SYNDROME or SLEEP-RELATED LARYNGOSPASM.

Nolan, J.B., Troyer, W.G., Collins, W.F., Silverman, T., Nichols, C.R., McIntosh, H.D., Estes, E.L. and Bogdonoff, M.D., "The Association of Nocturnal Angina Pectoris with Dreaming," *Annals of Internal Medicine* 63 (1965): 1040–1046.

sleep-related enuresis See SLEEP ENURESIS.

sleep-related epilepsy Epilepsy is a disorder characterized by the sudden occurrence of an excessive cerebral electric discharge. Epilepsy has a very specific relationship with the sleep-wake cycle, which can lead to epilepsy being exacerbated during sleep.

The generalized seizures (grand mal), the partial or focal motor seizures, and complex partial seizures are three forms of epilepsy that can occur during sleep. Although epilepsy can produce sleep disruption and lead to a complaint of INSOMNIA, in general the primary complaint is of abnormal movement activity during sleep. Episodes of sudden awakening with movements or walking raise a possibility that the episode is due to epilepsy, particularly if there is associated confusion.

Because sleep is a powerful activator of epilepsy, sleep is used for diagnostic purposes.

Electroencephalography (see ELECTROENCEPHALOGRAM) is often performed after a night of SLEEP DEPRIVATION so that the effects of either sleep loss or the subsequent sleep episode can be utilized to enhance detection of abnormal epileptic activity. Sometimes HYPNOTICS such as chloral hydrate are given to the patient, when epilepsy is suspected, to enhance the detection of epileptic discharges during sleep.

The form of epilepsy that causes the most difficulty in its differentiation from other sleep disorders, such as SLEEPWALKING, is the partial complex seizure. In this particular seizure type, a patient may awaken from sleep, pick at the bedclothes, have lip-smacking, get out of bed and walk around and appear to be unaware of other people in the environment. Usually the walking is performed in a semi-purposeful manner; however, the individual may be difficult to awaken and may go back to bed without assistance. If the person does awaken there is generally confusion followed by lethargy. What distinguishes this seizure disorder from sleepwalking episodes is the presence of the automatic and repetitive type of limb movements and lip-smacking behavior.

In generalized tonic-clonic seizures that occur during sleep, there is little difficulty in diagnosis because of the repetitive jerking of the limbs and associated urinary or fecal incontinence. The patient is also typically confused following the episode.

A focal epilepsy characterized by small jerking movements of one part of the body needs to be distinguished from other forms of movement disorder, such as PERIODIC LIMB MOVEMENT DISORDER. Sometimes a whole body jerk can occur at SLEEP ONSET, due to epilepsy, that is difficult to differentiate from SLEEP STARTS; however, such episodes usually recur during sleep, whereas sleep starts are present only at sleep onset.

A patient who presents with a single epileptic seizure during sleep may not proceed to have further episodes; however, most patients will develop not only sleep-related epileptic seizures but also daytime episodes. In the initial stages, a daytime electroencephalogram may help diagnose epilepsy. Polysomnographic monitoring with extensive electroencephalographic recording during sleep is necessary in some patients to confirm the diagnosis.

Sometimes epileptic seizures are heralded by a loud cry, followed by a generalized tremor, and such an episode may be difficult to differentiate from sleep terrors. However, other behavioral manifestations of epilepsy are usually present, such as repetitive movements like lip-smacking or jerking of the limbs, and there is the absence of the intense fear and panic that is characteristic of sleep terrors.

The diagnosis of epilepsy is confirmed if a specific electroencephalographic pattern is seen during the behavioral event. For tonic-clonic epilepsy, generalized spike and wave activity occurring bilaterally and in a synchronous manner is diagnostic. These spike and wave episodes occur with a frequency that is generally in the delta range (2 to 4 Hz), lasting up to five seconds in duration in the interictal period. Repetitive spike activity, called polyspikes, is also frequently seen during non-REM sleep in patients with generalized seizure disorders. Abnormal EEG activity is often suppressed during REM sleep. Polysomnographic monitoring of patients for seizure disorders is aided by using an extensive electroencephalographic array (arrangement or montage) with 12 to 16 channels of information, coupled to simultaneous audiovisual monitoring.

Treatment of the epilepsy depends upon the underlying type of epilepsy, and usually one or more anticonvulsant medications are required. (See also RHYTHMIC MOVEMENT DISORDER.)

Degan, R. and Neidermeyer, E., eds., *Epilepsy, Sleep and Sleep Deprivation.* Amsterdam: Elsevier, 1984.

sleep-related gastroesophageal reflux A disorder characterized by a reflux (backward flow) of acid from the stomach into the esophagus during sleep. Usually this disorder will cause the patient to awaken with a discomfort or pain in the chest or an awareness of a sour, acid taste in the mouth. The pain that is experienced is usually in the mid-chest behind the sternum and is often associated with a general tightness in the chest.

Gastroesophageal reflux can cause pharyngitis (inflammation of the throat), laryngospasm and difficulty in swallowing because of the acid irritation. Although episodes of gastroesophageal reflux can occur during the day, episodes occur more frequently at night. Ulcers and inflammation of the esophageal mucosa can occur that may progress to a complete constriction of the esophagus. Long-standing gastroesophageal reflux may lead to the development of an abnormal lining to the lower esophagus, which may be a premalignant condition.

Approximately 7% to 10% of the general population has HEARTBURN due to gastroesophageal reflux. It is a more common disorder in persons over the age of 40 years.

Gastroesophageal reflux may be precipitated by the OBSTRUCTIVE SLEEP APNEA SYNDROME, which causes an increased intra-abdominal pressure due to the increasing respiratory muscle activity. Reflux of acid may lead to pulmonary aspiration with subsequent pneumonia.

Sleep-related gastroesophageal reflux can be demonstrated by 24-hour esophageal acid (pH) monitoring. An acid-sensitive probe is placed through the nose and into the lower esophagus where changes in the acid content of the lower esophagus are detected. Concurrent polysomnographic monitoring demonstrates whether a physiological event, such as an obstructive sleep apnea, is associated with the precipitation of an episode of sleep-related gastroesophageal reflux.

Treatment of gastroesophageal reflux is primarily by weight reduction in those patients who are overweight. Prilosec is the drug of choice. Antacids and inhibitors of acid secretion such as rantidine (Zantac) or cimetidine (Tagamet) may be prescribed. Small meals taken at two- to three-hour intervals during the day may be useful in reducing gastroesophageal reflux; large meals should be avoided before going to bed at night. (See also OBESITY.)

Orr, William C., Johnson, L. and Robinson, M.G., "The Effect of Sleep on Swallowing, Esophageal Peristalsis, and Acid Clearance," *Gastroenterology* 8 (1984): 814–819.

sleep-related headaches The headache forms that are most likely to occur during sleep are MIGRAINE, CLUSTER HEADACHE and CHRONIC PAROXYSMAL HEMICRANIA.

These three headache forms appear to have a common pathophysiological basis in that they are all associated with autonomic (involuntary neurological system concerned with involuntary functions) features, especially cluster headache and chronic paroxysmal hemicrania. Polysomnographic monitoring has demonstrated that these headache forms are more likely to occur in REM SLEEP, and chronic paroxysmal hemicrania is more closely tied to REM sleep than the other two.

These headaches need to be differentiated from the group of headaches termed muscle contraction or tension headaches, which may be associated with ANXIETY or HYPERTENSION. Tension headaches typically occur upon awakening in the morning and do not usually cause an abrupt awakening from sleep.

Treatment of sleep-related headaches depends upon the particular headache form involved and may require the use of medications such as cafergot, Midrin, beta-blockers, calcium channel blockers or morphine derivative analgesics, in the case of migraine headaches. Cluster headaches may be treated by steroids, methysergide or oxygen therapy.

Muscle contraction headaches that occur upon awakening in the morning may be helped by relaxation therapy, amitriptyline (see ANTIDEPRESSANTS) or anxiolytic agents. Muscle contraction headaches need to be differentiated from headaches that occur upon awakening in the morning due to the OBSTRUCTIVE SLEEP APNEA SYNDROME, which respond to specific treatment for that syndrome.

sleep-related hemolysis See PAROXYSMAL NOCTURNAL HEMOGLOBINURIA.

sleep-related laryngospasm Condition characterized by an abrupt awakening from sleep with an intense inability to breathe and the development of stridor (a high-pitched inspiration sound). Stridor is characterized by a high-pitched sound made when trying to inspire through a partially closed upper airway. Patients with this disorder are abruptly awakened from sleep and typically will jump out of bed in intense fear and panic of dying. The patient will clutch his throat and try to inspire and often produce a loud and rather frightening gasping sound. Bed partners are always awoken by the event, which is very dramatic, and the patient may be seen to be slightly cyanotic (blue in color). Typically the episode will subside within five minutes; sometimes the individual requires a drink to speed the resolution of the episode. Following the episode of stridor, there may be hoarseness of the voice, and the anxiety and panic gradually subsides and the individual returns to sleep. Episodes usually occur only once a night and are very rare, recurring only two to three times a year.

In most patients, the cause of the episodes is unknown. However, episodes can occur with gastroesophageal reflux of acid. Sleep-related laryngospasm is also known to occur in patients who have the OBSTRUCTIVE SLEEP APNEA SYNDROME, usually as a result of associated gastroesophageal reflux. Patients with gastroesophageal reflux and laryngospasm will usually be aware of an acid taste in the mouth at the time of the awakening.

The cause of the stridor is believed to be vocal cord spasm; however, endoscopic evaluations immediately following the episodes have failed to show any abnormality of this laryngeal region.

The episodes of inability to breathe need to be distinguished from other causes of respiratory difficulty during sleep, such as the obstructive sleep apnea syndrome. The intense panic and anxiety associated with the episode requires one to distinguish it from SLEEP TERRORS or a panic attack due to a PANIC DISORDER. The SLEEP CHOKING SYNDROME is characterized by a sensation of an inability to breathe, but stridor and cyanosis do not occur in sleep choking syndrome, nor do episodes of the sleep choking syndrome disrupt the bed partner. Episodes of sleep choking syndrome, unlike sleep-related laryngospasm, occur on numerous occasions, often more than once at night. The SLEEP-RELATED ABNORMAL SWALLOWING SYNDROME, which is also associated with choking during sleep, can be differentiated by its typical clinical features, which include "gurgling" sounds during sleep.

Many patients with daytime stridor have been demonstrated to have the stridor as a result of psychogenic factors. Such patients can voluntarily induce stridor during wakefulness. The occurrence of stridor during sleep in such patients has not been reported to occur. Treatment of the sleep-related laryngospasm is dependent upon the discovery of an underlying cause, if one can be established. Usually sleep-related laryngospasm does not require treatment due to its very infrequent occurrence.

sleep-related neurogenic tachypnea Disorder characterized by a sustained increase in respiratory rate that occurs during sleep as compared with wakefulness. The respiratory rate increase is not due to alterations in blood gases that might result from cardiac or respiratory factors; it appears to be of central nervous system origin. Some patients with sleep-related neurogenic tachypnea have been reported to have EXCESSIVE SLEEPINESS during the day that appears to be related, at least in part, to the underlying tachypnea.

Neurological disorders have been associated with sleep-related neurogenic tachypnea, particularly lesions of the brain stem, such as the lateral medullary syndrome and multiple sclerosis. An idiopathic (without a known cause) form of the disorder can occur.

There have been only a few reports of this disorder and its exact cause is not understood. Polysomnographic monitoring has demonstrated sleep fragmentation, which appears to be related to the respiratory rhythm. Although excessive sleepiness would be expected, sleep latency testing has not been reported in this disorder.

Sleep-related neurogenic tachypnea must be differentiated from other SLEEP-RELATED BREATHING DISORDERS, such as OBSTRUCTIVE SLEEP APNEA SYNDROME, CENTRAL SLEEP APNEA SYNDROME and CENTRAL ALVEOLAR HYPOVENTILATION SYNDROME. These disorders can all produce an increase of respiratory rate during sleep. Left-sided heart failure and PAROXYSMAL NOCTURNAL DYSPNEA can result in an increase of respiratory rate during sleep.

No specific treatment is known for this disorder.

sleep-related painful erections Condition where penile erections occurring at night are very painful. All males, from infancy to old age, have erections during REM sleep, and the occurrence of a partial or full erection may be associated with intense pain that awakens the person during sleep. The frequent interruptions of sleep can cause the sufferer to have daytime tiredness and fatigue.

Typically erections during wakefulness are not painful. Some disorders, such as Peyrone's disease and phymosis, can be present concurrently with painful erections, but these disorders are not the cause of the discomfort.

This disorder is rare and typically will occur in the age group over 40, although it can occur at an earlier age. It tends to become more severe with increasing age. No clear penile pathology has been shown to explain this disorder.

Polysomnographic studies will demonstrate an awakening during an episode of sleep-related penile tumescence accompanied by the complaint of penile pain.

Treatment of the disorder is usually symptomatic, although medications such as tricyclic ANTIDEPRESSANTS, which impair sleep-related erections, may be effective. (See also IMPAIRED SLEEP-RELATED PENILE ERECTIONS.)

Karacan, I., "Painful Nocturnal Penile Erections," *Journal of the American Medical Association* 215 (1971): 1831.

Matthews, B.J. and Crutchfield, M.B., "Painful Nocturnal Penile Erections Associated with Rapid Eye Movement Sleep," *Sleep* 10 (1987): 184–187.

sleep-related penile erections All healthy males from infancy to old age have penile erections during sleep. The erections occur with each REM sleep episode, that is, approximately five times in a night, each erection lasting about 30 minutes in duration. The total amount of time that the penis is erect decreases slightly with age to a total of approximately 100 minutes in the elderly.

Erections during sleep have their onset in infants between three and four months of age. They are usually not produced by sexual excitement, but are an automatic response generated by the nervous system. However, some erections during sleep occur in association with sexual dreams, and NOCTURNAL EMISSIONS ("wet dreams") during sleep are always associated with sexual dreaming.

An assessment of normal penile erectile ability during sleep can be used to determine whether a complaint of IMPOTENCE has an organic or psychological cause. Patients with an organic cause of the impotence have an inability to obtain adequate erections during sleep. This form of testing, termed NOCTURNAL PENILE TUMESCENCE TESTING, is often used to determine the cause of the impotence before the patient is referred either for implantation of an artificial penile prosthesis or for psychiatric or sex therapy. (See also IMPAIRED SLEEP-RELATED PENILE ERECTIONS, IMPOTENCE, SLEEP-RELATED PAINFUL ERECTIONS.)

sleep-related penile tumescence See SLEEP-RELATED PENILE ERECTIONS.

Sleep Research Online (SRO) A sleep research journal published online by the SLEEP RESEARCH SOCIETY. There are no subscription fees for Sleep Research Online. Individuals may download and print single copies for the noncommercial purpose of scientific or educational advancement. Reprints for each article in SRO may be requested directly and automatically from the author by simply clicking on the web site's "Reprint Request" button. In the near future, reprints for articles that are cited in the list of references at the end of each SRO article may be requested, automatically, in a similar fashion. In addition, a special command will allow individuals to print any SRO article, formatted as it would appear in a traditional print journal. Sleep Research Online will also be printed in an annual volume which will include all articles that were published electronically during the preceding year. The printed volume will be distributed, free of charge, to libraries worldwide and on a subscription basis to individuals.

For further information, contact Sleep Research Online, c/o WebSciences, 10911 Weyburn Avenue, Suite 348, Los Angeles, California 90024. E-mail: sro@sro.org; Web: http://www.sro.com.

Sleep Research Society (SRS) Originally founded in Chicago in 1961 as the ASSOCIATION FOR THE PSYCHOPHYSIOLOGICAL STUDY OF SLEEP. In 1983, the association changed its name to the Sleep Research Society, in part because the society no longer primarily concerned itself with the psychophysiological aspects of sleep research.

The Sleep Research Society joined with the American Sleep Disorders Association (see AMERI-

CAN ACADEMY OF SLEEP MEDICINE) to form the federation called the ASSOCIATION OF PROFESSIONAL SLEEP SOCIETIES which holds a combined annual meeting of sleep research.

sleep restriction therapy A treatment for patients with INSOMNIA based upon the recognition that excessive time spent in bed often perpetuates insomnia. Typically, patients with insomnia go to bed on some nights earlier than usual in order to obtain more sleep, or to counteract feelings of daytime tiredness and fatigue. In addition, patients may stay in bed longer in the morning to make up for lost sleep at night, or because of feelings of tiredness or fatigue. Because sleep is often spread out over a longer portion of the 24-hour day, often as much as 12 hours, sleep becomes fragmented, with frequent intervals of wakefulness. Maintaining a consolidated nighttime sleep and a full episode of wakefulness for the rest of the day is most helpful in promoting normal and strong circadian rhythms.

Sleep restriction therapy involves reducing the amount of time spent in bed by one or more hours and ensuring that sleep occurs only during the set BEDTIME and awake times. In that way, sleep becomes more consolidated after one or two days on the new pattern. In some cases, the total time recommended for sleep may be as little as 4.5 hours, but typically it is on the order of 6 to 7.5 hours. Once the sleep restriction produces an increased consolidation of sleep with less wakefulness and more continuous and longer durations of sleep, the total time available for sleep may be increased slightly by 15 or 30 minutes. In this manner, an initial restricted pattern of 4.5 hours may be increased to 5 hours after one week, and then to 5.5 hours one week later, with sequential increases until a point is reached where allowing additional time contributes only to increased wakefulness at night.

People who undergo sleep restriction therapy may notice an increased tendency for sleepiness in the first few days, often because the reported TOTAL SLEEP TIME is less than the actual sleep and therefore there may be an element of SLEEP DEPRIVATION. However, as sleep fills the available time for sleeping, and the time for sleeping is extended, the tendency for daytime sleepiness reduces.

This therapy improves sleep by consolidating sleep and also by reducing the number of disrupting factors associated with sleep disturbance. Maintaining regular SLEEP ONSET and wake times and the occurrence of sleep at the time of the maximum circadian phase for sleep are some of the features that make sleep restriction therapy effective. In addition, because the patient knows that sleep onset will occur rapidly as a result of the sleep restriction, there is less concern and worry over being able to fall asleep at night. As the amount of sleep is predictable from night to night, the individual has less concern over having a night with no sleep. As the sleep restriction pattern is continued, the patient becomes conditioned to improved sleep, and the heightened anxiety and arousal related to sleep dissipates, allowing the individual to sleep peacefully.

Sleep restriction therapy has been shown to be useful for young and middle-aged adults; however, recent studies have shown that this form of treatment may be less effective in geriatric patients. Sleep restriction therapy has some similarities with STIMULUS CONTROL THERAPY, which has a similar basis of encouraging the reduction of the amount of wakefulness spent in bed.

Case History

A 48-year-old research scientist at a medical school had a lifelong history of sleeping difficulties, which had deteriorated even further several years prior to her presentation at the sleep disorders center. The presentation was related to a recent increase in anxiety that accompanied changing her employment. She occasionally would take a benzodiazepine hypnotic to help her sleep, although she preferred to avoid taking medications. She would awaken several times at night and would go to the bathroom each time but generally would stay in bed between the hours of 10 P.M. and 7 A.M. Sleep onset times were variable and she often would not go to bed until she was very tired and sleepy. On other occasions, following a night of very poor sleep, she would go to sleep a little earlier than usual. She regarded herself as slightly tense and anxious, although she denied any evidence of depression. She had undergone relaxation exercises in the past and occasionally would play a relaxation tape, which would somewhat help her to sleep.

She had visited a number of physicians, and had undergone a number of unorthodox treatments for her sleep disturbance. She had seen a nutritionist, an acupuncturist, a chiropractor and a homeopath. All these treatments had produced slight improvement but none had produced any consistent benefit. She received a number of diagnoses that included hypoglycemia (low blood sugar), hypothyroidism (low blood thyroid hormone) and infectious mononucleosis, although there was no strong evidence for the presence of any of those disorders.

The initial impression was one of a psychophysiological insomnia exacerbated by elements of underlying anxiety and depression. However, a psychiatric diagnosis of anxiety disorder or depression could not be established.

It was recommended that she be placed on a strict pattern of sleep restriction with a bedtime of 11 at night and an awake time of 6 in the morning. She was advised to restrict her use of hypnotic medication and to complete a sleep log, which would assist in determining any change in her sleeping pattern.

The strict adherence to the regular pattern of going to bed later and awakening at a fixed time in the morning produced a major benefit in her overall sleep. From having sleep times that could vary between 3 hours and 7.5 hours, she developed a consistent pattern of sleeping 6.5 to 7 hours on a regular basis. During this treatment program, she took a trip across time zones and although her stay in the new time zone was only a few days and she tried to keep to her new schedule, she found that her sleep deteriorated. Upon returning to her original environment, she reduced her total time in bed by half an hour so she would awaken at 5:30 in the morning. This brought about a resolution of the exacerbation produced by the time-zone travel.

After several weeks, she was able to return to her more usual pattern of going to bed at 11 P.M. and arising at 6 A.M., and her sleep pattern was significantly improved. (See also CIRCADIAN RHYTHMS, FATIGUE, SLEEP PATTERN.)

Spielman, Arthur J., Saskin, P. and Thorpy, Michael J., "Treatment of Chronic Insomnia by Restriction of Time Spent in Bed," *Sleep* 10 (1987): 45–56.

sleep schedule The pattern of sleep that occurs within a 24-hour day. Typically, the sleep schedule involves the sleep onset and awake times in relationship to the 24-hour clock time. The sleep schedule may vary if the times for sleep change, in which case an irregular sleep schedule may occur. However, a typical sleep schedule is one that has a regular sleep onset time at night and a regular awake time in the morning. (See also CIRCADIAN RHYTHMS, IRREGULAR SLEEP-WAKE PATTERN, NREM-REM SLEEP CYCLE, TOTAL SLEEP TIME.)

Sleep Society of Canada See CANADIAN SLEEP SOCIETY.

sleep spindles A pattern of electrical activity occurring during sleep that appears in an electroencephalographic recording. Sleep spindles are an identifying feature of stage two sleep. A sleep spindle consists of a spindle-shaped burst of 11 to 15 Hz waves that lasts for 0.5 to 1.5 seconds. Spindles can occur diffusely over the head and are of highest voltage over the central regions, with an amplitude that is usually less than 50 microvolts in adults. Sleep spindles, although characteristic of stage two sleep, may persist into deeper stages three and four sleep but usually are not seen in REM sleep. Reduction of spindle activity may be seen in the elderly, and an increase can be seen in association with disorders of the basal ganglia of the brain, such as dystonia, or as a result of medications, such as the BENZODIAZEPINES. Sleep disruption, if severe, can cause spindle activity to occur in other sleep stages, including REM sleep. (See also ELECTROENCEPHALOGRAM, HYPNOTICS, SIGMA RHYTHM, SLEEP STAGES.)

sleep stage demarcation Term that refers to the specific changes that mark the boundary between one sleep stage and another, or a sleep stage and wakefulness. Typically the boundary between one sleep stage and another is very clearly defined; however, in some sleep disorders sleep may become very fragmented and features of one sleep stage may occur with another and therefore the demarcations may become very blurred. A similar situation can occur in individuals who are taking MEDICATIONS, such as HYPNOTICS. (See also SLEEP STAGES.)

sleep stage episode An interval of sleep that represents a specific sleep stage in the non-REM/REM cycle. For example, the first REM sleep episode is the first interval of REM sleep that occurs in the major sleep episode and will comprise a part of the NREM-REM SLEEP CYCLE. Typically, four to six recurring cycles of non-REM-REM sleep occur, therefore four to six discrete stage episodes of non-REM and REM sleep will occur. (See also SLEEP STAGES.)

sleep stage period See SLEEP STAGE EPISODE.

sleep stages Following the development of the ELECTROENCEPHALOGRAM (or EEG) in 1930 by Hans Berger, sleep was recognized to consist of changes in the electroencephalographic activity of the brain. Based on these electroencephalographic patterns, sleep was originally classified into four stages, sometimes characterized by letters of the alphabet, excluding REM sleep, which was not discovered for another two decades. With the discovery of REM sleep in 1953 by NATHANIEL KLEITMAN, Eugene Aserinsky and WILLIAM DEMENT, sleep was recognized to be a continuous state of alternating rhythm with very pronounced physiological changes. REM sleep was occasionally termed stage five sleep, or D sleep. The electroencephalographic pattern of REM sleep was also termed desynchronized sleep, compared with the synchronized EEG activity of non-REM or SLOW WAVE SLEEP.

In 1968 a group of researchers headed by ALAN RECHTSCHAFFEN and ANTHONY KALES developed a standardized method of sleep scoring, and sleep was divided into four stages, plus REM sleep. The four stages of sleep came to be called NREM or non-REM sleep. In order to standardize the scoring of sleep, the record was divided into epochs of 20 or 30 seconds in duration. The electroencephalogram is performed at a slower rate of 10 or 15 millimeters per second than the more typical EEG speed of 30 millimeters per second. In addition to the electroencephalogram, electrodes placed to record eye movements and muscle tone are required to more adequately determine sleep stages.

The electroencephalogram electrode placement is at either C3 or C4 position. Eye movements are detected by electrodes placed at the outer CANTHUS of each eye and referred to a reference electrode, and the ELECTROMYOGRAM is typically recorded by electrodes placed over the muscles at the tip of the chin.

Stage One Sleep

Stage one sleep occurs right after the awake stage and comprises 4% to 5% of TOTAL SLEEP TIME. It is characterized by medium amplitude, mixed frequency activity that is mainly theta and comprises more than 20% of an epoch. During this stage there may be SLOW ROLLING EYE MOVEMENTS in contrast to the RAPID EYE MOVEMENTS seen during wakefulness. There are no SLEEP SPINDLES, K-COMPLEXES or REMs.

Stage Two Sleep

Stage two sleep is characterized by sleep spindles and K-complexes; it accounts for 45% to 50% of total sleep time. The sleep spindles are 11 to 15 Hz activity occurring in episodes greater than .5 second in duration and reaching 25 microvolts in amplitude. K-complexes consists of a negative vertex, sharp wave followed by a positive slow wave and are frequently seen accompanied by sleep spindles.

Electrode EEG studies, in which the electrodes are inserted directly through the scalp into the brain, performed concurrently with scalp electrode recordings suggest that spindle activity appears first in the thalamic nucleic of the brain and undergoes a certain degree of synchronization before it is detectable at the scalp EEG electrodes. Superior frontal regions appear to be the starting point for the spindle activity.

Stage Three Sleep

A deep level of sleep that comprises 4% to 6% of total sleep time. This stage is sometimes combined with stage four into NREM stages three and four because of the physiological similarities between the two stages, and called slow wave sleep. Stage three is present when between 20% and 50% of the epoch contains delta waves of .5 to 2.5 Hz, which are 75 microvolts or greater in amplitude. Typically eye movement activity is absent during this stage.

Stage Four Sleep

Stage four sleep is scored when over 50% of the epoch contains delta waves of the same frequency and amplitude as those seen in stage three sleep. Although rarely, sleep spindles may occur in stage four sleep. This stage, the deepest sleep of the four non-REM stages, is synonymous with slow wave sleep and usually comprises 12% to 15% of total sleep time. It is during this stage that SLEEP TERRORS or SLEEPWALKING may occur. Sometimes stage four is combined with stage three into NREM stages three and four because the stages are so similar.

Rapid Eye Movement Sleep (REM)

REM sleep is characterized by rapid eye movement (hence its name, REM), loss of muscle tone (or REM ATONIA) and a mixed frequency, low voltage EEG pattern with occasional bursts of "sawtooth" theta waves of 5 to 7 Hz. Dreaming occurs during REM sleep. (See also DREAMS, POLYSOMNOGRAPHY.)

sleep starts Also known as hypnagogic jerks, predormital myoclonus or hypnic jerks. Sleep starts are sudden, shocklike sensations that involve most of the body, particularly the lower limbs. They usually consist of a solitary, generalized contraction that occurs spontaneously or is caused by a stimulus. Sleep starts bring the individual to wakefulness, and a sensation of falling or a visual flash, dream or hallucination may be experienced at this time. Rarely the individual may call out with the acuteness of the episode. Multiple episodes can occur at SLEEP ONSET, and SLEEP ONSET INSOMNIA may develop. Not infrequently, individuals will have multiple episodes that do not induce a full awakening. Such episodes may not be remembered by the individual but will be reported by a bed partner.

It is thought that most people experience sleep starts at some time in their life, and only a few have frequent episodes. There is some evidence to suggest that the ingestion of stimulant agents, such as CAFFEINE, or the use of NICOTINE may exacerbate the occurrence of sleep starts. Physical exercise and emotional STRESS have also been reported to be associated with such episodes.

Sleep starts may occur at any age, although most typically they are reported in adulthood. There does not appear to be any gender or familial tendency.

Polysomnographic monitoring of sleep starts demonstrates a brief (generally 75–250 millisecond), high amplitude muscle potential that can be associated with an arousal pattern seen on the EEG. There may be accompanying increased heart rate following an episode, but usually the heart rate returns to normal and sleep resumes rapidly.

Sleep starts must be distinguished from hyperexplexia syndrome in which a generalized body jerk can occur during wakefulness or during sleep. The association of hyperexplexia with full wakefulness differentiates that disorder from sleep starts. An epileptic form of myoclonus can produce similar generalized body jerks; however, abnormal EEG activity can help differentiate that disorder. RESTLESS LEGS SYNDROME is not likely to be confused because the leg movements are slower and not associated with a whole body jerk. PERIODIC LEG MOVEMENTS, as with restless legs syndrome, generally have more prolonged muscle episodes and do not have the shocklike, brief character of the sleep start. Periodic movements occur in a repetitive manner during sleep and do not usually occur solely at sleep onset.

Treatment of sleep starts is usually unnecessary as they are an infrequent occurrence and usually are not associated with any great concern. However, in some individuals sleep starts may be a cause of sleep onset insomnia, in which case benzodiazepine muscle relaxants (see BENZODIAZEPINES), such as triazolam, may be useful in suppressing episodes and in allowing sleep onset to be initiated.

Oswald, I., "Sudden Bodily Jerks Upon Falling Asleep," *Brain* 82 (1959): 92–93.

sleep state misperception A disorder where there is a complaint of insomnia, yet the major sleep episode is objectively normal. This disorder has also been called "subjective DIMS complaint without objective findings," "pseudoinsomnia" or "sleep hypochondriasis," but sleep state misperception is the preferred term. Patients with this disorder present a very convincing history of sleep disturbance and insomnia and typically will awaken feeling unrefreshed. When studied polysomnographically in the sleep laboratory, sleep is normal in duration, sleep stages and sleep efficiency, yet the patient will awaken and report having had no sleep at all.

The cause of the misperception of sleep is unknown; however, it does appear to be an exaggeration of a normal phenomenon. Healthy individuals who have been asleep for only a few minutes often will report not having slept at all. As the duration of sleep increases, the awareness of having slept also increases. However, patients with sleep state misperception, despite having prolonged periods of good quality sleep, misperceive sleep as being a time of no sleep.

This disorder must be differentiated from individuals who report a lack of sleep in order to obtain MEDICATIONS. Such patients are often drug abusers, and the report of no sleep is usually not a convincing or honest report (see MALINGERERS.) This disorder also needs to be differentiated from other causes of insomnia, such as PSYCHOPHYSIOLOGICAL INSOMNIA or insomnia related to a mental disorder. Sleep fragmentation, reduced total sleep time and reduced sleep efficiency are characteristically seen in patients with insomnia due to these other causes. (See also DISORDERS OF INITIATING AND MAINTAINING SLEEP, PSYCHIATRIC DISORDERS.)

Carskadon, M., Dement, W., Mitler, M., Guilleminault, C., Zarcone, V. and Spiegel, R., "Self Report Versus Sleep Laboratory Findings in 122 Drug Free Subjects with a Complaint of Chronic Insomnia," *Annual Journal of Psychiatry* 133 (1976): 1382–1388.

sleep surface The sleep surface has been subject to investigation over the years to determine its role in the maintenance of good quality sleep. Most of the research has tended to demonstrate that the quality of sleep is independent of the surface on which a person sleeps; however, a change in the sleeping surface can disrupt sleep. The inhabitants of some countries typically sleep on a hard surface yet appear to sleep as well as people who sleep on soft, innerspring mattresses. Adaptation to the new surface needs to occur if someone changes from a hard to a soft surface, or vice versa. Many different sleeping surfaces have been produced; hard mattresses have been marketed particularly for people who have back complaints, whereas softer surfaces, such as water BEDS, appear to have more appeal to young adults.

Whether to change the sleeping surface should depend solely on comfort. If a mattress is too soft or too hard, a change may be beneficial to sleep. For most people, however, the sleeping surface plays a small role in the cause or maintenance of sleep disturbance. (See also INSOMNIA.)

sleep talking Also known as somniloquy. Sleep talking is the production of utterances of speech or other sounds during a sleep episode. Typically, individuals suffering from sleep talking are unaware of the content of their speech, which is reported afterward. The utterances may take the form of comprehensible speech, isolated words, parts of sentences, moans or other nonverbal sounds. Typically sleep talking is devoid of emotional content; however, it can be associated with intense emotional stress, at which time calling out, crying, screaming or cursing may occur.

Sleep talking is often a temporary phenomenon, although it may be a repetitive occurrence in those who suffer from SLEEP TERRORS or somnambulism (see SLEEPWALKING). It also is seen in individuals who have significant psychopathology, emotional stress or medical illness, such as febrile (feverish) illness, in which case it is related to that illness. It appears to be more common in males than females and a slight familial tendency is reported.

Sleep talking has been demonstrated to occur during all stages of sleep, including REM SLEEP. The majority of episodes, in fact, have been reported out of REM sleep, with the next most common being sleep stage two, followed by slow wave sleep. Individuals who have somnambulism or sleep terrors are more likely to have sleep talking out of slow wave sleep, whereas individuals who have the REM SLEEP BEHAVIOR DISORDER are more likely to have episodes out of REM sleep. (See also CONFUSIONAL AROUSALS, SLEEP STAGES.)

Arkin, A.M., "Sleep Talking: A Review," *Journal of Nervous Mental Disorders* 143 (1966): 101–122.

sleep terrors Considered one of the disorders of arousal as described by ROGER J. BROUGHTON in 1968. These episodes also go under the name of night terrors and they have occasionally been called pavor nocturnus (derived from the Latin *pavor,* for "terror," and *nocturnus,* for "at night") in children and INCUBUS in adults.

Sleep terror episodes are characterized by an arousal during the first third of the night from deep stage three/four sleep (see SLEEP STAGES), and are heralded by a loud, piercing scream along with intense fear and panic. An individual experiencing a sleep terror will typically sit up abruptly in bed with an agitated and confused expression. Following the intense and loud scream, there may be other features of panic and fear, such as rapid breathing, rapid heart rate, dilation of the pupils and profuse sweating. The individual will usually flee from the bedroom in an intense panic and is often inconsolable until the episode subsides. Most episodes last less than 15 minutes; sleep usually follows very rapidly, and the individual is unable to recall the episode the next morning.

The cause of the episodes is unknown, but it appears to be a benign and maturational behavior frequently seen in children. Up to 6% of prepubescent children will have recurrent episodes of night terrors, with the peak frequency of the behavior being around six years of age. Episodes then decrease in frequency and generally cease in early adolescence.

The frequency in adults is typically less than 1% and episodes usually persist from childhood, although episodes may occur for the first time in adulthood. Episodes occur equally in males and females, and there are no racial or cultural differences in the prevalence. However, there is a marked familial incidence of the disorder, with up to 96% of individuals having a family history of the disorder.

Episodes may be precipitated in susceptible individuals by fatigue, emotional stress and febrile illness. Adults with the disorder may also have evidence of psychopathology characterized by psychoasthenia (weakness and reduced motivation), DEPRESSION and schizophrenia.

Children with sleep terror episodes either concurrently have SLEEPWALKING episodes or develop sleepwalking episodes subsequently. Sleep terror episodes rarely occur in adulthood after the fifth decade.

Because of the intense fear and anxiety, sleep terror episodes are differentiated from more typical NIGHTMARES or DREAM ANXIETY ATTACKS. Nightmares usually occur in the later half of the night, more typically during REM sleep. Nightmares also have a less intense scream at their onset than sleep terrors, and usually the individual comes to full alertness, whereas the sufferer of night terrors does not usually become fully awake during an episode. Rarely does an epileptic seizure produce an episode similar to sleep terror; other features of epilepsy would typically be present in such individuals.

Some features of sleep terrors and sleepwalking overlap, and it appears that there is a spectrum of disorders of which CONFUSIONAL AROUSAL appears to be the most mild form, with sleepwalking episodes being a more severe form of AROUSAL DISORDERS, and sleep terrors being the most extreme form.

Treatment of sleep terrors is usually not necessary in the young child, but the child should be reassured. In older children, a psychological cause should be explored, and appropriate psychiatric treatment instituted, if warranted. Medications, such as the BENZODIAZEPINES, have been shown to be useful, as well as tricyclic ANTIDEPRESSANTS, such as imipramine. However, these agents are best reserved for children or adults with the most severe form of the disorder.

Since injuries might occur during the intense fleeing from the bedroom, objects liable to cause injury should be removed and appropriate steps made to secure the bedroom.

Case History

A 28-year-old woman came to a SLEEP DISORDER CENTER with the primary complaint of episodes of suddenly awakening and screaming. These episodes had occurred about once every month over the prior five years and had begun when she was in college, causing her considerable distress and embarrassment. The screaming would be frightening to those who slept around her as she would suddenly jump out of bed and rush to the door or window. The rapid attempt to flee the bed and bedroom resulted in her knocking into furniture and injuring herself on several occasions. Typically, during the episodes she would not remember any dream content, but was aware of being intensely frightened and panicky, as if she were about to die. The immediate reaction was to flee from the bed, although there was no clear comprehension of where she was going. Very often, her roommates were unable to console her during these episodes. However, eventually she would gradually settle down and when taken back to bed would fall asleep easily. Occasionally she would have abrupt episodes with screaming and immediately go back to sleep, only to be told about the episodes the next morning.

Polysomnographic monitoring failed to reveal a clinical episode; however, she did show frequent and abrupt arousals from SLOW WAVE SLEEP with a rapid change in heart rate. The arousals were considered to be minor and subclinical manifestations of the sleep terror episodes.

A psychological evaluation failed to reveal any evidence of psychopathology and psychotherapeutic intervention was not considered to be useful.

The patient was prescribed triazolam, initially 0.125 milligram, which improved the episodes but did not terminate them. This dosage was increased to 0.25 milligram and the episodes did not reoccur.

Five years later, the patient continued to remain free of episodes so long as she took the medication. However, attempts at reducing the medication led to the return of the sleep terror episodes. It is expected that in time, probably before her mid-30s, the episodes will spontaneously subside.

Broughton, R., "Sleep Disorders: Disorders of Arousal?" *Science* 159 (1968): 1070–1078.

Fisher, C., Kahn, E., Edwards, A. et al., "A Psycho-physiological Study of Nightmares and Night Terrors," *Journal of Nervous and Mental Disease* 157 (1973): 75–98.

Thorpy, Michael J. and Glovinsky, P.B., "Parasomnias," *Psychiatric Clinics of North America* 10 (1987): 623–639.

sleep therapy Term related to a treatment that employs the inducement of sleep in order to treat various medical disorders. In its simplest form, sleep therapy can be viewed as treatment by rest—required by situations that promote fatigue. Sleep therapy may also involve the inducement of sleep by MEDICATIONS and drugs, the use of HYPNOSIS to induce prolonged sleep, or the application of electrical current, which has been termed ELECTROSLEEP, ELECTRONARCOSIS or electroanesthesia.

Sleep therapy has been used to treat a variety of disorders, most commonly the mental disorders, but also cardiovascular, gastrointestinal, central nervous system and infective disorders.

The majority of studies on sleep therapy occurred around the turn of the century, and little objective documentation of their effectiveness has been presented. Electrosleep is still performed in some European countries and is administered in a variety of different manners. Electrodes may be applied to the forehead and a limb, and then the electrical current gradually increased to the amount of approximately three-quarters of a milliamp, at which time the patient can feel a tingling sensation through his head, which is believed to induce sleep. The majority of publications on electrosleep come from the Russian literature.

The usefulness of sleep therapy is believed to be limited at best. There is a need for more research and documentation of its effectiveness before it can be widely recommended.

Williams, R.L. and Webb, W.B., *Sleep Therapy.* Springfield, Ill.: Charles C. Thomas, 1966.

sleep-wake cycle See NREM-REM SLEEP CYCLE.

sleep-wake disorders center This term is occasionally used to describe a facility that evaluates patients who have disorders of sleep and wakefulness. The hyphenated term was used initially to emphasize the importance of disorders of both sleep and wakefulness, such as the disorders that produce EXCESSIVE SLEEPINESS. The shorter term, SLEEP DISORDER CENTERS, is more commonly used. (See also ACCREDITATION STANDARDS FOR SLEEP DISORDER CENTERS, AMERICAN ACADEMY OF SLEEP MEDICINE, ASSOCIATION OF SLEEP DISORDER CENTERS.)

sleep-wake schedule disorders See CIRCADIAN RHYTHM SLEEP DISORDERS.

sleep-wake transition disorders A subgroup of the PARASOMNIAS, as listed in the INTERNATIONAL CLASSIFICATION OF SLEEP DISORDERS, consisting of RHYTHMIC MOVEMENT DISORDER, SLEEP STARTS, SLEEP TALKING, and NOCTURNAL LEG CRAMPS. These disorders occur mainly during the transition from wakefulness to sleep, or during the transition from one SLEEP STAGE to another. Some of these disorders may occur during sleep, but the predominant activity occurs in the transition to and from sleep.

sleepwalking Episodes characterized by movement that occurs while the subject is still asleep and in a partially aroused state. This disorder, which is also known as somnambulism, typically occurs during deep SLOW WAVE SLEEP in the first third of the night. The behavior is often seen in prepubescent children, although it can persist or start anew in adulthood.

A typical sleepwalking episode is characterized by the individual sitting up in bed, usually with a vacant and unresponsive look. Repetitive movements, such as picking at the bedclothes, may occur prior to the individual rising from the bed and walking around the room. Episodes last minutes or hours at most. Frequently the individual will open doors and walk out of the bedroom, or sometimes walk out of the house. During the sleepwalking episode, there is a limited capacity to appreciate environmental stimuli, and there is an impaired ability to fully awaken. Occasional utterances may occur during sleepwalking, but verbalizations usually do not occur, and rarely is any cognitive or mental content expressed. Although unresponsive to environmental stimuli, the individual is able to negotiate objects without difficulty, although occasional stumbling or banging into walls or furniture may occur. Attempts at restraining a sleepwalker are usually met with some resistance. Sleepwalking episodes may involve dangerous activities, such as opening windows and climbing onto fire escapes, and serious falls have been reported. There are occasional reports of violent behavior during sleepwalking being directed toward a specific individual. Following a period of ambulation, the sleepwalker usually returns to bed and rapidly returns to sleep. The next morning, the individual is typically unable to recall the episode and is often surprised by the accounts of others.

Sleepwalking episodes usually occur in children in the prepubescent age group, and the peak frequency is around 10 years of age. According to ANTHONY KALES et al., up to 30% of healthy children are said to have sleepwalked at least once in their lives, and up to 5% of healthy children are reported to have frequent episodes.

Following puberty, episodes decrease in frequency, and usually children have outgrown them by the age of 15. It is estimated that approximately 1% of adults sleepwalk, the majority having done so since childhood. Usually, episodes in adulthood resolve by the fifth decade.

Elderly persons who walk around a house at night may be mistaken for sleepwalkers. They may be suffering from a brain dysfunction, such as DEMENTIA, and are typically awake when they walk about, although confused about their behavior.

Sleepwalking occurs equally in males and females, and there is little evidence for any cultural or racial differences in the tendency to sleepwalk. However, there is a strong pattern of inheritance, with a high rate of sleepwalking activity seen in relatives of sleepwalkers.

The cause of sleepwalking is unknown; however, sleepwalking can be provoked by arousing sleepwalking-prone individuals and standing them on their feet when they are in a deep sleep. Excessive fatigue can precipitate episodes as can febrile (feverish) illness. Episodes of sleepwalking behavior have been reported in association with mediations such as LITHIUM and triazolam (see BENZODIAZEPINES), or other HYPNOTICS.

Polysomnographically, the episodes are characterized by an abrupt arousal that occurs during the deep stage three/four sleep (see SLEEP STAGES). The slow wave activity appears to persist throughout the walking episode with some faster rhythms, such as theta and alpha activity. Individuals who sleepwalk may demonstrate abrupt arousals from deep sleep in the absence of full sleepwalking episodes.

Sleepwalking in children is not associated with any psychopathology, but Anthony Kales has reported a clear association between psychopathology and sleepwalking episodes in adults. Such individuals are reported to be more aggressive, hypomanic and have a tendency for acting out.

Sleepwalking episodes may be very similar to episodes of psychomotor epilepsy with ambulation. However, repetitive automatisms are more common during epileptic seizures and there is more confusion upon awakening.

Recently a form of episodic nocturnal wandering has been reported to occur in young adults in association with abnormal electroencephalographic activity on a daytime, awake ELECTROENCEPHALOGRAM. Such patients respond to anticonvulsant therapy, which may suggest that these individuals have a form of epilepsy and not true sleepwalking.

Sleepwalking episodes can be differentiated from psychogenetic fugues, which usually occur in individuals with severe psychopathology. Fugues consist of episodes of wandering that usually last for hours and days and are often associated with complex behaviors that are more typically seen during wakefulness. REM SLEEP BEHAVIOR DISORDER has similarities to sleepwalking in that motor activity can occur during sleep, but such individuals are usually elderly and the activity more clearly represents acting out of dream content. In addition, in REM sleep behavior disorder the abnormal features are seen during REM sleep and not slow wave sleep. OBSTRUCTIVE SLEEP APNEA SYNDROME can produce nocturnal wanderings that may simulate sleepwalking, although other typical features of obstructive sleep apnea, such as snoring and episodes of cessation of breathing, usually allow an easy differentiation from more typical sleepwalking episodes.

The child who infrequently sleepwalks requires no specific treatment other than making sure that the bedroom is secure to prevent the child from injury. It may be necessary to place locks on windows or doors for the child who walks excessively at night. The older individual and adult should be evaluated for underlying psychopathology, and the appropriate psychiatric treatment should be instituted. There have been good reports of response to psychotherapy and psychiatric management. In many situations sedatives, including imipramine, diazepam or flurazepam, can be helpful in suppressing episodes, particularly if an individual sleeps away from home.

Case History

A 26-year-old woman sought help at a SLEEP DISORDER CENTER because of sleepwalking episodes that had been occurring since she was 10 years of age. When the episodes began, they were infrequent and were regarded as being typical for childhood sleepwalking in that she would be found by her parents walking in the corridor and returned to her bedroom where she would go back to sleep without any difficulty. During the walking episodes, she was unaware of the environment although she did not walk into objects or injure herself.

At age 13, the episodes became less frequent until age 16, when they again increased in frequency. Over the following years, she would have episodes of sleepwalking that caused her considerable embarrassment, particularly when staying at the homes of friends. She would often have some DREAM CONTENT along with the episodes and get up and start to walk around the house. On one occasion she picked up some keys, put them in her pocket and walked out the front door. She was found by a friend sleepwalking outside the house.

With some of the episodes, she would awaken and become aware of having been sleepwalking. On other occasions, she would be returned to her bedroom by friends or family only to be told about the episodes the next morning.

The sleepwalking episodes appeared to occur less often when she was not in her usual environment. There was an increase in the frequency of the episodes if she became very tired, fatigued or was ill with a fever. There was no evidence of underlying psychopathology except for one short-lasting episode of DEPRESSION that had occurred several years prior to her presentation at the sleep disorder center. She would see a psychologist intermittently in order to help her cope with everyday stress, but not because of any psychiatric disturbance. She was successful in her occupation as a clerical administrator and outwardly was a bright and energetic woman who was involved in many social activities.

Polysomnographic evaluation during sleep did not reveal any sleepwalking episodes, and there was no evidence of any epileptic activity. However, she had frequent, abrupt awakenings from stage four sleep.

She was commenced on triazolam, 0.25 milligram taken on a nightly basis, and this completely suppressed the episodes. After six months, she attempted to gradually withdraw from the medication in the hope that the episodes would no longer occur. However, as the dose was reduced she had a return of the sleepwalking episodes and then recommenced the medication for a longer period of time. Five years after being placed on medication, she was free of sleepwalking episodes so long as she continued to take the medication. However, several additional attempts to withdraw from the medication were associated with a recurrence of episodes. She no longer had embarrassment or fear at staying over at other people's homes, and she felt more secure and confident of having a sound night of sleep.

If she ever decides to raise a family, she will need to consider coming off the medication prior to and during pregnancy. The decision to continue medication in the pregnancy will need to be balanced against her potential for harm from the sleepwalking episodes at that time. It is likely that her tendency for sleepwalking will gradually lessen in time.

Kales, A., Jacobsen, A., Paulson, M.J., Kales, J.D. and Walter, J.D. "Somnambulism: Psychophysiological Correlates," *Archives of General Psychiatry* 14 (1966): 586–594.

Thorpy, Michael J. and Glovinsky, P.B., "Parasomnias," *Psychiatric Clinics of North America* 10 (1987): 623–639.

slow rolling eye movements Movements that occur with the entrance into stage one non-REM sleep (see SLEEP STAGES). The eye movements begin a slow sinusoidal (cyclical) pattern of movement on a horizontal plane while other EEG (ELECTROENCEPHALOGRAM) and EMG (ELECTROMYOGRAM) features of stage one sleep are present. As the individual passes from stage one into deeper stage two and three sleep, the eye movements become less active. The presence of slow eye movements marks the onset of sleep from the rapid eye movements that are typically seen during wakefulness and helps distinguish stage one sleep from REM SLEEP, which is also characterized by rapid eye movements. Chin muscle activity is usually lower in stage one sleep than in wakefulness but is much higher than the muscle activity seen during REM sleep.

slow wave sleep (SWS) Sleep that is characterized by electroencephalographic waves of a frequency less than 8 Hz; typically comprises stages three and four sleep combined. Slow wave sleep usually comprises approximately 20% of the sleep of the young adult; however, greater percentages are seen in prepubertal children. Gradual reduction in the total amount of slow wave sleep is seen with aging so that after the age of 60 years, there is little slow wave sleep. Slowing of the EEG (see ELECTROENCEPHALOGRAM), with increased amounts of slow wave sleep, can be seen in several situations.

During partial SLEEP DEPRIVATION, the amount of stage three/four sleep (see SLEEP STAGES) is usually reduced. Following the sleep deprivation, slow wave sleep rebounds so that a greater percentage of slow wave sleep can be seen on the subsequent sleep episode. In addition, disorders that affect the cerebral hemispheres, such as a cerebral vascular accident, can be associated with an increased amount of slowing and therefore an increased amount of slow wave sleep. Drug effects, such as the use of HYPNOTICS or other central nervous system depressants, can also increase EEG slowing and lead to a greater amount of slow wave sleep. Lithium is a known cause of increased slow wave sleep.

smoking Smoking cigarettes can have an important effect upon INSOMNIA and the OBSTRUCTIVE SLEEP APNEA SYNDROME. Cigarettes contain NICOTINE, a stimulant that causes central nervous system arousal and therefore can contribute to difficulty in initiating sleep. People who suffer from insomnia are advised not to smoke prior to bedtime, and it is counterproductive to smoke cigarettes during nighttime awakenings.

Smoking can also exacerbate the obstructive sleep apnea syndrome by irritating the pharyngeal tissues, thereby contributing to increasing erythema and swelling. The carbon monoxide in smoke can contribute to impaired blood gas exchange, and the smoke can irritate the large pulmonary airways with production of mucus, thereby leading to chronic bronchitis that can further worsen the obstructive sleep apnea syndrome.

Smoking in bed at night is a major cause of fires, many of which are fatal. People with sleep disorders, or those who have ingested ALCOHOL or drugs, may have difficulty in remaining alert while smoking. If sleep occurs, cigarettes will be dropped and can set fire to bedclothes or other materials. Patients with obstructive sleep apnea syndrome are at particular risk, because of their severe lethargy, of accidentally starting a fire if they smoke in bed at night. (See also SLEEP HYGIENE, STIMULANT MEDICATIONS.)

snoring A noise produced by vibration of the soft tissue of the back of the mouth. Most typically the soft palate and the anterior and posterior pillar of fauces, which surround the tonsil, vibrate, causing the sounds. Snoring is associated with obstruction of the upper airway that occurs during sleep. Some snorers have only a very slight degree of UPPER AIRWAY OBSTRUCTION, and snoring will be rhythmical and regular on a breath to breath basis; lung ventilation is not compromised. Alternatively, if the upper airway obstruction is more severe, there may be a complete inability to inspire air, and consequently the oxygen in the lung will decrease, causing blood HYPOXEMIA. When snoring is severe, with associated hypoxemia, the disorder of OBSTRUCTIVE SLEEP APNEA SYNDROME most likely is present. This disorder is characterized by repetitive episodes of upper airway obstruction, loud snoring and EXCESSIVE SLEEPINESS during the day. Individuals with obstructive sleep apnea syndrome are at risk of developing cardiac irregularity during sleep and sudden death.

There is some evidence to suggest that snoring may be associated with elevated blood pressure, even in the absence of obstructive sleep apnea syndrome. Other epidemiological studies, which have not differentiated simple snoring from that associated with the obstructive sleep apnea syndrome, have shown a correlation of snoring with ischemic heart disease and stroke.

In addition to the direct cardiorespiratory consequences of snoring, the noise of snoring may be a social annoyance and handicap. A spouse's snoring may be the cause of marital discord that leads to the snorer having to sleep in a separate bed, or even in another room. Not only can snoring affect a spouse, it can also affect other people who are sleeping nearby. Snoring can be particularly disturbing to roommates who have to share rooms, such as on business trips, in the armed forces or at summer camp. Snoring has been measured at up to 80 decibels, a level that can be potentially harmful to hearing.

Some 300 mechanical devices have been patented in the United States to reduce or eliminate snoring. However, the majority are ineffective. Very few effective treatments are available for snoring, and, because most loud snorers will tend to have some degree of obstructive sleep apnea syndrome, a medical evaluation may be necessary.

Snoring may be affected by a number of factors, such as increased body weight, alcohol consumption, body position, respiratory tract infections and central nervous depressant medications, such as HYPNOTICS. Sleeping on the back is liable to induce snoring in a person who otherwise does not snore when sleeping on the side or stomach. However, most loud snorers will tend to snore in any position.

Treatment of snoring, if required, may encompass weight reduction, avoidance of alcohol, avoidance of depressant medications and training to sleep on the side rather than on the back. When these measures are ineffective, or if obstructive sleep apnea syndrome is present, then other forms of treatment may be necessary, such as surgical or mechanical treatment (see SURGERY AND SLEEP DISORDERS).

The most effective surgical treatment for loud snoring is removal of the upper airway obstructive lesion. Children who can be loud snorers with severe obstructive sleep apnea syndrome most typically will have upper airway obstruction due to enlarged tonsils or adenoids, which, when surgically removed will eliminate the snoring (see TONSILLECTOMY AND ADENOIDECTOMY). However, enlarged tonsils or adenoids are rarely the cause of snoring in adults, who more typically have an increase in the soft tissues of the pharynx, such as an elongated soft palate and excessive pillars of fauces. An operative procedure termed UVULOPALATOPHARYNGOPLASTY (UPP) is usually very effective in reducing the sound of snoring. UPP consists of the removal of the uvula and the lower portion of the soft palate as well as the removal of the tissue associated with the pillar of fauces. In general, this operation is not indicated for people who have snoring in the absence of obstructive sleep apnea syndrome because of the very slight risk that general anesthesia presents. However, this procedure may be performed on some snorers, but more commonly is performed on patients with obstructive sleep apnea syndrome in whom the snoring is associated with medically important upper airway obstruction. Two new forms of uvulopalatoplasty have been developed: LASER UVULOPALATOPLASTY and radiofrequency uvulo palatoplasty (see SOMNOPLASTY). Laser uvulopalatoplasty is a procedure that can be performed within 20 minutes in a physician's office. It is primarily done to eliminate snoring. Radiofrequency uvulopalatoplasty involves inserting a needle into the tissues of the soft palate and exposing the tissues to high-frequency radio waves. It is a less painful procedure than laser uvulopalatoplasty. Careful polysomnographic documentation of the presence and severity of the sleep apnea is essential before surgery is undertaken.

Alternative treatments of snoring can involve the use of mechanical devices, such as CONTINUOUS POSITIVE AIRWAY PRESSURE (CPAP) devices or airway patency devices such as the TONGUE RETAINING DEVICE (TRD) or other ORAL APPLIANCES. These appliances may be useful in treating some patients who have snoring; however, with the exception of the CPAP, these other mechanical devices have generally not been effective for the treatment of obstructive sleep apnea syndrome.

socially or environmentally induced disorders of the sleep-wake schedule This term has been applied to the CIRCADIAN RHYTHM SLEEP DISORDERS, which are induced by external or behavioral factors such as TIME ZONE CHANGE (JET LAG) SYNDROME and SHIFT-WORK SLEEP DISORDER. It can be applied to DELAYED SLEEP PHASE SYNDROME, ADVANCED SLEEP PHASE SYNDROME, and NON-24-HOUR SLEEP-WAKE SYNDROME when the cause of the disorder is induced by social or environmental factors. Examples of social or environmental factors include social isolation, extremes of light exposure such as that seen in the polar regions, or excessive activity late at night.

Sominex See OVER-THE-COUNTER MEDICATIONS.

somniferous Term meaning "causing or inducing sleep." The word is derived from the Latin word *somnus,* for "sleep."

somniloquy See SLEEP TALKING.

somnoendoscopy Procedure performed during sleep so the upper airway can be observed; involves placing a fiberoptic endoscope (see FIBEROPTIC ENDOSCOPY) through the nose into the upper airway and observing the changes that occur in a sleeping patient. Somnoendoscopy is most commonly performed on patients with the OBSTRUCTIVE SLEEP APNEA SYNDROME to determine the exact site of UPPER AIRWAY OBSTRUCTION during sleep.

Somnoendoscopy is a difficult procedure because the presence of the fiberoptiscope can be uncomfortable and disturb sleep; it is hard for someone to sleep through the procedure, and even harder for patients with the obstructive sleep apnea syndrome because of the frequent arousals associated with the apneic events. (See also ENDOSCOPY.)

somnofluoroscopy Term that refers to a fluoroscopic evaluation of the upper airway during sleep. This radiological procedure typically involves placement of barium in the upper airway to outline the upper airway cavity. When the patient falls asleep, the barium outlines the upper airway so the radiographic images enable the dynamic changes of the upper airway to be visualized. Somnofluoroscopy is rarely performed in patients with the

OBSTRUCTIVE SLEEP APNEA SYNDROME due to patients' difficulty in falling asleep during the radiological procedure. An alternative means of evaluating the upper airway is by SOMNOENDOSCOPY or by the use of FIBEROPTIC ENDOSCOPY during wakefulness. (See also UPPER AIRWAY OBSTRUCTION.)

somnolence See EXCESSIVE SLEEPINESS.

somnologist Term applied to sleep specialists. The word is derived from the Latin *somnus,* for "sleep." The term SLEEP DISORDER SPECIALIST is preferred. (See also ACCREDITED CLINICAL POLYSOMNOGRAPHER, SLEEP DISORDERS MEDICINE.)

somnology Word meaning the study of sleep, derived from the Latin *somnus,* for "sleep," and *ology,* meaning "the study of."

somnoplasty A surgical method that uses radiofrequency heating to create targeted tissue ablation to reduce tissue volume; also known as radiofrequency thermal ablation. The procedure uses very low levels of radiofrequency energy to create small, finely necrotic lesions in soft tissue structures. The necrosis leads to scar formation and retraction of tissue. This method has been applied to the soft palate of snorers to reduce soft palate tissue and thereby reduce SNORING. The procedure has been used successfully in clinical trials; patients experience a minimal amount of pain, mainly from the insertion of the needle into the soft palate to administer the local anesthesia. The procedure uses temperatures of less than 100 degrees centigrade, much less than those used in laser surgery (over 600 degrees centigrade).

The effectiveness of radiofrequency ablation has not been reported in patients with OBSTRUCTIVE SLEEP APNEA SYNDROME; however, the procedure appears to be effective in reducing tongue-based soft tissue in animal studies and therefore could be an effective treatment for human obstructive sleep apnea syndrome. Further research is required. (See also LASER UVULOPALATOPLASTY, SURGERY AND SLEEP DISORDERS, UPPER AIRWAY OBSTRUCTION, UVULOPALATOPHARYNGOPLASTY.)

Somnus The ancient Roman god of sleep, who was the son of night and the brother of death. The words "somnambulism" (SLEEPWALKING) and "somnolent" (sleepy) were derived from the Latin *somnus.* (See also HYPNOS.)

Sonata See HYPNOTICS.

soporific Term derived from Latin *sopor,* meaning "a deep sleep," and *ferre,* "to bring," that refers to the induction of a deep sleep, typically by the use of drugs. MEDICATIONS that can induce a deep sleep-like state are the HYPNOTICS and anesthetic agents, which include the BENZODIAZEPINES, BARBITURATES and opiate derivatives. These agents in high doses will produce a slowing of the ELECTROENCEPHALOGRAM and the patient will be difficult to arouse. (See also COMA, NARCOTICS.)

SOREMP See SLEEP ONSET REM PERIOD.

spindle See SLEEP SPINDLES.

SRS Distinguished Scientist Award An award presented by the SLEEP RESEARCH SOCIETY (SRS) to "recognize work of the highest distinction in the field of basic sleep research." The recipient is selected by the SRS Distinguished Scientist Award Committee, and the award is presented by the committee chairperson at the annual meeting. A plaque and cash prize are given by the SRS in the awardee's name to subsidize the attendance of a trainee at the annual meeting. Deadline for applications is March 1st of the year of the award, and applications should be sent to: Sleep Research Society, 6301 Bandel Road, Suite 101, Rochester, Minnesota 55901.

SRS Young Investigator Award A plaque and a travel honorarium of $750 are given to an author whose paper or abstract in the field of basic sleep research is recognized for its scientific excellence. The awardee must be younger than 36 years of age, have received a doctoral degree within five years before the award and be the first or sole author of the paper or abstract; abstracts submitted to the annual meeting of the ASSOCIATION OF PROFESSIONAL SLEEP SOCIETIES are eligible. Applicants must be a member of the SLEEP RESEARCH SOCIETY or include a membership application and fee with the award application. For further eligibility requirements and application procedures, contact: Sleep Research Society, 6301 Bandel Road, Suite 101, Rochester, Minnesota 55901.

stage A sleep One of five sleep stages (A to E) that were first classified in the 1930s by E. Newton Harvey, Alfred L. Loomis and Garret Hobart, according to their electroencephalographic pattern (see ELECTROENCEPHALOGRAM). This sleep stage classification was replaced by the method of ALAN RECHTSCHAFFEN and ANTHONY KALES in 1968 following the discovery of REM SLEEP. Stage A sleep is equivalent to presleep drowsiness and has no exact correlation with the new sleep stage classification system.

Stage A sleep consists of an interrupted alpha EEG, which is typically found in relaxed wakefulness or drowsiness. (See also SLEEP STAGES.)

stage B sleep The second stage of the original sleep classification devised by E. Newton Harvey, Alfred L. Loomis and Garret Hobart in the 1930s. It consists of a low-voltage EEG pattern without alpha activity. This pattern represents the onset of sleep and is reflective of stage one sleep of the Alan Rechtschaffen and Anthony Kales scoring method, which replaced the Harvey and Loomis method. (See also SLEEP STAGES.)

stage C sleep One of the five sleep stages first classified in the 1930s by E. Newton Harvey, Alfred L. Loomis and Garret Hobart, and now replaced by the Alan Rechtschaffen and Anthony Kales scoring method. Stage C sleep is characterized by the presence of SLEEP SPINDLE activity and is indicative of the stage of sleep that is now currently called stage two sleep. (See also SLEEP STAGES.)

stage D sleep Sleep according to the classification of E. Newton Harvey, Alfred L. Loomis and Garret Hobart; replaced by the Alan Rechtschaffen and Anthony Kales method of sleep scoring. Stage D sleep consists of a pattern of spindle activity with small waves of high amplitude and is consistent with stage three sleep. (See also SLEEP STAGES.)

Harvey, E.N., Loomis, A.L. and Hobart, G.A., "Cerebral States During Sleep: A Study by Human Brain Potential," *Science Monthly* 45 (1937): 191–192.

stage E sleep Stage of sleep according to the classification of E. Newton Harvey, Alfred L. Loomis and Garret Hobart, replaced by the Alan Rechtschaffen and Anthony Kales method of sleep scoring. Stage E sleep consists mainly of small high-amplitude EG waves and the absence of sleep spindle activity and is synonymous with stage four sleep. (See also SLEEP STAGES.)

stage four sleep See SLEEP STAGES.

stage one sleep See SLEEP STAGES.

stage three sleep See SLEEP STAGES.

stage two sleep See SLEEP STAGES.

Stanford Sleepiness Scale (SSS) A subjective measure of alertness developed at Stanford University in 1973. Individuals rate themselves according to one of several statements that most closely describes their level of ALERTNESS or SLEEPINESS. In order to achieve a spectrum of sleepiness across a day, the Stanford Sleepiness Scale is administered at two-hour intervals, most commonly across the waking part of the day. It is often completed immediately before and after the NAPS during a MULTIPLE SLEEP LATENCY TEST.

The Stanford Sleepiness Scale is as follows:

1. Feeling active, vital, alert, wide awake.
2. Functioning at a high level but not at peak. Able to concentrate.
3. Relaxed, awake, but not fully alert, responsive.
4. A little foggy, let down.
5. Foggy, beginning to lose track. Difficulty in staying awake.
6. Sleepy, prefer to lie down, woozy.
7. Almost in reverie, cannot stay awake, sleep onset appears imminent.

Hoddes, E., Zarcone, V., Slythe, H. et al., "Quantification of Sleepiness: A New Approach," *Psychophysiology* 10 (1973): 431–436.

status cataplecticus Continuous state of CATAPLEXY that occurs in a patient with NARCOLEPSY. The continuous cataplectic state can be induced by a persistence of the stimulus causing cataplexy, such as laughter, elation or anger. During the state of cataplexy the individual generally is paralyzed and, at most, can make moaning sounds. The episode may last several minutes and rarely can last up to one hour. The condition can also be precipitated by a sudden withdrawal of anticataplectic medications, such as the tricyclic ANTIDEPRESSANTS, in an individual with a diagnosis of narcolepsy.

stimulant-dependent sleep disorder Disorder characterized by a reduction in the ability to fall asleep at night, produced by the use of central nervous system stimulants, or an increase in drowsiness during the day, following drug abstinence. The central nervous system stimulants encompass a wide variety of medications that include amphetamines (see STIMULANT MEDICATIONS), COCAINE, thyroid hormones, CAFFEINE, methylxanthines (see RESPIRATORY STIMULANTS), bronchodilators and antihypertensives. Many OVER-THE-COUNTER MEDICATIONS also contain stimulants such as decongestants, cough mixtures or diet suppression medications. Typically these medications are associated with difficulty in the ability to fall asleep, especially when treatment with the medications is first started. After a period of time, TOLERANCE to this effect develops so that sleep initiation difficulties are less frequent. However, upon withdrawal of the medication, symptoms of sleepiness, irritability, tiredness and fatigue are common. The recurrence of daytime symptoms on withdrawal of the stimulant medications often leads to a cyclical pattern of administration. This can lead the individual to believe that the medication is required in order to maintain full daytime ALERTNESS.

Individuals can be oblivious to the pattern of medication use because it is not regarded as a problem. However, others may become aware of the relationship of the stimulant medication to changes in behavior that include periods of excessive acting out with high activity, sometimes with paranoid ideas and repetitive behaviors. In the case of high doses of cocaine, for example, generalized convulsions can occur; with the amphetamines, a severe psychiatric state of psychosis may develop. Abnormal movement disorders can also occur with toxic levels of amphetamines. Addiction to stimulant medications can develop, with severe DEPRESSION and often suicidal ideation and hallucinations.

The pattern of behavior associated with excessive stimulant ingestion often leads to denial of drug use, which may be detected only by means of urinary and screening tests.

Severe addiction to stimulants may lead to intravenous administration, which increases the possibility of contacting infectious hepatitis, acquired immune deficiency syndrome (AIDS) or a systemic arteritis. Infection with the AIDS virus is a real possibility for intravenous stimulant abusers. Acute severe toxicity of the medications may result in death from cardiac ARRHYTHMIAS, brain hemorrhages, convulsions and respiratory arrest.

Stimulant abuse is most common in adolescents and young adults, and it appears to be equal among the sexes. The effects of stimulant abuse may be seen on polysomnographic testing as a prolonged SLEEP LATENCY, reduced TOTAL SLEEP TIME and an increased number of awakenings. REM SLEEP is often reduced and fragmented. Upon withdrawal of the stimulants, there may be a REM REBOUND, with an increased amount of REM sleep. The chronic use of stimulants may give a picture on the MULTIPLE SLEEP LATENCY TEST suggestive of NARCOLEPSY. A one- to two-week withdrawal period from all medications may need to be documented before an accurate diagnosis of EXCESSIVE SLEEPINESS can be given.

Stimulant abusers may attempt to obtain stimulant medications from physicians by falsely giving a history of another sleep disorder (see MALINGERERS), such as narcolepsy. Polysomnographic monitoring of patients to confirm a bona fide diagnosis of a sleep disorder is necessary prior to the long-term administration of stimulant medications.

Patients who have stimulant dependency should embark upon a program of drug withdrawal under medical supervision and, if necessary, appropriate psychiatric therapy. Individuals who suffer from severe drug dependency may require treatment in a specialized drug detoxification clinic.

Nausieda, P.A., "Central Stimulant Toxicity," in Vinken, P.J. and Bruyn, G., eds., *Handbook of Clinical Neurology.* Amsterdam: Elsevier North Holland, 1979. pp. 223–297.

Oswald, I., "Sleep and Dependence on Amphetamine and Other Drugs," in Kales, Anthony, ed., *Sleep Physiology and Pathology.* Philadelphia: Lippincott, 1969. pp. 317–330.

stimulant medications This term applies to drugs that stimulate the central nervous system. It includes methylxanthines, the amphetamines and the RESPIRATORY STIMULANTS, such as doxypram and nikethimide, as well as other miscellaneous medications, such as pemoline and methylphenidate hydrochloride.

In sleep disorders medicine, the stimulant medications are primarily used for the improvement and relief of EXCESSIVE SLEEPINESS, and the most commonly used medications are the amphetamines, methylphenidate and pemoline.

The major disadvantage of the stimulant medications is that they produce general body stimulation and therefore can induce ANXIETY and cardiac stimulation, leading to HYPERTENSION or tachycardia (abnormally rapid heartbeat). There may also be gastrointestinal stimulation with resulting diarrhea.

Amphetamines

Stimulant medications that are derived from the sympathomimetic amines and consist of a benzene and an ethylamine group. The amphetamines have powerful central nervous system stimulant effects, and therefore are used to produce ALERTNESS in disorders associated with excessive sleepiness during the day. Most often, they are used for the treatment of NARCOLEPSY and related conditions. Due to their stimulant effects, these drugs can also be abused and illegally used for recreational purposes to provoke central nervous system excitement.

Amphetamines were first used for the treatment of narcolepsy in the 1930s and were found to be an effective agent for improving daytime sleepiness. However, the powerful side effects were also recognized, such as elevated blood pressure and greater incidence of cardiac ARRHYTHMIAS. The central nervous system effects can also provoke agitation, confusion, anxiety, irritability, DELIRIUM and DEPRESSION. However, in appropriate doses, amphetamines are very helpful in the treatment of narcolepsy, improving patients' functioning during the daytime.

Other forms and derivatives of amphetamines have been used more recently in the treatment of narcolepsy because they have less tendency for adverse reactions. Methamphetamine (Desoxyn) was also used to improve alertness but, like amphetamine, caused side effects and has largely been replaced by dextroamphetamine sulfate (Dexedrine).

Dextroamphetamine is available in 5-, 10- and 15-milligram tablets, a 5 milligram per 5 milliliter Elixir, and in 5-, 10- and 15-milligram slow-release spansules. Initial doses are typically 5 milligrams, three times a day, but may need to be increased to as much as 100 milligrams per day. The tablets have a duration of action of three to four hours, whereas the spansules have a duration of action up to 12 hours. Some patients find that a background dose of the longer-acting form of the medication, such as a 15-milligram Dexedrine spansule, can be used with the extra stimulant effect of the shorter-acting tablets.

The adverse effects of dextroamphetamine are similar to those of the other amphetamines except there is less peripheral stimulant effect. But because of the potential for cardiac and mental stimulation, disorders of daytime sleepiness, such as narcolepsy, are now more frequently treated with methylphenidate hydrochloride (Ritalin) or pemoline (Cylert).

Amphetamine users develop a TOLERANCE to the drug; consequently, prescribed dosages are increased in order to maintain improved alertness. Sudden cessation of medication will induce a level of sleepiness that is greater than baseline levels, thereby promoting the continued use of the medication. An amphetamine psychosis and abnormal movements have been reported to be associated with toxic doses of amphetamines.

Anorectics

Anorectics are the appetite suppressant medications. Anorectics typically are comprised of two groups, amphetamines and the non-amphetamines. As the amphetamines have stimulant effects, they are also used for the treatment of excessive sleepiness. When prescribed in appropriate dosages, they can be useful for the treatment of narcolepsy or IDIOPATHIC HYPERSOMNIA. However, some disorders that can produce daytime sleepiness, such as the OBSTRUCTIVE SLEEP APNEA SYNDROME, may be adversely affected by the use of amphetamines. These medications can be dangerous in the sleep apnea syndromes due to their cardiac stimulant effect. Also, the amphetamine anorectic medications are liable for abuse because of their general stimulant properties.

Anorectics, because of their stimulant effects, can produce an impaired ability to sleep at night. SLEEP ONSET and sleep maintenance difficulties are common. A STIMULANT-DEPENDENT SLEEP DISORDER may result from their chronic ingestion. They can also produce a feeling of fatigue or sleepiness when not taken, thereby leading to repeated ingestion to maintain full alertness.

Some non-amphetamine anorectic agents are available, such as phentermine, mazindol or diethylpropion. These agents are generally less effective than the amphetamines in producing weight reduction. Mazindol (see below) can be helpful in improving alertness in some patients with narcolepsy.

L-tyrosine

A naturally occurring stimulant agent, this amino acid has been shown to be effective in the treatment of narcolepsy. It is given in the dose of 100 milligrams per kilogram, and the beneficial effect upon cataplexy is seen within the first few days of use. The beneficial effects upon sleepiness take somewhat longer to occur. L-tyrosine is currently recommended only as a dietary supplement; in high doses it can cause alteration of blood pressure, nausea, vomiting and headaches.

The initial reports of the beneficial effects of L-tyrosine need to be confirmed before this medication can be recommended for the routine treatment of narcolepsy.

Mazindol

This is an imidazoline chemical produced mainly as a weight reduction medication. It has similar pharmacological effects to the amphetamines, but has less central nervous system stimulation and also less peripheral stimulant effects, such as tachycardia, tremor or gastrointestinal stimulation. But side effects, such as dry mouth, transient irritability and headaches, may occur. Mazindol is sometimes used in the treatment of disorders of excessive sleepiness, including narcolepsy. It has some similar effects to the tricyclic ANTIDEPRESSANTS, in that it blocks the uptake (ability to absorb) of the catecholamines, norepinephrine and dopamine.

Sanorex, the trade name for mazindol, is available in 1- and 2-milligram tablets, and the usual dosage is 1 milligram, three times a day. Usually doses of 2 to 12 milligrams per day are required for the treatment of sleepiness in narcolepsy. Unlike the amphetamine stimulants, mazindol has also been shown to be effective in the treatment of cataplexy.

Mazindol is less effective in treating excessive daytime sleepiness than pemoline or methylphenidate.

Methylphenidate Hydrochloride

This agent, a piperidine derivative, was first introduced by Dan Daly and Robert Yoss in 1956 as the treatment of choice for narcolepsy. The reduced tendency for central nervous system stimulation and peripheral stimulation, compared to amphetamines, was considered advantageous for the treatment of sleepiness in narcolepsy. Methylphenidate is still the treatment of choice for patients with severe narcolepsy, although patients with mild cases of narcolepsy are more typically treated with pemoline.

Methylphenidate is usually given in divided doses, two to three times a day. It has a relatively short duration of action, from four to six hours. Although most patients can be controlled with a dose of about 20 milligrams per day, doses of up to 60 milligrams may be required in some patients. Due to its poor absorption when taken with food, patients are instructed to take the medication on an empty stomach.

This drug is available in 5-, 10- and 20-milligram tablets and is also available in a sustained-release form of 20 milligrams (Ritalin-SR). Ritalin is the trade name for methylphenidate. Although some patients find the sustained-release form effective, others prefer the intermittent use of the shorter-acting form of the medication.

Pemoline

This is an oxizolidinone derivative stimulant that is quite different structurally from the amphetamines or methylphenidate hydrochloride. It is used for central nervous system stimulation to improve arousal in patients with narcolepsy or other disorders of excessive daytime sleepiness. It has fewer peripheral stimulant effects than the amphetamines or methylphenidate. It also has a longer duration of action, approximately 12 hours. It is available in 18.75-, 37.5- and 75-milligram tablets. Cylert is the trade or pharmaceutical name for pemoline.

Pemoline has a slow onset of action over several hours; initially, soon after ingestion, some patients may notice a worsening of their excessive sleepiness, which then dissipates. The clinical effects of pemoline may take several days or even weeks to occur. Because of its slow onset of action, and long half-life, there can be a tendency for drug buildup, with a consequent development of excessive central nervous system stimulation.

There is less tendency for tolerance with pemoline than with other central nervous system stimulants. Objective studies have shown that pemoline does not reduce the tendency or the ability to fall asleep; however, it does improve the ability to remain awake. This effect is demonstrated by an individual's ability to fall asleep in a situation conducive to sleep after having taken pemoline. However, tasks requiring alertness are improved when the individual tries to remain awake.

Pemoline can produce liver impairment, and therefore intermittent monitoring of blood liver enzymes is required for patients who chronically take the medication.

Over-the-Counter Medications

A number of nonprescription OVER-THE-COUNTER MEDICATIONS are available for weight reduction or stimulant purposes. These include phenylpropanolamine, which is sometimes given in combination with CAFFEINE. The use of these medications is controversial as they may be ineffective yet dangerous to individuals, particularly those with hypertension or cardiac disease.

Flitman, S.S., "Tranquilizers, Stimulants, and Enhancers of Cognition," *Physical Medicine and Rehabilitation Clinics of North America* 10, no. 2 (1999): 463–472.

stimulus control therapy BEHAVIORAL TREATMENT of INSOMNIA that counteracts the development of negative conditioning in someone who lies in bed awake at night, allowing the insomnia to persist. (Lying in bed awake at night heightens the ANXIETY for insomnia patients and further disrupts sleep and prevents its onset.)

Stimulus control instructions, ensuring that wakeful activities are kept away from the bedroom, are as follows: 1) go to bed only when sleepy; 2) if not asleep within 10 minutes of getting into bed, get out of bed and, after returning to bed, if sleep does not occur within 10 minutes, again leave the bed; 3) an alarm should be set so that awakening occurs at the same time every morning and the taking of NAPS should be avoided; 4) the bed should not be used for wakeful activities other than sexual activity. (See also SLEEP RESTRICTION THERAPY.)

Bootzin, R., "A Stimulus Control Treatment for Insomnia," *Proceedings of the American Psychological Association* 1 (1972): 395–396.

Bootzin, R. and Nicassio, P.M., "Behavioral Treatments for Insomnia," in *Progress in Behavior Modification*, vol. 6. New York: Academic Press, 1978. pp. 1–45.

strain gauge A mercury-filled tube that acts as a transducer for movement; most commonly used for the measurement of respiratory movements or penile tumescence (erection) during sleep. Strain gauges may be applied to the chest or abdomen in several places in order to detect respiratory movement.

The main disadvantage of strain gauges is that they need to be taped to the skin and may break, with resulting leakage of mercury. Many sleep disorder centers therefore utilize chest electromyography, bellows, pneumobelts or respitrace for the detection of abdominal or chest movement.

Strain gauges are commonly used for determining penile tumescence, with one strain gauge being applied to the base of the penis and the other to the tip. A commercially-produced device, the RIGISCAN, has supplanted the use of strain gauges in the determination of nocturnal penile tumescence in some sleep laboratories. However, the Rigiscan may be uncomfortable for some patients due to its method of action, which involves an intermittent constriction of bands around the penis. (See also NOCTURNAL PENILE TUMESCENCE TEST, POLYSOMNOGRAPHY.)

stress Term applied to the body's physical or psychological response to an unexpected or unpleasant environmental or emotional stimulus, such as marital problems, pressure at work, upcoming examinations, or even changes in everyday patterns, such as spending the night away from home or having to make a public speech. The term is most commonly used in SLEEP DISORDERS MEDICINE for the cause of a disturbed sleep pattern that occurs due to a marital, financial or employment situation. Typically, the sleep disorder, termed ADJUSTMENT SLEEP DISORDER, is a result of the psychological stress produced by such events. When the event produces a greater degree of stress, an overt ANXIETY DISORDER may result. (See also INSOMNIA, SHORT-TERM INSOMNIA.)

stupor A state of altered consciousness characterized by unresponsiveness to strong stimuli. Such patients are usually perceived as being in a deep sleep, and electroencephalographic studies may indicate slow wave activity. However, unlike in COMA, individuals can be awakened and become aware of the environment, but they usually return rapidly to the unresponsive state.

Stupor may be produced by metabolic or pharmacologic insults to the central nervous system. However, this condition can also be seen in severe psychiatric illness, such as that seen with catatonic schizophrenia or severe DEPRESSION. (See also DELIRIUM, OBTUNDATION.)

subjective DIMS complaint without objective findings See SLEEP STATE MISPERCEPTION.

subvigilance syndrome See SUBWAKEFULNESS SYNDROME.

subwakefulness syndrome Also known as the subvigilance syndrome; a chronic disorder that is characterized by a complaint of EXCESSIVE SLEEPINESS without objective evidence of impaired sleep at night or excessive sleepiness during the day. Twenty-four-hour polysomnographic monitoring of patients shows a tendency for intermittent, light stage one sleep and, rarely, stage two sleep occurring throughout the daytime (see SLEEP STAGES). An abnormality in the neurophysiological mechanism for maintaining ALERTNESS is postulated as its cause.

The complaints of DROWSINESS and SLEEPINESS are usually linked to a decreased ability to maintain full concentration and to carry out work and social activities.

This disorder needs to be differentiated from other disorders of excessive sleepiness, such as IDIOPATHIC HYPERSOMNIA, NARCOLEPSY, RECURRENT HYPERSOMNIA, INSUFFICIENT SLEEP SYNDROME, hypersomnia related to PSYCHIATRIC DISORDERS, and tiredness and fatigue related to other causes of INSOMNIA.

In view of the difficulty in objectively documenting any pathological features of this disorder, there is some question as to whether this truly represents a disorder in its own right or whether it is an atypical form of one of the disorders to be considered in the differential diagnosis.

Roth, B., *Narcolepsy and Hypersomnia.* Basel: Karger A.G., 1980.

sudden infant death syndrome (SIDS) The term used for the death of an otherwise healthy infant who dies suddenly and in whom a postmortem examination fails to reveal a cause of death. The majority (over 80%) of SIDS infants die during sleep.

Less than 5% of children who die of sudden infant death syndrome have been known to have some respiratory disturbance during sleep. However, the cause of the sudden infant death syndrome is unknown. Recent evidence suggests that it is not directly related to any prior respiratory irregularity.

There appear to be some predisposing factors, derived from epidemiological studies, that indicate that premature infants, infants with low birth weight, infants that are twins or of a multiple birth, and siblings of another child who has died of SIDS are at greater risk. Sleeping on the stomach is also a major factor. In addition, there are a number of maternal factors that appear to predispose some children to the development of SIDS: for example, infants born to mothers who are substance abusers of agents such as COCAINE or heroin. It does appear that SIDS is more common in lower socioeconomic and minority groups, such as American blacks and American Indians. Sudden infant death syndrome has a prevalence of between one and two per 1,000 live births, with the peak onset around three months of age, and up to 90% of cases occur before the sixth month of age. There is a slightly increased male to female ratio.

After death, autopsy examinations have demonstrated a number of features that suggest that the infant may have suffered from an acute upper respiratory tract obstruction. There are petechiae and evidence of pulmonary congestion and edema. Also, pathological abnormalities have been reported in the brain stem, suggesting a prior central nervous system insult, such as HYPOXIA.

Polysomnographic investigations are rarely useful. Although originally there was some suggestion that short apneic episodes may be predictive of SIDS, subsequent research has not confirmed this finding. Infants who have significant apneic events, such as those with APNEA OF PREMATURITY, or infants requiring assisted ventilation following an apneic event, do have a higher risk for sudden infant death syndrome, although this risk is less than 5%.

Having an infant sleep on the back is the most effective preventative measure a parent or caregiver can take. (See also AGE, CENTRAL ALVEOLAR HYPOVENTILATION SYNDROME, CENTRAL SLEEP APNEA SYNDROME, INFANT SLEEP APNEA, INFANT SLEEP DISORDERS, OBSTRUCTIVE SLEEP APNEA SYNDROME.)

Blatt, S.D. et al., "Sudden Infant Death Syndrome, Child Sexual Abuse, and Child Development," *Current Opinion in Pediatrics* 11, no. 2 (1999): 175–186.

Naeye, R.L., "Sudden Infant Death," *Scientific American* 242 (1980): 42–56.

Hoppenbrouwers, T. and Hodgman, J.E., "Sudden Infant Death Syndrome (SIDS)," *Public Health Reviews* 11 (1938): 363–390.

Scragg, R.K. et al., "Side Sleeping Position and Bed Sharing in the Sudden Infant Death Syndrome," *Annals of Medicine* 30, no. 4 (1998): 345–349.

sudden unexplained nocturnal death syndrome (SUND) Syndrome primarily recognized in people of Southeast Asian descent who die unexpectedly during sleep. It occurs in healthy young adults without any prior history of cardiac or respiratory disease. Typically there will be a sudden awakening with a choking or gasping sensation and difficulty in breathing. Cardiorespiratory arrest occurs with a fatal outcome. In very rare situations, patients have been successfully resuscitated and found to have cardiac irregularity called VENTRICULAR ARRHYTHMIAS.

This rare and unusual syndrome primarily affects persons between the ages of 25 and 45 who are of Laotian, Kampuchean (Cambodian), or Vietnamese origin. It is primarily a male disorder, although rare cases have been reported in females, and most of the reported cases have been described in refugees who have immigrated to the United States. However, the disorder has been recognized for a long time, and the Laotian term for the disease is *non-laita,* in Tagalog, *bangungut,* and in Japanese, *pokkuri.*

Investigations have failed to reveal any specific cause for the disorder either clinically or by autopsy. There has been no evidence of exposure to either biological or chemical toxins, or the use of drugs or alcohol.

Many of the victims of SUND have been reported to have had prior SLEEP TERROR episodes with a sudden awakening and screaming. It has been suggested that the sudden death during sleep may be due to a severe form of terror episode in which the heart is so stimulated that it goes into a fatal arrhythmia.

Most of the reported cases in the United States have been in the ethnic subgroup called the Hmong, from the highlands of northern Laos. The incidence of the disorder in the Hmong refugees in the United States is reported at 92 per 100,000. It is slightly less common in Laotian refugees at 82 per 100,000; it is 59 per 100,000 in Kampuchean (Cambodian) refugees.

Although SUND cannot be predicted, healthy young adults with cardiorespiratory arrest during sleep need to be examined for any underlying cardiorespiratory disorder. A sleep-related disorder, such as OBSTRUCTIVE SLEEP APNEA SYNDROME or REM SLEEP-RELATED SINUS ARREST, may be the cause of the arrest.

Baron, R.C., Thacker, S.B., Gorelkin, L., Vernon, A.A., Taylor, W.R. and Choi, I., "Sudden Death Among Southeast Asian Refugees," *Journal of American Medical Association* 250 (1983): 2947–2951.

SUND See SUDDEN UNEXPLAINED NOCTURNAL DEATH SYNDROME.

Sunday night insomnia Difficulty in initiating and maintaining sleep that commonly is seen on Sunday nights. This form of insomnia occurs due to the tendency to go to bed later on Friday and Saturday nights than during the week (because of social events). Typically the awake time on Saturday and Sunday mornings is later than usual, thereby causing the sleep pattern to be slightly delayed on the weekends compared to that of weekdays. Consequently, many people will attempt to fall asleep at an early time on Sunday night in order to achieve an adequate amount of sleep for work or school on Monday. Because the time of going to bed on Sunday night is much earlier than that of the previous two nights, there often can be difficulty in falling asleep, which is characterized by a long period of time spent in bed awake. If the time of falling asleep on Sunday night is similar to the later time of initiating sleep that occurs on the Friday and Saturday nights, then individuals may find that they are sleep deprived upon awakening for work or school on Monday morning. This will lead to a degree of SLEEP DEPRIVATION that is often termed MONDAY MORNING BLUES.

In order to prevent Sunday night insomnia, an individual should maintain a regular time of going to bed seven days a week and not allow the time to be significantly later on Friday or Saturday nights.

sundown syndrome See DEMENTIA.

suprachiasmatic nucleus (SCN) Cells that are located at the bottom of the third ventricle in the hypothalamus. This is believed to be the prime central nervous system site that determines endogenous circadian rhythms, the so-called ENDOGENOUS CIRCADIAN PACEMAKER. The suprachiasmatic nucleus (SCN) has connections with the eye by means of the retino-hypothalamic pathway, which is composed of fibers that pass from the optic nerves to the hypothalamus. By means of the retino-hypothalamic tract (RHT), light and dark influence the circadian pacemaker and act as entraining (maintaining a regular 24-hour) stimuli for our circadian rhythms. Other connections pass to local areas of the central nervous system, as well as through the brain stem and up to the pineal gland, causing the release of the hormone MELATONIN in darkness. Destruction of the suprachiasmatic nucleus has produced loss of the circadian rhythmicity of various CIRCADIAN RHYTHMS.

Moore, R.Y. et al., "Suprachiasmatic Nucleus Organization," *Chronobiology International* 15, no. 5 (1998): 475–487.

Silver, R. et al., "The Suprachiasmatic Nucleus and Circadian Function: An Introduction," *Chronobiology International* 15, no. 5 (1998): vii–x.

surgery and sleep disorders Surgery is a primary treatment form considered for patients who have the OBSTRUCTIVE SLEEP APNEA SYNDROME. Patients with this syndrome have UPPER AIRWAY OBSTRUCTION that occurs at the back of the mouth in the region from the nose to the larynx. Surgical procedures that remove excessive tissue or localized lesions in the upper airway have been shown to be effective in the treatment of some patients with this syndrome.

Obstructive sleep apnea may be due to enlarged tonsils or adenoids, craniofacial abnormalities including retrognathia (posterior-positioned lower jaw) or micrognathia (small lower jaw), or generalized soft tissue enlargement, particularly at the level of the soft palate. Various forms of surgery have been devised in order to improve the upper airway so that obstruction during sleep does not occur.

Surgical treatment of obstructive sleep apnea is still widely performed; however, most patients with this disorder are now treated by means of CONTINUOUS POSITIVE AIRWAY PRESSURE (CPAP) devices, a treatment that has very few complications. The CPAP device provides a low pressure of air to the back of the throat, thereby preventing its collapse during sleep. However, some patients do not find this device suitable for use, and surgery may be the only effective treatment available.

The most common form of surgery used in children with obstructive sleep apnea syndrome is tonsillectomy with or without an adenoidectomy (see TONSILLECTOMY AND ADENOIDECTOMY). Enlarged tonsils are a common cause of obstructive sleep apnea in prepubertal children. Children with enlarged tonsils may also have craniofacial abnormalities that contribute to the upper airway obstruction, such as an altered mandibular relationship to the skull with or without retrognathia. In such patients, MANDIBULAR ADVANCEMENT SURGERY can allow the tissues of the tongue to come forward, thereby preventing pharyngeal obstruction. An experimental surgical procedure involves the release of the hyoid muscles (see HYOID MYOTOMY). These muscles fasten the base of the tongue to the skull and their release allows the tongue to be moved forward to open up the posterior pharyngeal air space.

Patients who have a long soft palate, an enlarged uvula and narrow pillar of fauces may be suitable for the UVULOPALATOPHARYNGOPLASTY (UPP) operation, which is a soft tissue surgical procedure performed at the back of the mouth. This procedure is effective for patients with either the obstructive sleep apnea syndrome or simple SNORING; however, only 40% to 50% of patients have a successful result by means of this surgery. Two new forms of palatoplasty are LASER UVULOPALATOPLASTY and radiofrequency palatoplasty (see SOMNOPLASTY). CEPHALOMETRIC RADIOGRAPHS and FIBEROPTIC ENDOSCOPY aid in selecting patients for the uvulopalatopharyngoplasty procedure, thereby leading to improved surgical results.

TRACHEOSTOMY is a procedure that was the primary form of treatment for obstructive sleep apnea in the past, but it has largely been replaced by the use of mechanical treatments or the UPP operation. However, it is still an effective and commonly performed procedure. A hole is created in the trachea (windpipe) so that breathing occurs through the hole and the upper airway is bypassed during sleep. This procedure is very effective; however, the social problems associated with tracheostomy prevent it from being commonly performed today. (Patients are unable to swim with a tracheostomy and its appearance can be undesirable.) In some patients, tracheostomy can produce dramatic improvement in symptoms and features of the obstructive sleep apnea syndrome and can be lifesaving.

Sher, A.E., "Surgical Management of Obstructive Sleep Apnea," *Progress in Cardiovascular Diseases* 41, no. 5 (1999): 387–396.

sweating There can be an increase of sweating during sleep; if it is a regular occurrence it is called SLEEP HYPERHIDROSIS. An increase in sweating can be due to febrile illness, specific neurological disorders, such as stroke, or pregnancy. (See also PREGNANCY-RELATED SLEEP DISORDERS.)

synchronized sleep Term used to denote NON-REM-STAGE SLEEP, particularly in ontogenetic or phylogenetic sleep research. It is derived from the synchronized patterns of EEG (see ELECTROENCEPHALOGRAM) activity that are commonly seen in non-REM sleep, and it reflects the slowing of the EEG. The term is best avoided if other features of non-REM sleep can be determined. A more specific statement of the stage of sleep (see SLEEP STAGES), such as stage two or three sleep, should be given, if possible.

systemic desensitization Behavioral technique occasionally used to treat INSOMNIA, particularly in patients who have insomnia due to anxiety or negatively-conditioned associations. The patient is required to make a list of various situations that are likely to contribute to the sleep disturbance, and then concentrate upon those items while coupling them with more restful thoughts. The aim of the treatment is to try to turn the unpleasant associations into pleasant ones so they no longer contribute to the disturbed sleep. Systemic desensitization is sometimes used in conjunction with RELAXATION EXERCISES procedures. (See also AUTOGENIC TRAINING, BEHAVIORAL TREATMENT OF INSOMNIA, BIOFEEDBACK, COGNITIVE FOCUSING, PARADOXICAL TECHNIQUES, PROGRESSIVE RELAXATION.)

T

Tegretol See CARBAMAZEPINE.

temazepam See BENZODIAZEPINES.

temperature Body temperature decreases during sleep and reaches its minimum level before awakening. It reaches its maximum level during the middle of the period of wakefulness that typically occurs during the daytime. A fluctuation of 1.5 degrees Fahrenheit is usually seen between the low point and the highest point during any 24-hour period. The lowest point of body temperature is about three hours before awakening, typically between 3 A.M. and 5 A.M., and then rapidly rises during the time of awakening. Chronobiological studies have demonstrated that normal-sleeping individuals in time isolation will awaken 85% of the time during the rising phase of the body temperature cycle.

There is some evidence to suggest that exercise and WARM BATHS may be beneficial to nighttime sleep by raising the body temperature prior to sleep onset. However, elevation of the temperature of the sleeping environment is generally not helpful to good sleep and can be an environmental stimulus that contributes to INSOMNIA. Persons who sleep in hot tropical areas can sleep well as long as the environmental temperature is constant and the person has adapted to it. A sudden change in the environmental temperature during the sleeping hours can lead to a disturbed night of sleep. (See also CHRONOBIOLOGY, CIRCADIAN RHYTHMS, EXERCISE AND SLEEP, THERMOREGULATION.)

temporal isolation In 1962, MICHEL SIFFRE spent 59 days in an underground cavern in the French-Italian Alps and discovered that his sleep-wake cycle had a period length of just over 24 hours as a result of being isolated from ENVIRONMENTAL TIME CUES. In 1962, Jules Ashchoff developed a research facility in a German bunker and demonstrated that with isolation from social and temporal cues, many biological rhythms with a 24-hour cycle would free run (see FREE RUNNING) with a PERIOD LENGTH of just over 24 hours. Internally-generated rhythms were termed CIRCADIAN RHYTHMS by FRANZ HALBERG in 1959. Additional studies on humans were performed by ELLIOT WEITZMAN at Montefiore Hospital in New York where healthy subjects were studied in an environment free of time cues for periods of up to six months. From such experiments much was learned about the human circadian timing system and the effect of environmental and time cues in influencing circadian rhythms.

terminal insomnia See EARLY MORNING AROUSAL.

terrifying hypnagogic hallucinations Terrifying HYPNAGOGIC HALLUCINATIONS, also known as sleep onset nightmares, are terrifying DREAMS that occur at the beginning of sleep. These dreams are similar to NIGHTMARES; however, nightmares usually occur during REM SLEEP, well after sleep onset. The affected person will become drowsy, start to fall asleep, and then see images that become very terrifying. The images cause a sudden awakening, with anxiety and fear; the content of the nightmare can be recalled. Sometimes the associated movement activity in sleep can be very excessive, with calling out and screaming.

Terrifying hypnagogic hallucinations occur in disorders of disturbed REM sleep, such as in NARCOLEPSY, where a SLEEP ONSET REM PERIOD can occur, or following the acute withdrawal of REM-suppressant medications, such as the tricyclic ANTIDEPRESSANTS.

Terrifying hypnagogic hallucinations need to be differentiated from other forms of hallucinatory behavior, such as that seen in more typical hypnagogic hallucinations where the dream content is not terrifying. SLEEP TERRORS occur during SLOW WAVE SLEEP, well after sleep onset, and the terror episodes are associated with fear and anxiety but little dream recall. Rarely, a mental disorder can produce nocturnal hallucinatory behavior; however, the occurrence only at sleep onset would be atypical.

Treatment of terrifying hypnagogic hallucinations involves treatment of the underlying disorder, either narcolepsy or other causes of sleep onset REM episodes, and may involve the use of REM-suppressant medications, such as the tricyclic antidepressant medications.

Broughton, Roger, "Human Consciousness and Sleep-Wake Rhythms: A Review and Some Neuropsychological Considerations," *Journal of Clinical Neuropsychology* 4 (1982): 193–218.

theophylline See RESPIRATORY STIMULANTS.

thermistor Heat-sensitive device used to measure airflow at the nostrils or mouth. The thermistor responds to variations in temperature by changing its resistance when connected to an electrical current. The signal that is produced is amplified by the polysomnograph (see POLYSOMNOGRAPHY) and a record of airflow is obtained on the POLYSOMNOGRAM.

Thermistors are used in polysomnographic monitoring to detect whether airflow occurs during sleep, so that differentiation may be made between obstructive (see OBSTRUCTIVE SLEEP APNEA SYNDROME) and central apneas (see CENTRAL SLEEP APNEA SYNDROME). Thermistors are used in conjunction with measures of respiratory effort that are placed at both the chest and abdominal levels. (See also SLEEP-RELATED BREATHING DISORDERS.)

thermoregulation The body's ability to control body TEMPERATURE within a narrow range. Changes in body temperature and environmental temperature can have important effects upon sleep. The body maintains body temperature within a close range and usually varies it by no more than 1.5 degrees throughout the day. Body temperature falls during sleep, reaching a low point approximately three hours before the time of awakening. Even sleep during the daytime can cause body temperature to fall slightly. Therefore, sleep and circadian factors are important in the control of body temperature.

During sleep, there are specific effects of the sleep state upon the control of body temperature, which is under the control of the preoptic and anterior hypothalamic nuclei (POAH). Thermoregulation changes reduce body temperature during NON-REM-STAGE SLEEP in association with the reduction in the metabolic rate. During REM SLEEP, body temperature in humans increases slightly; however, studies in animals have tended to show that the metabolic rate and body temperature typically are reduced in REM sleep. The slight increase in humans may be related to the increased central nervous system activity. Reduced muscle activity is likely to be responsible for the reduction of metabolic rate and body temperature that is seen in animals.

The control of body temperature varies between sleep states so that the control mechanisms are intact during non-REM sleep and are inhibited during REM sleep. Sweating does not occur during REM sleep, and usual body responses to cold, such as shivering, are not seen during REM sleep. The body's temperature is largely under the control of the environment temperature during the REM sleep state.

Changes in the environmental temperature also have an effect on sleep itself. The amount of SLOW WAVE SLEEP and REM sleep is maximal at an environmental temperature of 29 degrees Celsius (84.2 degrees Fahrenheit); as the body temperature changes, the amount of each sleep stage reduces. In addition, there are changes in the quality of sleep with increased arousals and number of awakenings, and an increased sleep latency. However, a person's adaptation to the environmental temperature influences the effects on sleep that are seen.

Artificial changes in body temperature can have an effect on the quality of sleep. An increase in body temperature prior to the major sleep episode will lead to an increase in non-REM sleep (see WARM BATHS).

The control of body temperature may have important effects upon the infant during its development. Because of the prevalence of SUDDEN INFANT DEATH SYNDROME, the possibility has been raised that an abnormality in the control of thermoregulation during sleep stages may predispose an infant to apneic episodes. Hypothermia has been shown to cause laryngeal hyperexcitability, which can lead to UPPER AIRWAY OBSTRUCTION. Body temperature changes are also useful for the determination of circadian rhythmicity, as they are a marker of the phase of the circadian rhythm. Body temperature changes are commonly recorded in the investigation of shift work and jet-lag effects. (See also CIRCADIAN RHYTHMS, EXERCISE AND SLEEP, SHIFT-WORK SLEEP DISORDER, SLEEP LATENCY, TIME ZONE CHANGE (JET LAG) SYNDROME.)

Glotzbach, S.F. and Heller, H.C., "Thermoregulation," in Kryger, M.H., Roth, T. and Dement, W.C., eds., *The Principles and Practices of Sleep Disorders Medicine.* Philadelphia: Saunders, 1989. pp. 300–309.

theta activity EEG (ELECTROENCEPHALOGRAM) activity with a frequency of 4 to 8 Hz that is generally maximal over the central and temporal areas. Theta activity is commonly seen in lighter stages of NON-REM-STAGE SLEEP but also is present in REM SLEEP. A specific form of theta activity called SAW-TOOTH WAVES is characteristic of REM sleep.

tidal volume The amount of air usually taken into the lungs during a normal breath at rest. It is typically 500 cubic centimeters of air.

time zone change (jet lag) syndrome Syndrome associated with complaints of difficulty in maintaining sleep and EXCESSIVE SLEEPINESS; typically associated with rapid travel across multiple time zones. The sleep-wake pattern has to be temporarily shifted to another time, the difference in time depending upon the number of time zones crossed. In addition to disturbance of the sleep-wake pattern, there are changes in alertness and performance and general feelings of malaise. The severity and duration of these symptoms is dependent upon not only the number of time zones crossed but also the direction of travel. Adaptation to time zone change is usually quicker following westward travel, where the onset of a new sleep episode is delayed in relation to the prior sleep episode. The tendency for improved adaptation after westward travel is thought to be due to the natural tendency to delay the onset of the sleep episode, the same tendency seen if one is placed in an environment free of time cues.

Once the individual is in the new time zone, adaptation occurs rapidly, with the symptoms of sleep disturbance diminishing with each day in the new environment. Typically, the sleep episode in the new time zone is of shorter duration and may be of lesser quality than that prior to the travel, and this produces a tendency to SLEEP DEPRIVATION and consequent excessive sleepiness. As there is a greater ability to delay our sleep onset than to advance the sleep onset, travel to the east, where sleep is scheduled to occur at a time earlier than the prior sleep onset time, is associated with a greater SLEEP ONSET difficulty.

The disruption in the sleep episode and excessive sleepiness produced by time zone change may induce reduced work performance and interfere with social and occupational activities, but the sleep disturbance usually rapidly abates upon adaptation in the new environment. However, for business persons who frequently travel and have limited time to adapt to the time zone changes, chronic sleep disturbance and impaired work performance may be of particular concern. Airline crews are particularly susceptible to the effects of time zone change.

Polysomnographic studies following time zone change have shown a greater number of arousals and increased stages of lighter sleep with a consequent reduction in SLEEP EFFICIENCY. SLOW WAVE SLEEP generally occurs in normal amounts but there may be reduced REM sleep.

Time zone change sleep disorder can occur in individuals of any age; however, the elderly are believed to be more likely to suffer from symptoms due to their difficulty in maintaining a regular and highly efficient sleep-wake cycle.

JET LAG may be exacerbated by the use of HYPNOTICS. Treatment is directed toward maintaining a regular pattern of sleep in the new environment. A regular sleep onset time and wake time is recommended, with an appropriate sleep duration. An attempt to adapt to the new environmental time is preferable for individuals who plan to be in the new time zone for episodes of one or more weeks. However, if staying in the new time zone for only a few days, maintenance of the prior sleep-wake pattern, even though it is not coordinated with the new environmental time, is preferable.

If a delay in the sleep episode is to be expected in the new environment, attempts to adapt may involve initiating a gradual delay in the original environment prior to travel so the sleep episode is partially adapted.

Daytime flights are said to be preferable to nighttime flights, so the night sleep can occur in a more acceptable environment. Studies have shown that hypnotics use can be beneficial for the first one or two nights in the new time zone in order to enhance the efficiency of the sleep episode. (See also ARGONNE ANTI-JET-LAG DIET, CIRCADIAN RHYTHM SLEEP DISORDERS, ENVIRONMENTAL TIME CUES, PHASE ADVANCE, PHASE DELAY, PHASE RESPONSE CURVE.)

Tofranil See ANTIDEPRESSANTS.

tolerance Term used when greater dosages of medication are required to obtain the original effect. Certain MEDICATIONS, such as the amphetamines (see STIMULANT MEDICATIONS), induce a resistance to the drug so that greater dosages are necessary to achieve the initial results. In that way, tolerance to a drug necessitates the escalation of the dose in order to maintain the drug's effect, such as improved ALERTNESS in the case of the amphetamines. Since sudden cessation of the medication will often worsen the original problem that was being corrected, such as sleepiness, continued (and escalated) use of the medication is often inadvertently promoted.

tongue retaining device (TRD) Dental appliance designed to hold the tongue forward to prevent SNORING. The mouthpiece, which is inserted into the mouth and fitted over the upper and lower teeth, contains a compartment that holds the tongue in a forward position by suction. The tongue retaining device works on the principle that the position of the tongue contributes to UPPER AIRWAY OBSTRUCTION, thereby adding to snoring. It is particularly effective for patients who snore while lying in a supine position.

Polysomnographic studies have demonstrated that the TRD can be useful for treating mild OBSTRUCTIVE SLEEP APNEA SYNDROME, especially in patients who are unable either to use a nasal CONTINUOUS POSITIVE AIRWAY PRESSURE (CPAP) device or undergo UVULOPALATOPHARYNGOPLASTY. However, many patients find the device uncomfortable and are unable to tolerate it for more than 50% of the night. In addition, the device appears to be less successful in patients who are more than 50% overweight. (See also ORAL APPLIANCES.)

Cartwright, R., Stefoski, D., Caldarelli, D., Kravitz, H., Knight, S., Lloyd, S. and Samelson, D., "Toward a Treatment Logic for Sleep Apnea: The Place of the Tongue Retaining Device," *Behavioral Research Therapy* 26 (1988): 121–126.

tonsillectomy and adenoidectomy Tonsillectomy, with or without an adenoidectomy, is a surgical procedure that is performed for the relief of the OBSTRUCTIVE SLEEP APNEA SYNDROME. This procedure is most commonly performed in children because tonsil enlargement is common in the prepubertal age group. However, some adults can also have very enlarged tonsils, or enlarged adenoids, which contribute to UPPER AIRWAY OBSTRUCTION and therefore may need to undergo this surgery. Many patients treated by a UVULOPALATOPHARYNGOPLASTY (UPP) operation also have removal of tonsils or adenoids if they are enlarged at the time of the UPP surgery.

Tonsillectomy involves removal of the enlarged lymphoid tissue situated between the anterior and posterior pillar of fauces. This tissue is involved in the immune response to infections in childhood but gradually regresses and is of little functional importance in adulthood. Removal of the tonsils is a simple procedure in children, but it assumes greater likelihood of complications, such as excessive bleeding, in adults.

In the majority of children with enlarged tonsils and obstructive sleep apnea, tonsillectomy entirely relieves the obstructive sleep apnea. However, some patients who have craniofacial abnormalities may continue to have obstructive sleep apnea following removal of the tonsils or adenoids. Postoperative polysomnographic monitoring for obstructive sleep apnea is required for patients with severe obstructive sleep apnea who appear to be symptomatic following surgery. Other surgical procedures, for example, MANDIBULAR ADVANCEMENT SURGERY, may be required, or the use of a CONTINUOUS POSITIVE AIRWAY PRESSURE (CPAP) device. (See also CRANIOFACIAL DISORDERS, HYOID MYOTOMY, SURGERY AND SLEEP DISORDERS, TRACHEOSTOMY.)

total recording time (TRT) The duration of time from sleep onset (lights out) to the end of the final awakening. The total recording time comprises the TOTAL SLEEP TIME, including stages non-REM and REM sleep, and episodes of wakefulness and movement time that occur until the lights are on; arousal time; or ARISE TIME.

total sleep episode The duration of the major sleep episode, which usually occurs at night. This is the total amount of time available for sleep, and typically it is approximately eight hours in duration. The total sleep episode includes REM SLEEP and NON-REM-STAGE SLEEP, as well as periods of WAKEFULNESS that occur during the time available for sleep. (See also TOTAL RECORDING TIME, TOTAL SLEEP TIME.)

total sleep time (TST) The amount of actual sleep that occurs during a sleep episode; consists of the sum of the total amount of non-REM plus REM sleep. The total sleep time varies according to age, being greatest in infancy with a gradual reduction as one gets older. (See also SLEEP DURATION, TOTAL RECORDING TIME, TOTAL SLEEP EPISODE.)

toxin-induced sleep disorder A sleep disorder characterized by either INSOMNIA or EXCESSIVE SLEEPINESS; produced by the ingestion of toxic agents such as heavy metals or organic toxins. The poisoning due to the repeated ingestion of these agents produces central nervous system effects, such as stimulation and agitation, and can also produce depression-causing sleepiness and even COMA. Other symptoms such as cardiac stimulation, respiratory depression, and gastrointestinal upset can occur with the ingestion of the toxic agents. Liver, renal and cardiac poisoning can occur.

This type of sleep disorder is most commonly seen in industrial workers who are exposed to toxic chemicals. It can also be seen in children, who may ingest lead in paint or be excessively exposed to the exhaust fumes of leaded gasoline.

The treatment of the sleep disturbance involves removal of exposure to the offending agent as well as providing good SLEEP HYGIENE measures in order to prevent continuation of the sleep disturbance.

trace alternant An encephalographic pattern that is characterized by bursts of slow waves intermixed with sharp waves alternating with periods of relative low amplitude activity. This particular EEG pattern is characteristically seen in the sleep of newborns. (See also INFANT SLEEP.)

tracheostomy Regarded as the most effective surgical treatment for OBSTRUCTIVE SLEEP APNEA SYNDROME; involves placing a hole in the trachea and inserting a tube so that the upper airway is bypassed when the individual breathes. The tracheostomy typically is closed during the daytime and open at night so that sleep-related UPPER AIRWAY OBSTRUCTION does not occur.

Tracheostomy is reserved for patients with severe sleep apnea syndrome who are unable to be treated effectively by medical and nonsurgical means. The most effective alternative nonsurgical treatment is by means of a CONTINUOUS POSITIVE AIRWAY PRESSURE (CPAP) device. Some patients, for varying reasons, are unable to use such a system, and tracheostomy is considered if their obstructive sleep apnea is severe enough.

Immediately following the placement of the tracheostomy, patients with severe obstructive sleep apnea notice a dramatic improvement in terms of the quality of sleep at night and relief of daytime sleepiness. There are improved objective clinical features, such as improved oxygen saturation during sleep, reduced cardiac ARRHYTHMIAS, improved quality of sleep and objective evidence of improved daytime alertness.

The complications of tracheostomy are primarily the social difficulties of having a hole at the base of the neck. (Patients are unable to swim or go into small boats where they might fall into the water.) The complications of tracheostomy include recurrent infections, development of granulation tissue at the site of the tracheostomy, and recurrent irritation or cough. More severe problems, such as tracheomalacia (a weakness of the tracheal cartilage) may rarely occur. However, despite the potential complications, tracheostomy can be a dramatically effective and lifesaving treatment for many patients. (See also HYOID MYOTOMY, MANDIBULAR ADVANCEMENT SURGERY, UVULOPALATOPHARYNGOPLASTY, SURGERY AND SLEEP DISORDERS.)

tranquilizers Term introduced in the early 1950s to characterize the calming effect of the medication reserpine. The tranquilizers are often divided into two groups, the major and the minor tranquilizers.

The major tranquilizers include medications, such as phenothiazines, that are often used to treat the major psychiatric disorders. The minor tranquilizers are those that have lesser mind-altering effects and are primarily used for reducing anxiety, such as the BENZODIAZEPINE antianxiety agents. As the term *tranquilizer* can apply to agents with very marked effects on mood and thought, or can apply to agents with very mild effects, the term is best avoided. The terms *antipsychotic* and *antianxiety* mediations are preferred. (See also ANXIETY DISORDERS, HYPNOTICS, PSYCHIATRIC DISORDERS.)

transient insomnia Insomnia that is differentiated from SHORT-TERM and LONG-TERM INSOMNIA. These terms were generally publicized as a result of a National Institutes of Health consensus development conference that was convened by the National Institute of Mental Health and the Office of Medical Applications of Research in November of 1983. The summary statement of the conference suggested that the term "transient insomnia" be applied to normal sleepers who experience acute stress or situational changes that lead to sleep disturbance that is temporary, lasting only a few days. The term is synonymous with ADJUSTMENT SLEEP DISORDER and situational insomnia.

transient psychophysiological insomnia See ADJUSTMENT SLEEP DISORDER.

triazolam See BENZODIAZEPINES.

triclofos See HYPNOTICS.

tricyclic antidepressants See ANTIDEPRESSANTS.

Tripp, Peter A 32-year-old New York City radio disc jockey who stayed awake for eight consecutive days as a fund-raising event for the March of Dimes birth defects organization. Each day he performed his regular three-hour broadcasts, but he went without any sleep. By the fifth day, Tripp began hallucinating and became increasingly paranoid. At the end of his ordeal, Tripp slept for 13 consecutive hours. Although his psychotic-like thinking cleared up after he slept, Tripp was slightly depressed for several months, possibly linked to his SLEEP DEPRIVATION ordeal. (See also SLEEP NEED.)

TRT See TOTAL RECORDING TIME.

trypanosomiasis See SLEEPING SICKNESS.

tryptophan See HYPNOTICS.

TST See TOTAL SLEEP TIME.

tumescence Term used for the engorgement of the penis that occurs in relationship to sexual excitement or REM SLEEP at night. A measure of the ability of the penis to obtain adequate tumescence is used for a better understanding of the cause of IMPOTENCE. (See also IMPAIRED SLEEP-RELATED PENILE ERECTIONS, NOCTURNAL PENILE TUMESCENCE TEST, SLEEP-RELATED PAINFUL ERECTIONS, SLEEP-RELATED PENILE ERECTIONS.)

twitch A very small body movement such as a foot or finger jerk. A body twitch during sleep is not usually associated with an arousal but is consistently detected either visually or by electromyographic recordings. Body twitches are common during normal sleep, particularly of infants. These movements are often myoclonic jerks, and when they occur in great frequency in neonates the disorder BENIGN NEONATAL SLEEP MYOCLONUS may be present. In adults, twitches can occur at sleep onset and are then termed SLEEP STARTS, particularly if they are associated with a whole body movement.

type-1 oscillator See ENDOGENOUS CIRCADIAN PACEMAKER.

U

ulcer See PEPTIC ULCER DISEASE.

ultradian rhythm Rhythms that have a cycle length of less than 24 hours in duration. The term is used for biological rhythms that occur with a higher frequency than the 24-hour sleep-wake cycle, such as respiratory or cardiac rhythms. Biological rhythms that have a period length greater than 24 hours (such as the MENSTRUAL CYCLE) are known as *infradian rhythms*. (See also CHRONOBIOLOGY, CIRCADIAN RHYTHMS.)

unconsciousness A mental state in which there is loss of responsiveness to sensory stimuli. States of unconsciousness can be produced by metabolic, pharmacologic or intracerebral lesions. Patients who are unconscious are usually in COMA; however, impaired levels of consciousness may be present with intact sleep-wake cycling and retention of some responses to stimuli.

The term "clouding of consciousness" is often applied to reduced states of wakefulness and awareness in which the patient may be responsive to external stimuli but has a variation in the level of attention, with hyperexcitability and irritability, that alternates with episodes of drowsiness. More advanced degrees of clouding of consciousness can produce a confusional state in which there is difficulty in following commands. A state of DELIRIUM is characterized by disorientation, fear, irritability and a misperception of stimuli. Such patients frequently will have visual hallucinations that can alternate with periods when the mental state appears intact.

The term OBTUNDATION often applies to an impairment of full consciousness where the individual has some reduction in level of alertness, with decreased awareness of the environment. Such patients may have EXCESSIVE SLEEPINESS or DROWSINESS.

The term STUPOR is often applied to a loss of responsiveness in which the individual can be aroused only by very strong and vigorous stimuli. The patient may be in deep sleep with slow wave activity from which it is difficult to be aroused. After arousal, such subjects typically will lapse back into the unresponsive state. This condition is often associated with organic cerebral dysfunction; however, severe schizophrenia or DEPRESSION can lead to a similar state. (See also DEMENTIA, PSYCHIATRIC DISORDERS.)

Unisom See OVER-THE-COUNTER MEDICATIONS.

upper airway obstruction Term applied to obstruction that typically occurs during sleep and is associated with the OBSTRUCTIVE SLEEP APNEA SYNDROME. Obstruction can occur anywhere from the nose to the larynx and may not be evident during wakefulness. Causes of such obstruction include a very narrow nasal airway, enlarged adenoids or tonsils, an elongated soft palate, and obstruction at the base of the tongue by tongue tissues, including the lingual tonsil (tonsil sometimes found at the base of the tongue). Predisposing conditions to upper airway obstruction include skeletal abnormalities such as a posterior-placed lower jaw (retrognathia).

Surgery or appliances, such as a CONTINUOUS POSITIVE AIRWAY PRESSURE (CPAP) device, can relieve the upper airway obstruction during sleep and resolve the clinical features associated with the obstructive sleep apnea syndrome. (See also HYOID MYOTOMY, MANDIBULAR ADVANCEMENT SURGERY,

ORAL APPLIANCES, SURGERY AND SLEEP DISORDERS, TONSILLECTOMY AND ADENOIDECTOMY, TRACHEOSTOMY, UVULOPALATOPHARYNGOPLASTY.)

upper airway resistance syndrome (UARS) A disorder consisting of an increased effort of breathing during sleep which produces an arousal that results in sleep fragmentation and subsequent daytime sleepiness. These arousals occur in the absence of APNEAS, HYPOPNEAS and oxygen desaturation. The presence of frequent arousals in a patient complaining of EXCESSIVE SLEEPINESS who does not have apneas and hypopneas should raise suspicion that upper airway resistance syndrome is present.

The best way to document the pressure change is by esophageal pressure monitoring. However, in the absence of pressure monitoring an increased number of arousals (more than 10 per hour) during sleep is typically associated with this syndrome. Approximately 10% of all breaths have negative intrathoracic pressures (less than -10 centimeters of water). Ten percent of all breaths involve an increased effort that is greater than two standard deviations of the value monitored during quiet relaxed breathing. (See also OBSTRUCTIVE SLEEP APNEA SYNDROME.)

upper airway sleep apnea See OBSTRUCTIVE SLEEP APNEA SYNDROME.

uvulopalatopharyngoplasty (UPP) A surgical procedure that was developed by Tanenosuke Ikematsu in 1964. This surgical procedure was first used in Japan for the treatment of SNORING and was introduced into the United States by Shiro Fujita in 1979 as an alternative to TRACHEOSTOMY for the treatment of the OBSTRUCTIVE SLEEP APNEA SYNDROME. The surgical procedure for uvulopalatopharyngoplasty involves the removal of redundant and excessive tissue from the pharynx in order to prevent UPPER AIRWAY OBSTRUCTION during sleep. This surgical procedure shortens the soft palate and removes the uvula and the anterior and posterior pillar of fauces that attach to the soft palate. The tonsils, if present, are usually removed.

UPP is a widely used procedure for the treatment of snoring and the obstructive sleep apnea syndrome. However, studies have demonstrated that only 40% to 50% of an unselected group of patients with obstructive sleep apnea syndrome will respond to this procedure. Patients who have been screened by means of upper airway studies have an increased operative success; however, the procedure is ideal for only 20% to 30% of all patients who are evaluated for the obstructive sleep apnea syndrome.

Potential complications of the surgical procedure include insufficiency of the palate closure so that fluids being swallowed may be regurgitated into the nose. (But this complication rarely occurs if the patient is well screened beforehand and an excessive amount of tissue is not removed.) Other complications of uvulopalatopharyngoplasty are those related to anesthesia and other nonspecific surgical complications. Two new forms of palatoplasty have been developed: LASER UVULOPALATOPLASTY and radiofrequency palatoplasty (see SOMNOPLASTY). These procedures have the advantage of being able to be performed in a physician's office without the need for general anesthesia. (See also HYOID MYOTOMY, MANDIBULAR ADVANCEMENT SURGERY, SURGERY AND SLEEP DISORDERS, TONSILLECTOMY AND ADENOIDECTOMY, TRACHEOSTOMY.)

Fujita, S., Conway, W., Zorck, F. and Roth, Thomas, "Surgical Correction of Anatomic Abnormalities in Obstructive Sleep Apnea Syndrome: Uvulopalatopharyngoplasty," *Otolaryngal Head Neck Surgery* 89 (1981): 923–934.

Sher, A.E., Thorpy, Michael J., Shprintzen, R.J., Spielman, Arthur J., Burack, B. and McGregor, P.A., "Predictive Value of Muller Maneuver in Selection of Patients for Uvulopalatopharyngoplasty," *Laryngoscope* 95 (1985): 1483–1487.

V

Valium See BENZODIAZEPINES.

VAS See VISUAL ANALOGUE SCALE.

vasointestinal polypeptide (VIP) A peptide isolated in 1972 that contains 28 amino acid residues. It is a naturally occurring peptide that is released into the cerebrospinal fluid. Studies have shown VIP to be associated with an increase in wakefulness; however, in high doses it appears to be able to induce REM SLEEP.

VIP is present in several regions in the central nervous system and is located with the neurons that contain ACETYLCHOLINE. The effects of vasointestinal polypeptide are similar to the effects of acetylcholine in inducing wakefulness and REM sleep. (See also SLEEP-INDUCING FACTORS.)

ventilation Movement of air in and out of the lungs. Ventilation can be impaired by a number of disorders that affect the central nervous system, and the nerves and muscles involved in the chest mechanics. Several SLEEP-RELATED BREATHING DISORDERS, such as OBSTRUCTIVE SLEEP APNEA SYNDROME, CENTRAL SLEEP APNEA SYNDROME, CENTRAL ALVEOLAR HYPOVENTILATION SYNDROME and CHRONIC OBSTRUCTIVE PULMONARY DISEASE, can affect ventilation. Ventilation abnormalities during sleep can lead to ALVEOLAR HYPOVENTILATION (abnormal arterial blood gases during the daytime, with HYPOXEMIA and HYPERCAPNIA). Relief of the sleep-related breathing disorder can lead to resolution of these daytime blood gas impairments. Other disorders, such as KYPHOSCOLIOSIS and intrinsic lung disease, can also have impaired ventilation during sleep.

Treatment of sleep-related breathing disorders may involve weight reduction (see OBESITY), assisted ventilatory devices, such as a positive pressure ventilator or CONTINUOUS POSITIVE AIRWAY PRESSURE (CPAP) device, or upper airway surgery, such as TRACHEOSTOMY or UVULOPALATOPHARYNGOPLASTY. (See also SURGERY AND SLEEP DISORDERS.)

ventricular arrhythmias Also known as ventricular premature contractions, ventricular tachycardia, ventricular flutter and ventricular fibrillation. Ventricular arrhythmias are commonly seen in association with SLEEP-RELATED BREATHING DISORDERS, particularly at the end of an apneic episode when tachycardia (abnormally rapid heartbeat) is seen. The ventricular arrhythmias can reduce in frequency or be eliminated following the treatment of the sleep-related breathing disorder. Studies have demonstrated that the frequency of ventricular arrhythmias in sleep can vary; some reports show a decrease of ventricular arrhythmias during sleep, and others an increase in frequency of such episodes.

Studies on patients with chronic obstructive respiratory disease have demonstrated that ventricular arrhythmias seen during sleep can be reduced by the administration of supplemental oxygen, suggesting that HYPOXEMIA is directly related to these arrhythmias. The effect of hypoxemia in inducing cardiac arrhythmias may be by a direct mechanism of ischemia upon the cardiovascular system, or may be indirect, through the stimulation of catecholamines such as adrenaline. Also, RESPIRATORY STIMULANTS may exacerbate the cardiac ARRHYTHMIAS seen in patients with CHRONIC OBSTRUCTIVE PULMONARY DISEASE.

Ventricular arrhythmias of the ventricular tachycardia, flutter or fibrillation type are medical emergencies that require active intervention. Antiarrhythmic medications, such as beta-blockers, verapamil, or quinidine-like medications, may be useful in suppressing or preventing such arrhythmias. Because of the increased incidence of ventricular arrhythmias in patients with sleep-related breathing disorders, stimulant medications should not be given to treat the excessive sleepiness. (See also DEATHS DURING SLEEP, EXCESSIVE SLEEPINESS, OBSTRUCTIVE SLEEP APNEA SYNDROME, SLEEP-RELATED CARDIOVASCULAR SYMPTOMS, VENTRICULAR PREMATURE COMPLEXES.)

ventricular fibrillation See VENTRICULAR ARRHYTHMIAS.

ventricular flutter See VENTRICULAR ARRHYTHMIAS.

ventricular premature complexes Also known as premature ventricular contractions; very common arrhythmias that occur in patients with or without heart disease. These complexes are commonly seen during polysomnographic monitoring of patients. In those patients without cardiorespiratory disease, the premature ventricular contractions are usually benign and not associated with any increased incidence in mortality or morbidity.

However, ventricular premature complexes can commonly occur in association with SLEEP-RELATED BREATHING DISORDERS, such as OBSTRUCTIVE SLEEP APNEA SYNDROME. Typically, a pattern of bradycardia (slow heart rate), followed by tachycardia (fast heart rate), is seen in these disorders. The tachycardia phase occurs at the end of the apneic episode, during the hyperventilation portion of the apnea. The ventricular premature complexes seen at this time can also be associated with the tachyarrhythmias of ventricular tachycardia, which is defined as three or more consecutive ventricular contractions. Ventricular tachycardia imposes an increased risk of sudden death. Usually the ventricular premature contractions that are associated with sleep-related breathing disorders resolve once the breathing disorder has been treated, and therefore additional treatment is not required. However, the presence of frequent ventricular premature contractions, or the inability to completely resolve the sleep-related breathing disorder, may make treatment with antiarrhythmic medications necessary. Medications used in this setting could include the beta-adrenergic blockers. Other medications that may be required include quinidine or quinidine-like medications. (See also CENTRAL SLEEP APNEA SYNDROME, DEATHS DURING SLEEP, MYOCARDIAL INFARCTION, SLEEP-RELATED CARDIOVASCULAR SYMPTOMS.)

ventricular premature contractions See VENTRICULAR ARRHYTHMIAS.

ventricular tachycardia See VENTRICULAR ARRHYTHMIAS.

ventrolateral preoptic nucleus A nucleus believed to be important in the control of CIRCADIAN RHYTHMS. There are two groups of neurons responsible: the intergeniculate leaflet (IGL) and the dorsal SUPRACHIASMATIC NUCLEUS (SCN); and the cells in the ventrolateral preoptic area (VLPO).

It appears that sleep-activated VLPO neurons innervate the tuberomammillary nucleus of the posterior hypothalamus to modulate arousal. The neurons of the VLPO innervate cell bodies and proximal dendrites of histaminergic cells in the ipsilateral tuberomammillary nucleus (TMN). These histaminergic neurons are involved in the posterolateral hypothalamic arousal system. They are tonically active during waking, become less active during SLOW WAVE SLEEP, and cease firing in REM sleep. It is believed that the histaminergic system is inhibited during sleep by GABA-ergic input from the VLPO. Recent research has suggested that the medication MODAFINIL, which is used for the treatment of NARCOLEPSY, may act by means of VLPO.

vertex sharp transients Rapid ELECTROENCEPHALOGRAM (EEG) waves that occur either spontaneously during sleep or in response to a sensory stimulus. They are characterized by a sharp negative potential, which is maximal at the vertex of the head. The amplitude of these negative potentials varies but rarely exceeds 250 microvolts. *Vertex sharp transient* is preferred to *vertex sharp wave*.

vertex sharp wave See VERTEX SHARP TRANSIENTS.

vigilance Term first proposed by Henry Head in 1923 to refer to the physiological state of the central nervous system. With the development of an understanding of the reticular activating system, the term became indicative of the level of arousal. Vigilance is now used synonymously with ALERTNESS and is the opposite of SLEEPINESS.

Impaired vigilance may be due to reduced central nervous system functioning as a result of increased sleepiness brought about by reduced quality or quantity of nighttime sleep. Disorders of unknown cause, such as NARCOLEPSY and IDIOPATHIC HYPERSOMNIA, are associated with impaired vigilance and EXCESSIVE SLEEPINESS.

Tests of vigilance can be made either by performance measures, such as the WILKINSON AUDITORY VIGILANCE TEST, or by means of electroencephalographic testing for patterns consistent with sleepiness or DROWSINESS, such as the MULTIPLE SLEEP LATENCY TEST. (See also AROUSAL, ASCENDING RETICULAR ACTIVATING SYSTEM, SUBWAKEFULNESS SYNDROME.)

vigilance testing Tests of vigilance to assess the level of alertness during the period of wakefulness as applied in clinical or research settings. Tests may be subjective, by rating scales such as the STANFORD SLEEPINESS SCALE or the VISUAL ANALOGUE SCALE. However, most vigilance testing involves some physiological measure, such as the determination of pupil diameter by PUPILLOMETRY. (The pupil is very sensitive to changes in ALERTNESS and becomes smaller as the level of alertness decreases.)

Other tests involve reaction time tests, such as flicker fusion (rapid alternating pattern of light flashes) studies and letter sorting tasks. These tests determine the ability to concentrate and adequately perform the task at hand.

Other electrophysical means of determining alertness include MULTIPLE SLEEP LATENCY TESTING (MSLT) and MAINTENANCE OF WAKEFULNESS TESTING (MWT), which involve five nap opportunities and measure SLEEP LATENCY on each nap. Evoked potential (an electroencephalographic wave response) measurements by means of an auditory stimulus show changes consistent with alterations in levels of alertness. Computerized electroencephalography with analysis by power spectra can determine the presence of electroencephalographic slowing consistent with a change in the level of alertness.

viloxazine See NARCOLEPSY.

VIP See VASOINTESTINAL POLYPEPTIDE (VIP).

visual analogue scale (VAS) Scale that gives a quick subjective assessment of ALERTNESS or SLEEPINESS. The visual analogue technique has been used in research since the 1920s and is frequently administered for rating sleepiness or alertness in sleep research. The analogue scale consists of a straight line that represents the range of alertness from very sleepy, at one end, to very alert, at the other. Subjects mark on the line the position that adequately represents their status at a particular time. The distance from the left end of the line is measured and recorded in arbitrary units for comparison with the patients' state at another point in time.

The VAS scale of alertness is frequently used in studies of shift work, time of day effects, sleep loss and in chronobiological research. (See also CHRONOBIOLOGY.)

Vivactil See ANTIDEPRESSANTS.

Vivarin See OVER-THE-COUNTER MEDICATIONS.

VPCs See VENTRICULAR PREMATURE COMPLEXES.

W

wakefulness A brain state that occurs in the absence of sleep in an otherwise healthy individual. It is the state of being awake that is characterized by EEG wave patterns dominated by ALPHA RHYTHM, or electrocortical activity, between 8 Hz and 13 Hz. This alpha activity is most pronounced when the eyes are closed and the subject is relaxed. Infants tend to have a slower rhythm of about 4 Hz at four months of age, and this increases in frequency with age. The wakefulness rhythm is about 6 Hz at about 12 months of age, 8 Hz at three years of age, and reaches 10 Hz to 13 Hz at 10 years of age. The alpha rhythm remains stable in adults; however, there is often a decline in the elderly, particularly in those with some degree of cerebral pathology. The amplitude varies from person to person, but most often amplitudes of 20 to 60 microvolts are found (rarely, amplitudes above 100 microvolts can be seen). This wakefulness rhythm is thought to be of cortical origin.

In addition to the characteristic alpha activity of wakefulness, there are also BETA RHYTHMS, which occur particularly with increased ALERTNESS, motor activity and in response to environmental stimuli. Wakefulness is often subdivided into quiet wakefulness, where an individual is resting in a relaxed condition, compared with a period of active wakefulness, when the individual is more alert and may be engaged in talking or other motor activities.

wake time The total time that is scored as wakefulness during a polysomnographic recording. This period of wakefulness usually occurs between SLEEP ONSET and the final wake-up time.

warm baths Taking a warm bath just before sleep may improve sleep, according to some scientific studies. The beneficial effect of a warm bath is attributed to raising both the core body TEMPERATURE and the more peripheral skin temperature.

Webb, Wilse B. Dr. Webb (1920–) received his Ph.D. in experimental psychology in 1947 from the State University of Iowa; in 1957 he published his first paper on sleep. Using rats, he attempted to predict the rate of sleep onset as a function of several experimental variables. Beginning in 1961, at the University of Florida and in collaboration with Robert Agnew, Robert Williams, and students, Dr. Webb began work on human sleep. Over the following decades, his sleep research has concerned temporal variations, shift work, time-free environments, short and long sleepers, the role of stage four sleep, and the aging of sleep, among other topics. Since 1969, he has been a graduate research professor at the University of Florida. Dr. Webb was awarded the Distinguished Service Award of the Sleep Research Society in 1992.

Webb, Wilse B., ed., *Biological Rhythms, Sleep and Performance.* Chichester, England: John Wiley, 1982.

Webb, Wilse B., *Sleep: An Experimental Variable.* New York: Macmillan, 1968.

———, *Sleep: The Gentle Tyrant.* Englewood Cliffs, N.J.: Prentice-Hall, 1975.

weight Weight plays an important part in exacerbating some sleep disorders. OBSTRUCTIVE SLEEP APNEA SYNDROME more commonly occurs in persons who are overweight, and weight reduction can be associated with an improvement in the symptoms of the syndrome. However, the amount of weight loss required for improvement varies greatly. Some individuals may lose 100 pounds without there being any significant effect, whereas in others, five or 10 pounds of weight loss may produce improvement. Most of the sleep-related breathing disorders are worsened by weight gain.

The NOCTURNAL EATING (DRINKING) SYNDROME is a sleep disorder often associated with increasing body weight. People with this disorder will awaken during the night with a compulsion to eat or drink; most of the day's caloric intake may be taken during the hours of sleep. Those with the disorder often seek help in preventing the awakenings to eat in the hope that this will lead to a reduction of body weight. (See also CENTRAL ALVEOLAR HYPOVENTILATION SYNDROME, DIET AND SLEEP, OBESITY, OBESITY HYPOVENTILATION SYNDROME, SLEEP-RELATED BREATHING DISORDERS.)

Weitzman, Elliot D. One of the founders of the ASSOCIATION OF SLEEP DISORDER CENTERS, Dr. Weitzman (1929–1983) was largely responsible for writing its first policy guideline, the *Certification Standards and Guidelines*.

Dr. Weitzman was chairman of the Department of Neurology and director of the Sleep/Wake Disorders Center at Montefiore Medical Center. He founded its sleep disorders center, the first to be accredited, in 1977, by the Association of Sleep Disorder Centers. He also founded and directed the Institute of Chronobiology at New York Hospital-Cornell Medical Center and was professor of neurology in psychiatry, Cornell University Medical College.

He was editor of the eight-volume series of books entitled *Advances in Sleep Research*, published by SP Medical and Scientific Books. Weitzman is credited with being an outspoken advocate for the disciplines of SLEEP DISORDERS MEDICINE and CHRONOBIOLOGY. An annual award is given in his name by the ASSOCIATION OF POLYSOMNOGRAPHIC TECHNOLOGISTS (APT).

Weitzman, E.D., Schaumburg, H. and Fishbein, W., "Plasma 17-hydroxy-corticosteroid Levels During Sleep in Man," *Journal of Clinical Endocrinology* 26 (1966): 121–127.

Editors of *Sleep*, "In Memoriam: Elliot D. Weitzman," *Sleep* 6 (1983): 291–292.

wet dream See NOCTURNAL EMISSION.

White, David P. Dr. White (1949–) received his B.S. degree from Washington and Lee University in 1971 and his M.D. degree from Emory University School of Medicine in 1975. He is a past president (1996–97) of the American Sleep Disorders Association (renamed the AMERICAN ACADEMY OF SLEEP MEDICINE). He is the chair of the External Advisory Board of the National Center on Sleep Disorders Research for the National Heart, Lung and Blood Institute. Dr. White's sleep research has been centered on sleep-disordered breathing. In 2000, Dr. White, who is at the Sleep Disorders Program, Circadian, Neuroendocrine and Sleep Disorders Section, of Brigham and Women's Hospital in Boston, received the NATHANIEL KLEITMAN DISTINGUISHED SERVICE AWARD.

Wilkinson auditory vigilance testing Proven to be one of the most sensitive performance tests in documenting ALERTNESS and EXCESSIVE SLEEPINESS during the day. In this test, the subject listens through headphones to a recording of a repetitive series of timed pips. These pips of sound are 500 milliseconds in duration, have a regular stimulus interval of 1.5 seconds, and occur on a background of "gray" noise. Occasionally, at unpredictable intervals, one of the tone pips is slightly shorter in duration than the rest (approximately 400 milliseconds). The subject has the task of detecting the shorter signals and indicating their presence by pressing a button. The test continues for 30 minutes and is analyzed in terms of the signals correctly detected, the number of erroneously pushed buttons, and the reaction time from the presentation of the stimulus to the response.

This test is mainly used for research purposes to determine levels of alertness and has little clinical applicability.

World Federation of Sleep Research Societies Founded in 1989 by the EUROPEAN SLEEP RESEARCH SOCIETY, the JAPANESE SLEEP RESEARCH SOCIETY, the LATIN AMERICAN SLEEP RESEARCH SOCIETY, and the SLEEP RESEARCH SOCIETY (of the United States). International meetings are held every two years. The first congress was held in 1991.

Programs include a sleep training workshop, a training fellowship program, and an equipment and general exchange program. The first president was MICHAEL H. CHASE, PH.D., of the United States. For further information visit the federation's web site at: www.wfsrs.org.

X

Xanax See BENZODIAZEPINES.

xanthines See RESPIRATORY STIMULANTS.

X-oscillator See ENDOGENOUS CIRCADIAN PACEMAKER.

Y

yawning An involuntary movement of the mouth that occurs in humans as well as in such animals as dogs, cats, crocodiles, snakes, birds, and even some fish. A yawn begins with a slow inhalation of air followed by a quicker expiration. Yawns may signify sleepiness as well as stress or boredom.

Z

zaleplon (Sonata) See HYPNOTICS.

zeitgeber See ENVIRONMENTAL TIME CUES.

zimelidine See ANTIDEPRESSANTS.

zolpidem See HYPNOTICS.

zopiclone See HYPNOTICS.

APPENDIXES

I. Sources of Information

II. AASM-Member Sleep Centers and Laboratories

III. The International Classification of Sleep Disorders

IV. Diagnostic Classification of Sleep and Arousal Disorders

APPENDIX I
SOURCES OF INFORMATION

Since addresses, websites, and even names of associations, organizations or information resources may change at any time, accuracy of these listings cannot be guaranteed. Furthermore, a listing does not imply an endorsement of that information resource nor should omission from this listing have any implications.

American Sleep Apnea Association
2025 Pennsylvania Avenue NW
Suite 905
Washington, DC 20006
www.sleepapnea.org

American Academy of Sleep Medicine (AASM)
6301 Bandel Road NW
Suite 101
Rochester, MN 55901
www.aasmnet.org

Association for the Study of Dreams (ASD)
P.O. Box 1166
Orinda, CA 94563
http://www.asdreams.org

Better Sleep Council (of the National Association of Bedding Manufacturers) (BSC)
501 Wythe Street
Alexandria, VA 22314
www.bettersleep.org

British Sleep Society
P.O. Box 247
Huntingdon PE28 3UZ
United Kingdom
http://www.bss.org

Center for Sleep Research
Clinical Development Research Centre
The Queen Elizabeth Hospital
Woodville Road
Woodville, South Australia 5011 Australia
www.unisa.edu.au/sleep

Good Sleep and Circadian Learning Center
Circadian Information, Inc.
125 Cambridge Park Drive
Cambridge, MA 02140
E-mail: info@circadian.com
http://www.circadian.com
http://www.goodsleep.com

Narcolepsy Institute
Sleep-Wake Disorders Center
Montefiore Medical Center
111 East 210th Street
Bronx, NY 10467

Narcolepsy Network
10921 Reed Hartman Highway
Cincinnati, OH 45242
www.narcolepsynetwork.org

National Center for Sleep Disorders Research
National Institutes of Health
NHLB1, Building 31, Room 4A11
9000 Rockville Pike
Bethesda, MD 20892
http://www.nhlbi.nih.gov/about/ncsdr/index.htm

National Sleep Foundation
1522 K Street NW
#500
Washington, DC 20005
www.sleepfoundation.org

Restless Legs Syndrome Foundation, Inc.
P.O. Box 7050
Department CP
Rochester, MN 55903-7050
www.rls.org

Sleep Medicine Home Page
http://www.userscloud9.net/~thorpy

Sleep Research Online
c/o WebSciences
10911 Weyburn Avenue
Suite 348
Los Angeles, CA 90024
http://www.sro.org

Sleep Research Society
6301 Bandel Road NW
Suite 101
Rochester, MN 55901
http://www.srssleep.org

Sleep-Wake Disorders Center
Montefiore Medical Center
111 East 210th Street
Bronx, NY 10467
718-920-4841

The Sleep Well
http://www.stanford.edu/~dement/
http://www.SleepQuest.com

Society for Light Treatment and Biological Rhythms
P.O. Box 591687
San Francisco, CA 94159-1687
www.sltbr.org

World Federation of Sleep Research Societies (WFSRS)
http://www. wfsrs.org/homepage.html

APPENDIX II

AASM-MEMBER SLEEP CENTERS AND LABORATORIES

Sleep disorders include problems with sleeping, staying awake, and troublesome behavior during sleep. The American Academy of Sleep Medicine (AASM) is dedicated to maintaining high medical standards in the diagnosis and treatment of these difficulties. The following is a listing of sleep disorders centers and laboratories that have been accredited by and maintain membership in the American Academy of Sleep Medicine. Member centers provide the diagnosis and treatment of all types of sleep-related disorders, and member laboratories (identified by *) specialize only in sleep-related breathing disorders. The most up-to-date listing may be obtained from the American Academy of Sleep Medicine on the Internet at http://www.aasmnet.org.

ALABAMA

Sleep Disorders Laboratory*
Northeast Alabama Regional Medical Center
400 East 10th Street
P.O. Box 2208
Anniston, AL 36202
William J. Ferguson, M.D., Medical Director
D. Larry Cash, RRT, Director
Louise Cosper, RPSGT, Lead Technician
256-235-5077

Princeton Sleep/Wake Disorders Center
Baptist Medical Center Princeton
701 Princeton Avenue SW
P.O. Box II, Suite 50
Birmingham, AL 35211-1399
Stuart Padove, M.D., Medical Director
Regina McClain, RPSGT, Director,
Patsy Stanberry, Secretary
Herb Caillouet, Administrative Vice-President
Janet Carlisle, CRT, CPAP Manager
205-783-7378

Sleep Disorders Center of Alabama, Inc.
790 Montclair Road
Suite 200
Birmingham, AL 35213
Vernon Pegram, Ph.D.
Robert C. Doekel, M.D.
205-599-1020
Website: www.sleepsciences.com

Sleep-Wake Disorders Center
University of Alabama at Birmingham
1713 6th Avenue South
CPM Building, Room 270
Birmingham, AL 35233-0018
Susan Harding, M.D.
Vernon Pegram, Ph.D.
John McBurney, M.D.
Len Shigley, RPSGT, Technical Director
205-934-7110

Sleep Disorders Center
Children's Hospital
1600 Seventh Avenue South
Birmingham, AL 35233
Christopher Makris, M.D.
Juanita C. Bishop, RPSGT
205-939-9386

Brookwood Sleep Disorders Center
Brookwood Medical Center
2010 Brookwood Medical Center Drive
Birmingham, AL 35209
Robert C. Doekel, M.D.
B.J. Slonneger, RPSGT
205-877-2403

Sleep Disorders Lab*
Carraway Methodist Medical Center
1600 Carraway Boulevard
Birmingham, AL 35234
Kuruvilla George
Aneshia Williams
205-502-6164

Breathing Related Sleep Disorders Center*
Marshall Medical Center South
P.O. Box 758
601A Corley Avenue
Boaz, AL 35957
Lori Johnson, RPSGT, Coordinator
Robert Doekel Jr., M.D.
256-593-1226

Sleep Disorders Center/ Neurodiagnostic Lab
Cullman Regional Medical Center
1912 Alabama Highway 157
Cullman, AL 35056-1108
G. Scott Warner, M.D., Medical Director
Lisa Nelson Barnett, RPSGT, Administrative Director
256-737-2140
Website: http://www.crmc-bhs.com/services/sleep/sleep.htm

Decatur General Sleep Disorders Center
1201 7th Street SE
Decatur, AL 35601
Edward M. Turpin, M.D.
Marc A. Hays, RRT
256-340-2558

Sleep-Wake Disorders Center
Flowers Hospital
4370 West Main Street
P.O. Box 6907
Dothan, AL 36305
Ronald C. Kornegay, RPSGT
Ann B. McDowell, M.D.
Alan Purvis, M.D.
David Davis, M.D.
334-793-5000 ext. 1685

Thomas Hospital Sleep Services*
Thomas Hospital
188 Hospital Drive
Suite 201
Fairhope, AL 36532
William E. Goetter, M.D., FCCP
James J. Griffin, M.D.
334-990-1940

ECM Sleep Disorders Lab*
Eliza Coffee Memorial Hospital
205 Marengo Street
P.O. Box 818
Florence, AL 35631
Felix Morris, M.D.
Byron Jamerson, RPSGT
256-768-9153

Sleep Diagnostics of Northeast Alabama for Breathing Related Disorders at Gadsden Regional Medical Center*
1007 Goodyear Avenue
Gadsden, AL 35903
Denise J. Barton, RRT, RPSGT, Lead Technologist
Stephen Coleman, M.D., Medical Director
256-494-4551
Website: www.gadsdenregional.com

The Sleep Center at Huntsville Hospital
911 Big Cove
Huntsville, AL 35801
Paul LeGrand, M.D.
Parke Keith
256-517-8553

The Crestwood Center for Sleep Disorders
250 Chateau Drive
Suite 235
Huntsville, AL 35801
Robert A. Serio, M.D.
Richard M. Sneeringer, M.D.
256-880-4710

Southeast Regional Center for Sleep/Wake Disorders
Springhill Memorial Hospital
3719 Dauphin Street
Mobile, AL 36608
Lawrence S. Schoen, Ph.D.
334-460-5319

USA Knollwood Sleep Disorders Center
University of South Alabama Knollwood Park Hospital
5644 Girby Road
Mobile, AL 36693-3398
William A. Broughton, M.D.
334-660-5757

Sleep Disorders Center
Mobile Infirmary Medical Center
P.O. Box 2144
Mobile, AL 36652
Robert Dawkins, Ph.D., M.P.H.
Emerson Kerr, BS, RRT
334-435-5559 or 800-422-2027
Website: www.mimc.com/sleep.html

Sleep Apnea Center*
Providence Hospital
6801 Airport Boulevard
Mobile, AL 36608
James Hunter, M.D.
Nancy Whiteley, RPSGT
334-639-2876

Jackson Sleep Disorders Center
Jackson—MedSouth
1722 Pine Street
Suite 300
Montgomery, AL 36106
Cary Evans, RPSGT
888-454-9067

Sleep Disorders Center
Baptist Medical Center South
2105 East South Boulevard
Montgomery, AL 36116-2498
David P. Franco, M.D.
Tammy Taylor, RPSGT
334-286-3252

Sleep Disorders Lab*
East Alabama Medical Center
2000 Pepperell Parkway
Opelika, AL 36801-5452
Gina White, RRT, RPSGT
Steven E. Dekich, M.D.
334-705-2404
Website: www.eamc.org

Sleep Disorders Lab*
Helen Keller Hospital
P.O. Box 610
Sheffield, AL 35660
Larry Carmichael, M.D.
Ronda Hood, RRT
256-386-4191

Tuscaloosa Clinic Sleep Center
701 University Boulevard East
Tuscaloosa, AL 35401
Richard M. Snow, M.D., FCCP
205-349-4043

ALASKA

Sleep Disorders Center
Providence Alaska Medical Center
3200 Providence Drive

P.O. Box 196604
Anchorage, AK 99519-6604
Anne H. Morris, M.D., Medical Director
Gerald Trodden, RPSGT, Clinical Manager
907-261-3650

ARIZONA

Banner Regional Sleep Disorders Program
Thunderbird Samaritan Medical Center in Glendale
5555 West Thunderbird Road
Glendale, AZ 85306-4622
Bernard E. Levine, M.D.
Stephen Anthony, M.D.
Connie Boker, RPSGT
602-588-4800
Website: http://bannerhealthaz.com/services/sleep/sleep.html

Banner Regional Sleep Disorders Program
Desert Samaritan Medical Center
1400 South Dobson Road
Mesa, AZ 85202
Paul Barnard, M.D.
Tom Munzlinger, BS, RPSGT
480-835-3684
Website: http://bannerhealthaz.com/services/sleep/sleep.htm l

Banner Regional Sleep Disorders Program
Good Samaritan Regional Medical Center
1111 East McDowell Road
Phoenix, AZ 85006
Bernard Levine, M.D.
David Baratz, M.D.
Connie Boker, RPSGT
602-239-5815
Website: http://bannerhealthaz.com/services/sleep/sleep.html

Sleep Disorders Center at Scottsdale Healthcare
Scottsdale Healthcare Shea
9003 East Shea Boulevard
Scottsdale, AZ 85260
Jeffrey S. Gitt, D.O.
Sharon E. Cichocki, RPSGT
480-860-3200

Sleep Disorders Center
University of Arizona
1501 North Campbell Avenue
Tucson, AZ 85724
Stuart F. Quan, M.D.
520-694-6112 or 520-626-6115

ARKANSAS

Sleep Disorders Center
Washington Regional Medical Center
1125 North College Avenue
Fayetteville, AR 72703
David L. Brown, M.D., Director
William A. Rivers, RPSGT, Coordinator
501-713-1272

Pediatric Sleep Disorders
Arkansas Children's Hospital
800 Marshall Street
Little Rock, AR 72202-3591
May Griebel, M.D.
Linda Rhodes, EMT, RPSGT
501-320-1893

Sleep Disorders Center
Baptist Medical Center
9601 I-630, Exit 7
Little Rock, AR 72205-7299
David Davila, M.D.
Buddy Marshall, CRTT, RPSGT
501-202-1902
Website: www.baptist.health.com

CALIFORNIA

Southern California Sleep Disorders Specialists
1101 South Anaheim Boulevard
Anaheim, CA 92805
Clyde Dos Santos, M.D., Medical Director
Deborah Kerr, Director
714-491-1159
Website: www.Tenethealth.com/westernmedical/

Sleep Center
Mercy San Juan Hospital
6401 Coyle Avenue
Suite 109
Carmichael, CA 95608
Janice K. Herrmann, RPSGT, MA
Richard Stack, M.D.
916-864-5874

Sleep Disorders Institute
St. Jude Medical Center
1915 Sunny Crest Drive
Fullerton, CA 92835
Louis J. McNabb, M.D.
Justine Petrie, M.D.,
Robert Roethe, M.D.
Bruce Tammelin, M.D.
Margaret H. White, Ph.D.
714-446-7240

Glendale Adventist Medical Center Sleep Disorders Center
Glendale Adventist Medical Center
1509 Wilson Terrace
Glendale, CA 91206
David A. Thompson, M.D.
Kathy Cavander
818-409-8323

Sleep Disorders Center
Grossmont Hospital
P.O. Box 158
La Mesa, CA 91944-0158
Ellie Hoey, RPSGT
619-644-4488

Loma Linda Sleep Disorders Center
Loma Linda University Community Medical Center
25333 Barton Road
Loma Linda, CA 92354
Ralph Downey III, Ph.D.
Joanne MacQuarrie, RRT, RPSGT
909-478-6344
Website: www.llu.edu/llumc/sleep

Sleep Disorders Center
Long Beach Memorial Medical Center
2801 Atlantic Avenue
P.O. Box 1428
Long Beach, CA 90801-1428
Stephen E. Brown, M.D.
Monir Kashani, RRT, RPSGT, Technical Coordinator
877-536-3314

UCLA Sleep Disorders Center
24-221 CHS, Box 957069
Los Angeles, CA 90095-7069
Frisca Yan-Go, M.D.
310-206-8005

Clinical Monitoring Center, Inc.
Sleep Disorders Center
555 Knowles Drive
Suite 218
Los Gatos, CA 95032
Tom Pace, RPSGT, Clinical Coordinator
Laughton Miles, M.D., Ph.D.
408-341-2080
Website:
http://www.sleepscape.com

Mercy Hospital Sleep Laboratory*
Mercy Hospital and Health Services
2740 M Street
Merced, CA 95340
A. Adam Williams, RRT, MBA
Sunit Patel, M.D.
209-384-4726

Sleep Disorders Institute
27800 Medical Center Road
Suite 210
Mission Viejo, CA 92691
Louis McNabb, M.D.
Justine Petrie, M.D.
Robert Roethe, M.D.
Bruce Tammelin, M.D.
Margaret White, Ph.D.
949-347-7400

Sleep Disorders Center
Community Hospital of the Monterey Peninsula
880 Cass Street
Suite 106
Monterey, CA 93940
Daniel Ehnstrom
Barbara Barrett, CRTT, RPSGT
831-641-0136

Sleep Disorders Center
Hoag Memorial Hospital Presbyterian
One Hoag Drive
P.O. Box 6100
Newport Beach, CA 92658-6100
Catherine L. Rain, Coordinator
Paul A. Selecky, M.D.
949-760-2070
Website: www.hoag.org

Sleep Evaluation Center
Northridge Hospital Medical Center
18300 Roscoe Boulevard
Northridge, CA 91328
Jeremy Cole, M.D.
David Brandes, M.D.
Dennis McGinty, Ph.D.
Ron Szymusiak, Ph.D.
818-885-5344

California Center for Sleep Disorders
3012 Summit Street
5th Floor, South Building
Oakland, CA 94609
Jerrold Kram, M.D.
Glenn Roldan, BS, RPSGT
510-834-8333
Website: www.sleepsmart.com

St. Joseph Hospital Sleep Disorders Center
1310 West Stewart Drive
Suite 403
Orange, CA 92868
Sarah Mosko, Ph.D.
714-771-8950

Sleep Disorders Center
University of California, Irvine
101 The City Drive, Route 23
Orange, CA 92868
Peter A. Fotinakes, M.D.
714-456-5105

Premier Diagnostics, Inc.
1851 Holser Walk,
Suite 210
Oxnard, CA 93030
Jerry Harris, RCP, RRT
Rebecca Palmieri, RCP, RRT, RN, BS
George Yu, M.D.
805-485-2633
Website:
www.sleep.diagnostics.com

Sleep Disorders Center
Huntington Memorial Hospital
100 West California Boulevard
P.O. Box 7013
Pasadena, CA 91109-7013
Steven Lenik, RPSGT
Charles A. Anderson, M.D.
Richard A. Shubin, M.D.
626-397-3061

Sleep Disorders Center
Doctors Medical Center—Pinole
2151 Appian Way
Pinole, CA 94564-2578
Geoffrey Hux, RPSGT
Frederick Nachtwey, M.D.
Richard Sankary, M.D.
510-741-2525 and 800-640-9440
Website: www.tenethealth.com

Sleep Disorders Center
Pomona Valley Hospital Medical Center
1798 North Garey Avenue
Pomona, CA 91767
Dennis Nicholson, M.D.
Fares Elghazi, M.D.
Robert Jones, M.D., FCCP
909-865-9587

The Center for Sleep Apnea*
Redding Medical Center
2701 Old Eureka Way
Suite II
Redding, CA 96001
Everett Trevor, M.D.
Jean Amari-Melancon, RPSGT
530-242-6821

Sequoia Sleep Disorders Center
Sequoia Health Services
170 Alameda de las Pulgas
Redwood City, CA 94062-2799
J. Al Reichert, RPSGT
Bernhard Votteri, M.D., Medical Director
650-367-5137
Website:
http://www.sleepscene.com

Sutter Sleep Disorders Center
650 Howe Avenue
Suite 910
Sacramento, CA 95825
David J. Groza, RPSGT, RCP, EEE

Lydia Wytrzes, M.D.
James N. Nishio, M.D.
916-646-3300

UCDMC Sleep Disorders Center
University of California Davis Medical Center
2315 Stockton Boulevard
Room 5305
Sacramento, CA 95817
Masud Seyal, M.D., Ph.D.
William Bonekat, D.O.
916-734-0256

Inland Sleep Center
401 East Highland Avenue
Suite 552
San Bernardino, CA 92404
Sunil Arora, M.D.
909-883-8058

Sleep Disorders Center
Scripps Mercy Hospital
4077 Fifth Avenue
San Diego, CA 92103-2180
Alex Mercandetti, M.D., FCCP, Medical Director
Cheryl L. Spinweber, Ph.D., Clinical Director
619-260-7378
Website: www.scrippshealth.org

San Diego Sleep Disorders Center
1842 Third Avenue
San Diego, CA 92101
Renata Shafor, M.D.
619-235-0248

Stanford Health Services
Sleep Clinic in San Francisco
3700 California Street
San Francisco, CA 94118
Bruce T. Adornato, M.D.
Christopher R. Brown, M.D.
Rowena Korobkin, M.D.
Alex Clerk, M.D.
Clete Kushida, M.D., Ph.D.
Anstella Robinson, M.D.
Rafael Pelayo, M.D.
415-750-6336

Sleep Disorders Center at Mount Zion
University of California, San Francisco
1600 Divisadero Street
San Francisco, CA 94115
David M. Claman, M.D.
Kimberly A. Trotter, MA, RPSGT
415-885-7886
Website: http://mzweb.his.ucsf.edu/clin_departments/medicine/pulmonary/sleep/sleep.html

The Sleep Disorders Center of Santa Barbara
2410 Fletcher Avenue
Suite 201
Santa Barbara, CA 93105
Andrew S. Binder, M.D.
Laurie Laatsch, RPSGT
805-898-8845

St. John's Medical Plaza Sleep Disorders Center
1301 20th Street
Suite 370
Santa Monica, CA 90404
Paul B. Haberman, M.D.
310-828-2293

Sleep Disorders Clinic
Stanford University Medical Center
401 Quarry Road
Suite 3301-A
Stanford, CA 94305
Jed Black, M.D.
650-725-5917

Southern California Pulmonary and Sleep Disorders Medical Center
2230 Lynn Road
Thousand Oaks, CA 91360
Ronald A. Popper, M.D.
805-495-1066

Torrance Memorial Medical Center
Sleep Disorders Center
3330 West Lomita Boulevard
Torrance, CA 90505
Lawrence W. Kneisley, M.D.
310-517-4617

Sleep Disorders Laboratory*
Kaweah Delta District Hospital
400 West Mineral King Avenue
Visalia, CA 93291
William R. Winn, M.D.
Gregory C. Warner, M.D.
David Akins, RPSGT, Clinical Coordinator
559-624-2338

West Valley Sleep Disorders Center
7320 Woodlake Avenue
Suite 140
West Hills, CA 91307
Gordon Dowds, M.D., Medical Director
Pamela Pierce, Director
818-715-0096

Sleep Disorders Center
Woodland Memorial Hospital
1325 Cottonwood Street
Woodland, CA 95695
Richard A. Beyer, M.D.
Marie Kearney, Manager
530-669-5555

COLORADO

Sleep Health Centers at National Jewish Medical Center
1400 Jackson Street
A200
Denver, CO 80206
Robert D. Ballard, M.D.
303-270-2708

Sleep Center of Southern Colorado
Parkview Medical Center
400 West 16th Street
Pueblo, CO 81003
James Pagel, M.D., Medical Director
Craig Shapiro, M.D., Associate Director
George Juszynski, BS, RPSGT, Program Coordinator
719-584-4659
Website: www.parkviewmc.com/sleep.htm

CONNECTICUT

Danbury Hospital Sleep Disorders Center
Danbury Hospital
24 Hospital Avenue
Danbury, CT 06810
Arthur Kotch, M.D.
Arthur Spielman, Ph.D.
David Oelberg, M.D.
Stuart Moses, RPSGT, RRT
203-731-8033

Gaylord/Fairfield Sleep Services
1495 Black Rock Turnpike
Fairfield, CT 06430
Debra Pollack, M.D.
Paul Trigilia, RRT, MPH
203-624-3140
Website: www.gaylord.org

Sleep Disorders Laboratory*
Manchester Memorial Hospital
Haynes Street
Manchester, CT 06040
Richard M. Shoup, M.D., FCCP
Tom Farrell, BS, RPSGT, RPFT, CRT
860-647-6881

Yale Center for Sleep Disorders
Yale University School of Medicine
333 Cedar Street
P.O. Box 208057
New Haven, CT 06520-8057
Vahid Mohsenin, M.D.
203-737-5556
Website: info.med.yale.edu/intmed/sleep

The Sleep Disorders Center
Norwalk Hospital
Maple Street
Norwalk, CT 06856
Edward B. O'Malley, Ph.D., D,ABSM
Judith Odell
203-855-3632

Gaylord/New Haven Sleep Services
Gaylord Hospital Inc.
P.O. Box 400
Wallingford, CT 06492
Debra Pollack, M.D.
Paul Trigilia, RRT, MPH
203-624-3140
Website: www.gaylord.org

Gaylord/Wallingford Sleep Services
Gaylord Hospital
Gaylord Farms Road
Wallingford, CT 06492
Carlos A.V. Fragoso, M.D.
Thomas Whelan, RPSGT
203-284-2853
Website: www.gaylord.org

DELAWARE

Sleep Disorders Center
Christiana Care Health Systems
4755 Ogletown-Stanton Road
P.O. Box 6001
Newark, DE 19718
John B. Townsend III, M.D.
Thomas C. Mueller, M.D.
Mary Rose Hancock
302-428-4600

Sleep Disorders Center
Christiana Care Health Services
Wilmington Hospital
501 West 14th Street
Wilmington, DE 19899
John B. Townsend III, M.D.
Thomas C. Mueller, M.D.
302-428-4600

DISTRICT OF COLUMBIA

Sibley Memorial Hospital Sleep Disorders Center
5255 Loughboro Road NW
Washington, DC 20016
David N.F. Fairbanks, M.D.
Samuel J. Potolicchio, M.D.
202-364-7676

Sleep Disorders Center, 5 Main Hospital
Georgetown University Hospital
3800 Reservoir Road NW
Washington, DC 20007-2197
Marilyn L. Faucette, RPSGT
Anne O'Donnell, M.D.
Kenneth Plotkin, M.D.
Richard E. Waldhorn, M.D., Medical Director
202-784-3610

FLORIDA

Boca Raton Sleep Disorders Center
899 Meadows Road
Suite 101
Boca Raton, FL 33486
Natalio J. Chediak, M.D.
Sheila R. Shafer, CMA
561-750-9881

Florida Hospital Celebration
Florida Hospital
400 Celebration Place
Celebration, FL 34747
Morris T. Bird, M.D.
Robert S. Thornton, M.D.
Martha McNamara
407-303-4002

Mayo Sleep Disorders Center
Mayo Clinic Jacksonville
4500 San Pablo Road
Jacksonville, FL 32224
Paul Fredrickson, M.D.
Joseph Kaplan, M.D.
904-953-7287

Watson Clinic Sleep Disorders Center
The Watson Clinic, LLP
1600 Lakeland Hills Boulevard
P.O. Box 95000
Lakeland, FL 33804-5000
Eberto Pineiro, M.D.
941-680-7627

Atlantic Sleep Disorders Center
1401 South Apollo Boulevard
Suite A
Melbourne, FL 32901
Dennis K. King, M.D.
David R. Schneider, RPSGT
407-952-5191
Website: http://doctor.medscape.com/DennisKingMD

Sleep Disorders Center
Mt. Sinai Medical Center
4300 Alton Road
Miami Beach, FL 33140
Alejandro D. Chediak, M.D.
305-674-2613

University of Miami School of Medicine, JMH and VA Medical Center Sleep Disorders Center
Department of Neurology (D4-5)
P.O. Box 016960
Miami, FL 33101
Bruce Nolan, M.D.
305-324-3371
Website: www.miami.edu/neurology/centers/sleep.html

Sleep Disorders Center
Miami Children's Hospital
6125 Southwest 31st Street
Miami, FL 33155
Marcel J. Deray, M.D.
305 669 7136

Orlando Sleep Disorders Center
1118 South Orange Avenue
Suite 102
Orlando, FL 32806
Barry Decker, M.D.
Geri Lockhart, BS, RPSGT, RRT
407-649-6869

Florida Hospital Sleep Disorders Center
601 East Rollins Avenue
Orlando, FL 32803
Morris T. Bird, M.D.
Robert S. Thornton, M.D.
407-303-1558

Health First Sleep Disorders Center
Palm Bay Community Hospital
1425 Malabar Road NE
Suite 250
Palm Bay, FL 32907
John Jessup, M.D.
Anna Barker, BA, RPSGT
321-434-8087

Baptist Hospital Sleep Disorders Center
Baptist Hospital
1000 West Moreno Street
Pensacola, FL 32501
Thomas B. Williams, M.D.
Novie A. Jenkins, RPSGT
850-469-7042

Sleep Disorders Center
West Florida Regional Medical Center
8383 North Davis Highway
Pensacola, FL 32514
Robert Dawkins, Ph.D., MPH
Jane Wilkinson, Director
850-494-4850

Sleep Disorders Center
Charlotte Regional Medical Center
733 East Olympia Avenue
Punta Gorda, FL 33950
Carlos E. Maas, M.D., FACP, Medical Director
Mary Darling, RPSGT, Coordinator
941-637-3141

Sleep Disorders Center
Sarasota Memorial Hospital
1700 South Tamiami Trail
Sarasota, FL 34239
Glenn D. Adams, M.D., Medical Director
941-917-2525

St. Petersburg Sleep Disorders Center
Palms of Pasadena Hospital
1501 Pasadena Avenue South
St. Petersburg, FL 33707
Neil T. Feldman, M.D.
813-360-0853 and
800-242-3244 (in Florida)

Tallahassee Sleep Disorders Center
1304 Hodges Drive
Suite B
Tallahassee, FL 32308-4613
George F. Slade, M.D.
800-662-4278 ext. 4 or
850-878-7271

The Sleep Center
University Community Hospital
3100 East Fletcher Avenue
Tampa, FL 33613
Daniel J. Schwartz, M.D.
David Bollinger, RPSGT, REEGT
813-979-7410
Website: www.uch.org

GEORGIA

Sleep Disorders Center of Georgia
5505 Peachtree Dunwoody Road
Suite 370
Atlanta, GA 30342
D. Alan Lankford, Ph.D.
James J. Wellman, M.D.
404-257-0080
Website: sleepsciences.com

Sleep Disorders Center
Northside Hospital
5780 Peachtree Dunwoody Road
Suite 150
Atlanta, GA 30342
Russell Rosenberg, Ph.D.
Michael Lacey, M.D.
David Westerman, M.D.
404-851-8135
Website: www.nshsleep.com

Sleep Disorders Center
Children's Healthcare of Atlanta
1001 Johnson Ferry Road
Atlanta, GA 30097
Lesa Kervin, RRT, RPSGT
Gary L. Montgomery, M.D.
404-250-2096

Atlanta Center for Sleep Disorders
303 Parkway Drive
Box 44
Atlanta, GA 30312
Patrick Merrill, RPSGT
Francis Buda, M.D.
Jonne Walter, M.D.
Robert Schnapper, M.D.
404-265-3722

The Sleep Center at Piedmont Hospital
1968 Peachtree Road NW
Atlanta, GA 30309
Reba Pearson
Walter S. James, M.D.
404-605-4278

Sleep Disorders Center
Wellstar Cobb Hospital
3950 Austell Road
Austell, GA 30106
Susan T. Keller, Coordinator
Mark Letica, M.D.
Aris Iatridis, M.D., Medical Director
770-732-2250

Sleep Disorder Center
DeKalb Medical Center
2665 North Decatur Road
Suite 435
Decatur, GA 30033
Mark T. Pollock, M.D., FCCP, Medical Director
Michael J. Breus, Ph.D., Clinical Director
404-501-5927

Central Georgia Sleep Disorders Center
777 Hemlock Street
Second Floor
P.O. Box 1035
Macon, GA 31202
Charles C. Wells, M.D., Medical Director
Todd Jones, Technical Director
912-633-7222

Sleep Disorders Center
Wellstar Kennestone Hospital
677 Church Street
Marietta, GA 30060
William Dowdell, M.D.
David Lesch, M.D.
Susan T. Keller, RPSGT
770-793-5353

Savannah Sleep Disorders Center at Saint Joseph's Hospital
1 St. Joseph's Professional Plaza
11706 Mercy Boulevard
Savannah, GA 31419
Anthony M. Costrini, M.D., D,ABSM
912-927-5141
Website: www.drsleepwell.com

Sleep Disorders Center
Memorial Health University Medical Center
4700 Waters Avenue
Savannah, GA 31403
Herbert F. Sanders, M.D.
Stephen L. Morris, M.D.
912-350-8327

Department of Sleep Disorders Medicine
Candler Hospital
5353 Reynolds Street
Savannah, GA 31405
James A. Daly III, M.D., Medical Director
Pamela Rockett, RPSGT, RRT
912-692-6673

HAWAII

Orchid Isle Sleep Disorders Laboratory*
1404 Kilauea Avenue
Hilo, HI 96720
Gilbert J. Ransley, RRT, Technical Director
John P. Dawson, M.D., MPH, Medical Director
808-935-6105

Queen's Medical Center Sleep Laboratory*
The Queen's Medical Center
1301 Punchbowl Street
Honolulu, HI 96813
Bruce A.G. Soll, M.D.
Jamil Sulieman, M.D.
808-547-4396

Sleep Disorders Center of the Pacific
Straub Clinic & Hospital
888 South King Street
Honolulu, HI 96813
James W. Pearce, M.D.
Linda Kapuniai, Dr. P.H.
808-522-4448

Orchid Isle Sleep Disorders Laboratory*
Waimea Town Plaza
64-1061 Mamalahoa Highway 105
Kamuela, HI 96743
Gilbert J. Ransley, RRT, Technical Director
John P. Dawson, M.D., MPH, Medical Director
808-885-9681

IDAHO

Idaho Sleep Disorders Center-Boise
St. Luke's Regional Medical Center
190 East Bannock Street
Boise, ID 83712
Brett Troyer, M.D.
David K. Merrick, M.D.
Stephen W. Asher, M.D.
Mary R. Gable, RPSGT
208-381-2440

SJRMC Sleep Lab
St. Joseph Regional Medical Center
415 Sixth Street
Lewiston, ID 83501
Luke A. Pluto, M.D.
Bob Rosselle, RRT
Patty Morgan, RPSGT
Joanne Bruegeman, RPSGT
Cheryl Wagoner, RPSGT
208-799-5484

Idaho Sleep Disorders Center-Nampa
Mercy Medical Center
1512 12th Avenue Road
Nampa, ID 83686
Brett E. Troyer, M.D.
David K. Merrick, M.D.
Mary R. Gable, RPSGT
208-463-5820

Idaho Diagnostic Sleep Lab*
526-C Shoup Avenue West
Twin Falls, ID 83301
Ron Fullmer, M.D.
Richard Hammond, M.D., Medical Director

Brian Fortuin, M.D.
Diana Lincoln-Haye, RRT, RCP
Robin Baggett, John Williams, RPSGT
208-736-7646

ILLINOIS

Sleep Disorders Center
Northwestern Memorial Hospital
201 East Huron
Galter 7th Floor
Chicago, IL 60611
Phyllis C. Zee, M.D., Ph.D., Director
Steve Baker, M.D.
Glenn Clark, RPSGT
312-926-8120

Sleep Medicine Center
Children's Memorial Hospital
2300 Children's Plaza, Box 43
Chicago, IL 60614-3394
Stephen Sheldon, D.O.
Laura Becke, RPSGT, Team Leader
Michelle Arrizola, RN, Administrator
773-880-8230

Sleep Disorder Service and Research Center
Rush-Presbyterian-St. Luke's Medical Center
1653 West Congress Parkway
Chicago, IL 60612
Rosalind Cartwright, Ph.D.
312-942-5440
Website: http://www.rush.edu/Med/Psych/sleep.html

Sleep Disorders Center
The University of Chicago Hospitals
5841 South Maryland
MC2091
Chicago, IL 60637
Jean-Paul Spire, M.D., Clinical Director
Wallace B. Mendelson, M.D., Research and Training Director
Helene Rubeiz, M.D.
773-702-1782

Center for Sleep and Ventilatory Disorders
University of Illinois at Chicago
1740 West Taylor Street
Room 536E
M/C 722
Chicago, IL 60612
Deborah E. Sewitch, Ph.D.
Maureen Smith, RPSGT
312-996-7708

Sleep Disorders Center
Alexian Brothers Medical Center
810 Biesterfield Road
Suite 409
Elk Grove Village, IL 60007
Robert W. Hart, M.D.
Clifford A. Massie, Ph.D.
847-981-5926

Sleep Disorders Center
Evanston Hospital
2650 Ridge Avenue
Evanston, IL 60201
Richard S. Rosenberg, Ph.D.
847-570-2567

Sleep Disorders Center
Hinsdale Hospital
120 North Oak Street
Hinsdale, IL 60521
Peter Freebeck, M.D., Medical Director
Lisa Paauwe, Manager
630-856-3901

Carle Regional Sleep Disorders Center/Mattoon Branch
200 Lerna Road South
Mattoon, IL 61938
Daniel Picchietti, M.D.
Donald A. Greeley, M.D.
217-383-3198

Sleep Disorders Center
Lutheran General Hospital
1775 Dempster Street
Parkside Center, Suite B06
Park Ridge, IL 60068
Barry Weber, M.D.
Wayne Rubinstein, M.D.
Lauren Witcoff, M.D.
847-723-7024

C. Duane Morgan Sleep Disorders Center
Methodist Medical Center of Illinois
221 Northeast Glen Oak Avenue
Peoria, IL 61636
Arthur W. Fox, M.D., Medical Director
309-672-4966 or 309-671-5136

Sleep Disorders Laboratory*
Rockford Health System
2400 North Rockton Avenue
Rockford, IL 61103
Theodore S. Ingrassia III, M.D.
815-971-5595

SIU School of Medicine/Memorial Medical Center
Sleep Disorders Center
Memorial Medical Center
701 North First
Springfield, IL 62781
Joseph Henkle, M.D.
Steven Todd, RRT, RPSGT
217-788-4269

Carle Regional Sleep Disorders Center
Carle Foundation Hospital
611 West Park Street
Urbana, IL 61801-2595
Daniel Picchietti, M.D.
Donald A. Greeley, M.D.
217-383-3364

Sleep Disorders Center
Central Du Page Hospital
Robert McCormick Pavilion, Entrance E, 3rd Floor
25 North Winfield Road
Winfield, IL 60190
Robert Hart, M.D.
Linda Klora, RPSGT
630-933-2975

INDIANA

Sleep Disorders Center
St. Francis Hospital and Health Centers
1500 Albany Street
Suite 1110
Beech Grove, IN 46107
Dianna L. Miller, RPSGT

Manfred P. Mueller, M.D., FCCP
317-783-8144

St. Joseph Sleep Disorders Center
St. Joseph Medical Center
700 Broadway
Fort Wayne, IN 46802
James C. Stevens, M.D.
Thomandram Sekar, M.D.
219-425-3552

Sleep/Wake Disorders Center
Community Hospitals Indianapolis
1500 North Ritter Avenue
Indianapolis, IN 46219
Hany W. Haddad, M.D.
Marvin E. Vollmer, M.D.
317-355-4275

Methodist Sleep Disorders Center
Clarian Health
I-65 at 21st Street
P.O. Box 1367
Indianapolis, IN 46206-1367
Thomas Sullivan, M.D.
Tom Ehle, Manager
317-929-5706

Sleep Disorders Center
St. Vincent Hospital and Health Services
8401 Harcourt Road
Indianapolis, IN 46260-0160
Albert Wauquier, Ph.D.
Thomas Cartwright, M.D.
Praveen Vohra, M.D.
317-338-2152
Website: www.stvincent.org

Sleep/Wake Disorders Center
Winona Memorial Hospital
3232 North Meridian Street
Indianapolis, IN 46208
Kenneth N. Wiesert, M.D.
317-927-2100

Center for Sleep Disorders
Indiana University School of Medicine
550 North University Boulevard
Room S450
Indianapolis, IN 46202
Brian H. Foresman, D.O., FCCP
Richard A. Fiero, M.D.
317-274-2136

Sleep Alertness Center
Lafayette Home Hospital
2400 South Street
Lafayette, IN 47904
Frederick Robinson, M.D.
765-447-6811 ext. 2840

IOWA

Sleep Disorders Center
Mary Greeley Medical Center
1111 Duff Avenue
Ames, IA 50010
Selden Spencer, M.D., Director
Mark Hislop, RRT, RPSGT
515-239-2353

Genesis Sleep Disorders Center
Genesis Medical Center
1227 East Rusholme
Davenport, IA 52803
Akshay Mahadevia, M.D.
Carol Everson, MBA, RPSGT, REEG/EPT
319-421-1525

Sleep Center at Mercy
Mercy Medical Center
1111 Sixth Avenue
Des Moines, IA 50314-2611
Donald Burrows, M.D.
Jolee Fisk, RPSGT
515-247-3171

Sleep Disorders Center
The Department of Neurology
The University of Iowa Hospitals and Clinics
Iowa City, IA 52242
Mark Eric Dyken, M.D.
319-356-3813

KANSAS

Sleep Disorders Center
Hays Medical Center
201 East Seventh Street
Hays, KS 67601
Suzanne Bollig, RRT, RPSGT, REEGT
785-623-5373

Sleep Disorders Center
Overland Park Regional Medical Center
10500 Quivira Road
P.O. Box 15959
Overland Park, KS 66215
Michael W. Anderson, Ph.D.
John B. Nelson, M.D.
913-541-5641

Sleep Disorders Center
St. Francis Hospital and Medical Center
1700 Southwest Seventh Street
Topeka, KS 66606-1690
Ted W. Daughety, M.D.
David D. Miller, RPSGT
785-295-7900

Sleep Medicine Center of Kansas
Wichita Clinic
818 North Carriage Parkway
Wichita, KS 67208
Thomas J. Bloxham, M.D.
Robert Hendrickson, RPSGT
316-651-2250
Website: http://www.wichitaclinic.com

Sleep Disorders Center
Wesley Medical Center
550 North Hillside
Wichita, KS 67214-4976
Janice Oeltjenbruns, REEG/EPT, RPSGT
Emilio D. Soria, M.D.
316-688-2663

KENTUCKY

Physicians' Center for Sleep Disorders
Graves-Gilbert Clinic
1555 Campbell Lane
P.O. Box 90025
Bowling Green, KY 42102-9007
Michael Zachek, M.D.
Randall Hansbrough, M.D., Ph.D.
Douglas Thomson, M.D., MPH
502-781-5111

Sleep Disorders Center
Greenview Regional Hospital

1801 Ashley Circle
Bowling Green, KY 42101
Gul K. Sahetya, M.D.
Steven Zeller, RPSGT
502-793-2175

Sleep Disorders Center
St. Luke Hospital West
7380 Turfway Road
Florence, KY 41042
Steven Scheer, M.D.
606-525-5347

The Sleep Disorder Center of St. Luke Hospital
St. Luke Hospital, Inc.
85 North Grand Avenue
Fort Thomas, KY 41075
Steven Scheer, M.D.
606-572-3535

Methodist Hospital Sleep Lab*
Methodist Hospital
1305 North Elm Street
Henderson, KY 42420
Steven G. Hollowell, BS, RRT
270-827-7474

Sleep Apnea Center*
Jennie Stuart Medical Center
320 West 18th Street
Hopkinsville, KY 42240
Sanjay Chavda, M.D.
Manoj H. Majmudar, M.D.
Mark L. Pierce, RRT, RPSGT
502-887-0410

Sleep Center
Samaritan Hospital
310 South Limestone
Lexington, KY 40508
Barbara Phillips, M.D., MSPH, FCCP
Gary King, RRT, Director
606-226-7006
Website: www.KYSS.org or SamaritanHospital.org

Sleep Disorders Center
St. Joseph's Hospital
One St. Joseph Drive
Lexington, KY 40504
James Thompson, M.D.
Kathryn Hansen, BS
606-313-1855

Sleep Disorders Center
Baptist Hospital East
4000 Kresge Way
Louisville, KY 40207
Kenneth C. Anderson, M.D.
Vasudeva G. Iyer, M.D.
Karen Bell, RRT, Director
Marilee Burnside, RPSGT
502-896-7612

Sleep Disorders Center
Norton Audubon Hospital
One Audubon Plaza Drive
Louisville, KY 40217
Pamela McCullough, ARNP
David Winslow, M.D.
502-636-7459
Website: www.nortonhealthcare.com or www.kyss.org

Caritas Sleep Apnea Center*
Caritas Medical Center
1850 Bluegrass Avenue
Louisville, KY 40215
Pete Moore, M.D.
William Lacy, M.D.
Richard Baker, M.D.
502-361-6555

Sleep Disorders Center
University of Louisville Hospital
530 South Jackson Street
Louisville, KY 40202
Barbara J. Rigdon, RPSGT, R.EEG.T.
Vasudeva G. Iyer, M.D.
Eugene C. Fletcher, M.D.
502-562-3792
Website: www.ulh.org

Sleep Medicine Specialists
1169 Eastern Parkway
Suite 3357
Louisville, KY 40217
David H. Winslow, M.D., Director
Diania Alsager, RPSGT, Clinical Manager
502-454-0755

Regional Medical Center Lab for Sleep-Related Breathing Disorders*
900 Hospital Drive
Madisonville, KY 42431
Thomas Gallo, M.D.
Frank Taylor, M.D.
502-825-5918

OMHS Sleep Laboratory
Owensboro Mercy Health System
811 East Parrish
Owensboro, KY 42303
Robert N. Pope, M.D.
Kelly A. Morris, R.N., M.S.N.
270-688-2078

Diller Regional Sleep Disorders Center
Lourdes Hospital
1530 Lone Oak Road
Paducah, KY 42001
James Metcalf, M.D.
Rick Irvan, R.EEG.T., RPSGT, Manager
502-444-2660

The Sleep Lab*
9 Linville Drive
Paris, KY 40361
Pamela Combs, M.D.
Bruce Carter, RPSGT, CRT
606-987-1127

Breathing Disorders Sleep Lab*
Pikeville Methodist Hospital
911 South Bypass Road
Pikeville, KY 41501
Ramanarao V. Mettu, M.D., FACP, FCCP, Medical Director
Sally Compton, RRT, Director
Linda Greer, CRTT, Manager
Kathy Shaunessy, COO
606-437-3989

P.A.C. Sleep Disorders Lab*
Pattie A. Clay Hospital
P.O. Box 1600
801 Eastern Bypass
Richmond, KY 40475
Rajan Joshi, M.D., FCCP
Tom Grant
David Broughton
606-625-3334

The Medical Center Sleep Center
456 Burnley Road
Scottsville, KY 42164

Walter Warren, M.D.
Chris A. Barnett, RRT, RPSGT
270-622-2865
Website: www.mcbg.org\scottsville\sleep

LOUISIANA

The Neurology and Sleep Clinic
2205 East 70th Street
Shreveport, LA 71105
Nabil A. Moufarrej, M.D.
Annette Berry, RPFT, RPSGT
318-797-1585

Lourdes Sleep Disorders Center
Our Lady of Lourdes Regional Medical Center
611 St. Landry
Lafayette, LA 70506
Christine Soileau, RPSGT, R.EEG.T.
337-289-2858
Website: www.lourdes.net

Tulane Sleep Disorders Center
1415 Tulane Avenue
Box HC17
New Orleans, LA 70112
Denise Sharon, Ph.D.
504-584-1657

Memorial Medical Center Sleep Disorders Center
2700 Napoleon Avenue
New Orleans, LA 70115
Gregory S. Ferriss, M.D.
Li Yu, M.D.
504-896-5439

LSU Sleep Disorders Center
Louisiana State University Health Sciences Center
P.O. Box 33932
Shreveport, LA 71130-3932
Andrew L. Chesson Jr., M.D.
318-675-5365

Sleep Disorder Lab*
Slidell Memorial Hospital and Medical Center
1001 Gause Boulevard
Slidell, LA 70458
Hans E. Schuller, M.D., FCCP, D,ABSM
Craig Gravley, RPSGT
504-643-2200 ext. 2501

NSRMC Sleep Disorders Center
North Shore Regional Medical Center
100 Medical Center Drive
Slidell, LA 70461
Anwant Chawla, M.D.
Mary B. Jones, BS, MT, RPSGT
504-646-5711

MAINE

St. Mary's Sleep Disorders Laboratory*
St. Mary's Regional Medical Center
97 Campus Avenue
Lewiston, ME 04240
Ralph V. Harder, M.D.
Peter J. Leavitt, RRT
207-777-8959

Maine Institute for Sleep Breathing Disorders*
930 Congress Street
Portland, ME 04102
George E. Bokinsky Jr., M.D.
207-871-4535

MARYLAND

The Johns Hopkins Sleep Disorders Center
Asthma and Allergy Building, Room 4B50
Johns Hopkins Bayview Medical Center
5501 Hopkins Bayview Circle
Baltimore, MD 21224
Philip L. Smith, M.D.
Alan Schwartz, M.D.
410-550-0571

Maryland Sleep Disorders Center
Greater Baltimore Medical Center
6701 North Charles Street
Suite 4100
Baltimore, MD 21204-6808
Thomas E. Hobbins, M.D.
410-494-9773

Frederick Sleep Disorders Center
Frederick Memorial Hospital
400 West Seventh Street
Frederick, MD 21701
Marc Raphaelson, M.D.
Konrad W. Bakker, M.D.
Garland McDonald
301-698-3802

The Sleep-Breathing Disorders Center of Hagerstown*
12821 Oak Hill Avenue
Hagerstown, MD 21742
Abdul Waheed, M.D.
Shaheen Iqbal, M.D.
Johny Alencherry, M.D.
301-733-5971

Shady Grove Sleep Disorders Center
14915 Broschart Road
Suite 102
Rockville, MD 20850
Jean Neuenkirch, RPSGT
301-251-5905

Washington Adventist Sleep Disorders Center
7525 Carroll Avenue
Takoma Park, MD 20912
Marc Raphaelson, M.D.
Konrad W. Bakker, M.D.
301-891-2594

MASSACHUSETTS

Sleep Disorders Center
Beth Israel Deaconess Medical Center
330 Brookline Avenue, KS430
Boston, MA 02215
Jean K. Matheson, M.D.
Janet Mullington, Ph.D.
617-667-3237

Sleep Disorders Center
Lahey Clinic
41 Mall Road
Burlington, MA 01805
Paul T. Gross, M.D.
David A. Neumeyer, M.D.
Susan M. Dignan, RPSGT
781-744-8251

Sleep Disorders Institute of Central New England
St. Vincent Hospital
25 Winthrop Street
Worcester, MA 01604
Jayant G. Phadke, M.D.
508-798-6066 (Office) or
508-798-1485 (Lab)

MICHIGAN

Sleep Disorders Center
St. Joseph Mercy Hospital
P.O. Box 995
Ann Arbor, MI 48106
Thomas R. Gravelyn, M.D.
Sharon S. Potoczak, RPSGT
734-712-4651

Sleep Disorders Center
University of Michigan Hospitals
1500 East Medical Center Drive
UH8D 8702, Box 0117
Ann Arbor, MI 48109-0117
Brenda Livingston, Coordinator
Michael S. Aldrich, M.D.
Ronald Chervin, M.D.
Beth Malow, M.D.
Alon Avidan, M.D.
Alan Eiser, Ph.D.
Timothy Hoban, M.D.
734-936-9068

Sleep Disorders Center
Bay Medical Center
1900 Columbus Avenue
Bay City, MI 48708
John M. Buday, M.D.
Mary K. Taylor, RPSGT, RRT
517-894-3332

Sleep Disorders Center at Hutzel Hospital
Hutzel Hospital
4707 St. Antoine, 1 Center
Detroit, MI 48201
James A. Rowley, M.D.
David Calahan, RRT
313-745-9009

Sleep Disorders Center
Sinai-Grace Hospital
6071 West Outer Drive
Detroit, MI 48235
313-966-3091

Sleep/Wake Disorders Laboratory (127B)
VA Medical Center
4646 John R. Street
Detroit, MI 48201-1916
Sheldon Kapen, M.D.
M. Safwan Badr, M.D.
Greg Koshorek
313-576-3663

McLaren Sleep Diagnostic Center
McLaren Regional
Medical Center
401 South Ballenger
Flint, MI 48532
Joseph Varghese, M.D., Medical Director
Kent Matthews, RRT, Manager of Pulmonary Services
810-342-4980

Sleep Disorders Center at Spectrum Health
4100 Lake Drive
Suite 100
Grand Rapids, MI 49546
Lee Marmion, M.D.
Ronald Van Drunen, RPSGT
616-391-3759

Sleep Disorders Center
Borgess Medical Center
1521 Gull Road
Kalamazoo, MI 49001
Sue Cammarata, M.D.
Thomas Wittenberg, RRT
Sheri Dillon, RRT
616-226-7081

Ingham Regional Medical Center
Sleep/Wake Center
2025 South Washington Avenue
Suite 300
Lansing, MI 48910-0817
Pamela Minkley, RRT, RPSGT
Gauresh Kashyap, M.D., FACP, FCCP
517-372-6444

Sparrow Sleep Center
Sparrow Hospital
1200 East Michigan Avenue
Suite 455
P.O. Box 30480
Lansing, MI 48909-7980
Alan M. Atkinson, D.O.
David K. Young, D.O.
517-364-5370

Sleep & Respiratory Associates of Michigan
28200 Franklin Road
Southfield, MI 48034
Harvey W. Organek, M.D.
248-350-2722

Munson Sleep Disorders Center
Munson Medical Center
1105 Sixth Street
MPB Suite 307
Traverse City, MI 49684-2386
David A. Walker, D.O., FCCP, Medical Director
Leon R. Olewinski, RRT, Director
Marcia Rinal, CRTT, RPSGT, Manager
800-358-9641 or 231-935-6600

Sleep Disorders Institute
44199 Dequindre
Suite 311
Troy, MI 48098
R. Bart Sangal, M.D.
248-879-0707
Website:
www.sleep-attention.com

MINNESOTA

Duluth Regional Sleep Disorders Center
St. Mary's Duluth Clinic
Health System
407 East Third Street
Duluth, MN 55805
Peter K. Franklin, M.D.
Paul J. Windberg, M.D.
Mary Carlson, RPSGT
218-726-4692

Fairview Sleep Center
Fairview Southdale Hospital
6401 France Avenue South
Edina, MN 55435
John E. Trusheim, M.D.
612-924-5053

Sleep Disorders Center
Abbott Northwestern Hospital
800 East 28th Street at Chicago Avenue
Minneapolis, MN 55407
Wilfred A. Corson, M.D.
612-863-4516
Website: www.mnsleep.com

Minnesota Regional Sleep Disorders Center, #867B
Hennepin County Medical Center
701 Park Avenue South
Minneapolis, MN 55415
Mark Mahowald, M.D.
612-347-6288

Mayo Sleep Disorders Center
Mayo Clinic
200 First Street SW
Rochester, MN 55905
Lois E. Krahn, M.D., Administrative Director
John W. Shepard Jr., M.D.
Suresh Kotagal, M.D.
507-266-8900

Sleep Disorders Center
Methodist Hospital
6500 Excelsior Boulevard
St. Louis Park, MN 55426
Barb Feider, RPSGT
Salim Kathawalla, M.D.
952-993-6083

Health East Sleep Care
St. Joseph's Hospital
69 West Exchange Street
St. Paul, MN 55102
Thomas Mulrooney, M.D.
651-232-3682

MISSISSIPPI

Sleep Disorders Center
Forrest General Hospital
6051 Highway 49
P.O. Box 16389
Hattiesburg, MS 39404-6389
Geoffrey B. Hartwig, M.D.
John R. Harsh, Ph.D.
Dennis Kramer
601-288-1994 or 800-280-8520
Website: www.forrestgeneral.com/sleepdisorders.htm

Sleep Disorders Center and Division of Sleep Medicine
University of Mississippi Medical Center
2500 North State Street
Jackson, MS 39216-4505
Howard Roffwarg, M.D., D,ABSM, Director
Alp Sinan Baran, M.D., D,ABSM, Medical Director
Allen Richert, M.D., D,ABSM, Staff Specialist
601-984-4820

Sleep Disorder Center of Mississippi
Mississippi Baptist Medical Center
1225 North State Street
Jackson, MS 39202
William D. Frazier, M.D.
Sallye Wilcox, Ph.D.
601-968-1157

Sleep Disorder Center
Baptist Memorial Hospital—North Mississippi
2301 South Lamar
Oxford, MS 38655
Jeff Evans, M.D.
Kevin Buie, RPSGT, RRT
662-232-8146

MISSOURI

Unity Sleep Medicine and Research Center
St. Luke's Hospital
232 South Woods Mill Road
Chesterfield, MO 63017
James K. Walsh, Ph.D.
Gihan Kader, M.D.
314-205-6030

University of Missouri Sleep Disorders Center
M-741 Neurology
University Hospital and Clinics
One Hospital Drive
Columbia, MO 65212
Pradeep Sahota, M.D.
573-884-SLEEP or 800-ADD-SLEEP

Sleep Disorders Center
St. Luke's Hospital
4400 Wornall Road
Kansas City, MO 64111
Ann M. Romaker, M.D.
816-932-3207

Sleep Disorders Center
Research Medical Center
2316 East Meyer Boulevard
Kansas City, MO 64132-1199
Jon D. Magee, Ph.D.
816-276-4334
Website: www.healthmidwest.org

Cox Regional Sleep Disorders Center
3800 South National Avenue
Suite LL 150
Springfield, MO 65807
Edward Gwin, M.D.
417-269-5575

St. John's Sleep Disorders Center
St. John's Regional Health Center
1235 East Cherokee
Springfield, MO 65804
John Brabson, M.D., Medical Director
Terry M. Yarnell, REEGT, RCPT, Administrative Director
417-885-5464

St. Joseph Health Center Sleep Disorders Laboratory*
St. Joseph Health Center
300 First Capitol Drive
St. Charles, MO 63301
Thomas M. Siler, M.D.
Susan Townsley, RPSGT, Laboratory Coordinator
636-947-5165
Website: www.ssmhc.com

Sleep Disorders & Research Center
Forest Park Hospital of Tenet Health System
6150 Oakland Avenue
St. Louis, MO 63139
Sidney D. Nau, Ph.D.
Korgi V. Hegde, M.D.
314-768-3100

MONTANA

Sleep Disorders Center
Deaconess Billings Clinic

2800 10th Avenue North
P.O. Box 37000
Billings, MT 59107
Terry Padgett, RPSGT, RRT
Robert K. Merchant, M.D.
406-657-4075
Website: www.billingsclinic.org

The Sleep Center at St. Vincent Hospital
St. Vincent Hospital and Health Center
1233 North 30th Street
Billings, MT 59101
William C. Kohler, M.D.
Karen Y. Allen, CRT, RPSGT
406-238-6815

St. Patrick Hospital Sleep Center
St. Patrick Hospital
500 West Broadway
Missoula, MT 59802
Stephen F. Johnson, M.D.
Richard B. Wall, R.EEG T.
406-329-5650
Website: www.saintpatrick.org

NEBRASKA

Great Plains Regional Sleep Physiology Center
Bryan LGH Medical Center West
2300 South 16th Street
Lincoln, NE 68502
Timothy R. Lieske, M.D.
Leigh Heithoff, RPSGT, R.EEG.T.
402-481-5338

Adult and Pediatric Sleep Related Breathing Disorders Laboratory*
Bryan LGH Medical Center East
1600 South 48th Street
Lincoln, NE 68506
Debra Bailey, RN, Clinical Manager
William M. Johnson, M.D., Medical Director
402-481-3950

Sleep Disorders Center
Methodist Hospital
2566 St. Mary's Avenue
Omaha, NE 68105
Robert J. Ellingson, Ph.D., M.D.
402-354-6305 or 402-354-6309

Sleep Disorders Center
Nebraska Health System
987546 Nebraska Medical Center
Omaha, NE 68198-7546
Carie L. Smith, RRT, RPSGT
Stephen B. Smith, M.D.
402-552-2286

NEVADA

Mountain Medical Sleep Disorders Center
Mountain Medical Associates, Inc.
710 West Washington Street
Carson City, NV 89703-3826
Robert L. McDonald, M.D.
John T. Zimmerman, Ph.D.
775-882-2106 or 775-882-4139

The Sleep Clinic of Nevada St. Rose Dominican Hospital
102 East Lake Mead Drive
Henderson, NV 89105
John F. Pinto, M.D.
Darlene Steljes, CEO
702-893-0020

Regional Center for Sleep Disorders
Sunrise Hospital and Medical Center
3131 LaCanada
Suite 107
Las Vegas, NV 89109
Paul Saskin, Ph.D., D,ABSM
Dory Markling, RPSGT
702-731-8365

The Sleep Clinic of Nevada
1012 East Sahara Avenue
Las Vegas, NV 89104
Darlene Steljes, CEO
702-893-0020

Washoe Sleep Disorders Center and Sleep Laboratory
Sleep Management, Inc., EYE-COM, Inc.
Washoe Professional Building and Washoe Medical Center
75 Pringle Way
Suite 701
Reno, NV 89502
William C. Torch, M.D., MS
Paul Binks, Ph.D.
775-329-4060

Pulmonary Medical Associates Sleep Center
Pulmonary Medicine Associates
236 West Sixth Street
Suite 100
Reno, NV 89503
Donna K. Bybee, CMPE
775-329-1597

NEW HAMPSHIRE

Sleep Disorders Center
Dartmouth-Hitchcock Medical Center
One Medical Center Drive
Lebanon, NH 03756
Michael Sateia, M.D.
603-650-7534

Center for Sleep Evaluation
Elliot Hospital
One Elliot Way
Manchester, NH 03103
Jeanetta C. Rains, Ph.D., Clinical Director
Peter E. Corrigan, M.D., Medical Director
603-663-6680

NEW JERSEY

SleepCare Center of Cherry Hill
457 Haddonfield Road
Suite 520
Cherry Hill, NJ 08002
James La Russo, Chief Executive Officer
John D. Miladin, President/Chief Operating Officer
Kathleen L. Ryan, M.D., FCCP, FACP
800-753-3779
Website: sleepcarecenter.com

Center for Sleep Medicine
Saint Clare's Hospital
400 West Blackwell Street
Dover, NJ 07801
Mark J. Atkins, M.D.
Sandy Fitzgerald, Coordinator
973-989-3477

Website: www.saintclares.org or mjatkins.salu.net

Institute for Sleep/Wake Disorders
Hackensack University Medical Center
30 Prospect Avenue
Hackensack, NJ 07601
Hormoz Ashtyani, M.D.
Sue Zafarlotfi, Ph.D.
201-996-3732

Sleep Disorder Center
Morristown Memorial Hospital
95 Mount Kemble Avenue
Morristown, NJ 07962
Robert A. Capone, M.D., FCCP
Pamela Wolfsie, RPSGT
973-971-4567
Website: www.atlantichealth.org

SleepCare
Virtua Health
175 Madison Avenue
Mount Holly, NJ 08060
Kathleen L. Ryan, M.D.
Jack Miladin
800-753-3779
Website: sleepcarecenter.com

Comprehensive Sleep Disorders Center
Robert Wood Johnson University Hospital/UMDNJ
Robert Wood Johnson Medical School
One Robert Wood Johnson Place
P.O. Box 2601
New Brunswick, NJ 08903-2601
Richard A. Parisi, M.D.
Raymond Rosen, Ph.D.
732-937-8683

Sleep Disorders Center
Newark Beth Israel Medical Center
201 Lyons Avenue
Newark, NJ 07112
Monroe Karetzky, M.D.
973-926-6668
Website: www.njsleephelp.com

Sleep Disorders Center of New Jersey
2253 South Avenue
Suite 7
Scotch Plains, NJ 07076
David S. Goldstein, M.D.
Michael Lahey, RPSGT
908-789-4244
Website: www.SleepNJ.com

Mercer Sleep Disorders Center
Capital Health System
446 Bellevue Avenue
Trenton, NJ 08607
Debra DeLuca, M.D.
Rita Brooks, R.EEG/EP.T, RPSGT, CNIM
609-394-4167

Snoring and Sleep Apnea Center*
Capital Health System
750 Brunswick Avenue
Trenton, NJ 08638
Marcella Frank, D.O.
Rita Brooks, R.EEG/EP T., RPSGT, CNIM
609-278-6990
Website: www.capitalhealth.org

NEW MEXICO

University Hospital Sleep Disorders Center
4775 Indian School Road NE
Suite 303
Albuquerque, NM 87110
Rose Mills, Manager
Amanda A. Beck, M.D., Ph.D., Medical Director
505-272-6111

New Mexico Center for Sleep Medicine
Lovelace Health Systems
4700 Jefferson NE
Suite 800
Albuquerque, NM 87109
Lee K. Brown, M.D., Medical Director
Nancy L. Polnaszek, Director of Medical Group Operations
505-872-6000 or
Toll Free: 887-805-REST
Website: www.lovelace.com

NEW YORK

Capital Region Sleep/Wake Disorders Center
St. Peter's Hospital
Pine West Plaza #1
Washington Avenue Extension
Albany, NY 12205
Aaron E. Sher, M.D.
Paul B. Glovinsky, Ph.D.
518-464-9999
Website: MERCYCARE.COM

Sleep/Wake Disorders Center
Montefiore Medical Center
111 East 210th Street
Bronx, NY 10467
Michael J. Thorpy, M.D.
718-920-4841
Website: www.cloud9.net/~thorpy/mmc/

Sleep Disorders Center
New York Methodist Hospital
506 6th Street
Brooklyn, NY 11215
Gerard Lombardo, M.D., Medical Director
John M. Cunningham, RPSGT, Administrator
718-780-3017

Sleep Disorder Center of Western New York
Kaleida Health
3 Gates Circle
Buffalo, NY 14222
Daniel Rifkin, M.D.
Edward Snusz, RRT, RPSGT
Barbara Simonian
716-88-SLEEP (887-5337)

Bassett Healthcare Sleep Disorders Center
Bassett Healthcare
One Atwell Road
Cooperstown, NY 13326
Lee C. Edmonds, M.D.
Robert C. Reese, RRT, RPSGT
607-547-6979
Website: www.bassetthealthcare.org

St. Joseph's Hospital Sleep Disorders Center
St. Joseph's Hospital
555 East Market Street
Elmira, NY 14902
Kathleen R. Reilly, BS, RRT
Paula Cook, RPSGT, RRT
607-737-7008

Parkway Hospital Sleep Disorders Center
The Parkway Hospital
70-35 113th Street
Forest Hills, NY 11375
Jang B.S. Chadha, M.D.
718-990-4590
Website: www.phsdc.com

Sleep Disorders Laboratory*
St. James Mercy Health
411 Canisteo Street
Hornell, NY 14843
Randall L. Clark II, Director, Respiratory Care
Joseph E. Modrak, M.D., Medical Director, Sleep Laboratory
607-324-8781

Sleep Disorders Center
Winthrop-University Hospital
222 Station Plaza North
Mineola, NY 11501
Michael Weinstein, M.D.
Maritza Groth, M.D., FCCP
Claude Albertario, RPSGT
516-663-3907

Sleep-Wake Disorders Center
Long Island Jewish Medical Center
270-05 76th Avenue
New Hyde Park, NY 11042
Harly Greenberg, M.D.
Jane Luchsinger, MS
718-470-7058

The Sleep Disorders Center
Columbia-Presbyterian Medical Center
161 Fort Washington Avenue
New York, NY 10032
Neil B. Kavey, M.D.
212-305-1860 and 914-948-0400

Sleep-Wake Disorders Center
The New York Presbyterian Hospital—Cornell Campus
520 East 70th Street
New York, NY 10021
Gabriele M. Barthlen, M.D., Director, Cornell Campus
Daniel Wagner, M.D., Medical Director
Margaret Moline, Ph.D., Director
212-746-2623

Sleep Disorders Institute
1090 Amsterdam Avenue
New York, NY 10025
Gary K. Zammit, Ph.D.
212-523-1700 or 888-SLEEPNY
Website: www.sleepny.com

Sleep Disorders Center of Rochester
2110 Clinton Avenue South
Rochester, NY 14618
Robert H. Israel, M.D.
716-442-4141

Sleep Apnea Center*
Staten Island University Hospital
375 Sequine Avenue
Staten Island, NY 10309
R. Ciccone, M.D., Medical Director
T. Kilkenny, D.O., Associate Medical Director
Nicholas Caruselle, Administrator
Steve Grenard, RRT, Program Director
800-333-6533 or 718-226-2331

The Sleep Laboratory
St. Joseph's Hospital Health Center
945 East Genesee Street
Suite 300
Syracuse, NY 13210
Edward T. Downing, M.D.
Stephen F. Swierczek, RPSGT
315-475-3379
Website: www.sjhsyr.org

The Sleep Center
Community General Hospital
Broad Road
Syracuse, NY 13215
Robert E. Westlake, M.D.
Antonio Culebras, M.D.
Bruce D. Hall, RPSGT, RRT
315-492-5877
Website: www.cgh.org

The Mohawk Valley Sleep Disorders Center
St. Elizabeth Medical Center
2209 Genesee Street
Utica, NY 13501
Steven A. Levine, D.O., FCCP
Mark Cassidy, RPSGT
315-734-3484

Sleep-Wake Disorders Center
The New York Presbyterian Hospital—Westchester Division
21 Bloomingdale Road
White Plains, NY 10605
Daniel R. Wagner, M.D., Medical Director
Margaret L. Moline, Ph.D., Director
914-997-5751

The Sleep Disorders Center—White Plains
Columbia-Presbyterian Medical Center
185 Maple Avenue
White Plains, NY 10601
Neil B. Kavey, M.D.
914-948-0400

NORTH CAROLINA

Mission/St. Joseph's Sleep Center
445 Biltmore Avenue
Suite 404
Asheville, NC 28801
Charles O'Cain, M.D.
James McCarrick, M.D.
Jean C. Hardy, RPSGT
828-213-4670

Carolinas Sleep Services
University Hospital
P.O. Box 560727

8800 North Tyron Street
Charlotte, NC 28256
Mindy B. Cetel, M.D., Medical Director
Michael Stolzenbach, RPSGT, Manager
704-548-5855 and 877-2SLEEPEZ

Carolinas Sleep Services
Mercy Hospital South
16028 Park Road
Charlotte, NC 28210
William C. Sherrill, M.D.
Scott Lindblom, M.D.
Mary Susan Esther, M.D.
Mindy Beth Cetel, M.D.
Michael Stolzenbach, RPSGT, Manager
704-543-2213

Sleep Disorders Center
Moses Cone Health System
1200 North Elm Street
Greensboro, NC 27401-1020
Clinton D. Young, M.D.
Reggie Whitsett, RPSGT
336-832-7406

Sleep Medicine Center of Salisbury
911 West Henderson Street
Suite L30
Salisbury, NC 28144
Dennis L. Hill, M.D.
Sharon Leach, RPSGT
704-637-1533

Sleep Disorders Center
North Carolina Baptist Hospital
Wake Forest University School of Medicine
Medical Center Boulevard
Winston-Salem, NC 27157
W. Vaughn McCall, M.D.
Linda Quinlivan, RPSGT
336-716-5288
Website: www.wfubmc.edu or www.wfubmc.edu/neurology/department/diagneur.html

Summit Sleep Disorders Center
160 Charlois Boulevard
Winston-Salem, NC 27103
J. Baldwin Smith III, M.D.
Richard Doud Bey, M.D.
336-765-9431

NORTH DAKOTA

No Accredited Member Centers

OHIO

Cincinnati Regional Sleep Center
2123 Auburn Avenue
Suite 341
Cincinnati, OH 45219
Bruce C. Corser, M.D.
Joseph W. Zompero, RPSGT
513-721-4680
Website: www.sleeptonight.com

TriHealth Sleep and Alertness Center
Good Samaritan Hospital
375 Dixmyth Avenue, 7H
Cincinnati, OH 45220-2489
Virgil D. Wooten, M.D.
513-872-4000
Website: www.trihealth.org

The Tri-State Sleep Disorders Center
1275 East Kemper Road
Cincinnati, OH 45246
Martin B. Scharf, Ph.D.
513-671-3101

Cincinnati Regional Sleep Centers West
5049 Crookshank Road
Suite G-3
Cincinnati, OH 45238
Bruce Corser, M.D.
James Armitage, M.D.
Joe Zompero
513-347-0220

University Hospitals Sleep Center
University Hospitals of Cleveland
Department of Neurology
11100 Euclid Avenue
Cleveland, OH 44106
Carl Rosenberg, M.D., MBA
Lucica Buzoianu
216-844-1301

Sleep Disorders Program
MetroHealth Medical Center
2500 MetroHealth Drive
Cleveland, OH 44109
David W. Hudgel, M.D.
Kristina Port, RPSGT, R EEG/EPT
216-778-5985

PMA Cardiopulmonary Sleep Laboratory*
Pulmonary Medicine Associates, Inc.
15805 Puritas Avenue
Cleveland, OH 44135
Paul C. Venizelos, M.D., FCCP
Babu M. Eapen, M.D., FCCP
Petra Podmore, RPSGT, REEGT
216-267-5933

Sleep Disorders Center
The Cleveland Clinic Foundation
9500 Euclid Avenue
Desk S-51
Cleveland, OH 44195
Nancy Foldvary, D.O., Director
216-444-2165

Regional Sleep Disorder Center
Columbus Community Hospital
1430 South High Street
Columbus, OH 43207
Allen Nicholson, Clinical Coordinator
Robert W. Clark, M.D., Medical Director
614-437-7800
Website: www.thesleepsite.com

Samaritan North Sleep Center*
9000 North Main Street
Suite 225
Dayton, OH 45415
Rajesh C. Patel, M.D., FCCP, Medical Director
Joyce E. Gray, Manager
937-567-6180

The Center for Sleep & Wake Disorders
Miami Valley Hospital

One Wyoming Street
Suite G-200
Dayton, OH 45409
James Graham, M.D.
Kevin Huban, Psy.D.
937-208-2515

Sleep Disorders Center
Kettering Medical Center
3535 Southern Boulevard
Dayton, OH 45429-1295
Donna Arand, Ph.D.
937-296-7805

Sleep Disorders Center
Grady Memorial Hospital
561 West Central Avenue
Delaware, OH 43015
Suzanne M. Holt, BS, RPSGT, RRT, RCP
Steven M. Hirsch, M.D.
740-368-5330

Marymount Hospital Sleep Disorders Center
Marymount Hospital
12300 McCracken Road
Garfield Heights, OH 44125
Raymond J. Salomone, M.D.
A. Romeo Craciun, M.D.
Gary L. Foreman, BS, RRT, RCP
216-587-8151

St. Rita's Sleep Disorders Lab
St. Rita's Medical Center
730 West Market Street
Lima, OH 45801
Jeffrey E. Godwin, M.D., R.Ph., FCCP
Mary L. Reed
419-226-9397

Sleep Disorders Center
St. Luke's Hospital
5901 Monclova Road
Maumee, OH 43537
E. Tomas Calderon, M.D., Medical Director
Marty Ensman, RRT, Director
Larry Martin, RPSGT, Supervisor
419-897-8490
Website: www.stlukeshospital.com

Meridia Sleep Disorders Center
Meridia-Cleveland Clinic Health System
6780 Mayfield Road
Mayfield Heights, OH 44124
Daniel W. Sutton, BS, RRT, RCP
Raymond Salomone, M.D.
Eva Hu-Whittemore, M.D.
440-646-8090

MGH Sleep Related Breathing Disorders Lab*
Medina General Hospital
1000 East Washington Street
Medina, OH 44256
Robert Castele, M.D., Medical Director
Michael Neuendorff, Director of Sleep Lab
330-725-1000

Ohio Sleep Disorders Center
150 Springside Drive
Montrose, OH 44333
Jose Rafecas, M.D.
Frankie Roman, M.D.
Larry Saltis, M.D.
330-670-1290
Website: www.ohiosleep.com

Ohio Sleep Disorders Center—Green
5590 Lauby Road
North Canton, OH 44720
Jose Rafecas, M.D.
Michael Perry, RPSGT, R.EEG.T
330-498-5020

Northwest Ohio Sleep Disorders Center at Flower Hospital
5200 Harroun Road
Sylvania, OH 43560
Pamela K. Lang, Lead Therapist, RPSGT
Greg Stang, Director of Respiratory Care
419-824-1624

Sleep Improvement Lab*
Mercy Hospital Tiffin
P.O. Box 727
Tiffin, OH 44883-0727
Vijay K. Mahajan, M.D., Medical Director
Lynette Clifton, RPSGT, CEEGT, Clinical Coordinator
419-448-7666

Sleep Disorders Center
Riverside Mercy Hospital
1600 North Superior Street
Toledo, OH 43604
E. Tomas Calderon, M.D.
Cindy Miller, Director of Cardio-Pulmonary Services
419-729-8600

Sleep Disorders Center
St. Vincent Medical Center
3829 Woodley
Suite 1
Toledo, OH 43606
Michael J. Neeb, Ph.D.
419-251-0570

Northwest Ohio Sleep Disorders Center
The Toledo Hospital
Harris-McIntosh Tower, Second Floor
2142 North Cove Boulevard
Toledo, OH 43606
Pam Lang, RPSGT
Frank O. Horton, III, M.D.
419-471-5629

Sleep Disorders Center
Genesis Health Care System
Bethesda Hospital
2951 Maple Avenue
Zanesville, OH 43701
Roger J. Balogh, M.D.
Thomas E. Rojewski, M.D.
Robert J. Thompson, M.D.
740-454-4725

OKLAHOMA

Sleep Disorders Center of Oklahoma
Integris Health
4401 South Western Avenue
Oklahoma City, OK 73109
Jonathan R.L. Schwartz, M.D.

Elliott R. Schwartz, D.O.
Chris A. Veit, M.S.W., RPSGT
405-636-7700
Website:
www.integris-health.com

Sleep Disorders Center of Oklahoma
Integris Baptist Medical Center
3300 Northwest Expressway
Oklahoma City, OK 73112
Jonathan Schwartz, M.D.
Chris Veit
405-951-8333

OREGON

Sleep Disorders Center
Sacred Heart Medical Center
1255 Hilyard Street
P.O. Box 10905
Eugene, OR 97440
Connie Dunks, CRTT, RCP
Robert Tearse, M.D.
503-686-7224

Sleep Disorders Center
Rogue Valley Medical Center
2825 East Barnett Road
Medford, OR 97504
Eric Overland, M.D.
Michael Schwartz, RPSGT
Nic Butkov, RPSGT
Geoff Zanotto, RPSGT
541-608-4320

Pacific Sleep Program
Suite 202
1849 Northwest Kearney
Portland, OR 97209
Gerald B. Rich, M.D.
503-228-4414
Website: www.snoreweb.com

Sleep Disorders Center
Providence St. Vincent Medical Center
9205 Southwest Barnes Road
Portland, OR 97225
Lyn Miskowicz, Coordinator
Keith Hyde, Administrator
503-216-2010

Legacy Good Samaritan Sleep Disorders Center
Neurology, T-302
1015 Northwest 22nd Avenue
Portland, OR 97210
John J. Greve, M.D., Medical Director
Jan White, Manager
503-413-7540

Sleep Disorders Center
Providence Portland Medical Center
4805 Northeast Glisan Street
Portland, OR 97213-1967
Louis Libby, M.D.
Keith Hyde, MBA
503-215-6552

Salem Hospital Sleep Disorders Center
Salem Hospital
665 Winter Street SE
Salem, OR 97309-5014
Mark T. Gabr, M.D.
Stephen J. Baughman, RRT, RPSGT
503-370-5170

MCMC Sleep Studies Lab*
Mid-Columbia Medical Center
1700 East 19th Street
The Dalles, OR 97058
Michael Wacker
541-296-7724

PENNSYLVANIA

Sleep Disorders Center
Abington Memorial Hospital
1200 Old York Road
Second Floor, Rorer Building
Abington, PA 19001
B. Franklin Diamond, M.D.
Albert D. Wagman, M.D.
Kevin R. Booth, M.D.
215-481-2226
Website: www.AMH.org

Sacred Heart Sleep Disorders Center
Sacred Heart Hospital
421 Chew Street
Allentown, PA 18102-3490
William R. Pistone, D.O.
Ross Futerfas, M.D.
K. Alexander Haraldsted, M.D.
David J. Brooks, RRT, RPSGT
610-776-5333

Sleep Disorders Center
Lower Bucks Hospital
501 Bath Road
Bristol, PA 19007
Howard J. Lee, M.D.
215-785-9752

Penn Center for Sleep Disorders
800 West State Street
Doylestown, PA 18901
Richard J. Schwab, M.D.
Allan I. Pack, M.D., Ph.D.
Louis Metzger
215-345-5003

Sleep Disorders Center of Lancaster
Lancaster General Hospital
555 North Duke Street
Lancaster, PA 17604-3555
Harshadkumar B. Patel, M.D.
James M. O'Connor, RPSGT, MPA
717-290-5910

Saint Mary Sleep/Wake Disorder Center
Langhorne-Newtown Road
Langhorne, PA 19047
Howard J. Lee, M.D., Medical Director
James J. Burke, Administrative Director
215-741-6744

Sleep Medicine Services
Paoli Memorial Hospital
255 West Lancaster Avenue
Paoli, PA 19301
Mark R. Pressman, Ph.D.
Donald D. Peterson, M.D.
610-645-3400

Temple Sleep Disorders Center
Temple University Hospital
3401 North Broad Street
Seventh Floor, Parkinson Pavilion
Philadelphia, PA 19140
Samuel Krachman, D.O.
Grace R. Denault, BA, RPSGT
215-707-8163

Penn Center for Sleep Disorders
University of Pennsylvania Medical Center
3400 Spruce Street
11 Gates West
Philadelphia, PA 19104
Allan I. Pack, M.D., Ph.D.
Richard J. Schwab, M.D.
Louis F. Metzger
215-662-7772

Center for Sleep Medicine, Department of Neurology
MCP—Hahnemann University
3200 Henry Avenue
Philadelphia, PA 19129
June M. Fry, M.D., Ph.D., Director
215-842-4250

Sleep Disorders Center
Thomas Jefferson University
1015 Walnut Street
Suite 319
Philadelphia, PA 19107
Karl Doghramji, M.D.
215 955-6175

Pennsylvania Hospital Sleep Disorders Center
Pennsylvania Hospital
Eighth and Spruce Streets
Philadelphia, PA 19107
Charles R. Cantor, M.D.
Ronald L. Kotler, M.D.
215-829-7079

Northeast Sleep Disorders Center
Nazareth Hospital
2601 Holme Avenue
Philadelphia, PA 19152
John P. Mahan, M.D.
Timothy Flanagan, BS, RPSGT
215-335-6190

University Services Sleep Disorder Centers
6561 Roosevelt Boulevard
Philadelphia, PA 19149
Irvin M. Gerson, M.D.
Benjamin Gerson, M.D.
215-535-3335
Website: www.uservices.com

Sleep and Chronobiology Center
Western Psychiatric Institute and Clinic
3811 O'Hara Street
Pittsburgh, PA 15213-2593
Charles F. Reynolds III, M.D.
412-624-2246

Pulmonary Sleep Evaluation Laboratory*
University of Pittsburgh Medical Center
Montefiore University Hospital
3459 Fifth Avenue, S639
Pittsburgh, PA 15213
Nancy Kern, CRTT, RPSGT
Mark H. Sanders, M.D.
Patrick J. Strollo, M.D.
412-692-2880

University Services
1133 High Street
Pottstown, PA 19464
Irvin M. Gerson, M.D.
Benjamin Gerson, M.D.
610-326-6737
Website: www.uservices.com

Crozer Sleep Disorders Center at Taylor Hospital
175 East Chester Pike
Ridley Park, PA 19078
Calvin Stafford, M.D., Clinical Director
610-595-6272

Sleep Disorders Center
Community Medical Center
1822 Mulberry Street
Scranton, PA 18510
S. Ramakrishna, M.D., FCCP
570-969-8931

Sleep Disorders Center
Mercy Hospital
25 Church Street
Wilkes-Barre PA 18765
John Della Rosa, M.D.
570-826-3410

Sleep Medicine Services
The Lankenau Hospital
100 Lancaster Avenue
Wynnewood, PA 19096
Mark R. Pressman, Ph.D.
Donald D. Peterson, M.D.
610-645-3400

SOUTH CAROLINA

Roper Sleep/Wake Disorders Center
Roper Hospital
316 Calhoun Street
Charleston, SC 29401-1125
William T. Dawson Jr., M.D.
Wayne C. Vial, M.D.
Graham C. Scott, M.D.
John A. Mitchell, M.D.
Tim Fultz, MS, RRT, RPSGT
843-724-2246
Website: www.carealliance.com/sleep/index.html

Sleep Disorders Center of South Carolina
Baptist Medical Center
Taylor at Marion Streets
Columbia, SC 29220
Richard Bogan, M.D., FCCP
Sharon S. Ellis, M.D. Neonatologist
803-296-5847 or 800-368-1971
Website: www.sleepmed.md

Southeast Regional Sleep Disorders Center Easley
200 Fleetwood Drive
P.O. Box 2129
Easley, SC 29640
Freddie E. Wilson, M.D., Medical Director
Katrinka Scalise
864-855-7200

Sleep Disorders Center
Greenville Memorial Hospital
701 Grove Road
Greenville, SC 29605
Don McMahan
864-455-8916

Southeast Regional Sleep Disorders Center
440A Roper Mountain Road
Greenville, SC 29615

Freddie E. Wilson, M.D., Medical Director
Robin Brown, GRT, RPSGT, Clinic Coordinator
Katrinka Scalise, Facility Manager
864-627-5337

Sleep Disorders Center
Spartanburg Regional Medical Center
101 East Wood Street
Spartanburg, SC 29303
Shari Angel Newman, RPSGT
Bill Hazen, RN, CHT
864-560-6904

SOUTH DAKOTA

The Sleep Center
Rapid City Regional Hospital
353 Fairmont Boulevard
P.O. Box 6000
Rapid City, SD 57709
K. Alan Kelts, M.D., Ph.D.
Terry Anderson, BS, RRCP
605-341-8037

Sleep Disorders Center
Sioux Valley Hospital
1100 South Euclid
Sioux Falls, SD 57117-5039
Liz Grav
Richard Hardie, M.D., Co-Medical Director
Brian Hurley, M.D., Co-Medical Director
605-333-6302

TENNESSEE

Regional Sleep Center
Memorial Hospital
2525 DeSalles Avenue
Chattanooga, TN 37404
Michael Dunn, RRT, RPSGT
Robert L. Lindsey, RPSGT
423-495-8340
Website: www.memorial.org

Summit Center for Sleep Health
Summit Medical Center
5655 Frist Boulevard
MOB—Suite 401
Hermitage, TN 37076
Timothy L. Morgenthaler, M.D.
Lee Ann Covington, RRT, RPSGT
615-316-3495

Sleep Disorders Center
Ft. Sanders Regional Medical Center
1901 West Clinch Avenue
Knoxville, TN 37916
Thomas G. Higgins, M.D.
Bert A. Hampton, M.D.
C. Keith Hulse, Ph.D.
865-541-1375

Sleep Disorders Center
St. Mary's Medical Center
900 East Oak Hill Avenue
Knoxville, TN 37917-4556
Michael Eisenstadt, M.D., Medical Director
Steven C. Plenzler, Ph.D., Director
865-545-6746

BMH Sleep Disorders Center
Baptist Memorial Hospital
899 Madison Avenue
Memphis, TN 38146
Robert Schriner, M.D.
Sharon Burt, RPSGT
901-227-5337

Sleep Disorders Center
Methodist Hospitals of Memphis
1265 Union Avenue
Memphis, TN 38104
Kristin W. Lester, Manager
Jim Donaldson, Supervisor
Robert Neal Aguillard, M.D., Medical Director
Srinath Bellur, M.D., Assistant Medical Director
901-726-REST

Sleep Disorders Center
Middle Tennessee Medical Center
400 North Highland Avenue
Murfreesboro, TN 37130
Timothy J. Hoelscher, Ph.D.
William H. Noah, M.D.
615-849-4811

Baptist Sleep Center
Baptist Hospital
2000 Church Street
Nashville, TN 37236
J. Michael Bolds, M.D., Director
Stephen J. Heyman, M.D., Co-Director
615-284-7806

Sleep Disorders Center
Centennial Medical Center
2300 Patterson Street
Nashville, TN 37203
David A. Jarvis, M.D.
Marcie T. Poe, RPSGT
615-342-1670

Sleep Disorders Center
Saint Thomas Hospital
P.O. Box 380
Nashville, TN 37202
J. Brevard Haynes Jr., M.D.
Susan L. Snyder, Ph.D.
615-222-2068

TEXAS

NWTH Sleep Disorders Center
Northwest Texas Hospital
P.O. Box 1110
Amarillo, TX 79175
Marshall Bradshaw, M.D.
John Moss, CRTT
806-354-1954

Sleep Medicine Institute
Presbyterian Hospital of Dallas
8200 Walnut Hill Lane
Dallas, TX 75231
Philip M. Becker, M.D.
Andrew O. Jamieson, M.D.
Wolfgang Schmidt-Nowara, M.D.
214-345-8563
Website: www.sleepmed.com

Sleep Disorders Center for Children
Children's Medical Center of Dallas
1935 Motor Street
Dallas, TX 75235
Roya Tompkins
John Herman, Ph.D.
Joel Steinberg, M.D.
214-456-2793

Sleep Disorders Center
Del Sol Medical Center
10301 Gateway West
El Paso, TX 79925
Gonzalo Diaz, M.D.
Jean R. Joseph-Vanderpool, M.D.
Elizabeth Baird, RPSGT
915-594-5882
Website: www.SPHN.com

Sleep Disorders Center
Providence Memorial Hospital
2001 North Oregon
El Paso, TX 79902
Gonzalo Diaz, M.D., FCCP
Joseph Arteaga, RPSGT
915-577-6152

Sleep Consultants, Inc.
1521 Cooper Street
Fort Worth, TX 76104
Edgar Lucas, Ph.D.
Kristyna M. Hartse, Ph.D.
John R. Burk, M.D.
817-332-7433
Website:
www.sleepconsultants.com

Sleep Disorders Center
Hermann Hospital
6411 Fannin Street
Houston, TX 77030
Richard Castriotta, M.D.
713-704-2337
Website: www.salu.net/hermannsleep/

Sleep Disorders Center
Baylor College of Medicine and VA Medical Center
Room 6C344
2002 Holcombe Boulevard
Houston, TX 77030
Constance Moore, M.D., Director
Max Hirshkowitz, Ph.D., Co-Director
713 794-7563

Sleep Disorders Center
Scott and White Clinic
2401 South 31st Street
Temple, TX 76508
Francisco Perez-Guerra, M.D.
254-724-2554

UTAH

Intermountain Sleep Disorders Center of Murray
Cottonwood Hospital
5770 South, 300 East
Murray, UT 84106
James M. Walker, Ph.D.
Robert J. Farney, M.D.
John B. Krueger, M.D.
Patricia Nelson, M.D.
801-314-2015

Intermountain Sleep Disorders Center
LDS Hospital
8th Avenue & C Street
Salt Lake City, UT 84143
James M. Walker, Ph.D.
Robert J. Farney, M.D.
Tom V. Cloward, M.D.
801-408-3617

Sleep Disorders Center
University of Utah Hospitals and Clinic
50 North Medical Drive
Salt Lake City, UT 84132
Christopher R. Jones, M.D., Ph.D., Co-Medical Director
Kenneth R. Casey, M.D., FCCP, Co-Medical Director
Laura Czajkowski, Ph.D.
Linda Webster, R.EEG/EP T., RPSGT, Manager
801-581-2016

VERMONT

No Accredited Member Centers

VIRGINIA

Fairfax Sleep Disorders Center
3289 Woodburn Road
Suite 360
Annandale, VA 22003
Konrad W. Bakker, M.D.
Marc Raphaelson, M.D.
703-876-9870

Virginia-Carolina Sleep Disorders Center
159 Executive Drive
Suite D
Danville, VA 24541
Jacalyn A. Nelson, M.D., Medical Director
Kofi A. Doonquah, M.D.
Nancy Craig Williams, BS, RPSGT
Eileen Mullikin, RPSGT
804-792-2209

Sleep Disorders Center for Adults and Children
Eastern Virginia Medical School
Sentara Norfolk General Hospital
600 Gresham Drive
Norfolk, VA 23507
J. Catesby Ware, Ph.D.
Jeffery A. Scott, M.D.
Nancy Fishback, M.D.
A.J. Quaranta, M.D.
Robert D.Vorona, M.D.
757-668-3322
Website: www.evms.edu/sleep/

Sleep Disorders Center of Virginia
1800 Glenside Drive
Suite 103
Richmond, VA 23226
Richard A. Parisi, M.D.
Kathe G. Henke, Ph.D.
Read F. McGehee Jr., M.D.
804-285-0100
Website: www.sleepcenter.org

Sleep Disorders Center
Medical College of Virginia
2529 Professional Road
Richmond, VA 23235
Rakesh K. Sood, M.D.
804-323-2255

Sleep Disorders Center
Carilion Roanoke Community Hospital
P.O. Box 12946
Roanoke, VA 24029
William S. Elias, M.D.
540-985-8526

Sleep Disorders Center
Obici Hospital
1900 North Main Street
P.O. Box 1100
Suffolk, VA 23439-1100

Frances Davidson, RT, Administrative Director
Leah S. Pixley, CRT, REEGT, RPSGT, Clinical Manager
Hemang Shah, M.D., Medical Director
757-934-4450
Website: www.obici.com

Sleep Disorders Center
Sentara Virginia Beach General Hospital
1060 First Colonial Road
Virginia Beach, VA 23454
Bruce Johnson, M.D.
Yvonne Wright-Dunn, BA, RPSGT
757-395-8168

WASHINGTON

ARMC Sleep Apnea Laboratory*
Auburn Regional Medical Center
Plaza One
202 North Division
Auburn, WA 98001
Julie Holdaas, RPSGT
Leslie Cuiper, M.D., Medical Director
253-804-2809

St. Clare Sleep Related Breathing Disorders Clinic*
St. Clare Hospital
11315 Bridgeport Way SW
Lakewood, WA 98499
Arthur Knodel, M.D.
Erin Salsbury, RPSGT
253-581-6951

Sleep Disorders Center for Southwest Washington
Providence St. Peter Hospital
413 North Lilly Road
Olympia, WA 98506
Kim A. Chase, RPSGT
John L. Brottem, M.D.
360-493-7436

Sleep Center at Valley
Valley Medical Center
400 South 43rd Street
Renton, WA 98055
William J. DePaso, M.D., FCCP
425-656-5340
Website: www.valleymed.org

Richland Sleep Disorders Center
800 Swift Boulevard
Suite 260
Richland, WA 99352
A. Pat Hamner Jr., M.D.
509-946-4632
Website: www.richsleep.com

Columbia Sleep Lab*
780 Swift Boulevard
Suite 130
Richland, WA 99352
W.S. Klipper, M.D., FACCP
Claudia Havner, CRTT, NRT, PSGT
509-943-6166

Providence Sleep Disorders Center
500 17th Avenue
Department 4W
Seattle, WA 98122
Noel T. Johnson, D.O.
206-320-2575
Website: www.sleep.org

Highline Sleep Disorder Center
Highline Community Hospital
14212 Ambaum Boulevard SW
Suite 201
Seattle, WA 98166
William J. DePaso, M.D., Medical Director
John Lovelace, RRT
Lamont Porter, RCP
206-325-7396

Sleep Disorders Center, H10-SDC
Virginia Mason Medical Center
925 Seneca Street
Seattle, WA 98111
Daniel I. Loube, M.D., Director
Steven H. Kirtland, M.D.
Nigel J. Ball, D.Phil., Associate Director
206-625-7180

Swedish Sleep Medicine Institute Ballard
Swedish Medical Center/Ballard
5300 Tallman Avenue NW
Seattle, WA 98107-1507
Gary A. DeAndrea, M.D.
Richard P. Swanson, RPSGT, CRTT
206-781-6359
Website: www.swedish.org

Sleep Disorders Center
Sacred Heart Doctors Building
105 West Eighth Avenue
Suite 418
Spokane, WA 99204
Elizabeth Hurd, RPSGT
Jeffrey C. Elmer, M.D.
509-455-4895

Kathryn Severyns Dement Sleep Disorders Center
St. Mary Medical Center
401 West Poplar
P.O. Box 1047
Walla Walla, WA 99362
Richard D. Simon Jr. M.D.
Kevin Hurlburt, RPSGT
509-522-5845
Website: www.smmc.com/sleep

WEST VIRGINIA

Sleep Disorders Center
Charleston Area Medical Center
501 Morris Street
P.O. Box 1393
Charleston, WV 25325
George Zaldivar, M.D., FCCP
Karen Stewart, RRT, Manager
304-348-7507

St. Mary's Regional Sleep Center
St. Mary's Hospital
2400 First Avenue
Huntington, WV 25702
William R. Beam, M.D., FCCP
David Imhoff, RRT, RN, MBA
Kathy Johnson, R.EEG/EP T., RPSGT
304-526-1881

PM Sleep Medicine
3803 Emerson Avenue
P.O. Box 4179
Parkersburg, WV 26104
Michael A. Morehead, M.D.
M. Barry Louden, M.D.
304-485-5041

WISCONSIN

Sleep Disorders Center
Appleton Medical Center
1818 North Meade Street
Appleton, WI 54911
Kevin C. Garrett, M.D.
920-738-6460

Marshfield Clinic Sleep Disorders Center
Chippewa Center Sleep Laboratory
2655 County Highway I
Chippewa Falls, WI 54729
Mary Jacks, RPSGT, R.EEG.T.
Nancy Bender Hausman, M.D.
715-726-4136

Luther/Midelfort Sleep Disorders Center
Luther Hospital/Midelfort Clinic
Mayo Health System
1221 Whipple Street
P.O. Box 4105
Eau Claire, WI 54702-4105
Donn Dexter, M.D.
David Nye, M.D.
715-838-3165

St. Vincent Hospital Sleep Disorders Center
St. Vincent Hospital
P.O. Box 13508
Green Bay, WI 54307-3508
John Andrews, M.D.
John Stevenson, M.D.
Paula Van Ert, RPSGT
920-431-3041

Sleep Disorders Laboratory*
Bellin Hospital
744 South Webster Avenue
Green Bay, WI 54301
John Stevenson, M.D.
Lee Kvaley, RRT
920-433-7451

Franciscan Skemp Healthcare Sleep Laboratory*
Franciscan Skemp Medical Center
700 West Avenue South
La Crosse, WI 54601
Robert Gunnink, D.O., Medical Director
Becky Appenzeller, R.EEGT, RPSGT, Coordinator
608-785-0940 ext. 2871

Wisconsin Sleep Disorders Center
Gundersen Lutheran
1836 South Avenue
La Crosse, WI 54601
Alan D. Pratt, M.D.
608-782-7300 ext. 2870

Sleep Disorders Center
St. Marys Hospital Medical Center
707 South Mills Street
Madison, WI 53715
Steve Dalebroux
Kathryn L. Middleton, M.D.
608-258-5266

Comprehensive Sleep Disorders Center
D6/662 Clinical Science Center
University of Wisconsin Hospitals and Clinics
600 Highland Avenue
Madison, WI 53792
Steven M. Weber, Ph.D.
John C. Jones, M.D.
608-263-2387

Sleep Disorders Center Meriter Hospital
Meriter Hospital, Inc.
202 South Park Street
Madison, WI 53715
Lyman Riley, Manager
Mary Klink, M.D., Medical Director
608-267-5938

Marshfield Sleep Disorders Center
Marshfield Clinic
1000 North Oak Avenue
Marshfield, WI 54449
Jody Scherr, RPSGT/R.EEG.T.
Kevin Ruggles, M.D.
715-387-5397
Website: www.marshfieldclinic.org

St. Luke's Sleep Disorders Center
St. Luke's Medical Center
2801 West Kinnickinnic River Parkway
Suite 445
Milwaukee, WI 53215
David Arnold, RPSGT
Michael N. Katzoff, M.D.
414-649-5288

Milwaukee Regional Sleep Disorders Center
Columbia Hospital
2025 East Newport Avenue
Suite 426Y
Milwaukee, WI 53211
Marvin Wooten, M.D.
Joni Tombari, Program Director
414-961-4650

WYOMING

No Accredited Member Centers

APPENDIX III
THE INTERNATIONAL CLASSIFICATION OF SLEEP DISORDERS

	Recommended ICD-9-CM
1. DYSSOMNIAS	
A. Intrinsic Sleep Disorders	
1. Psychophysiological Insomnia	307.42-0
2. Sleep State Misperception	307.49-1
3. Idiopathic Insomnia	780.52-7
4. Narcolepsy	347
5. Recurrent Hypersomnia	780.54-2
6. Idiopathic Hypersomnia	780.54-7
7. Posttraumatic Hypersomnia	780.54-8
8. Obstructive Sleep Apnea Syndrome	780.53-0
9. Central Sleep Apnea Syndrome	780.51-0
10. Central Alveolar Hypoventilation Syndrome	780.51-1
11. Periodic Limb Movement Disorder	780.52-4
12. Restless Legs Syndrome	780.52-5
13. Intrinsic Sleep Disorder NOS	780.52-9
B. Extrinsic Sleep Disorders	
1. Inadequate Sleep Hygiene	307.41-1
2. Environmental Sleep Disorder	780.52-6
3. Altitude Insomnia	289.0
4. Adjustment Sleep Disorder	307.41-0
5. Insufficient Sleep Syndrome	307.49-4
6. Limit-setting Sleep Disorder	307.42-4
7. Sleep-onset Association Disorder	307.42-5
8. Food Allergy Insomnia	780.52-2
9. Nocturnal Eating (Drinking) Syndrome	780.52-8
10. Hypnotic-dependent Sleep Disorder	780.52-0
11. Stimulant-dependent Sleep Disorder	780.52-1
12. Alcohol-dependent Sleep Disorder	780.52-3
13. Toxin-induced Sleep Disorder	780.54-6
14. Extrinsic Sleep Disorder NOS	780.52-9
C. Circadian Rhythm Sleep Disorders	
1. Time-Zone Change (Jet Lag) Syndrome	307.45-0
2. Shift Work Sleep Disorder	307.45-1
3. Irregular Sleep-Wake Pattern	307.45-3
4. Delayed Sleep Phase Syndrome	780.55-0
5. Advanced Sleep Phase Syndrome	780.55-1
6. Non-24 Hour Sleep-Wake Disorder	780.55-2
7. Circadian Rhythm Sleep Disorder NOS	780.55-9

	Recommended
2. PARASOMNIAS	
A. Arousal Disorders	
1. Confusional Arousals	307.46-2
2. Sleepwalking	307.46-0
3. Sleep Terrors	307.46-1
B. Sleep-wake Transition Disorders	
1. Rhythmic Movement Disorder	307.3
2. Sleep Starts	307.47-2
3. Sleep Talking	307.47-3
4. Nocturnal Leg Cramps	729.82
C. Parasomnias usually associated with REM sleep	
1. Nightmares	307.47-0
2. Sleep Paralysis	780.56-2
3. Impaired Sleep-related Penile Erections	780.56-3
4. Sleep-related Painful Erections	780.56-4
5. REM Sleep-related Sinus Arrest	780.56-8
6. REM Sleep Behavior Disorder	780.59-0
D. Other Parasomnias	
1. Sleep Bruxism	306.8
2. Sleep Enuresis	780.56-0
3. Sleep related Abnormal Swallowing Syndrome	780.56-6
4. Nocturnal Paroxysmal Dystonia	780.59-1
5. Sudden Unexplained Nocturnal Death Syndrome	780.59-3
6. Primary Snoring	780.53-1
7. Infant Sleep Apnea	770.80
8. Congenital Central Hypoventilation Syndrome	770.81
9. Sudden Infant Death Syndrome	798.0
10. Benign Neonatal Sleep Myoclonus	780.59-5
11. Other Parasomnia NOS	780.59-9
3. SLEEP DISORDERS ASSOCIATED WITH MEDICAL/PSYCHIATRIC DISORDERS	
A. Associated with Mental Disorders	290-319
1. Psychoses	292-299
2. Mood Disorders	296-301
3. Anxiety Disorders	300
4. Panic Disorder	300
5. Alcoholism	303
B. Associated with Neurological Disorders	320-389
1. Cerebral Degenerative Disorders	330-337
2. Dementia	331
3. Parkinsonism	332-333
4. Fatal Familial Insomnia	337.9
5. Sleep-related Epilepsy	345

	Recommended
6. Electrical Status Epilepticus of Sleep	345.8
7. Sleep-related Headaches	346
C. Associated with Other Medical Disorders	
1. Sleeping Sickness	086
2. Nocturnal Cardiac Ischemia	411-414
3. Chronic Obstructive Pulmonary Disease	490-494
4. Sleep-related Asthma	493
5. Sleep-related Gastroesophageal Reflux	530.1
6. Peptic Ulcer Disease	531-534
7. Fibrositis Syndrome	729.1
4. PROPOSED SLEEP DISORDERS	
1. Short Sleeper	307.49-0
2. Long Sleeper	307.49-2
3. Subwakefulness Syndrome	307.47-1
4. Fragmentary Myoclonus	780.59-7
5. Sleep Hyperhidrosis	780.8
6. Menstrual-associated Sleep Disorder	780.54-3
7. Pregnancy-associated Sleep Disorder	780.59-6
8. Terrifying Hypnagogic Hallucinations	307.47-4
9. Sleep-related Neurogenic Tachypnea	780.53-2
10. Sleep-related Laryngospasm	780.59-4
11. Sleep Choking Syndrome	307.42-1

Reproduced by permission of the American Sleep Disorders Association. Diagnostic Classification Committee: Michael J. Thorpy, Chairman. *International Classification of Sleep Disorders: Diagnostic and Coding Manual.* (Rochester, Minnesota: American Sleep Disorders Association, 1990).

APPENDIX IV

DIAGNOSTIC CLASSIFICATION OF SLEEP AND AROUSAL DISORDERS

ASDC Code		Recommended ICD-9-CM Code
	A. DIMS: Disorders of Initiating and Maintaining Sleep (Insomnias)	
	1. Psychological	
A.1.a	a. Transient and Situational	307.41-0
A.1.b	b. Persistent	307.42-0
A.2	2. Associated with Psychiatric Disorders	
A.2.a	a. Symptom and Personality Disorders	307.42-1
A.2.b	b. Affective Disorders	307.42-2
A.2.c	c. Other Functional Psychoses	307.42-3
A.3	3. Associated with Use of Drugs and Alcohol	
A.3.a	a. Tolerance or Withdrawal from CNS Depressants	780.52-0
A.3.b	b. Sustained use of CNS Stimulants	780.52-1
A.3.c	c. Sustained Use or Withdrawal from Other Drugs	780.52-2
A.3.d	d. Chronic Alcoholism	780.52-3
A.4	4. Associated with Sleep-induced Respiratory Impairment	
A.4.a	a. Sleep Apnea DIMS Syndrome	780.51-0
A.4.b	b. Alveolar Hypoventilation DIMS Syndrome	780.51-1
A.5	5. Associated with Sleep-related (Nocturnal) Myoclonus and "Restless Legs"	
A.5.a	a. Sleep-related (Nocturnal) Myoclonus DIMS Syndrome	780.52-4
A.5.b	b. "Restless Legs" DIMS Syndrome	780.52-5
A.6	6. Associated with Other Medical, Toxic and Environmental Conditions	780.52-6
A.7	7. Childhood-Onset DIMS	780.52-7
A.8	8. Associated with Other DIMS Conditions	
A.8.a	a. Repeated REM Sleep Interruptions	307.48-0
A.8.b	b. Atypical Polysomnographic Features	307.48-1
A.8.c	c. Not Otherwise Specified	307.42-9 or 780.52-9
A.9	9. No DIMS Abnormality	
A.9.a	a. Short Sleeper	307.49-0
A.9.b	b. Subjective DIMS Complaint Without Objective Findings	307.49-1
A.9.c	c. Not Otherwise Specified	307.40-1

ASDC Code		Recommended ICD-9-CM Code
	B. DOES: Disorders of Excessive Somnolence	
B.1	1. Psychophysiological	
B.1.a	a. Transient and Situational	307.43-0
B.1.b	b. Persistent	307.44-0
B.2	2. Associated with Psychiatric Disorders	
B.2.a	a. Affective Disorders	307.44-1
B.2.b	b. Other Functional Disorders	307.44-2
B.3	3. Associated with Use of Drugs and Alcohol	
B.3.a	a. Tolerance to or Withdrawal from CNS Stimulants	780.54-0
B.3.b	b. Sustained Use of CNS Depressants	780.54-1
B.4	4. Associated with Sleep-induced Respiratory Impairment	
B.4.a	a. Sleep Apnea DOES Syndrome	780.53-0
B.4.b	b. Alveolar Hypoventilation DOES Syndrome	780.53-1
B.5	5. Associated with Sleep-related (Nocturnal) Myoclonus and "Restless Legs"	
B.5.a	a. Sleep-related (Nocturnal) Myoclonus DOES Syndrome	780.54-4
B.5.b	b. "Restless Legs" DOES Syndrome	780.54-5
B.6	6. Narcolepsy	347
B.7	7. Idiopathic CNS Hypersomnolence	780.54-7
B.8	8. Associated with Other Medical, Toxic and Environmental Conditions	780.54-6
B.9	9. Associated with Other DOES Conditions	
B.9.a	a. Intermittent DOES (Periodic) Syndromes	
B.9.a.i	i. Kleine-Levin Syndrome	780.54-2
B.9.a.ii	ii. Menstrual-associated Syndrome	780.54-3
B.9.b	b. Insufficient Sleep	307.49-4
B.9.c	c. Sleep Drunkenness	307.47-1
B.9.d	d. Not Otherwise Specified	307.44-9 or 780.54-9
B.10	10. No DOES Abnormality	
B.10.a	a. Long Sleeper	307.49-2
B.10.b	b. Subjective DOES Complaint Without Objective Findings	307.49-3
B.10.c	c. Not Otherwise Specified	307.40-2
	C. Disorders of the Sleep-Wake Schedule	
C.1	1. Transient	
C.1.a	a. Rapid Time Zone Change ("Jet Lag") Syndrome	307.45-0
C.1.b	b. "Work Shift" Change in Conventional Sleep-Wake Schedule	307.45-1
C.2	2. Persistent	
C.2.a	a. Frequently Changing Sleep-Wake Schedule	307.45-2
C.2.b	b. Delayed Sleep Phase Syndrome	780.55-0
C.2.c	c. Advanced Sleep Phase Syndrome	780.55-1
C.2.d	d. Non-24-hour Sleep-Wake Syndrome	780.55-2

ASDC Code		Recommended ICD-9-CM Code
C.2.e	e. Irregular Sleep-Wake Pattern	307.45-3
C.2.f	f. Not Otherwise Specified	307.45-9 or 780.55-9
	D. Dysfunctions Associated with Sleep, Sleep Stages or Partial Arousals (Parasomnias)	**307.47-0**
D.1	1. Sleepwalking (Somnambulism)	307.46-0
D.2	2. Sleep Terror (Pavor Nocturnus, Incubus)	307.46-1
D.3	3. Sleep-related Enuresis	307.46-2 or 780.56-0
D.4	4. Other Dysfunctions	
D.4.a	a. Dream Anxiety Attacks (Nightmares)	307.47-0
D.4.b	b. Sleep-related Epileptic Seizures	780.56-1
D.4.c	c. Sleep-related Bruxism	306.8
D.4.d	d. Sleep-related Headbanging (Jactatio Capitis Nocturna)	307.3
D.4.e	e. Familial Sleep Paralysis	780.56-2
D.4.f	f. Impaired Sleep-related Penile Tumescence	780.56-3
D.4.g	g. Sleep-related Painful Erections	780.56-4
D.4.h	h. Sleep-related Cluster Headaches and Chronic Paroxysmal Hemicrania	780.56-5
D.4.i	i. Sleep-related Abnormal Swallowing Syndrome	780.56-6
D.4.j	j. Sleep-related Asthma	780.56-7
D.4.k	k. Sleep-related Cardiovascular Symptoms	780.56-8
D.4.l	l. Sleep-related Gastroesophageal Reflux	780.56-9
D.4.m	m. Sleep-related Hemolysis (Paroxysmal Nocturnal Hemoglobinuria)	283.2
D.4.n	n. Asymptomatic Polysomnographic Finding	780.59
D.4.o	o. Not Otherwise Specified	307.47-9 or 780.56

Adapted from Association of Sleep Disorder Centers Classification Committee, *Diagnostic Classification of Sleep and Arousal Disorders* (New York: Raven Press, 1979);

BIBLIOGRAPHY

Aldrich, Michael S. *Sleep Medicine.* New York: Oxford University Press, 1999.

American Psychiatric Association. *Diagnostic and Statistical Manual of Mental Disorders.* 3rd ed. Washington, D.C.: American Psychiatric Association, 1982.

American Sleep Disorders Association (Diagnostic Classification Committee, Michael J. Thorpy, Chairman). *International Classification of Sleep Disorders: Diagnostic and Coding Manual.* Rochester, Minnesota: American Sleep Disorders Association, 1990, rev. 1997.

Anch, A. Michael, Browman, Carl P., Mitler, Merrill M. and Walsh, James K. *Sleep: A Scientific Perspective.* Englewood Cliffs, N.J.: Prentice-Hall, 1988.

Association of Sleep Disorder Centers, "Diagnostic Classification of Sleep and Arousal Disorders" (prepared by Sleep Disorders Classification Committee, H.P. Roffwarg, Chairman), *Sleep* 2 (1979): 1–137.

Barnes, C. and Orem, J. *Physiology in Sleep.* New York: Academic, 1980.

Beck, A.T., Rush, A.J., Shaw, B.F. and Emery, G. *Cognitive Therapy of Depression.* New York: Guilford Press, 1979.

Bixler, E.O., Kales, A. and Soldatos, C.R., "Sleep Disorders Encountered in Medical Practice: A National Survey of Physicians," *Behavioral Medicine* 6 (1979): 1–6.

Bootzin, R. and Nicassio, P.M., "Behavioral Treatment for Insomnia," in M. Hersen, R.M. Eissler, P.M. Miller, eds., *Progress in Behavior Modification.* New York: Academic Press, 1978. pp. 1–45.

Borbely, Alexander. *Secrets of Sleep.* New York: Basic Books, 1986.

Bradbury, John Buckley, "The Croonian Lectures on Some Points Connected With Sleep, Sleepiness, and Hypnotics," *The Lancet* (1899): 1685–1694.

Burros, Marian, "Eating Well" (L-tryptophan), *New York Times,* December 20, 1989, C8.

Carskadon, M.A., *Encyclopedia of Sleep and Dreams.* New York: Macmillan, 1993.

Carskadon, M.A., Brown, E.D. and Dement, W.C., "Sleep Fragmentation in the Elderly: Relationship to Daytime Sleep Tendency," *Neurology of Aging* 3 (1982): 321–327.

Carskadon, M.A. and Dement, W.C., "Cumulative Effects of Sleep Restriction in Daytime Sleepiness," *Psychophysiology* 18 (1981): 107–113.

Degen, R. and Neidermeyer, E., eds. *Epilepsy, Sleep and Sleep Deprivation.* Amsterdam: Elsevier, 1983.

Dement, William C. *Some Must Watch While Some Must Sleep.* New York: Norton, 1976.

Dement, William C. and Vaughan, Christopher. *The Promise of Sleep.* New York: Delacorte Press, 1999.

Diamond, Edwin. *The Science of Dreams.* Garden City, N.Y.: Doubleday, 1962.

Dinges, David F. and Broughton, Roger J., eds. *Sleep and Alertness: Chronobiological, Behavioral, and Medical Aspects of Napping.* New York: Raven Press, 1989.

Dobkin, Bruce H., "Sleep Pills," *New York Times Sunday Magazine* (Body and Mind), February 5, 1989, page 39.

Empson, Jacob. *Sleep and Dreaming.* London: Faber and Faber, 1989.

Erman, M.K., ed. *The Psychiatric Clinics of North America: Sleep Disorders.* Philadelphia: W.B. Saunders, 1987. pp. 517–724.

Fairbanks, D.N.F., Fumita, S., Ikematsu, T. and Simmons, F.B., eds. *Snoring and Obstructive Sleep Apnea.* New York: Raven Press, 1987.

Ferber, Richard. *Solve Your Child's Sleep Problems.* New York: Simon and Schuster, 1985.

Fletcher, E.C., ed. *Abnormalities of Respiration During Sleep: Diagnosis, Pathophysiology, and Treatment.* Orlando: Grune & Stratton, 1986.

Foster, Henry Hubbard, "The Necessity for a New Standpoint in Sleep Theories," *American Journal of Psychology* (1901): 145–177.

Garfield, Patricia. *Creative Dreaming.* New York: Ballantine Books, 1974.

Guilleminault, C. and Dement, W.C., eds. *Sleep Apnea Syndromes.* New York: Alan R. Liss, 1978.

Guilleminault, C. and Lugaresi, E., eds. *Sleep/Wake Disorders: Natural History, Epidemiology, and Long-Term Evolution.* New York: Raven Press, 1983.

Hartmann, E. *The Biology of Dreaming.* Springfield, Ill.: C.C. Thomas, 1967.

Hartmann, E., ed. *Sleep and Dreaming.* Boston: Little, Brown, 1970.

Hauri, Peter. *The Sleep Disorders.* 2nd edition. Kalamazoo, Mich.: Upjohn Company, 1982.

Hauri, Peter and Linde, Shirley J., *No More Sleepless Nights.* New York: Wiley, 1990.

Haymaker, Webb. *The Founders of Neurology.* Springfield, Ill.: Charles C. Thomas, 1953.

Hayward, Linda. *I Had A Bad Dream.* New York: Golden Book, 1985.

Horne, James. *Why We Sleep: The Function of Sleep in Humans and Other Mammals.* Oxford: Oxford University Press, 1988.

Johnson, L.C., "Psychological and Physiological Changes Following Total Sleep Deprivation," in Kales, A., ed., *Sleep: Physiology and Pathology.* Philadelphia: J.B. Lippincott, 1969.

Kales, Anthony, Cladwell, A.B., Preston, T.A., Healey, S. and Kales, J.D., "Personality Patterns in Insomnia," *Archives of General Psychiatry* 33 (1976): 1128–1134.

Kales, Anthony and Kales, Joyce D. *Evaluation and Treatment of Insomnia.* New York: Oxford University Press, 1984.

Kamei, R., Hughes, L., Miles, L. and Dement, W., "Advanced Sleep Phase Syndrome Studied in a Time Isolation Facility," *Chronobiologia* 6 (1979): 115.

Karacan, I., Williams, R.L., Little, R.C. and Salis, P., "Insomniacs: Unpredictable and Idiosyncratic Sleepers," in Levin, P. and Koella, W.P., eds., *Sleep Physiology, Biochemistry, Psychology, Pharmacology, Clinical Implications.* Basel: S. Karger, 1973. pp. 120–132.

Kaye, Marilyn. *Baby Fozzie Is Afraid of the Dark,* illustrated by Tom Brannon. New York: Muppet Press, 1986.

Kleitman, Nathaniel. *Sleep and Wakefulness.* Chicago: University of Chicago Press, 1939; revised, 1963.

Konner, Melvin, "Where Should Baby Sleep?" *New York Times Sunday Magazine,* January 8, 1989, pp. 39–40.

Kripke, D.F., Gillin, J.C., Mullaney, D.J., Risch, S.C. and Janowsky, D.S., "Treatment of Major Depressive Disorders by Bright White Light for 5 Days," in Halaris, E., ed., *Chronobiology and Psychiatric Disorders.* New York: Elsevier Sciences Publishing Company, 1987. pp. 207–218.

Kripke, D.F., Simons, R.N., Garfinkel, L. and Hammond, E.C., "Short and Long Sleep and Sleeping Pills: Is Increased Mortality Associated?" *Archives of General Psychiatry* 36 (1979): 103–116.

Krueger, James M. "No Simple Slumber," *Sciences,* May/June 1989, pp. 36–41.

Kryger, M., "Fat, Sleep, and Charles Dickens: Literary and Medical Contributions to the Understanding of Sleep Apnea," *Clinics in Chest Medicine* 6 (1985): 555–562.

———, "Sleep in Restrictive Lung Disorders," *Clinics in Chest Medicine* 6 (1985): 675–678.

Kryger, M., Roth, Thomas and Dement, W., eds. *The Principles and Practices of Sleep Disorders Medicine.* Philadelphia: W.B. Saunders, 1989, 1994.

Kupfer, D.J. and Thase, M.E., "The Use of the Sleep Laboratory in the Diagnosis of Affective Disorders," *Psychiatric Clinics of North America* 6, no. 1 (1983): 3–24.

Kutner, Lawrence, "Parent & Child," *New York Times* (Bedtime), June 22, 1989, page C8.

Lamberg, Lynne. *American Medical Association Guide to Better Sleep.* Revised edition. New York: Random House, 1984.

Leech, Judith A. *Falling Asleep in the Middle of Life.* Ogdensburg, N.Y.: AYD Medical Services, 1999.

Luce, Gay and Segal, Julius. *Sleep.* New York: Lancer, 1966.

Lyons, Albert S. *Medicine: An Illustrated History.* New York: Abradale Press, 1978.

Maas, James B. *Power Sleep.* New York: Harper Perennial, 1999.

MacKenzie, Norman. *Dreams and Dreaming.* New York: Vanguard Press, 1965.

Maneceine, Marie de. *Sleep: Its Physiology, Pathology, Hygiene and Psychology.* London. Walter Scott, 1897.

McGinty, D., Drucker-Colin, R., Morrison, A. and Parmeggiani, P. *Brain Mechanisms of Sleep.* New York: Raven Press, 1984.

McHenry, Lawrence C., Jr. *Garrison's History of Neurology.* Springfield, Ill.: Charles C. Thomas, 1969.

Mellinger, G.D., Balter, M.B. and Uhlenhuth, E.H., "Insomnia and its Treatment: Prevalence and Correlates," *Archives of General Psychiatry* 42 (1985): 225–232.

Mendelson, W.B. *Human Sleep: Research and Clinical Care.* New York: Plenum Press, 1987.

Monroe, L.J., "Psychological and Physiological Differences Between Good and Poor Sleepers," *Journal of Abnormal Psychology* 72 (1967): 255–264.

Moore-Ede, M.C., Sulzman, F.M. and Fuller, C.A. *The Clocks That Time Us.* Cambridge: Harvard University Press, 1982.

Morton, Leslie T. *A Medical Bibliography.* 4th edition. London: Gower, 1983.

Moruzzi, Giuseppe, "The Historical Development of the Deafferentation Hypothesis of Sleep," *Proceedings of the American Philosophical Society* 108 (1964): 19–28.

Moruzzi, G. and Magoun, H.W., "Brain Stem Reticular Formation and Activation of the EEG," *Electroencephalography and Clinical Neurophysiology* 1 (1949): 455–473.

Mullaney, D.J., Johnson, L.C., Naitoh, P., Freidman, J.K. and Globus, G.G., "Sleep During and After Gradual Sleep Reduction," *Psychophysiology* 14:3 (1977): 237–244.

Nicholson, A.N., "Hypnotics: Clinical Pharmacology and Therapeutics," in Kryger, M.H., Roth, T. and Dement, W.C., eds., *The Principles and Practices of Sleep Disorders Medicine.* Philadelphia: Saunders, 1989. pp. 219–227.

Oswald, Ian. *Sleep.* Middlesex, England: Penguin, 1966.

Overman, Stephenie, "Rise and Sigh," *HR Magazine,* May 1999, pp. 68–74.

Parkes, J.D. *Sleep and Its Disorders.* London: W.B. Saunders, 1985.

Pavlov, I.P. *Lectures on Conditioned Reflexes.* London: Lawrence & Wishart, 1928. Chapter 32.

Pieron, Henri. *Le Probleme Physiologique du Sommeil.* Paris: Masson et C., 1943.

Radulovacki, M., "Role of Adenosine in Sleep of Rats," *Review of Clinical and Basic Pharmacology* 5 (1985): 327–339.

Riley, T.L., ed. *Clinical Aspects, Sleep and Nap Disturbance.* London: Butterworth, 1985.

Rosner, Fred. *Julius Preuss' Biblical and Talmudic Medicine.* New York: Sanhedrin Press, 1978.

Seidel, W.F. and Dement, W.C., "Sleepiness in Insomnia: Evaluation and Treatment," *Sleep* 5 (1982): S182–S190.

Shepard, John F. *The Circulation and Sleep.* New York: MacMillan, 1914.

Shneerson, John. *Handbook of Sleep Medicine.* Oxford: Blackwell Science Ltd., 2000.

Siegel, Rudolph E., *Galen on the Affected Parts,* from the Greek, with explanatory notes. London: S. Karger, 1976.

Smolensky, Michael, and Lamburg, Lynne, *The Body Clock Guide to Better Health.* New York: Holt, 2000.

Sperling, Dan, "Sleep Disorders of the Kiddie Kind," *USA Today,* June 22, 1989, page 5D.

Spielman, A.J., "Assessment of Insomnia," *Clinical Psychology Review* 6 (1986): 11–25.

Spielman, A.J., Caruso, L. and Glovinsky, P., "A Behavioral Perspective on Insomnia Treatment," *Psychiatric Clinics of North America* 10, no. 4 (1987): 541–553.

Spielman, A.J., Saskin, P. and Thorpy, M.J., "Treatment of Chronic Insomnia by Restriction of Time Spent in Bed," *Sleep* 10, no. 1 (1987): 45–56.

Stepanski, E., Zorick, F., Roehrs, T., Young, D. and Roth, T., "Daytime Alertness in Patients with Chronic Insomnia Compared with Asymptomatic Control Subjects," *Sleep* 11 (1988): 54–60.

Sterman, M.B., Clemente, C.D. and Wyrwicka, W., "Forebrain Inhibitory Mechanisms: Conditioning of Basal Forebrain Induced EEG Synchronization and Sleep," *Experimental Neurology* 7 (1963): 404–417.

Sterman, M.B., Shouse, M.N. and Passouant, P., eds. *Sleep and Epilepsy.* New York: Academic Press, 1982.

Sweetwood, H.L., Kripke, D.F., Grant, I., Yager, J. and Gerst, M.S., "Sleep Disorder and Psychobiological Symptomatology in Male Psychiatric Outpatients and Male Nonpatients," *Psychosomatic Medicine* 38 (1976): 373–378.

Thorpy, Michael J., "Diagnosis, Evaluation and Classification of Sleep Disorders," in Karacan, I. and Williams, R.L., eds., *Sleep Disorders: Diagnosis and Treatment.* New York: Wiley, 1987.

Thorpy, Michael J. and Glovinsky, Paul B., "Jactatio Capitis Nocturna," in Kryger, M., Roth, T. and Dement, W., eds., *The Principles and Practices of Sleep Disorders Medicine.* Philadelphia: Saunders, 1987.

Thorpy, Michael J., ed. *Handbook of Sleep Disorders,* in Neurological Disease and Therapy Series (W. Koller, series editor). New York: Marcel Dekker, 1990.

Wagman, A. and Allen, R., "Effects of Alcohol Ingestion and Abstinence on Slow Wave Sleep of Alcoholics," in Gross, M.M., ed., *Alcohol Intoxication and Withdrawal, 2.* New York: Plenum Press, 1975. pp. 453–466.

Walsleben, Joyce A., and Baron-Faust, Ruth, *A Woman's Guide to Sleep.* New York: Crown, 2000.

Webb, Wilse B. *Sleep: The Gentle Tyrant.* Englewood Cliffs, N.J.: Prentice-Hall, 1975.

Weitzman, Elliot D., "Sleep and Aging," in Katzman, R. and Terry, R.D., eds., *The Neurology of Aging.* Philadelphia: F.A. Davis, 1983. pp. 167–188.

Williams, H.L. and Salamy, A., "Alcohol and Sleep," in Kissen, B. and Begleiter, H., eds., *The Biology of Alcoholism.* New York: Plenum Press, 1972. pp. 435–483.

Williams, R.L., Karacan, I. and Moore, C., eds. *Sleep Disorders: Diagnosis and Treatment.* 2nd edition. New York: John Wiley, 1988.

INDEX

Boldface page numbers indicate main headings.

N

O